Endoscopic Management of Gynecologic Disease

Endoscopic Management of Gynecologic Disease

Editors

G. David Adamson, M.D., F.R.C.S.C., F.A.C.O.G., F.A.C.S.

Clinical Associate Professor
Department of Gynecology and Obstetrics
Stanford University School of Medicine
Stanford, California;
Associate Clinical Professor
Department of Obstetrics, Gynecology, and Reproductive Sciences
University of California, San Francisco
San Francisco, California; and
Director
Fertility and Reproductive Health Institute of Northern California
Palo Alto, California

Daniel C. Martin, M.D.

Clinical Associate Professor
Department of Obstetrics and Gynecology
University of Tennessee, Memphis
and
Reproductive Surgeon
Baptist Memorial Hospital
Memphis, Tennessee

Lippincott - Raven
PUBLISHERS
Philadelphia • New York

Lippincott-Raven Publishers, 227 East Washington Square, Philadelphia, Pennsylvania 19106

Printed and bound in Hong Kong

Library of Congress Cataloging-in-Publication Data

Endoscopic management of gynecologic disease/[edited by] G. David Adamson, Daniel C. Martin.
p. cm.
Includes bibliographical references and index.
ISBN 0-7817-0281-X
1. Generative organs, Female—Endoscopic surgery. I. Adamson, G. David. II. Martin, Dan C.
[DNLM: 1. Genital Diseases, Female—surgery. 2. Surgery, Laparoscopic—methods. 3. Hysteroscopy—methods. WP 660 E567 1995]
RG104.7.E53 1995
618.1′059—dc20
DNLM/DLC
for Library of Congress
94-48584
CIP

The material contained in this volume was submitted as previously unpublished material, except in the instances in which some of the illustrative material was derived.

Great care has been taken to maintain the accuracy of the information contained in the volume. However, neither Lippincott-Raven Publishers nor the editors can be held responsible for errors or for any consequences arising from the use of the information contained herein.

9 8 7 6 5 4 3 2 1

This book is dedicated to my family:

My mother, for encouraging me to dream,
My father, for teaching me to work;

My children, Stephanie, Rebecca, and Eric,
for their patience and understanding;

My wife, Rosemary, for her constant love and support,
which make everything possible.

G. David Adamson

I would like to dedicate this book to:

My mother and father, for their encouragement
and for teaching me to be concerned for others;

My sons, Adam and Josh, and my wife, Glenn Ann,
for their continuing support.

Daniel C. Martin

Contents

Part IV. Preparation for Hysteroscopy

Part V. Surgical Technique: Hysteroscopy

Contributing Authors

G. David Adamson, M.D., F.R.C.S.C., F.A.C.O.G., F.A.C.S.
Clinical Associate Professor
Department of Gynecology and Obstetrics
Stanford University School of Medicine
300 Pasteur Drive
Stanford, California 94305; and
Associate Clinical Professor
Department of Obstetrics, Gynecology, and Reproductive Sciences
University of California, San Francisco
513 Parnassus Avenue
San Francisco, California 94143; and
Director
Fertility Physicians of Northern California
540 University Avenue
Suite 200
Palo Alto, California 94301

Stephen A. Agatson, M.D.
Diagnostic Radiologist
Presbyterian Hospital of Dallas
8320 Walnut Hill Lane
Suite 100
Dallas, Texas 75231

Philip G. Brooks, M.D.
Clinical Professor
Department of Obstetrics and Gynecology
UCLA School of Medicine; and
Attending Physician
Cedars Sinai Medical Center
8631 West 3rd Street
510E
Los Angeles, California 90048

Joel M. Childers, M.D.
Associate Professor of Clinical Obstetrics and Gynecology
Department of Obstetrics and Gynecology
University Medical Center
2625 North Craycroft Road
Suite 201
Tucson, Arizona 85712

Brian M. Cohen, M.D., M.B.Ch.B.
Clinical Professor
Department of Obstetrics and Gynecology
The University of Texas Southwestern Medical School; and
President, National Fertility Center of Texas
7777 Forest Lane
C-638
Dallas, Texas 75230

Mary Jane Carroll Collins, M.D.
Medical Director
Sereno Surgery Center
14601 South Bascom Avenue
Suite 100
Los Gatos, California 95032

Andrew S. Cook, M.D.
Omega Institute of Health
One Galleria Boulevard
Suite 810
Metairie, Louisiana 70001-2082

Stephen L. Corson, M.D.
Clinical Professor of Obstetrics and Gynecology
Section Head, Reproductive Endocrinology
Department of Obstetrics and Gynecology
University of Pennsylvania School of Medicine
Pennsylvania Hospital
815 Locust Street
Philadelphia, Pennsylvania 19107

Scott R. Crowgey, M.D., M.S.E.E.
Georgia Tech Research Institute
Georgia Institute of Technology
CND/ITL/GTRI
Atlanta, Georgia 30332

James F. Daniell, M.D.
Department of Obstetrics and Gynecology
Centennial Medical Center
2222 State Street
Suite A
Nashville, Tennessee 37203

Alan H. DeCherney, M.D.
Louis E. Phaneuf Professor and Chairman
Department of Obstetrics and Gynecology
Tufts University School of Medicine
New England Medical Center
750 Washington Street, Box 324
Boston, Massachusetts 02111

Michael P. Diamond, M.D.
Professor of Obstetrics and Gynecology
Director, Division of Reproductive Endocrinology and Infertility
Wayne State University
4707 St. Antoine Boulevard
Detroit, Michigan 48201

Joseph R. Feste, M.D.
Clinical Associate Professor
Department of Obstetrics and Gynecology
Baylor College of Medicine
University Health Science Center
7550 Fannin
Houston, Texas 77054

Harrith M. Hasson, M.D.
Associate Professor
Rush Medical College
P.O. Box 14898
Chicago, Illinois 60614-0898

David I. Hoffman, M.D.
Northwest Center for Infertility
Northwest Medical Plaza
5800 Colonial Drive
Suite 200
Margate, Florida 33063

Stephen H. Jackson, M.D.
Department of Anesthesiology
Good Samaritan Hospital of Santa Clara Valley
2425 Samaritan Drive
San Jose, California 95124

Grace M. Janik, M.D., F.A.C.O.G.
Director, Columbia IVF
Reproductive Specialty Center
2315 North Lake Drive
Suite 501
Milwaukee, Wisconsin 53211

D. Alan Johns, M.D.
Richland Medical Center
3700 Rufe Snow Drive;
GYN Laparoscopy Center
Harris Methodist; and
Department of Obstetrics and Gynecology
John Peter Smith Hospital
Forth Worth, Texas 76180

John F. Kerin, M.D., F.R.A.C.O.G., F.A.C.O.G.
Professor of Reproductive Medicine
Department of Obstetrics and Gynecology
Flinders University
Flinders Drive
Bedford Park
South Australia 5042

William R. Keye, Jr., M.D.
Associate Clinical Professor
Department of Obstetrics and Gynecology
University of Michigan
1301 Catherine Road
Ann Arbor, Michigan 48109; and
Director
Division of Reproductive Endocrinology
William Beaumont Hospital
3535 West Thirteen Mile Road
Suite 344
Royal Oak, Michigan 48073

Charles H. Koh, M.D., F.A.C.O.G., F.R.C.O.G.
Associate Clinical Professor
Reproductive Specialty Center
Medical College of Wisconsin
2315 North Lake Drive
Suite 501
Milwaukee, Wisconsin 53211

Bryan R. Kurtz, M.D.
Department of Obstetrics and Gynecology
Centennial Medical Center
2222 State Street
Suite A
Nashville, Tennessee 37203

Grace Lee, M.D.
Assistant Professor
Department of Obstetrics and Gynecology
Yale University School of Medicine
333 Cedar Street
New Haven, Connecticut 06510

John M. Leventhal, M.D.
Clinical Instructor
Department of Obstetrics and Gynecology
Harvard Medical School
Boston, Massachusetts 02115

Barbara S. Levy, M.D.
Clinical Assistant Professor
Department of Obstetrics and Gynecology
University of Washington School of Medicine
34509 Ninth Avenue South, #300
Federal Way, Washington 98003

Franklin D. Loffer, M.D.
Director, Division of Gynecologic Endoscopy
Department of Obstetrics and Gynecology
Maricopa Medical Center
2601 East Roosevelt
Phoenix, Arizona 85008

Anthony A. Luciano, M.D.
Professor
Department of Obstetrics and Gynecology
University of Connecticut School of Medicine
New Britain General Hospital
100 Grand Street
New Britain, Connecticut 06050

Charles M. March, M.D.
Professor
Department of Obstetrics and Gynecology
University of Southern California School of Medicine
1240 North Mission Road
Room L-1022
Los Angeles, California 90033

Daniel C. Martin, M.D.
Clinical Associate Professor
Department of Obstetrics and Gynecology
University of Tennessee, Memphis; and
Reproductive Surgeon
Baptist Memorial Hospital
910 Madison Avenue
Suite 805
Memphis, Tennessee 38103

Wayne S. Maxson, M.D.
Northwest Center for Infertility
Northwest Medical Plaza
5800 Colonial Drive
Suite 200
Margate, Florida 33063

Deborah A. Metzger, M.D., Ph.D.
Associate Clinical Professor
Department of Obstetrics and Gynecology
University of Connecticut Health Center
263 Farmington Avenue
Farmington, Connecticut 06030; and
Director, Reproductive Medicine
Institute of Connecticut
Hartford, Connecticut 06105

Dean M. Moutos, M.D.
Assistant Professor
Department of Obstetrics and Gynecology
The University of Arkansas
4301 West Markham, Mail Slot 518
Little Rock, Arkansas 72205

H. Preston Nelson, M.D.
Clinical Assistant Professor
Department of Obstetrics and Gynecology
University of California, San Francisco
San Francisco, California 94143
Fertility Physicians of Northern California
540 University Avenue
Suite 200
Palo Alto, California 94301

Farr Nezhat, M.D.
Clinical Professor
Department of Obstetrics and Gynecology
Stanford University
900 Welch Road
Suite 403
Palo Alto, California 94304

David L. Olive, M.D.
Associate Professor
Chief, Reproductive Endocrinology and Infertility
Department of Obstetrics and Gynecology
Yale University School of Medicine
333 Cedar Street
New Haven, Connecticut 06510

Steven J. Ory, M.D.
Associate Professor
Head, Division of Reproductive Endocrinology and Infertility
Department of Obstetrics and Gynecology
Mayo Clinic
200 First Street SW
Rochester, Minnesota 55905

David B. Redwine, M.D.
St. Charles Medical Center
2500 NE Neff Road
Bend, Oregon 97701

Harry Reich, M.D.
Chief
Advanced Laparoscopic Surgery
New Rochelle Hospital
New Rochelle, New York 10802; and
Advanced Laparoscopic Consultant
Wyoming Valley Health Care System
North River and Auburn Streets
Wilkes-Barre, Pennsylvania 18704

John A. Rock, M.D.
James Robert McCord Professor and Chairman
Department of Gynecology and Obstetrics
Emory University School of Medicine
P.O. Box 21246
Atlanta, Georgia 30322

Joseph S. Sanfilippo, M.D.
Professor
Department of Obstetrics and Gynecology
University of Louisville School of Medicine
550 South Jackson Street
Louisville, Kentucky 40292

Carmelo S. Sgarlata, M.D.
Private Practice
San José, California 95124
Stanford University School of Medicine
Stanford, California 94305

Fayek N. Shamma, M.D.
Assistant Professor
Department of Obstetrics and Gynecology
Michigan State University; and
Ann Arbor Reproductive Medicine Associates
4990 Clark Road
Ypsilanti, Michigan 48197

Cynthia Sherry, M.D.
Diagnostic Radiologist
Presbyterian Hospital of Dallas
8320 Walnut Hill Lane, Suite 100
Dallas, Texas 75231

Eric S. Surrey, M.D.
Assistant Clinical Professor
Department of Obstetrics and Gynecology
UCLA School of Medicine
Los Angeles, California 90024; and
Medical Director
Center for Reproductive Medicine and Surgery
9675 Brighton Way
Suite 420
Beverly Hills, California 90210

Mark W. Surrey, M.D.
Center for Reproductive Medicine and Surgery
9675 Brighton Way
Suite 420
Beverly Hills, California 90210

Thierry G. Vancaillie, M.D.
7940 Floyd Curl Drive
Suite 260
San Antonio, Texas 78229

Ellen E. Wilson, M.D.
7777 Forest Lane
Building C, Suite 638
Dallas, Texas 75230

Preface

Operative endoscopy has revolutionized gynecology in the span of one decade. It has been a great privilege to be able to participate as reproductive surgeons in this transformation of the surgical care of women.

We were very pleased when Lippincott-Raven Publishers asked us to be editors of an atlas of gynecologic endoscopy. The opportunity to contribute to our specialty and to the care of women through the publication of a textbook was, and is, exciting.

We have had several objectives for this atlas. First, we wanted to publish a book that represented the perspectives and experience of the leading endoscopists in North America. Although a few notables were not able to participate, we believe the authors who have written for this atlas do represent most of the leaders in the field of gynecologic endoscopy. Second, it was our purpose to write a comprehensive book. To achieve this goal, each author agreed to write a chapter that would cover all aspects of each unique topic, while contributing to a consistent and focused text. Despite the inherently disparate topics addressed, we believe this goal has been met. Third, we wanted not only to introduce the most recent advances in our field but also to address principles and applications of endoscopic surgery that are necessary for surgeons at any level of expertise. Therefore, we have described different techniques and principles in detail. Fourth, we wanted to provide balance and perspective. We have, therefore, discussed outcomes, complications, and limitations of endoscopic surgery, especially some of the more recent applications. Finally, it was our intention to create a teaching atlas using photographs and illustrations. We believe that the hundreds of excellent photographs and paired descriptive illustrations will achieve that end and help the technical aspects of the text come alive.

This atlas and textbook will be a valued resource for medical students, residents, fellows, and practicing surgeons. Ultimately, our greatest hope is that this atlas will improve the quality of endoscopic surgery provided to our patients in the years to come.

G. David Adamson, M.D.
Daniel C. Martin, M.D.

Acknowledgments

Many people are responsible for the publication of an atlas and textbook. The work involved is an order of magnitude greater than expected when the project is undertaken. A few very special people deserve recognition.

Kathey Alexander of Lippincott-Raven Publishers had the idea to publish this atlas, and we appreciate very much her asking us to do it. We are forever indebted to her for her patience and understanding in the writing of this book.

Associate Editor Mimi Wainwright provided the professional expertise on a daily basis needed to expedite the manuscript. Her professional, friendly, calm, yet relentless demeanor was instrumental in organizing, editing, and compiling chapters, photographs, and drawings from so many authors. We sincerely enjoyed our working relationship with her.

We thank all of the contributors for following the guidelines, editing their manuscripts, and finding photographs for the atlas. It was a pleasure working with them.

We thank our artist, Laura Duprey, for her accurate rendition of our photographs and her commitment to our atlas.

We acknowledge the operating room personnel who made it possible to perform endoscopic surgery. For Dr. Adamson, these include all the Sereno Surgery Center staff, especially Rhonda Ahearne, who was his first and most exuberant surgical assistant when he embarked on advanced endoscopic surgery. It also includes the operating room staff at Good Samaritan Hospital, especially Linda Harman and Karen Marberg. Dr. Martin thanks his staff at Baptist Memorial Hospital.

We thank our office staff, especially Mary Anne McNulty for her dedication and commitment to excellence in preparation of the manuscripts.

Dr. Adamson thanks his mentor, Emmet Lamb, M.D., for supporting his early interest in endoscopy and in the pursuit of clinical research and teaching. Dr. Martin thanks Bob Wheeless with whom he trained and Melvin Cohen and Richard Kleppinger for their teaching and support.

Finally, and most important, we thank our patients, without whom this atlas would not have happened and without whom it would not matter.

PART I

An Introduction to Endoscopic Surgery

Endoscopic Management of Gynecologic Disease,
edited by G.D. Adamson and D.C. Martin.
Lippincott-Raven Publishers, Philadelphia © 1996.

CHAPTER 1

How Endoscopy Transformed Gynecologic Surgery

Grace Lee and Alan H. DeCherney

The establishment of a dominant role for endoscopic surgery in gynecology was foreseen well before the 1990s (1), by which time gynecologic surgeons regarded the use of the laparoscope as commonplace. Since then, a myriad of endoscopic procedures have been fully integrated into the routine gynecologic care of the female patient and an ever increasing number of additional surgical procedures are being approached endoscopically. These procedures are both diagnostic and operative in nature, involving not only preservation but removal of pelvic organs. Today's gynecologist utilizes the laparoscope to visualize, to alleviate, and to prognosticate pelvic disease.

HISTORICAL PERSPECTIVE

In 1944, historian Victor Robinson welcomed operative advances in gynecology that promoted the field beyond darker periods, during which treatment merely added "the tortures of surgery to the blunders of nature" (2). Early endoscopists were restricted by the inability to transfer sufficient light distally into the body cavity, as well as the limited field of vision offered by the open tube. The development of endoscopy and the means by which it has transformed gynecology can thus be viewed literally as a path of light illuminating the darkness.

As early as the era of Hippocrates, primitive tube-like instruments for endoscopy were described (2). Mirrors served as the earliest means to illuminate body cavities, and the technique was developed by the Arabs before 1000 A.D. By 1806, Bozzini had developed a relatively sophisticated vaginal tube illuminated with a lamp. Candlelight illumination of cystoscopic and hysteroscopic procedures was reported by others in the same time period. In the late 1870s, Nitze developed the forerunner of the modern endoscope, which contained a lens system of his own design. Illumination in the Nitze cystoscope was originally achieved with an incandescent platinum wire loop, but by the early 1900s illumination was provided by a low-voltage light bulb.

With significant enhancement of distal illumination and expansion of the visual field, experimentation with endoscopy progressed. Modern operative laparoscopy was initiated by von Ott who in 1901 performed an open laparoscopy and by Kelling who in 1902 introduced the novel concept of filling the cavity with air for better visualization (3). Continuing advances in instrumentation popularized and increased the scope of laparoscopic surgery. In the 1930s, operative laparoscopy for tubal sterilization was introduced to the gynecologic surgeon. By the mid-1970s, an extensive list of operative laparoscopic procedures was reported by Semm.

ENDOSCOPY AND CONSERVATIVE SURGICAL PRACTICE

The endoscopic approach may be regarded as a modern standard for conservative gynecologic surgery. The concept of gynecologic conservatism was formally defined by Kelly in 1898 as "the effort to spare as much as possible of pelvic organs during an operation and to conscientiously avoid the removal of any organs" (4). This principle emphasizes the ideal of preserving the in-

G. Lee: Department of Obstetrics and Gynecology, Yale University School of Medicine, New Haven, Connecticut 06510.

A. H. DeCherney: Department of Obstetrics and Gynecology, Tufts University School of Medicine and New England Medical Center, Boston, Massachusetts 02111.

tegrity of body structures as the highest aim of surgery. In the ideal of conservatism, the endoscopist aims for the greatest relief of diseased tissue while maximally preserving organ structure and minimizing tissue trauma.

This principle is perhaps best exemplified by procedures such as tubal ectopic pregnancy removal by laparoscopic linear salpingostomy and hysteroscopic resection of uterine septa (5,6). With the availability of early measurements of human chorionic gonadotropin (HCG) titers and transvaginal ultrasonography, laparoscopic removal of the ectopic pregnancy has become a routine treatment in the hemodynamically stable patient. Tubal preservation is enhanced by early diagnosis and minimal trauma to the surgical site (7). After laparoscopic discrimination from a bicornuate uterus, a uterine septum may be resected by operative hysteroscopy without the previous sacrifice of myometrium dictated by metroplasty. Hysteroscopic resection of a septum provides equivalent pregnancy rates to metroplasty without mandating cesarean section as a future delivery mode (8). Thus, endoscopy gives the conservative surgeon an elegant means of achieving a favorable outcome.

With the advent of endoscopy, the gynecologist has acquired an invasive means of treatment that leaves less trace of tampering than earlier surgical methods. De novo adhesion formation has been shown to be decreased in laparoscopy (9). The abdominal cavity is not exposed to air, excessive tissue handling is avoided, and the packing of bowel for visualization is not necessary. In order to address the issue of reformation of adhesions, second-look laparoscopy has been advocated for evaluation of previous treatment and, if necessary, repeat lysis of adhesions (9,10). This is in marked contrast to laparotomy, where second-look procedures do not reduce adhesions. In any event, a repeat laparoscopic procedure is more likely to be acceptable to the patient than a repeat laparotomy.

ENDOSCOPY AND THE TREATMENT OF INFERTILITY

For the infertile patient, endoscopy offers diagnosis, treatment, and prognosis. Laparoscopy in conjunction with hysteroscopy is performed diagnostically in instances where the cause of infertility is not readily apparent. Laparoscopy is performed to assess tubal status, pelvic adhesive disease, presence of endometriosis, and resection of myomas, all of which are considered standard indications for endoscopy (11,12). Submucosal myomas, uterine synechiae, and congenital abnormalities can all be addressed by hysteroscopy. These procedures may afford not only diagnosis but the opportunity for concurrent treatment as well.

Endoscopic procedures also have developed concurrently with the emergence of assisted reproductive technologies, such as in vitro fertilization (IVF), gamete intrafallopian tube transfer (GIFT), and zygote intrafallopian tube transfer (ZIFT). If tubal disease is so severe as to prevent adequate repair by endoscopy, in vitro fertilization may provide an effective alternative therapy (13). Hence, endoscopy may serve as a predictor of the next course of treatment, or it may determine the likelihood of success. Prior to the advent of transvaginal aspiration, laparoscopic collection of follicles was performed for in vitro fertilization. In particular groups of patients, the laparoscopic route is preferred for transfer of gametes or embryos into the fallopian tube. Current gynecologic care of the infertile patient routinely involves endoscopy at critical points in the diagnostic and treatment algorithms.

LAPAROTOMY VS. ENDOSCOPY

Complete removal of pelvic structures is readily achieved with endoscopic assistance in the majority of patients. Thus, patients avoid the necessity for laparotomy despite the failure of conservation. Even gynecologic oncology procedures are being performed via an endoscopic approach. Ovarian cystectomy, oophorectomy, lymph node dissection, and hysterectomy have all been performed in selected patients (14,15). With the current universal acceptance of laparoscopy, the role of laparotomy has been redefined and decreased in breadth.

Laparotomy is reserved for cases in which an endoscopic approach cannot render safe or adequate care. Yet some procedures, which were previously categorized as such, are now considered appropriate for endoscopy. This is true for many cases of advanced endometriosis and severe tubal disease. Patients are given the opportunity for corrective surgery by endoscopy if possible, with the recourse of laparotomy if necessary. The gynecologist is at liberty to utilize endoscopic procedures to their utmost, since an appropriate laparotomy may serve to correct any lingering shortcomings of the endoscopic approach.

With regard to enhanced surgical benefits and decreased morbidity, endoscopy may in many cases be viewed as preferable to traditional laparotomy. In general, the choice of an endoscopic route means a shorter recovery period, outpatient management, and decreased cost (16). Furthermore, early ambulation in endoscopy leads to fewer respiratory complications and thromboembolic events. The typical gynecologic patient undergoing operative laparoscopy will not have an overnight hospital stay and will most probably return to work in several days. A similar procedure by laparotomy would mean several days of hospitalization and at least 4 weeks of convalescence. The endoscopic procedure permits the modern woman to minimize the disruption to her life from gynecologic disease.

THE FUTURE

Miniaturization and automation will advance current endoscopic practice to an even higher level of operative elegance (see the chapter by Keye, "Future Developments"). Technical advances in computer-enhanced imaging systems will most surely provide a means of overcoming difficulties associated with distance and limited space in surgical technique (17). Endoscopic surgery, enhanced by an expanded visual field and unhampered by spatial limitations, will constitute an even more refined means of delivering surgical treatment than it does today. Nevertheless, clinical efficacy will ultimately determine the appropriateness of any surgical procedure, regardless of delivery mode.

HIGHLIGHTS

Endoscopy has oriented gynecologic care toward minimally invasive treatments that preserve form while restoring function. Endoscopy permits diagnoses that were previously unavailable except by massive compromise of body integrity. In many instances, endoscopy is the preferential treatment approach. Most importantly, endoscopic findings often prognosticate the benefits and risks of further surgery.

REFERENCES

1. DeCherney A. The leader of the band is tired . . . *Fertil Steril* 1985;44:299.
2. Robinson V. Preface. In: Leonardo R, ed. *History of gynecology.* New York: Forben Press; 1944.
3. Harrison R. The development of modern endoscopy. *J Med Primatol* 1976;5:73.
4. Kelly H. *Operative gynecology.* New York: D Appleton; 1898.
5. Gomel V. Salpingostomy by laparoscopy. *J Reprod Med* 1977;18:265.
6. Chervenak F, Neuwirth R. Hysteroscopic resection of the uterine septum. *Am J Obstet Gynecol* 1981;141:351.
7. DeCherney A, Kase N. The conservative management of unruptured ectopic pregnancy. *Obstet Gynecol* 1979;54:451.
8. DeCherney A, Russell J, Graebe R, Polan M. Rectoscopic management of the mullerian fusion defects. *Fertil Steril* 1985;45:726.
9. Diamond MD, Daniell JF, Feste J, et al. Adhesion reformation and de novo adhesion formation following reproductive surgery. *Fertil Steril* 1987;47:864.
10. Jansen R. Early laparoscopy after pelvic operations to prevent adhesions: safety and efficacy. *Fertil Steril* 1988;49:26.
11. Grimes D. Frontiers of operative laparoscopy. *Am J Obstet Gynecol* 1992;166:1062.
12. Semm K. New methods of pelviscopy for myomectomy, ovariectomy, tubectomy, and adnectomy. *Endoscopy* 1979;2:85.
13. Holst N, Maltau JM, Forsdahl F, Hansen LJ. Handling of tubal infertility after introduction of in vitro fertilization. *Fertil Steril* 1991;55:140.
14. Hunt R, Martin D, eds. *Proceedings of the World Congress of Gynecologic Endoscopy,* 1993.
15. Kovac SR, Cruikshank SH, Retto HF. Laparoscopy assisted vaginal hysterectomy. *J Gyn Surg* 1990;6:185.
16. Azziz R, Steinkampf MP, Murphy A. Post-operative recuperation: relation to the extent of endoscopic surgery. *Fertil Steril* 1989;51:1061.
17. Grimson W, Mundy J. Computer vision applications. *Commun ACM* 1994;37:45.

Endoscopic Management of Gynecologic Disease,
edited by G.D. Adamson and D.C. Martin.
Lippincott-Raven Publishers, Philadelphia © 1996.

CHAPTER 2

Credentialing in Operative Endoscopy

John A. Rock and Dean M. Moutos

The introduction of endoscopy into the field of gynecology has revolutionized both the diagnosis and treatment of many gynecologic diseases. Although initially used as a diagnostic tool, technical advancements in fiberoptics, gas insufflation, and surgical instrumentation have allowed the transition from diagnostic to operative endoscopy to occur over a relatively short period of time. Today over half of all gynecologic operations that once required laparotomy can be performed endoscopically.

Endoscopic surgery has received much attention in the lay press and in the scientific literature and there is considerable pressure on physicians, by both patients and peers, to perform gynecologic procedures endoscopically. Just as ultrasonography and electronic fetal heart rate monitoring had to be mastered by those physicians who received their formal residency training prior to the introduction of these technologies, so too is the case with endoscopic surgery. There are few guidelines that address the issues of training and credentialing in operative endoscopy. The purpose of this chapter is to set forth some general guidelines for the initial training and ongoing evaluation of endoscopic surgeons.

GENERAL CONSIDERATIONS

Before an efficacious technique, such as laparotomy, is replaced by a new technique, such as operative endoscopy, the new technique should meet certain criteria. These include the following: (a) there must be an obvious advantage over the older technique, (b) results must be comparable or superior to those of the older technique, (c) there must be lower risk and/or greater benefit to the patient than the older technique, and (d) the new technique must be one that can be mastered by the practicing gynecologist. A list of gynecologic procedures that can be performed via the laparoscope or hysteroscope is given in Table 1. The fact that a surgical procedure can be performed endoscopically is an insufficient reason by itself to do so. The decision to perform a procedure endoscopically depends on multiple factors, including the expertise of the surgeon, the availability of the necessary equipment, the desires of the patient, and the surgical results one wishes to obtain.

The fact that all gynecologic surgeons perform diagnostic endoscopy does not necessarily qualify them to perform operative endoscopy. Expertise in operative endoscopy requires specific training and experience. Experience in operative endoscopy can be obtained through formal training during residency, postgraduate educational programs, preceptorships with experienced endoscopists, or fellowships in either reproductive endocrinology or reproductive surgery. According to the educational objectives set forth by the Council on Resident Education in Obstetrics and Gynecology (1), the resident should be able to perform both diagnostic and operative endoscopy. The amount of operative endoscopic experience obtained during residency or fellowship is highly variable and there is no agreement as to what constitutes an adequate experience.

GUIDELINES FOR CREDENTIALING IN OPERATIVE ENDOSCOPY

Currently there are no widely accepted standards for credentialing in operative endoscopy to which hospital credentialing committees may refer when granting hospital privileges for endoscopic surgery. Based on the standards proposed by the American Society for Laser Medicine and Surgery for the use of lasers in surgery, we suggest a similar set of guidelines for operative endoscopy (see following paragraphs). Because the laser is frequently utilized in the course of endoscopic surgery, the

J. A. Rock: Department of Gynecology and Obstetrics, Emory University School of Medicine, Atlanta, Georgia 30322.

D. M. Moutos: Department of Obstetrics and Gynecology, The University of Arkansas, Little Rock, Arkansas 72205.

TABLE 1. *Endoscopic procedures*

Laparoscopy	Hysteroscopy
Lysis of adhesions	Resection of submucous myoma
Tubal reconstruction	Removal of uterine polyps
Ovarian cystectomy/reconstruction	Removal of retained intrauterine device
Destruction of endometriosis	Lysis of uterine synechiae
Retroperitoneal dissection	Endometrial ablation
Presacral neurectomy	Sterilization
Removal of tubal ectopic pregnancy	
Myomectomy	
Oophorectomy	
Hysterectomy	
Uterosacral nerve interruption	
Salpingectomy	
Sterilization	
Uterine, ovarian suspension	
Appendectomy	

standards for lasers should also be met by all endoscopic surgeons who wish to use the laser.

1. Physicians requesting privileges to perform endoscopic surgery should have completed a residency in obstetrics and gynecology and be board-certified or an active candidate for board certification. The physician should also have privileges for the same procedures performed by laparotomy.
2. The physician should demonstrate an interest in performing endoscopic surgery by having reviewed the pertinent literature and having used appropriate audiovisual teaching aids. The physician should also have attended a formal course in advanced endoscopic surgical techniques. Such a course should include the following: (a) didactic sessions covering basic endoscopic techniques and instrumentation, (b) hands-on laboratory sessions for a minimum of 8–10 hr with endoscopic training models, such as the Pelvi-Trainer, utilizing tissue specimens such as a placenta or extirpated pelvic organs.
3. The physician should then serve a preceptorship under the guidance of an experienced endoscopist. During this time the physician will observe and assist the preceptor in endoscopic surgery. The physician should then become the primary surgeon with the preceptor assisting and critiquing his or her techniques.
4. Items 2 and 3 may be unnecessary if the physician has had advanced endoscopic training during an accredited residency or fellowship. This training should be documented by a letter from the residency director, who should outline the specific endoscopic procedures for which the applicant received training.

INSTRUMENTATION

The rapid progress in operative endoscopy is due in large part to the development of endoscopic equipment, including fiberoptics, high-flow gas insufflators, video-monitoring devices, lasers, endoscopic sutures, electrical current and heat-delivery systems, and a vast array of surgical instruments. This highly sophisticated equipment requires proper care and maintenance. Certain members of the operating team should have the responsibility of ensuring that the surgical instruments are working properly and that backup instruments are available. Each surgeon should be familiar with the assembly and use of the endoscopic instruments. Although the surgeon is not generally required to assemble the equipment, circumstances may arise that require the surgeon to do so. As new instruments are acquired, the surgeon and the rest of the operating team should become familiar with their use before employing them during surgery. In addition to the endoscopic instruments, the operating room should always have instruments and personnel readily available to perform a laparotomy.

OPERATING ROOM PROFESSIONAL TEAM

Successful endoscopic surgery is clearly a team effort, and the surgeon is but one member of this team. The anesthesiologist, scrub nurse, circulating nurse, and the technicians who maintain the surgical equipment complete the operating team. These members of the team should also have both didactic and clinical training in endoscopic procedures. Each member must have a clear understanding of the principles of operative endoscopy and the goals of each surgical procedure. The endoscopic surgeon is more dependent on other members of the team than he or she would be if the same procedure were performed through the open abdomen. The success of the endoscopic surgeon depends on how well the surgical team works together. Because operative endoscopy is an evolving field, new instruments and procedures are constantly being introduced. In-service programs should be scheduled periodically to keep the members of the operating team abreast of the latest developments. Some of the equipment used in endoscopic surgery is potentially dangerous to both the patient and the operating room personnel; therefore, safety issues should be reviewed periodically.

SURGICAL PROCEDURES

Before a patient undergoes endoscopic surgery, she should be thoroughly apprised of the risks and benefits of endoscopy vs. laparotomy for the specific procedure she is to undergo. The success of a surgical procedure depends to some degree on the experience of the surgeon. Results reported in the literature by experienced endoscopists may not necessarily be achieved by the novice endoscopist. The availability of endoscopic equipment is a necessary but insufficient prerequisite for a successful outcome. Patients should be given realistic expectations about what their surgeon can accomplish through the laparoscope. In some situations laparotomy may be preferred over laparoscopy despite the fact that the procedure can be performed endoscopically by others.

Endoscopic surgery may be frustrating at first. The learning curve for endoscopic procedures is a function of the innate hand–eye coordination of the surgeon and the complexity of the procedure being performed. Some procedures, such as removal of an unruptured tubal pregnancy, can be mastered relatively quickly, whereas more complex procedures, such as resection of deeply infiltrating endometriosis or retroperitoneal node dissection, may be mastered only after carefully supervised instruction. There are no guidelines to determine how many endoscopic procedures a surgeon must perform before he or she masters the technique. It is essential, however, that the initial portion of the learning curve occur under the auspices of an experienced endoscopist. Only in this manner can the trainee's endoscopic techniques be critically evaluated and modified.

PRIMARY CERTIFICATION AND COMPETENCE

Primary credentialing in operative endoscopy should require the successful completion of a training course in endoscopic surgery. The use of a video display is useful in learning and critiquing endoscopic surgery. When one is learning endoscopic surgery, experience and confidence should initially be gained with relatively simple endoscopic procedures. Once these simple procedures have been mastered, the more complicated techniques may be acquired.

It does not necessarily follow that a person credentialed to perform endoscopic surgery is credentialed to perform any procedure endoscopically. Just as a surgeon who performs laparotomies has privileges to perform only certain surgical procedures through the open abdomen, so should be the case for the endoscopic surgeon. Endoscopic surgical privileges should be granted for each procedure the surgeon wishes to perform and after the surgeon has presented evidence that he or she has had sufficient experience to perform that procedure.

OUTCOME ASSESSMENT AND CONTINUOUS QUALITY IMPROVEMENT

Once a physician has been credentialed in endoscopic surgery, there should be a system to monitor his or her performance periodically. This should be done for the recently credentialed endoscopist as well as for the experienced endoscopist. Quality assurance has been defined as an effort to enhance patient care through the ongoing, objective assessment of important aspects of patient care and the correction of identified problems (2). A well-organized quality assurance program not only improves patient care but helps to minimize medicolegal liabilities. Quality assurance may consist of a focused review of selected clinical indicators. A clinical indicator is a quantifiable clinical event, complication, or outcome for which data are collected. Examples of clinical indicators relevant to operative endoscopy include the following: (a) unplanned admission of an ambulatory surgery patient, (b) unplanned return to the operating room for surgery, (c) injury or repair of an organ during surgery, (d) initiation of postoperative antibiotics or occurrence of infection not present on admission, and (e) transfusion of blood products. The presence of one or more of these clinical indicators does not necessarily imply substandard care; it identifies potential problems that require further review. Peer review of the medical record will then determine whether or not the quality of care deviated significantly from the accepted norm. In this manner substandard care can be identified early and corrective action taken. Evaluation of the quality of care given by a physician is a sensitive issue. Patient and physician anonymity should be upheld as much as possible except when the information is needed to take corrective action or when it is required for recredentialing.

An equally important aspect in the monitoring of endoscopic surgery is an evaluation of surgical outcome, i.e., pain relief, pregnancy, indications for further surgery. Measurement of these outcomes requires long-term follow up but is essential to improving patient care. There are few studies that accurately compare endoscopic surgery to laparotomy. One should not automatically assume that an endoscopic procedure will yield better or even equivalent results to laparotomy. There is significant interphysician variability in the technique and results of endoscopic surgery, and it is essential that each physician carefully monitor his or her results for each type of endoscopic procedure. Only in this manner can unsuccessful procedures be identified and abandoned while successful ones are maintained and improved.

PRACTICAL ASPECTS OF CREDENTIALING IN HOSPITALS

Endoscopic surgery requires special training and experience. Each hospital should establish an endoscopy credentialing committee consisting of physicians who are actively involved in endoscopic surgery. Physicians requesting endoscopic surgical privileges should present their qualifications to this committee along with a list of the specific endoscopic procedures for which they are requesting privileges. We have attempted to set forth some general guidelines by which endoscopic surgeons should be credentialed, but each hospital must establish its own specific criteria. Whatever the mechanism, it is imperative that the physician present evidence of his or her competence in performing advanced endoscopic surgery. When a new or innovative endoscopic procedure is to be performed, the surgeon should present his or her rationale for performing the procedure along with a review of the published literature, if any, concerning this new procedure. The purpose of this is not to discourage the development of new surgical procedures but to ensure patient safety and provide peer review of new techniques.

We believe it is imperative that every hospital establish a formal credentialing process for gynecologic endoscopy. In addition to the initial credentialing process, there should be a periodic reassessment of all endoscopic surgeons. Physicians should take the initiative for monitoring and regulating their own actions and those of their peers. If physicians do not do this, outside agencies will certainly do it for them.

REFERENCES

1. Council on Resident Education in Obstetrics and Gynecology. *Educational objectives for residents in obstetrics and gynecology.* 1984: 101.
2. American College of Obstetricians and Gynecologists. *Quality assurance in obstetrics and gynecology.* 1989:73.

Endoscopic Management of Gynecologic Disease,
edited by G.D. Adamson and D.C. Martin.
Lippincott-Raven Publishers, Philadelphia © 1996.

CHAPTER 3

Electrosurgery and Endoscopic Energy

Principles and Risks

Thierry G. Vancaillie

There are many energy sources available for endosurgical procedures. These can be divided into two main groups: the cold energy group, including mechanical and hydraulic energy; and the hot energy group, which includes the direct application of heat, electrical current, and electromagnetic energy, i.e., laser.

In the cold energy group, the effects are direct, immediate, and simple. Force is applied to a structure until it breaks. The resistance to breakage of tissue depends on the elasticity and tensile strength of the tissue. Adhesions are generally less elastic than normal tissue. Their tensile strength is also lower. As a result, when force is applied, the adhesion will be the structure that breaks before the healthy tissue gives way.

Energy effects on tissue from the so-called hot energy group can be divided into two successive steps. The first step consists of tissue-specific energy absorption. This causes a rise in tissue temperature. The second step consists of heat propagation in tissue. Heat propagation in tissue is tissue-dependent, not energy source–dependent. The energy source that was originally used to create a temperature rise in tissue does not affect the wave of heat propagation through the tissue. The factors limiting or promoting heat propagation are, among others, fluid content of the tissue and the cooling effect of vascularization.

Heat transforms tissue, which in turn may influence the tissue specificity by which energy is absorbed. An example is the blanching of tissue when the proteic content is slowly heated (Fig. 1). Energy absorption, such as laser energy, may be color-dependent, and is impeded by this heat-induced change.

T. G. Vancaillie: Center for Gynecologic Endosurgery, San Antonio, Texas 78229.

The resting temperature of tissue is approximately 37°C. When tissues heat up somewhat slowly to approximately 45°C, one observes reversible changes, which can only be assessed by chemical means. So-called heat shock proteins are produced by the cells to protect themselves against the rise in tissue temperature.

Sustained tissue temperature increased beyond 45°C induces coagulation of the protein contents of the cell. Theoretically, the term *coagulation* is used correctly only in this context; however, in everyday language *coagulation* and *hemostasis* are often interchanged. In this text, an effort is made to use these terms correctly. Coagulated tissue is not compatible with survival. Vital stains show that the tissue is void of respiratory activity. However, the tissue framework remains intact, i.e., the cell membranes, the lamina propria, and the reticular supportive tissues remain in place. In tissues with high regenerative capacity, this thermal insult has little long-term effect.

Increasing the tissue temperature beyond 60°C starts the process of desiccation. During this process, the water content of the cell is driven out until there is complete dryness. As long as there is water available for evaporation, the tissue temperature remains below 100°C. This is the point of no return. The tissue framework is destroyed, although there is no loss of material except for vapor. The difference between coagulated tissue and desiccated tissue is similar to that between a worn-down building and a collapsed building. In both cases there is no loss of material, but a collapsed building and desiccated tissue cannot be salvaged. Desiccation is the optimal endpoint for thermal tissue destruction because hemostasis and irreversible tissue damage result. In addition to this, there are no long-term deleterious effects. Therefore, desiccation is the endpoint aimed for in energy transfer to tissue.

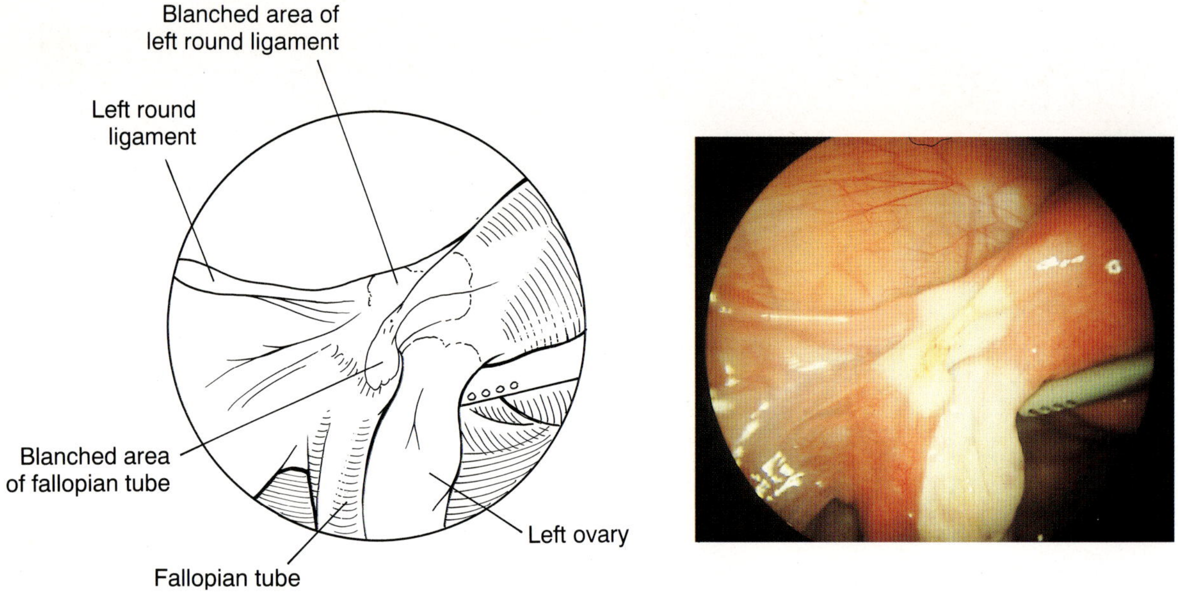

FIG. 1. Blanching of the mesosalpinx and the left round ligament are noted following a bipolar coagulation of the tube.

Once the tissue is completely dry or desiccated, continued heat transfer causes disintegration of the individual components of the cell into parts of oxygen, nitrogen, hydrogen, and other elements, including carbon. This is expressed visually in the blackening of the tissue, which is called *carbonization* (Fig. 2).

If energy transfer occurs fast and in huge amounts, these different steps of tissue transformation are shortcut. One observes vaporization or fulguration. In vaporization the fluids inside the cells heat up so fast that they cause explosion of the cell (Fig. 3). This occurs, for instance, with the CO_2 laser that is in optical resonance with water. In fulguration, the arc that generates up to 500°C of heat hits the tissue from the outside and causes explosion of the tissue (Fig. 4). In both circumstances, intact and viable particles of the cell are released into the atmosphere. This mixture of smoke and particles is called plume.

The efficiency of heat transfer to tissue depends on the amount of energy delivered to the tissue and on the cooling system available within the tissue. If an insufficient dose of energy is delivered to the tissue per unit of time,

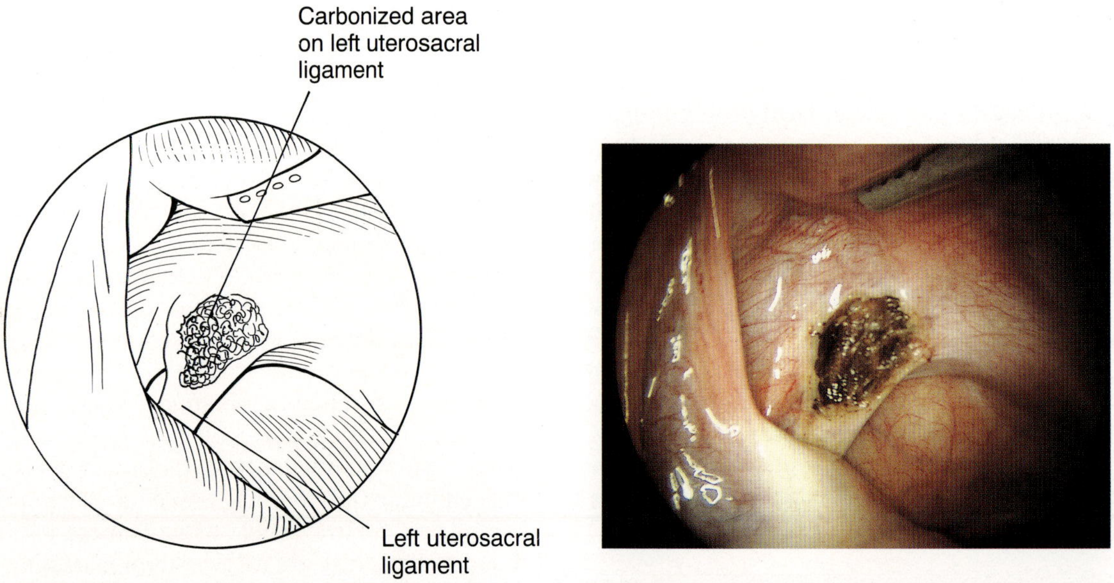

FIG. 2. Carbonization after using fulguration for hemostasis following resection of the left uterosacral ligament lesion.

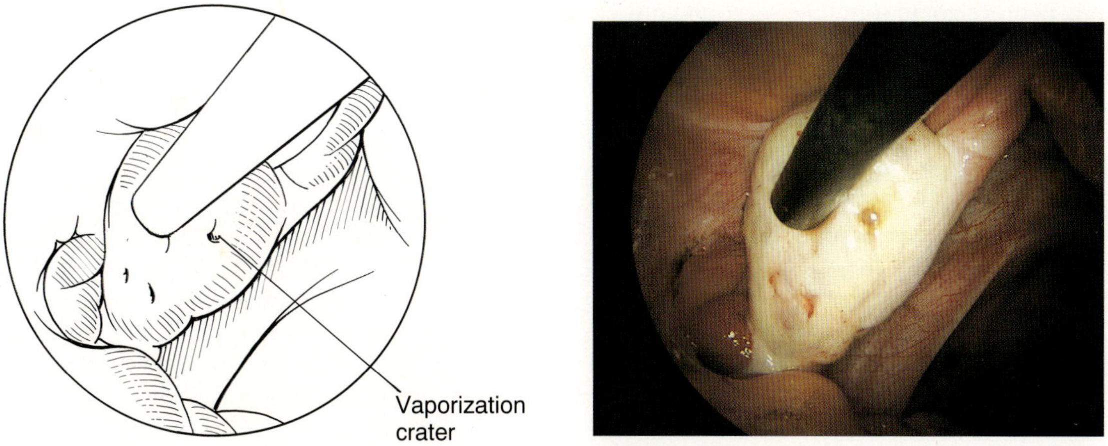

FIG. 3. Vaporization crater following vaporization of a small lesion of the left ovary.

a rise in temperature is somewhat difficult to obtain and maintain. On the other hand, if an excess of energy is delivered to the tissue within a short period of time, carbonization occurs; this situation is to be avoided because it will cause a foreign body reaction. Ideally, enough energy is delivered to the tissue to obtain desiccation.

PRINCIPLES OF "MONOPOLAR" ELECTROSURGERY (1)

Electrocautery is the indirect application of electrical current by heating a conductive element, which is then used to burn tissue. Electrosurgery is the direct application of electrical energy to the tissues. The patient is actually part of the electrical circuit.

When the electrical field is applied to tissue, elements of opposite charge are attracted to either a positive or a negative pole of the electric field. Tissue is composed of large negatively charged particles, i.e., the proteins, and small positively charged particles such as sodium and potassium. Because of the difference in mass, it is obvious that the sodium and potassium will move more readily than the large proteins. The result is an exit of sodium and potassium out of the cell, which causes the membrane potential to decrease, resulting in the formation of an action potential. This action potential causes nerve and muscle stimulation. If the electrical field is maintained, the sodium and potassium cannot reenter the cell and therefore paralysis will occur. This kind of application of electrical current is actually used in medicine for treatment of pain and is called diadynamic current. The depolarization of the cell membrane prevents stimulation and interrupts the signal that is responsible for pain sensation.

To avoid stimulation of the cell membrane, one can alternate the signs of the poles at a fast rate, so that there is no time for sodium and potassium to leave the cell physically. This is called high-frequency or radiofrequency electrical current. It has been shown that the number of cycles per second—in other words, the number of times the signs change—has to be 100,000 per sec-

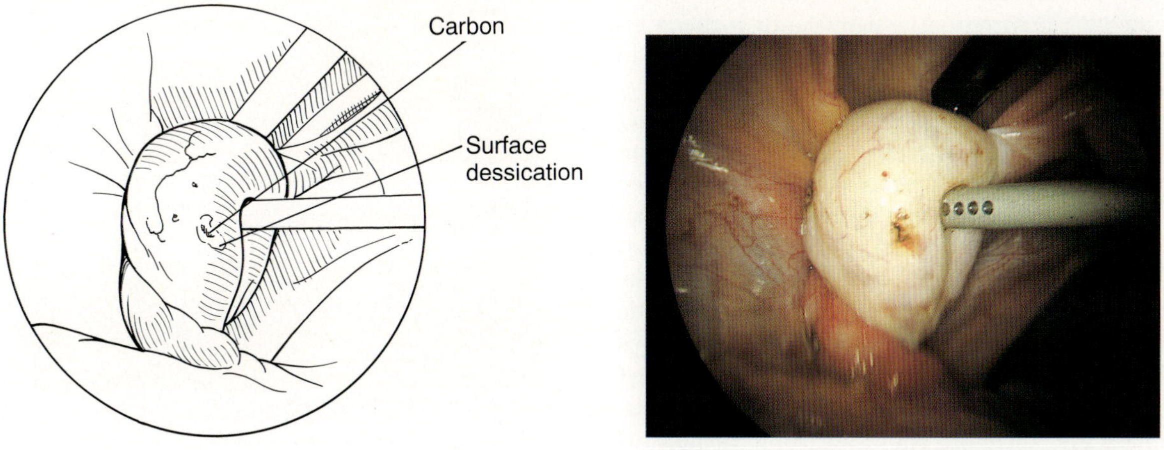

FIG. 4. Surface desiccation and carbon following fulguration of a surface lesion of a left ovary.

ond or more, in order not to stimulate nerve and muscle tissues. The electrosurgical units (ESUs) used in the operating room typically operate between 400,000 and 1 million cycles per second (Hertz).

The frequency at which alternating current is used in surgery can be modulated. Modulation means that the number of cycles per second is changed, as is the deflection of each cycle. Some typical modulations have been given names, such as cutting, fulguration, spray coagulation, blend, etc. It is important to note that these denominations are purely empirical. Employing one or the other modulation does not necessarily imply that cutting or fulguration will ensue. Neither does it imply that the other effect cannot take place. It probably is wishful thinking that denomination of the waveforms will one day return to a purely descriptive form, such as continuous, interrupted, or damped waveform. Some manufacturers are making an effort to increase our understanding of the different waveforms. However, they invariably fall in the trap of naming the waveform according to the expected bioeffect that its application is supposedly intended for. The use of electrical energy is far from the simplicity this nomenclature seems to foster.

Cutting current is a current with a continuous, sinusoidal waveform. A continuous current is used to desiccate or cut tissues. What used to be called coagulation waveform should be called fulguration or—better—damped waveform. In this waveform, the voltage is increased to, for instance, 5000 V and the time of exposure of the current to tissue is reduced to a short period of time, approximately 6%; in other words, the current is on 6% of the time and off 94% of the time. On average the amount of electrical energy delivered may actually be higher in the continuous mode than in the damped mode, because the continuous mode is on all the time whereas, the damped mode is on for a very short period of time.

A continuous current is a very smooth and soft current that causes fine, sharp cuts. In the damped mode, the electrical current is more powerful and abrupt and causes more tissue damage per unit of time the tissues are exposed to the current. The significantly higher voltage of the damped mode allows the current to jump a gap more easily than in the continuous mode.

Blend current has led to some confusion among physicians. In practical terms and in consideration of an electrosurgical unit in the operating room, the damped mode would be on the right and the continuous or desiccation mode would be on the left, and it is the latter that can be blended. Blending current does not mean that the output of the damped mode and the continuous mode are mixed. The blended mode means that the continuous mode is modified to look a little bit more like the damped mode. The voltage is increased, which provides more tissue damage and therefore allows for some hemostasis during cutting. The increased voltage is compensated for by interrupting the blend continuous mode for variable periods of time. Blending may vary from one electrosurgical unit to another but typically the current is interrupted for 25% or 50% to 75% of the time in successive degrees of blending.

One of the cardinal principles of electrosurgery is the difference between contact and noncontact modes (Fig. 5A and B). When contact is established between the electrode and tissue before the circuit is activated, the current can spread into the tissue immediately. Therefore a large volume of tissue is affected and the tissue temperature rises rather slowly over a large volume (Fig. 6). This is ideal when desiccation is desired. In the noncontact mode, the ESU is activated prior to establishing contact between the electrode and the tissue. In so doing, there is actually no current flowing through the tissue and the circuit is said to be open. A high-voltage difference is built up between the tissue and the electrode that has been activated. A spark, which is generated by this potential difference, hits the tissue and causes a very localized and superficial burn. Consequently, very little tissue is affected by the electrical current (Fig. 7).

Another important principle of electrosurgery is the relationship between time and intensity (Fig. 8A and B). It is a tendency of most surgeons to set the wattage as high as possible in order for them to move as quickly as possible through the tissue. A high-intensity current

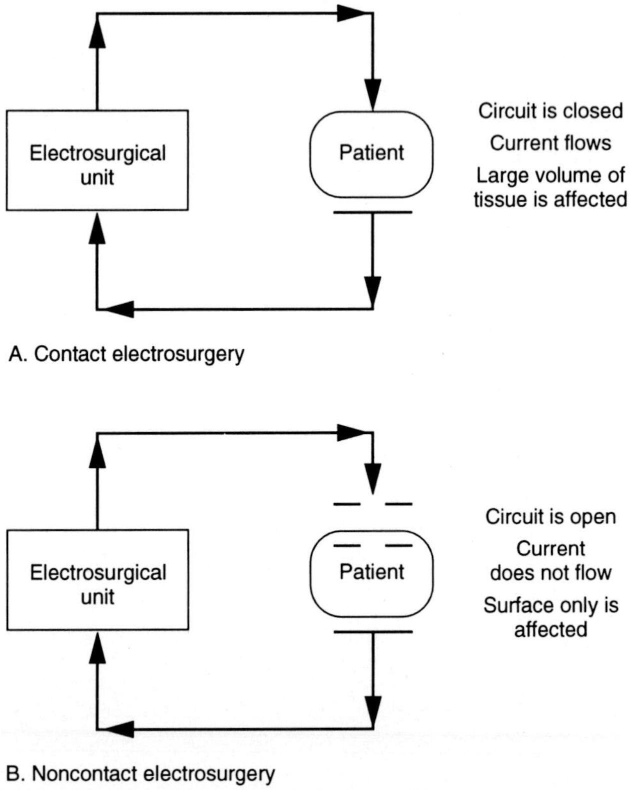

FIG. 5. Schematic representation of (**A**) contact vs. (**B**) noncontact electrosurgery. ESU, electrosurgical unit.

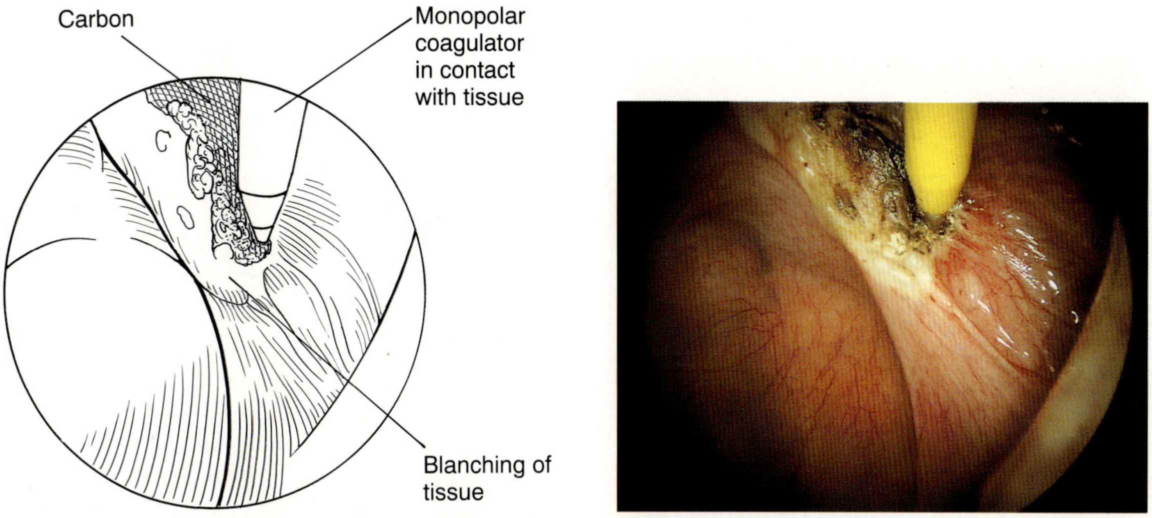

FIG. 6. Contact coagulation with monopolar used and blanching noted.

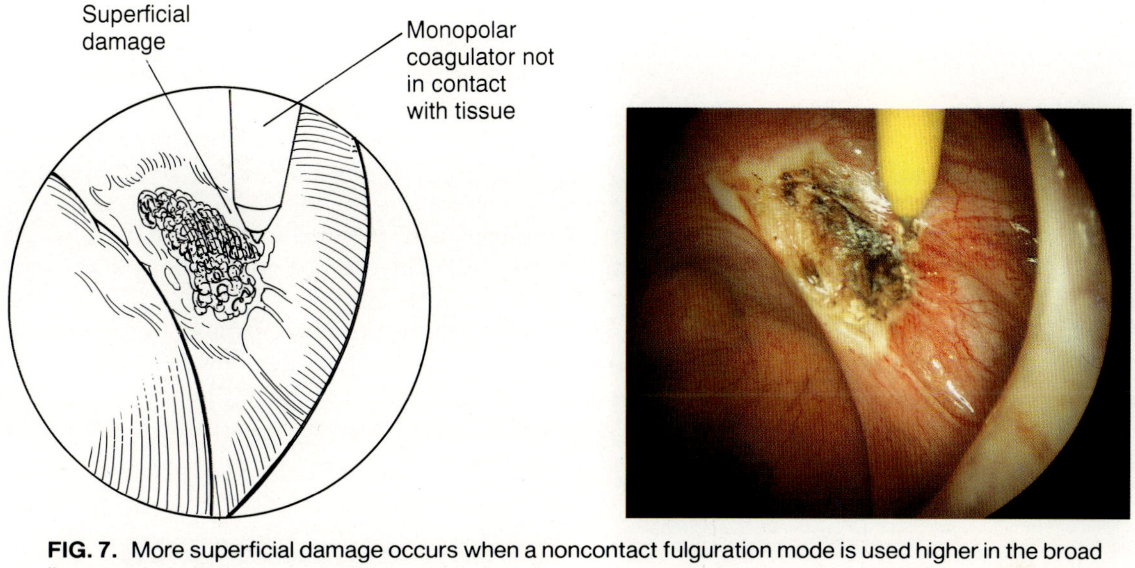

FIG. 7. More superficial damage occurs when a noncontact fulguration mode is used higher in the broad ligament.

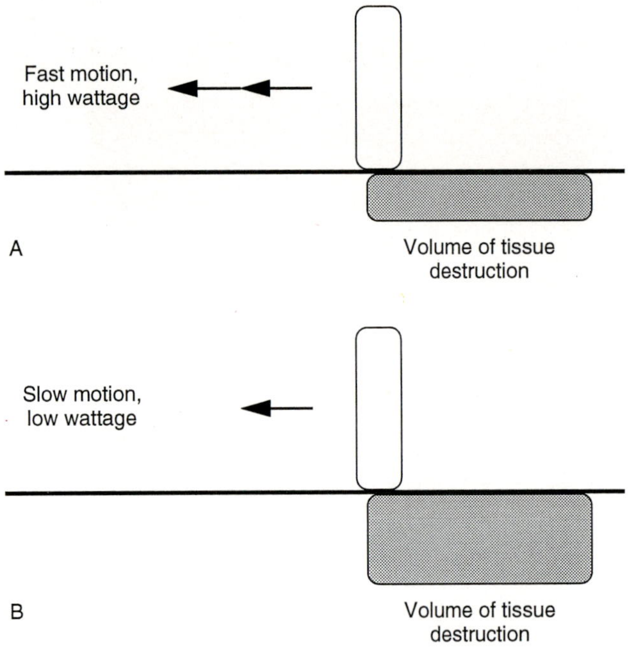

FIG. 8. Schematic representation of the difference in bioeffect caused by the relation of current intensity and speed. **A**: Fast motion, high wattage. **B**: Slow motion, low wattage.

indeed allows the surgeon to move the electrode quickly; however, this current affects the tissue only superficially. This may be the ideal method for cutting but not for desiccation. If the density is set at a low level and the electrode is moved slowly, then the current penetrates more deeply and affects larger volumes of tissues. This is the ideal handling of the electrode for desiccation purposes.

A third principle is that the electrode needs to remain as clean as possible. In some cases one should consider the electrode a disposable item. Buildup of char on the electrode (Fig. 9) forces the user to increase the intensity and voltage of the current used. A high-intensity, high-voltage current is more likely to produce stray currents, which may result in inadvertent burns (2). Frequent cleaning of the electrode during use is certainly advisable.

PRINCIPLES OF BIPOLAR ELECTROSURGERY

All electrosurgical systems used since the 1970s are bipolar in nature. Two poles are in contact in one fashion or another with the patient. However, because of the analogy between a ground plate and a return electrode, systems that use a large return electrode continue to be called monopolar. In strict physical terms this is not correct.

Bipolar systems are systems with two poles of identical electrical mass. In other words, each one of these electrodes has an equal power density. In what is erroneously called monopolar electrosurgery, the two electrodes have power densities that are significantly different. Future systems may make this differential definition obsolete, but for the time being such definition helps in understanding the difference in mechanism between a monopolar and bipolar system.

In a monopolar system, the entire patient is in between the two poles, which are physically separated far apart. In a bipolar system, the electrodes are close to each other and the tissue is brought in between these two electrodes (Fig. 10). The practical implications of the bipolar system are as follows.

Because the leads are parallel to each other, voltage differences have to be kept low to avoid shortcircuits. A low-voltage difference limits the spectrum of clinical ap-

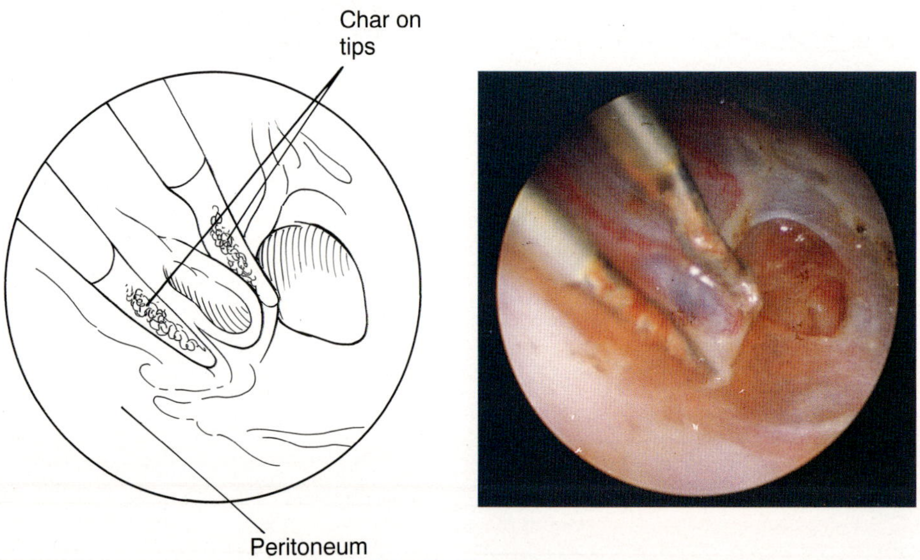

FIG. 9. Bipolar instrument with char on the tip.

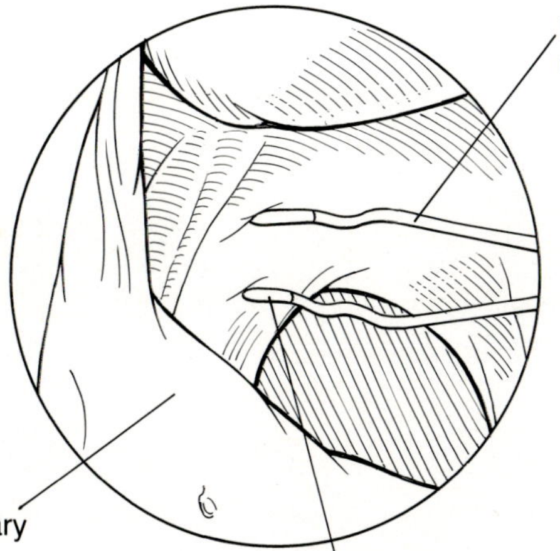

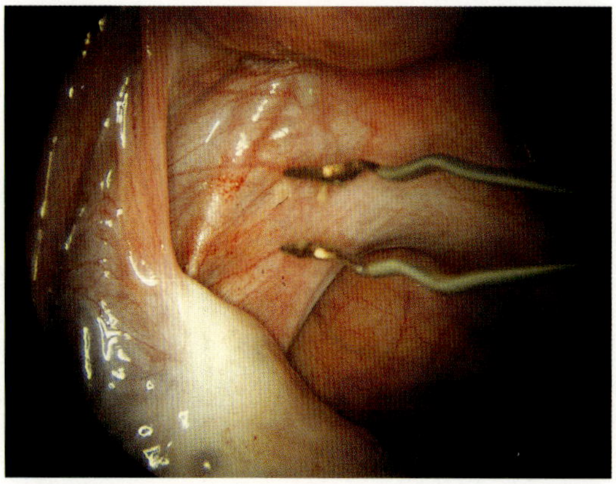

FIG. 10. Bipolar Kleppinger forceps.

plications. Although bipolar electrodes designed to cut tissue are available on the market, they certainly do not come close to the efficiency of monopolar electrodes. It is claimed that they are safer. I would personally disagree with this. The main safety factor in surgery is the surgeon, both through his or her knowledge of the instrumentation used and his or her ability to perform the technical aspects of the procedure. Nevertheless there are intrinsic differences between monopolar and bipolar systems, which make the bipolar safer. The two most important differences are the low voltage and the absence of capacitive coupling. The low voltage of bipolar systems is a physical requirement to avoid internal breakdown of the instrument by electrical shortcircuit. This leads to the reduced risk of direct coupling between the instrument and the tissue. However, this also leads to reduced ability to spark a gap. The latter physical effect is the one required to achieve bioeffects, such as cutting and spray coagulation. As a result, the bipolar instruments are inferior in performance when it comes to cutting tissue or arresting capillary bleeding by fulguration. Capacitive coupling is absent because the two poles are parallel to each other and the induced currents cancel each other out. An exception to this would occur in the event a significant amount of current leaks from one of the poles. Even in such an unusual event, the low voltage again plays in favor of the bipolar instrument because the amount of energy that can be coupled is a direct function of the voltage.

In summary, the bipolar instrument is safer because of the significant reduction of direct and capacitive coupling. However, the bipolar instrument is less effective in producing the energy required to cut or fulgurate efficiently. Therefore this instrument is ideally used for desiccation of tissue. In this latter function, the bipolar instrument is superior to the monopolar equivalent because the tissue to be desiccated can be placed precisely in between the prongs of the instrument.

The main disadvantage of the bipolar equipment is that the amount of energy transfer is more likely inadequate as compared to monopolar instruments. One does not fear excess but rather deficit of energy. The best known example is tubal sterilization with bipolar forceps. Failure rates as high as 10% have been reported from surgeons using bipolar electrosurgery as the method of tissue destruction (3).

PRACTICAL APPLICATIONS

The physical characteristics of the electrical current in relation to the desired bioeffect are given in Table 1.

Cutting

To obtain a smooth cutting of tissue, one uses a needle tip electrode that allows application of a high-power den-

TABLE 1. *Physical characteristics of the electrical current in relation to the desired bioeffect*

Characteristic	Cut	Desiccate	Fulgurate
Configuration (shape factor)	Needle	Spatula	Any
Waveform	Continuous	Continuous or interrupted	Damped
Contact vs. noncontact	Noncontact	Contact	Noncontact

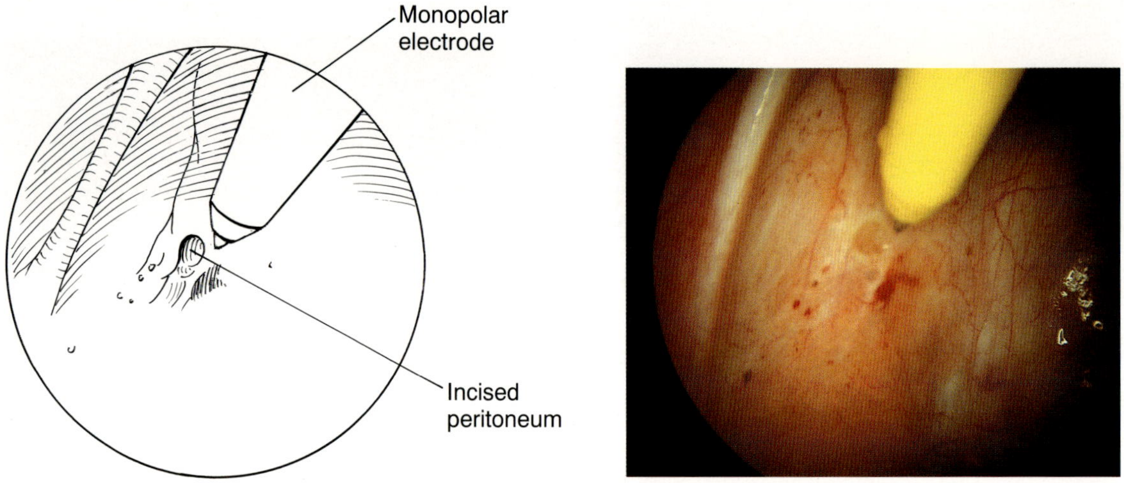

FIG. 11. Initial incision into the peritoneum to remove a left cul-de-sac lesion of endometriosis.

sity of electrical energy on the tissue. One uses a continuous low-voltage current to offer a smooth and continuous cut. The surgeon holds the electrode away from the tissue. Cutting is a *no-contact* mode; it could be said that the surgeon brushes over the surface with the electrode (Figs. 11 and 12). This brushing maneuver is done in short strokes to avoid inadvertent contact with tissue that is not intended for cutting. The smoothest cutting action is obtained with a continuous current at relatively high wattage. Actually, the speed by which the electrode can be moved directly depends on the wattage used. For surgery under water, as in transurethral resections or in operative hysteroscopy, high energy levels are required because of the higher impedance of the fluid medium. Underwater electrosurgery is the most demanding situation for the electrosurgical unit, and it is very important to use the appropriate machine.

Cutting and Coagulation

Simultaneous cutting and coagulation is actually a hybrid situation in which the surgeon wants to obtain hemostasis along with cutting. There is no electrosurgical modality that allows for optimal cutting and optimal hemostasis at the same time. Both tissue effects are diametrically opposite. To obtain some hemostasis while cutting, one needs to use an electrode that provides a low power density. This is achieved with a spatula-type electrode. The surgeon still activates the continuous mode of the generator and still brushes the tissue in a noncontact manner but, to allow for hemostasis, he now uses the interrupted continuous mode. In the interrupted continuous mode the voltage is higher and therefore causes more tissue destruction. However, the current is on for only a portion of time to compensate for the increased

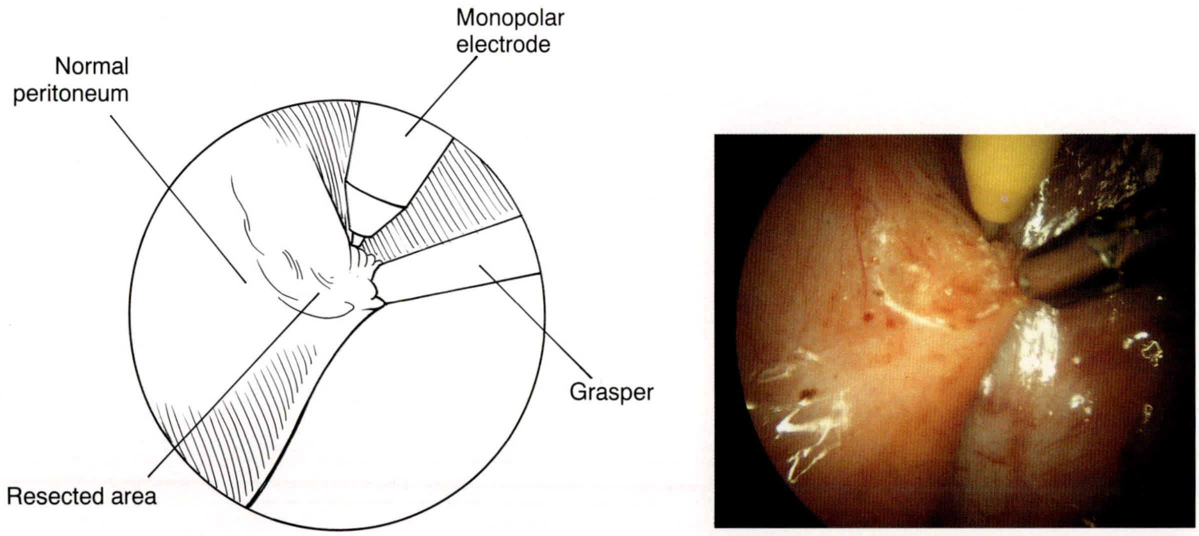

FIG. 12. The lesion of Fig. 11 has been grasped pulled medially. The monopolar electrode is used to dissect and remove the lesion.

voltage. This reduction in time allows cooling of the electrode in between bursts of energy. In the absence of such cooling periods, the active electrode could actually start melting. The wattage used in the blend mode again dictates how fast the surgeon can move the electrode. However, because the surgeon aims at obtaining simultaneous hemostasis, it is important to move the electrode relatively slowly and, therefore, to use a relatively low wattage.

Desiccation

The objective of dessication is to obtain destruction of tissue over a relatively large volume. This may be in the context of hemostasis or in the context of destruction of a particular type of tissue, such as the endometrium. To obtain desiccation, we use an electrode that lowers the power density, such as the ball-type electrode. They are the largest electrodes used currently in electrosurgery. Because the surgeon wants deep penetration into tissue, he or she uses a low-voltage current, i.e., a continuous or interrupted waveform. This is disconcerting for most surgeons because the electrical current is labeled as in cutting mode, whereas the surgeon aims at obtaining desiccation, often mistakenly thought of as coagulation. However, slow and deep penetration of current into tissue, affecting a large volume, can best be obtained using low-intensity continuous current. Two different tissue effects are obtained: cutting vs. desiccation, with one and the same waveform through differences in usage of the current. For desiccation, contact between the electrode and the tissue is established before activation of the electrode. For cutting, the electrode is activated before contact. The shape of the electrode is such that a low power density is obtained for desiccation and a high power density for cutting. With a spatula-type electrode, one can present the edge of the electrode for cutting and the large flat side for desiccation. With the same settings on the ESU, the difference in surface is sufficient to alter the power density and obtain different tissue effects. Both the continuous and interrupted mode are useful for desiccation. The choice between both depends primarily on the tissue type that is considered. Tissues that do not conduct electrical current very well, such as fat, require higher voltage to obtain the same effect as compared to tissues that conduct electrical current well. As far as wattage is concerned, the lowest wattage possible is the best to obtain maximum desiccation.

Bipolar Desiccation

A continuous current is the most effective for bipolar desiccation. A setting at approximately 25 W achieves the best results. It is important to remember that bipolar desiccation is a relatively slow process when compared to monopolar electrosurgery. However, the advantage of bipolar systems is that the tissue to be desiccated is held in between the two poles of the instruments. Damage at a distance is still possible but by thermal spread rather than by electrical current.

There are several important issues to discuss with regard to bipolar desiccation. First of all, because the poles are so close, there is a high risk for electrical shortcircuit and therefore inadequate delivery of the energy to the tissue. Shortcircuit can occur when fluid is absorbed within the sheath of the instrument. The law of least resistance dictates that the current will travel through the fluid and bypass the tissue. The fluid evaporates and only then does desiccation of tissue start, delaying the desired effect.

Some system models have built-in current intensity meters, which indicate when current ceases to flow. Supposedly this means that the tissue is adequately desiccated. This is an assumption, not a fact. The actual information provided to the surgeon is that the resistance to current flow is too high. It is implied that the electrosurgical generator is capable of overcoming the impedance of desiccated tissue. Therefore, if there is no further flow, a logical consequence of these assumptions is that the tissue between the branches of the instrument is indeed desiccated to the point that current cannot flow through it any longer. The impedance of the tissue, however, is not only dependent on the presence of fluid and electrolytes but on the amount of tissue between the prongs of the instrument. The forceps applied to the tissue will compress the tissue and ideally reduce the gap to 1 or 2 mm. The voltage applied to the instrument is then able to drive the current through this mass of tissue until it is completely void of conductive particles, i.e., a state of complete dryness is achieved. However, in the event approximation of the branches is not possible, e.g., the oviduct is significantly thickened, then the tissue presents an increased impedance to start with, and the voltage available will not be sufficient to reach complete desiccation because of the larger gap. This cannot be assessed by simple visual inspection. In this case the current meter indicates that there is no further flow of current, which is correct information. The tissue however is not completely desiccated and therefore not completely destroyed (Fig. 13). These restrictions taken into account, the availability of a current meter is valuable in the use of bipolar instrumentation and when the limiting factor that bulky clumps of tissue represent is known. Added information can be obtained by what I would call the biological meter. This applies for tubal sterilization in particular. After the surgeon obtains desiccation that appears adequate according to parameters such as visual inspection or by physical measurement of the current flow, the fallopian tube is transected. This allows the surgeon to inspect visually whether the actual endosalpinx has indeed been fully destroyed. Complete desicca-

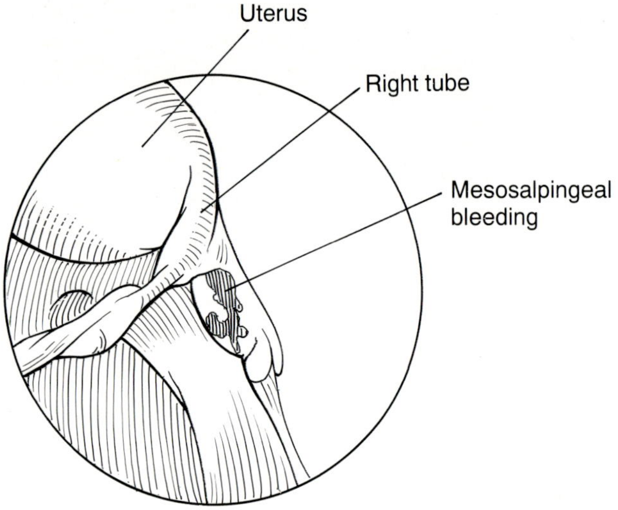

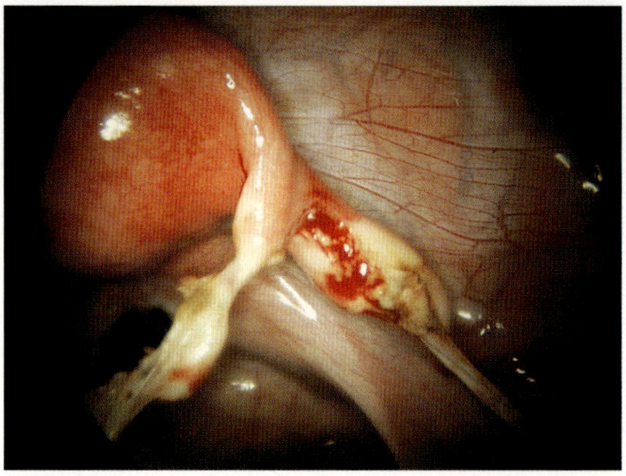

FIG. 13. Incomplete desiccation of the mesosalpingeal vessels has resulted in bleeding during removal of the right tube.

tion is marked by a complete absence of capillary bleeding from the section plane (Fig. 14). One may note that capillary bleeding can occur several minutes after the oviduct has been cut. This remains an indication of inadequate energy transfer.

Additional discussion of the safety of bipolar instrumentation is needed. One is familiar with the bubbling of tissue when bipolar forceps are applied (Fig. 15). It is also noted that, once this effect subsides, the blanching of the tissue seems to spread laterally (Fig. 16). The actual events are as follows. Fluid of the tissue evaporates, which is seen as bubbling. Evaporation provides cooling and prevents heat from propagating to neighboring tissues. Once all fluid evaporates, the generated heat cannot be contained any longer and spreads. This is seen clinically as a blanching of tissues away from the forceps, which seems to progress rapidly. Although this is not an electrical effect, it is damaging to healthy tissue. Temperatures at lethal levels have been recorded in tissue as far as 20 mm away from a bipolar instrument used in the usual fashion (4).

It is therefore somewhat inappropriate to state that bipolar instruments can be used close to vital structures, such as the ureter, without fear for complications. Thermal injuries are as lethal to tissue as electrical injuries.

Prevention of thermal injuries is relatively simple. First it is recommended to keep the instruments used for electrosurgery away from tissue not intended for destruction. Instruments for electrosurgery should be used only for that purpose. This includes not using an electrosurgical instrument to passively stabilize the bowel, in case it is unintentionally electrified. Also, one should not use the bipolar forceps as grasping forceps except when electrical current is to be applied.

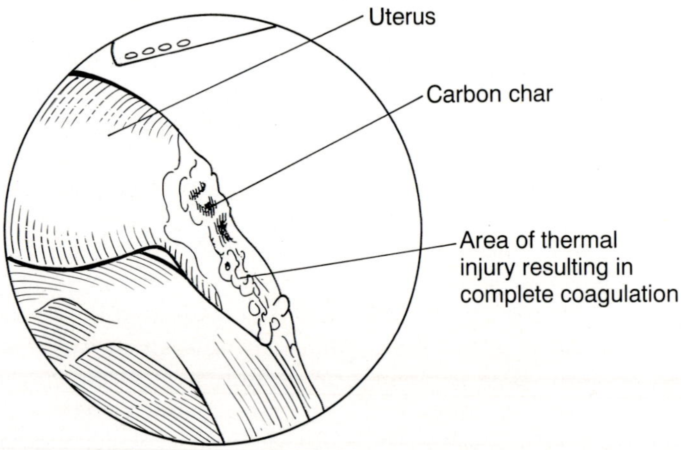

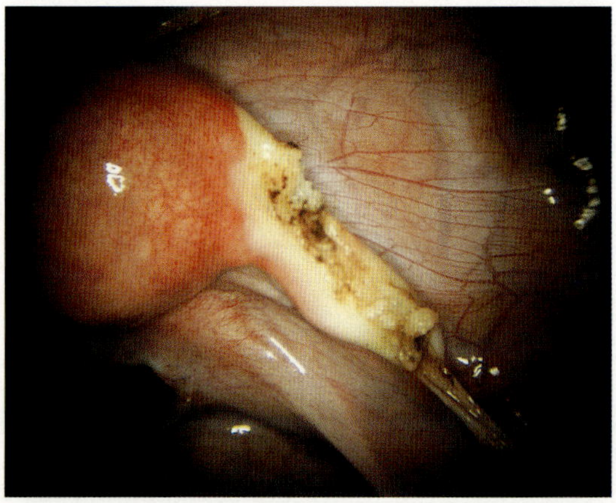

FIG. 14. Complete coagulation and full hemostasis in the patient of Fig. 13.

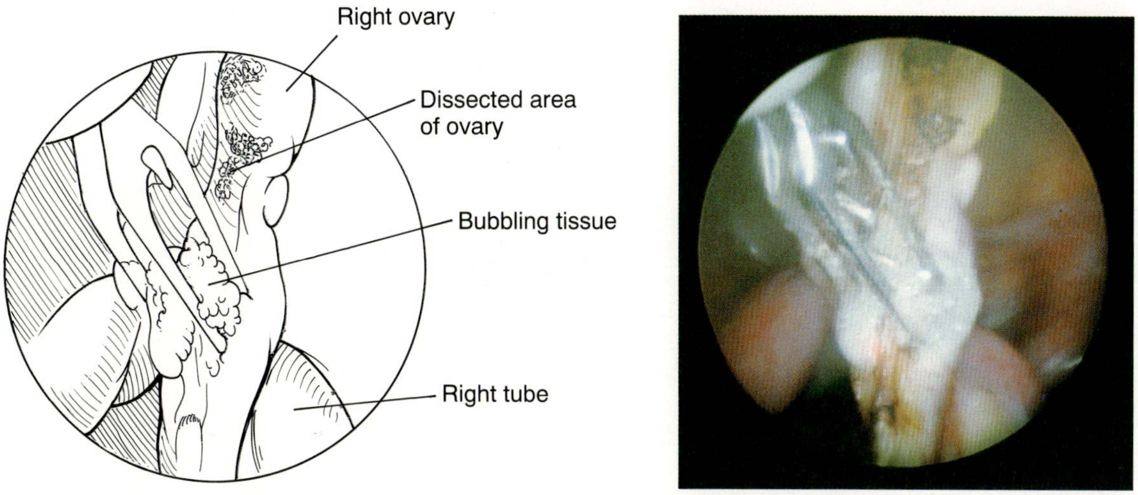

FIG. 15. Bipolar dessication initially results in bubbling of tissue.

Spread of thermal energy can be minimized by judicious use of irrigation. This applies to monopolar as well as to bipolar electrosurgery. Tissue destruction is the result of a balance between an external heat source and internal cooling. When it comes to protecting tissue not intended to be coagulated, one should support the existing cooling system. This can be done by irrigating the tissues surrounding the tissue being destroyed. The electrical forceps can be irrigated directly and continually in case of bipolar desiccation because the desiccation process is occurring between the branches. In case of monopolar application, it is recommended to irrigate at a short distance away from the electrode, because the desiccation process is primarily occurring at the edges of the instrument, rather than within its branches. Alternatively, the irrigation is executed in interrupted fashion. Cooling is maximized in a submersed field, such as in the transcervical resection of fibroids and/or endometrium. Under these circumstances, desiccation of tissue lasts considerably longer. When facing arterial bleeding in direct vicinity with the ureter, one may consider filling the pelvic cavity with nonconductive fluid and fulgurating the bleeding with a damped waveform. The fluid serves as a heat sink and absorbs the heat generated by the electrical arc. Therefore the thermal injury at distance from the target will be minimal.

Large Surface Desiccation

Large surface desiccation is a rather unusual clinical situation. It is used, for instance, in endometrial ablation with a roller ball or bar electrode. The difference between large surface desiccation and desiccation of a single ves-

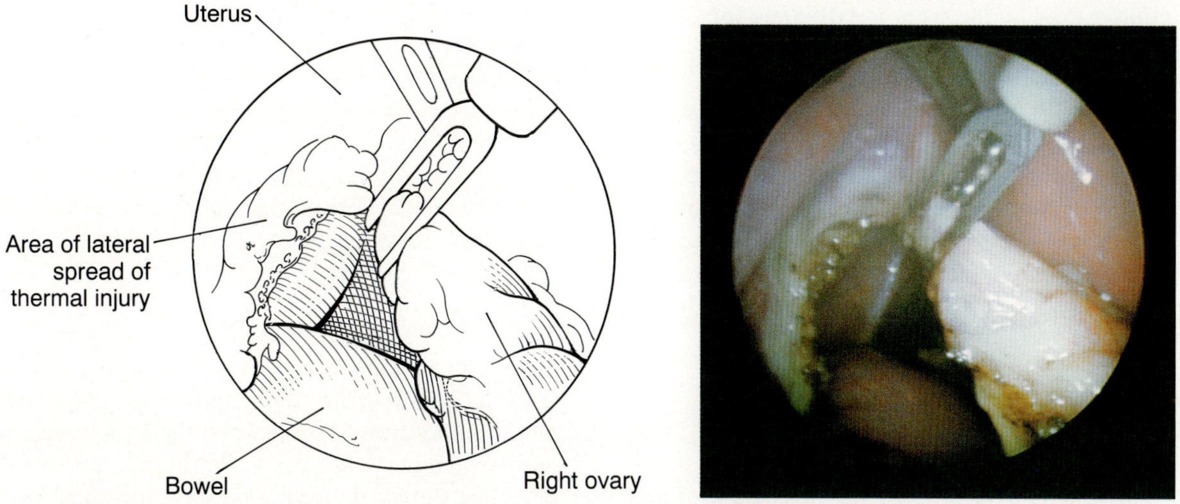

FIG. 16. The spread of thermal energy is limited during the bubbling phase. Following removal of all tissue water by evaporation, thermal injury can occur by lateral spread of heat by conduction.

sel, for instance, is that the electrode is dynamically moved in the first instance as opposed to the second clinical situation, in which the electrode is held in the same physical location for the duration of application of the current. This changes the physical conditions rather dramatically. Theoretically, to obtain desiccation, a continuous current is ideal. However, the continuous mode has a low potential. This means that continuous current is easily impeded from traveling through tissue with a high resistance. When a moving electrode is used to desiccate a large surface, the electrode at any given time is in contact with desiccated tissue, which becomes the gap through which the current must flow. Such flow is obtained by increasing the voltage. Experimental data are not available, but empirically one would say that an interrupted or damped mode would be more suitable for dynamic large surface desiccation. Clinically, the surgeon looks for indicators of thermal damage preceding the electrode, which is slowly moved over the surface. These indicators of thermal damage are, for all practical purposes, a ridge of blanching tissue and small gas bubbles escaping from the tissue in front of the electrode. As a general rule, for large surface desiccation, the electrode is moved extremely slowly and steadily.

Spray Coagulation

Spray coagulation is the original denomination of the damped side of the early electrosurgical units. This current was designed to jump a gap in the electrical circuit. Spray coagulation is extremely efficient in obtaining hemostasis of small vessels and capillaries ("oozing"). The principle of spray coagulation is based on building a high potential difference between an electrode of any shape and the tissue. At a particular voltage difference and at a particular distance between the electrode and the tissue—the gap—a spark is generated. That spark is approximately 500°C and creates hemostasis. The tissue destruction caused by the spark is extremely superficial, provided the application of the electrical energy is of short duration. Continued application of spray coagulation causes progressively more tissue damage at deeper levels. The wattage required to obtain sparking depends on the electrode used and the medium bridging the gap between the electrode and the tissue. Changing the medium in between the electrode and the tissue, such as the use of argon gas, greatly facilitates the generation of the spark and, under certain circumstances, makes the use of damped current more efficient.

COMPLICATIONS AND COMPLICATION PREVENTION

There are four areas of concern: the alternate site burn, the return electrode burn, direct coupling, and capacitive coupling.

Alternate Site Burn

Alternate site burn is the occurrence of an electrical burn at a site where electrical energy can be accumulated and cause damage beyond the control of the surgeon. The prototype site of such mishap is the electrocardiogram (ECG) electrode. These electrodes are conductors and can collect electrical energy, which is then led away to the ground. For an alternate site burn to occur, two conditions must be fulfilled: electrical energy must be collected in a small area and that energy must then be led away to allow flow of current. Flow of current through a small area then causes the burn.

The possibility of alternate site burns has been dramatically reduced if not eliminated by the introduction in 1972 of the isolated electrosurgical generators. These generators are not connected to ground anymore. A closed circuit is generated and the patient is an integral part. Since 1972, ground plates have been eliminated. The correct term is return electrode. Elimination of the necessity for a ground plate greatly reduces the risk for alternate site burns. Generators built before 1972 do not have that safety feature and are less suitable for use in laparoscopy.

Return Electrode Burn

The return electrode is truly an electrode. The patient is caught between two electrodes. The damage occurs primarily at the active electrode because that electrode is smaller than the return electrode. However, the skin underneath the return electrode will invariably heat up, fortunately only by a few degrees. If the return electrode happens to detach, the power density of the current flowing through goes up and causes more tissue damage. Because of the fact that the return electrode (even if partly detached) is large, the rise in tissue temperature is slow but steady. Damage to tissue may reach several centimeters into the patient's tissues and reach catastrophic proportions.

A system was designed some 10 years ago to monitor the function of the return electrode. REM (return electrode monitoring) is such a system. The principle of this system is relatively simple (Fig. 17). The return electrode is divided into two separate electrodes, which are electrically connected to each other by the skin of the patient. The ESU emits a low-intensity, continuous current through this return electrode. This intelligent current is expected to return to the ESU. If this does not happen, the ESU is shut down. Interruption of this low-intensity continuous current occurs when the return electrode detaches from the patient or when the skin underneath the plate heats up more than 2°C. Since introduction of this system, no more return electrode burns have been reported.

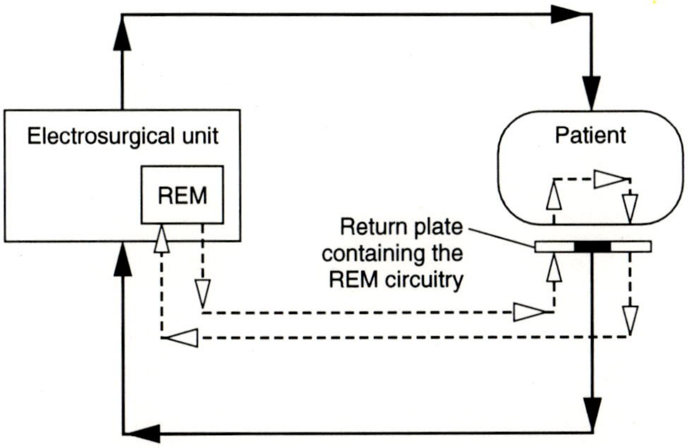

FIG. 17. Schematic representation of the working mechanism of the REM return electrode. ESU, electrosurgical unit; REM, return electrode monitoring.

Direct Coupling

Direct coupling is the inadvertent application of electrical current through a defect in the insulation of an instrument or through contact with a conducting instrument (Fig. 18A). The electrical current is, although unintentionally, directly applied to the tissues. This represents the most common and most dangerous complication derived from the use of electrical instruments in surgery.

When direct coupling occurs between an instrument and the metal sheath of the trocar through which it has been introduced, distinct events occur that should alert the surgeon: stray currents may cause the muscles of the abdominal wall to contract; a typical hissing sound may be heard; and, if the surgeon uses a video screen, interference in the form of lightening on the screen will be seen. It is advisable in all these circumstances to check the instrument used and, when in doubt, exchange it for another one.

There is currently no true defense against direct coupling, except for the Electroscope system (Electroscope, Boulder, CO), which was recently introduced. This system applies the principles of the REM to ancillary instruments. A sheath is slipped over the active electrode, which then monitors the occurrence of stray currents, analyzes them, and—in the presence of danger—shuts off the generator.

Capacitive Coupling

Capacitive coupling is the indirect application of electrical energy through the electromagnetic properties of

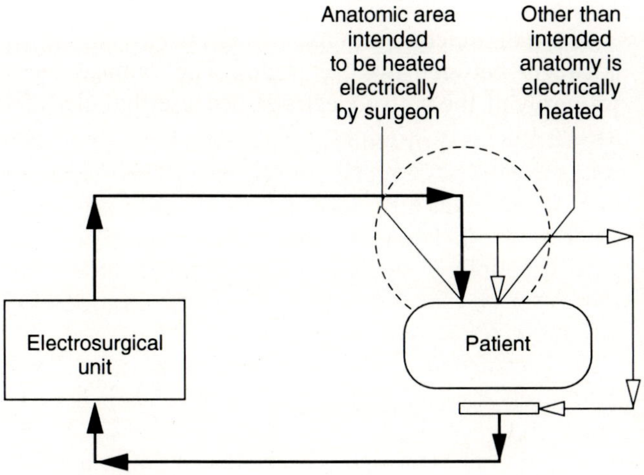

A. Direct coupling

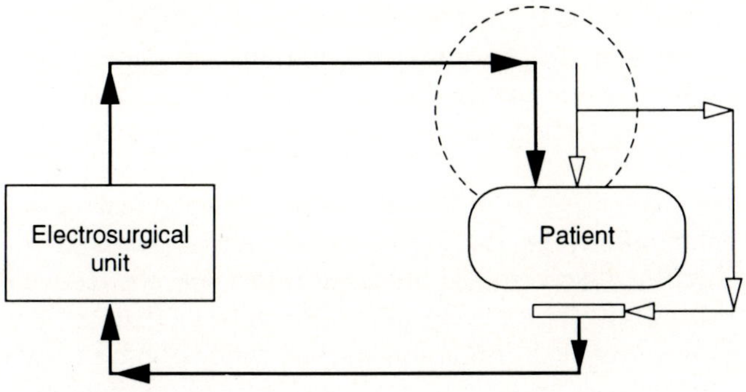

B. Capacitive coupling

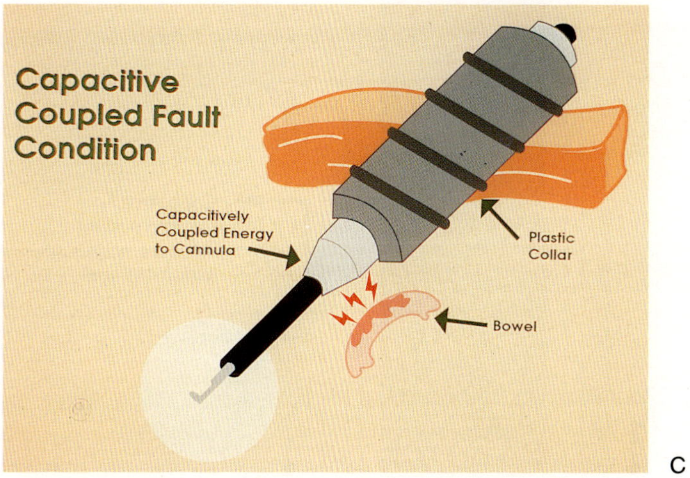

FIG. 18. Schematic representation of (**A**) direct and (**B** and **C**) capacitive coupling. ESU, electrosurgical unit.

conductors. Charged conductors induce currents in any conductor that happens to be in close proximity (Fig. 18B). Many factors influence the amount of energy coupled in this fashion: the length of conductor in parallel course, the distance between both conductors, the dielectric constant of the materials, the frequency of the alternating current, the voltage of the current, and so on. Capacitive coupling is always present, but it is not always dangerous. The true pitfall occurs when energy is coupled in an area isolated from the rest of the patient. An example is the conductive trocar, isolated from the patient by a plastic collar. When activating the electrical instrument, especially in the fulguration mode and prior to touching the target, there is a high amount of energy generated in the trocar sleeve. Contact between the sleeve and tissue invariably leads to irreversible damage. Typical sites for such a burn are the left lower trocar touching the sigmoid colon or the operative laparoscope touching the terminal ileum.

Capacitive coupling cannot be avoided. The damage caused by it can, however, be eliminated by using all conductive materials for the trocars. Problems arise when hybrid trocars are used. These hybrid trocars combine conductive and nonconductive materials, which can lead to complex electrical situations.

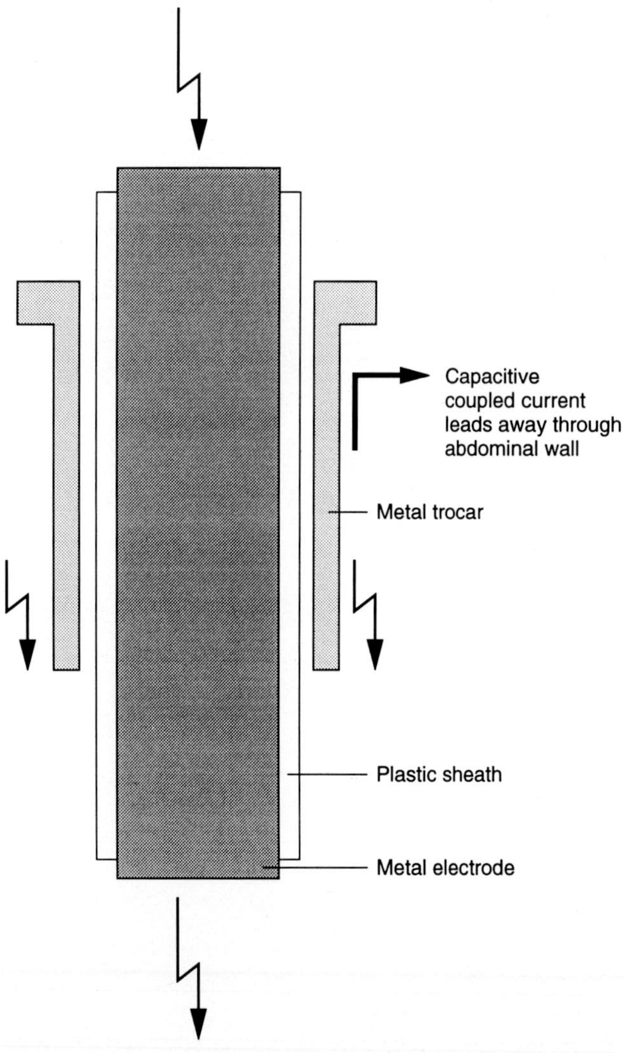

FIG. 19. Schematic representation of the rule of three layers.

TABLE 2. *Summary of precautions to limit electrosurgical accidents*

1. Increase available intraabdominal space by use of a bowel preparation, a nasogastric tube, and an indwelling catheter and by avoiding N_2O as anesthesia gas.
2. Use low-voltage current as much as possible.
3. Check instruments on a regular basis.

Even with all metal trocars, there may be situations in which capacitive coupling can cause damage. This occurs when an electrical instrument is introduced through a complex system of channels and sheaths. A simplified rule of the three layers (Fig. 19) is helpful to detect possible problems caused by capacitive coupling: the metal of the electrical instrument is considered the first layer; the insulation around the metal core is the second layer; and the metal of the trocar is the third layer. Under these circumstances there is minimal chance that the energy coupled in the trocar sheath will cause damage, because there is good contact with the abdominal wall of the patient, which leads the current back to the return electrode. Another safe example is one having the metal core of an instrument (layer 1), the insulation surrounding it (layer 2), a plastic cannula in which the instrument is channeled (part of layer 2), and the trocar through which the instrument is introduced (layer 3). However, a dangerous example is a metal core (layer 1), the insulation (layer 2), a metal introducer (layer 3), and a fiberglass trocar (layer 4). The metal introducer is charged by capacitive coupling and is isolated from the abdominal wall. When contact is established between tissue and the introducer, serious damage may ensue.

The Electroscope system also detects the presence of capacitively coupled energy and safely leads it back to the generator, or else it shuts the generator down. Safety in the use of electrosurgery is based on common sense. Even without sophisticated systems such as the Electroscope system, the surgeon should be able to increase the margin of safety by simple measures (Table 2).

The first of these simple precautions is to increase the volume of the intraabdominal space, which in turn reduces the risk of inadvertent contact between electrode and tissue. Increase of the intraabdominal space can be achieved with a combination of a mechanical bowel preparation and the use of a nasogastric tube and indwelling catheter. The intraabdominal space is reduced during surgery by accumulation of nitrous oxide in the bowel lumen. Elimination of this anesthesia gas is important so as to keep optimal access to all intraabdominal organs.

The second precaution is to limit the use of high-voltage current. The surgeon should suppress the natural tendency to use coagulation current for all purposes. The likelihood of both direct and capacitive coupling is significantly increased when using high-voltage current. In addition, it is in most instances unnecessary to use that particular kind of current; in some cases, it is even inappropriate. Judicious use of low-voltage current is safer.

Finally, it should be emphasized that electrical instruments should be tested on a regular basis. There is no particular equipment available to test electrical instruments. However, it is readily achieved using any piece of conductive material and applying, for example, 50 W of high-voltage current to the insulation. If sparking occurs, it is time to replace that particular piece of equipment. One should not be tempted to believe that disposable instruments are immune to insulation failure. The materials used for single-use instruments may not endure long-standing application of electrical current.

HIGHLIGHTS

The principles of electrosurgery are reviewed. Emphasis is placed on how to use this versatile energy source as effectively as possible to obtain the desired bioeffect. The risks of return plate injury, alternate site burn, direct coupling, and capacitive coupling are also discussed. A brief review is given of the latest technology involving active shielding of instruments used at laparoscopy.

REFERENCES

1. Odell RC. Electrosurgery in laparoscopy. *Infertil Reprod Med Clin North Am* 1993;4(2):289–304.
2. Tucker RD, Voyles CR, Silvis SE. Capacitive coupled stray currents during laparoscopic and endoscopic electrosurgical procedures. *Biomed Instrum Technol* 1992;26:303–311.
3. Stovall T, Ling FW, O'Kelley KR, Coleman SA. Gross histologic examination of tubal ligation failures in a residency training program. *Obstet Gynecol* 1990;76:461–465.
4. Phipps J. Thermometry studies with bipolar diathermy during hysterectomy. *Gynecol Endosc* 1994;3:5–8.

Endoscopic Management of Gynecologic Disease,
edited by G.D. Adamson and D.C. Martin.
Lippincott-Raven Publishers, Philadelphia © 1996.

CHAPTER 4

Endoscopic Energy

Laser

Scott R. Crowgey and G. David Adamson

Since development of the first laser in 1960, laser applications have rapidly grown and attained a significant role in many aspects of our society (1). In gynecology, lasers have had a particularly widespread application over the past 10 years (2–4). Since then they have also been an important factor spurring dramatic developments in other types of endoscopic surgery. One of the most important advantages of surgical lasers is their ability to control very precisely the degree and selectivity of thermal destruction of tissue without necessarily contacting the tissue. In achieving this goal, the laser surgeon is able to select from a variety of lasers (Table 1) that can produce different tissue effects and that can be controlled by means of a variety of different delivery systems.

PHYSICAL PROPERTIES OF LASER ENERGY

All light energy travels through space in the form of electromagnetic waves. Individual bundles of light energy are called photons. Normal light, produced by the spontaneous emission of radiation, is composed of many photons with many different wavelengths all traveling in many different directions at the same time. Photons with the longest wavelengths make up infrared light whereas photons with the shorter wavelengths make up ultraviolet light. Both types of light energy are invisible. Photons with wavelengths in between those of infrared and ultraviolet light energies make up the visible spectrum of light (5).

S. R. Crowgey: Georgia Technical Research Institute, Georgia Institute of Technology, Atlanta, Georgia 30332.

G. D. Adamson: Fertility Physicians of Northern California, Palo Alto, California 94301.

Laser light results from a process known as the stimulated emission of radiation, which produces waves of light that are coherent (all waves are in phase or traveling together in time and space), monochromatic (all waves have the same wavelength), and collimated (all waves are parallel to each other) (Fig. 1). These properties allow laser light to be focused into very confined beams or spots with high energy densities, producing predictable, controllable, and very precise tissue thermal damage at variable distances from the actual site of laser light production within the laser cavity.

When a beam of photons from any source strikes tissue, these photons are transmitted through the tissue (similar to light transmitted through glass), reflected by the tissue (similar to light reflected by a mirror), completely absorbed by the tissue (resulting in the production of heat), or scattered within the tissue (resulting in the deflection of photons away from the original straight path of transmission and a small amount of heat production with each deflection). The exact degree of transmission, reflection, absorption, and scattering (especially absorption and scattering) is dependent on the wavelength of the photons and the properties of the tissue (Fig. 2) (6–10).

Both absorption and scattering result in the production of heat within the tissue, although scattering is generally a less precise and slower means of heat production. Photon absorption generally results in the thermal destruction of tissue directly in the path of transmission to very shallow depths, with the width of destruction being approximately equal to the width of the laser beam. Photon scattering results in ball- or oval-shaped distributions of thermal destruction as the photons get bounced around within the tissue, with the total width of destruc-

TABLE 1. *Characteristics of different lasers*

Laser medium	Carbon dioxide	Neodymium: yttrium-aluminum-garnet	Potassium-trideuterium-phosphate	Argon
Abbreviation	CO_2	Nd:YAG	KTP	Ar
Wavelength (nm)	10,600	1064	532	488–511
Water absorption	High	Low	Low	Low
Pigment absorption	Low	Moderate	High	High
Tissue scattering	Low	Moderate	High	High
Penetration (mm)	0.1	4–10	0.3–3.0	0.4–4.0
Delivery system	Mirrors, lenses, waveguides	Fiberoptics, contact tips	Fiberoptics	Fiberoptics
Cutting	High	Low	Fair	Fair
Coagulation	Low	High	Fair	Fair

tion being proportional to but always somewhat greater than the spot size of the laser beam and approximately equal to the depth of destruction. The use of monochromatic laser energy photons during laser surgery allows precision and predictability in the amount of heat production by both absorptive and scattering processes, since the photons being produced are all exactly the same wavelength.

Far-infrared and far-ultraviolet wavelength photons are very well absorbed by a variety of materials (Fig. 3). In soft tissue, the primary component absorbing photons at these wavelengths is water. Therefore, with lasers operating at wavelengths far outside of the visible spectrum (such as the carbon dioxide and excimer lasers), photons do not penetrate very deeply and the high degree of water absorption results in significant heat production confined to very shallow depths below the surface of soft tissues with high water content.

Photons with wavelengths in the visible and near-visible spectrum are not well absorbed by water but instead are transmitted to significant depths, making water appear clear. The energy from lasers operating at visible and near-visible wavelengths are absorbed primarily by pigments, such as hemoglobin and melanin, allowing the fairly selective destruction of pathologic lesions containing large quantities of these pigments. However, pigment absorption with these lasers is not as great as water absorption with the far-infrared and far-ultraviolet lasers and tends to vary widely depending on the type of pigment, the quantity of pigment, and the wavelength of the laser. Therefore, photons from visible and near-visible lasers tend to penetrate more deeply into high-water-content, soft tissues, interacting with the collagen fibers and other constituents of opaque soft tissues and resulting in heat dissipation primarily through the process of scattering.

As with absorption, scattering also limits the depth of penetration of photons below the surface of the tissue, with the depth of penetration decreasing as wavelength shortens. Therefore, longer wavelength photons in the near-infrared and red portions of the spectrum (such as those produced by the Nd:YAG and ruby lasers) tend to

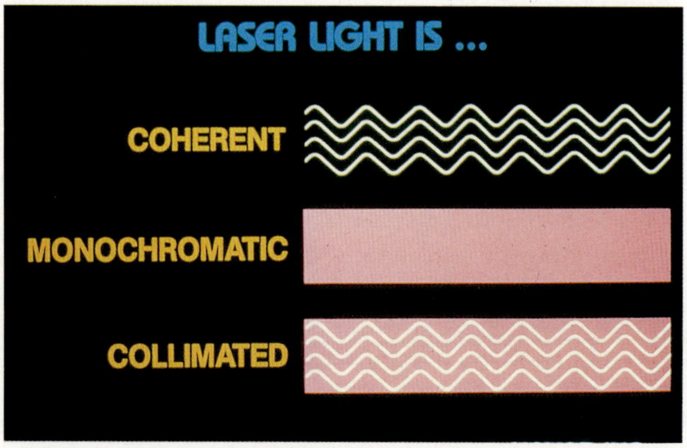

FIG. 1. The characteristics of laser light.

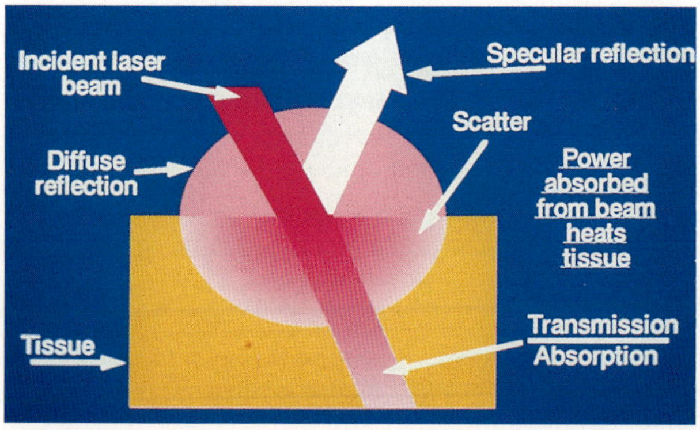

FIG. 2. The various interactions of laser light with tissue.

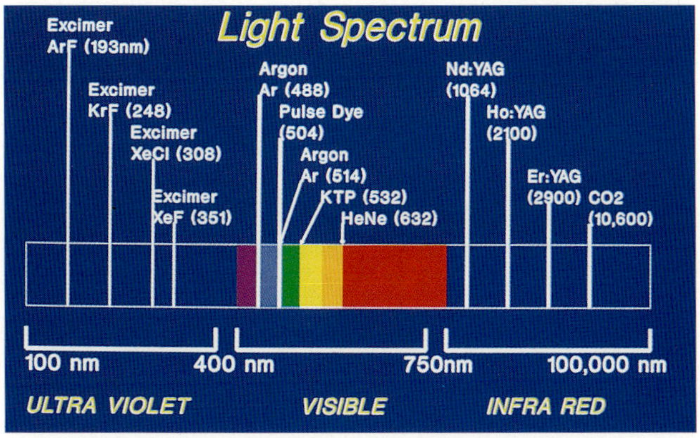

FIG. 3. The spectrum of light and laser energies.

penetrate more deeply than shorter wavelength photons in the blue and near-ultraviolet portions of the spectrum (such as those produced by the argon and some of the longer wavelength excimer lasers). In addition, most organic pigments tend to absorb photons best in the yellow, green, and blue portions of the spectrum, further confining the depth of thermal destruction to fairly shallow depths. Both absorption and scattering contribute to limiting the depth of photon penetration to a certain distance below the surface of the tissue known as the depth of penetration; a point at which approximately 63% of the energy is absorbed (Fig. 4). Distances at which approximately 86.5%, 95%, and 98% absorption of energy occurs are equivalent to two, three, and four times the depth of penetration, respectively.

THERMAL DESTRUCTION OF TISSUE

Laser surgery is primarily an accurate, precise, rapid, and efficient method of performing surgery by means of the thermal destruction of tissue. In tissue, exposure to temperatures in excess of 45°C over time results in vasodilatation, edema, endothelial damage, and eventual cell death. At temperatures above 60°C, protein denaturation and coagulation occur, even with extremely brief exposures, resulting in irreversible tissue injury. Between 60°C and 100°C, denatured collagen contracts causing blood vessel walls to constrict while the carbohydrate constituents of tissue melt forming a glue-like slurry. These events occurring within this narrow temperature range result in the most effective coagulative sealing of vessels and tissue, and are evidenced by the white blanching and puckering of tissue. Above 100°C, water converts to steam, resulting in either the vaporization and disruption of tissue with rapid heating or the gradual dehydration and cavitation of tissue with slow heating. Continued heating of dehydrated coagulum at temperatures much above 100°C results in the browning/burning of the carbohydrate portion of the coagulum and the loss of flexibility and strength in a coagulative seal. At some point between 300°C and 400°C, skin begins to carbonize, and then to "outgas" or smoke. At approximately 530°C and in the presence of atmospheric oxygen, skin burns and evaporates. Although these temperature-related effects are similar for all medical lasers once the energy is converted to heat, the differences in absorption and scattering of the various laser wavelengths by the various components of tissue and the related differences in spatial distribution of the laser energy make a great difference in the actual temporal process of heat conversion during laser surgery (11–14).

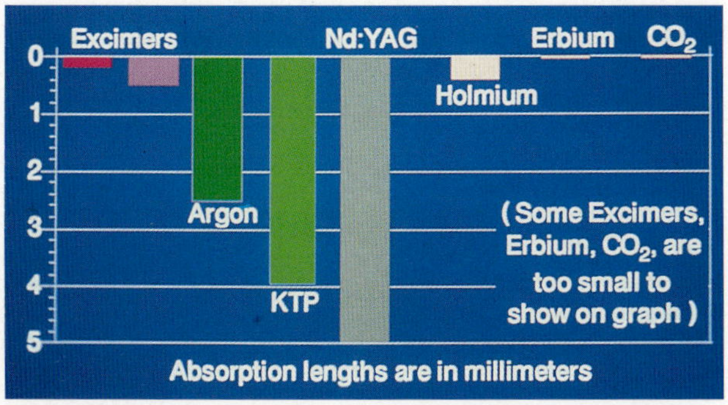

FIG. 4. The relative absorption lengths, or depths of penetration, of surgical laser energies in soft tissues.

The temperature achievable using the CO_2 laser (when tested on dry firebrick) may be as high as 1500°C [15]. However, because the absorption of this particular wavelength by water is so great, the temperature of the skin never achieves this level. Water selectively absorbs the CO_2 laser energy and immediately converts this energy to heat which in turn converts the water within the tissues into steam at a temperature of 100°C (16). The conversion of water to steam results in a 1000-fold increase in volume. This sudden and almost instantaneous expansion therefore results in cell disruption, which carries solid cellular material away and causes tissue separation (Fig. 5).

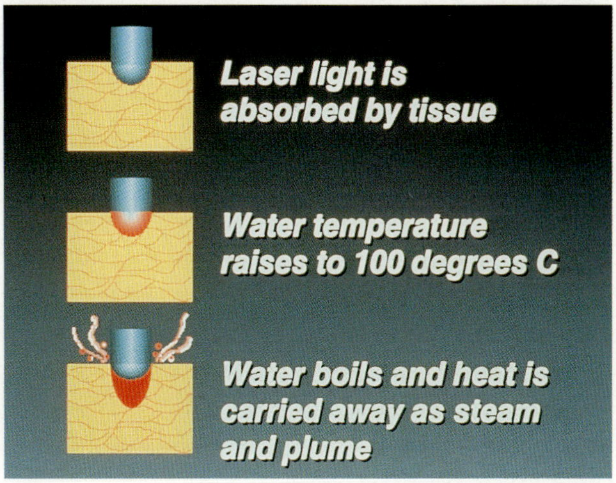

FIG. 5. The process of tissue vaporization by laser energy.

The large latent heat of vaporization of water acts as a tremendous energy sink, maintaining the temperature at 100°C at the tissue surface as long as water or steam is present. Any heat energy above that required to raise the temperature of the water to 100°C is spent in the conversion of that water to steam. Even if the conditions were just right for superheating of the cell water just prior to steam formation, the expansion of the steam would result in an immediate cooling of the tissue surface to 100°C. Thus, the formation of steam from cell water acts as a 100°C thermostat for the surface of the tissue and helps to prevent any high-temperature damage from occurring below the surgical surface. Dehydrated tissue, however, is very capable of heating to higher temperatures.

Carbonization and outgassing of biological tissues from the use of the CO_2 laser occurs only after the cellular particles released by this vaporization process, once devoid of insulating water, cross back through the CO_2 laser beam. This fact explains why the layer of carbonization following CO_2 laser surgery is so easily removed. The carbonization layer is primarily composed of tissue particles that have been released by the vaporization process, dehydrated, incinerated, and then redeposited on the surface of the laser wound. There is also a small ring of minimal tissue carbonization (Fig. 6) around the periphery of the laser lesion in the "tails" of the Gaussian distribution of the laser spot as the power density drops off.

Since the thermal destruction of tissue by visible and near-visible laser energies, such as the neodymium: yttrium-aluminum-garnet (Nd:YAG), potassium-trideuterium-phosphate (KTP) and argon, are dependent primarily on scattering by the protein constituents and secondarily on absorption by the pigmented constituents of biological tissue, the process of heat conversion occurs primarily within these tissue components. The actual laser surgery is therefore principally a process of heating of these tissue components rather than vaporization of water as with the CO_2 laser. Some vaporization may occur at very high power densities as the heated tissue components transfer the heat to inter- and intracellular water. However, heating in general occurs at a slower rate due to the less efficient energy conversion processes resulting in cell dehydration, coagulation, and eventual burning rather than vaporization.

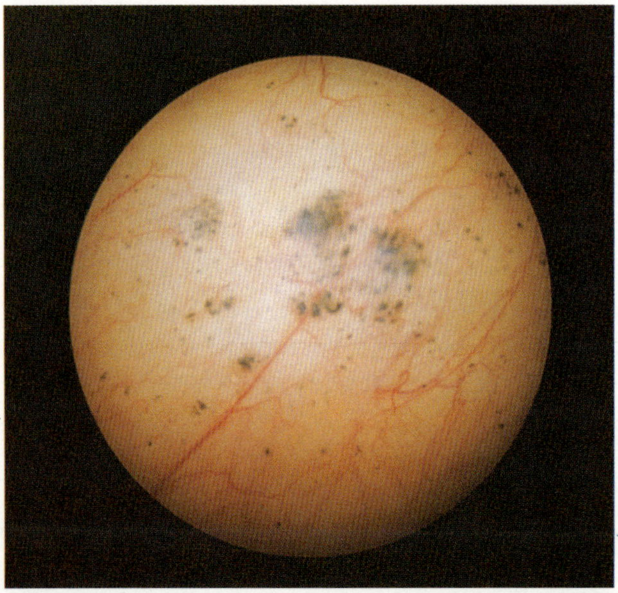

FIG. 6. The minimal carbonization remaining following CO_2 laser vaporization.

Heat coagulation of moist tissue is generally a slow process, gradually accelerating as the tissues become more dehydrated. Upon carbonization, energy absorption increases dramatically as does the rise in surface temperature. This is true for all types of thermal surgical energy since carbon is such a good absorber in virtually all portions of the electromagnetic spectrum. Thermal surgery should never be continued for very long on carbonized tissue. Carbon absorbs both laser and electrosurgical energy extremely well and can rapidly heat adjacent tissues to 300°–500°C. Surface temperatures this high significantly extend the zone of thermal necrosis underlying the tissue surface.

Not only does carbonized tissue heat to much higher temperatures faster than noncarbonized tissue, but carbon also conducts this heat extremely well to the surrounding noncarbonized tissue, continuing extension of the zone of thermal necrosis even after the laser energy has been discontinued. In the case of the CO_2 laser, the results of lasering even a thin layer of carbon and leaving it behind can completely eliminate the anticipated narrow zone of thermal necrosis that is one of this laser's primary advantages. Water, on the other hand, acts as a thermal insulator and is not very thermally conductive. The water content of hydrated tissue serves as a barrier to the secondary spread of thermal damage following thermal surgery, slowing the spread of injury by conduction and allowing surgically heated tissue to lose excess heat through other means.

This thermal conduction of heat from heated tissue to the surrounding tissue is a process common to all types of thermal surgery. Tissue, once heated above the normal skin temperature of 37°C, must dissipate this heat in some manner in order to return to normal skin temperature. Although surgically heated tissue may cool partially as a result of convection (loss of heat to moving air or fluid streams) and radiation (loss of heat to space), the primary means of cooling is by thermal conduction to the surrounding tissues. Thus, hemispheric, isothermal zones of heated tissue form below surgically heated tissue as it cools, slowly spreading the width and depth of thermal injury beyond the original limits of surgical thermal destruction (Fig. 7). This thermally conductive spread of

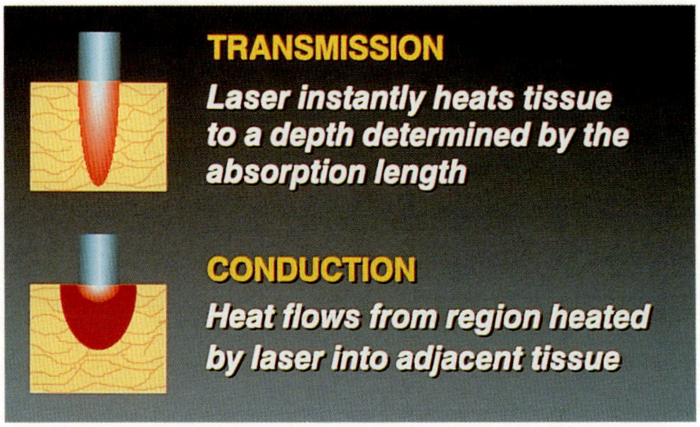

FIG. 7. Two of the principal mechanisms by which laser tissue heating occurs and the resultant patterns of tissue destruction. Heating as a result of laser transmission results in a columnar pattern of tissue damage, whereas heating as a result of secondary thermal conduction results in a hemispherical pattern of tissue damage.

thermal injury can be minimized by limiting the duration of exposure of the tissue to the source of surgical heating, limiting the surface temperature of the heated tissue, minimizing the formation of carbon and eliminating it when present, preserving near-normal tissue hydration, and encouraging the convective cooling of the site of thermal surgery as much as possible through the use of intermittent irrigation.

OPERATING PARAMETERS

The surgical heating of tissue is actually a volume heating process and not simply a surface heating process. Approximately 4 J (or W-sec) of energy is needed to heat 1 cm^3 of tissue by 1°C. The choice of laser wavelength and the composition of the tissue in question determines the depth to which heating occurs by the penetration depth of that wavelength in the tissue being lased. Assuming that this dimension is fixed for a given laser, the remaining operating parameters for the laser surgeon to control are primarily two-dimensional: the power of the laser beam, the surface area of contact for the laser beam, and the time over which the laser beam is applied (17–19).

Laser beam power, given in W, is typically the first and easiest of the operating parameters to determine, and is set using the power meter (watt meter) that is required on all lasers. A general rule-of-thumb is that the power setting should be the highest with which the laser surgeon is comfortable getting the surgery done as rapidly as is safely possible and minimizing time on target.

The second operating parameter is the area of laser beam contact. This is determined approximately by the spot size of the laser beam and is dependent primarily on the delivery device used to transport the laser beam from the laser cavity where the beam is produced to the tissue being lased. Since laser beams are characteristically circular, the diameter of this beam is all that is necessary to define this area of contact. All noncontact laser delivery devices have a minimum spot size specification, which is the effective beam diameter or beam width at the point from the device where the laser beam is most focused and concentrated. The effective diameter is the beam width within which 86% of the energy or power from the laser beam is contained. The actual area of laser interaction is somewhat larger than the effective diameter, as determined by the power distribution curve of the laser energy. However, most of the tissue reaction occurs within the circle described by this effective diameter. It is important to realize that the specified spot size for a delivery device occurs only at the effective focal point of the delivery device where the laser beam diameter is minimal. All noncontact delivery devices cause the laser beam to diverge eventually, permitting the delivery of less concentrated laser power (and less effective thermal destruction) at larger spot sizes.

Time is the third operating parameter of the laser and the most difficult to specify. In many ways, this parameter is determined by the skill and experience of the laser surgeon as well as the surgeon's speed of operation and reaction time. More precise control of this parameter is aided by the pulsing parameters of the laser. Pulsing of the laser beam allows the laser power to be repetitively delivered using specified on and off periods. A less experienced laser surgeon can, in this manner, safely use higher peak power levels during surgery for more effective thermal destruction without being as dependent on individual reaction times. However, the periodic off periods will slow the overall surgical process.

Power density, a parameter that combines two of the three operating parameters discussed above into one, is given in W/cm^2. Power density is calculated as the laser power setting divided by the surface area of contact between the laser beam and the tissue. One version of this formula is given below:

$$\text{Power density } (W/cm^2) = \frac{400 \times (\text{power, W})}{\pi \times (\text{spot diameter, mm})^2}$$

Low power densities result in the slow heating, coagulation, and dehydration of tissue whereas very high power densities result in the rapid vaporization and incision of tissue. Power density is directly proportional to power but inversely proportional to the square of the spot size. Therefore, relatively small changes in spot size have much greater effects on power density than changes in power.

The parameter known as energy density, given in J/cm^2, combines all three of the operating parameters into one and is more closely related to the actual thermal damage done to tissue during laser surgery. One joule is equivalent to 1 W of power delivered over 1 sec and can heat approximately 0.25 cm^3 of tissue by 1°C. Therefore, energy density is equal to power density multiplied by time.

It bears repeating that the operating parameters described above only determine the first two dimensions of a three-dimensional heating process. As stated previously, the surgical heating of tissue is a volume heating process and not simply a surface heating process. Power and energy densities cannot be easily compared between the various types of lasers or even between lasers and other surgical heating modalities because the penetration depths and volume distributions of the heating energy may be very different.

PULSING PARAMETERS

One means of better controlling the operating parameter of time and, ultimately, the energy density and resultant degree of thermal destruction of tissue is by pulsing the surgical laser beam (Fig. 8). Most surgical lasers can be operated in either a continuous mode or a normal (shuttered) pulse mode. Normal or shuttered pulsing is typically performed using an electromechanical shutter that passes back and forth in front of the continuous laser beam, effectively chopping the beam into pulses. Because of limits in the speed of electromechanical shutters, the shortest pulse widths (on times) as well as the shortest interpulse intervals (off times) are typically 50–100 msec. Lasers excited by radiofrequency energy can produce electronically enhanced pulses with pulse widths as short as 5–10 msec. Short pulse widths, as well as small spot sizes, are extremely useful in creating precise, small, and focal areas of thermal injury in sensitive tissues located in delicate areas. In addition, short pulse widths combined with long interpulse intervals limit the conductive spread of thermal injury to adjacent normal tissues and enhance interpulse tissue cooling.

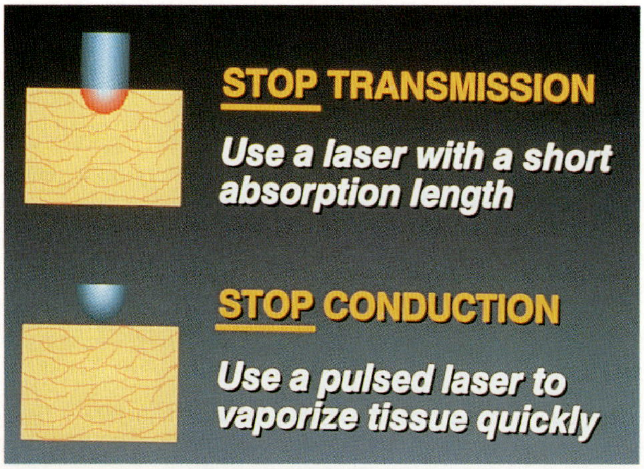

FIG. 8. The principles used in minimizing laser tissue damage, with emphasis on the advantage of laser beam pulsing to minimize the secondary destruction of tissue by thermal conduction.

Unfortunately, the combination of short pulse widths and long interpulse intervals also results in a decrease in average power over time, thus increasing the time required to perform surgery. Although instantaneous peak powers or pulse energies are related to the rate of penetration of the energy into tissue, the overall speed of performing a surgical procedure, as well as the degree of adjacent thermal damage, is proportional to the average power over time. Average power during pulsing is determined by the following equation:

$$\text{Average power} = (\text{peak power}) \times (\text{pulse width}) \times (\text{pulse repetition rate})$$

The production of very short pulses with very high instantaneous peak powers (high pulse energies) permits lasers to perform precise thermal tissue destruction with minimal adjacent thermal damage and without seriously affecting overall surgical time. However, not all lasers are capable of producing short, high-energy pulses. The long lifetimes of the CO_2 molecule's high-energy states permit special forms of pulsing, such as electronically phased pulsing, superpulsing, and, more recently, ultrapulsing with the CO_2 laser.

Superpulsing of the laser (20–22) allows the creation of extremely short pulses of laser energy with very high peak powers. The superpulse is created by using a combination of electrical and mechanical techniques to supercharge the laser cavity to a very high level of population inversion in a detuned state prior to rapidly creating a tuned cavity state, resulting in the sudden release of the stored energy in a burst of stimulated emission energy. The resultant burst of laser energy is extremely short but has a peak instantaneous power much higher than that which would have occurred with the laser operating in its continuous wave (CW) mode. Peak instantaneous powers of these pulses can easily be 4–20 times greater than the peak powers possible with the same laser operating in its CW mode, with the pulse widths typically lasting only a few μsec.

The superpulsing mode of a CO_2 laser is an excellent tool for optimizing the surgical cutting of tissues, since the brief, high-power pulses allow maximal delivery of laser power for vaporization while minimizing thermal spread to the surrounding tissues. Very fine incisions with decreased char are the result. However, in the superpulsed mode, slightly more oozing can result following incisions because less average power is available to coagulate the surrounding vessels. Thus, superpulsing is not as effective in ablating large lesions or in coagulating as is the CW or shuttered pulse mode.

Another limitation of superpulsed CO_2 lasers is the amount of average power that can be delivered to tissue. Super-pulsed CO_2 lasers are limited to very short pulse widths (with typical values ranging anywhere from 2 to 250 μsec, but with some lasers capable of up to 400 μsec) and usually very limited variability in the selection of the desired pulse width. Because of these limitations, average powers can only be increased by delivering the pulses at a more rapid rate (typically up to 1000 Hz), with average powers rarely exceeding more than half of the maximum power output of the laser when operating in its continuous mode. As already described above, any limitation in average power to tissue limits the speed with which the laser can operate. In addition, increasing the pulse repetition rate in an attempt to increase speed also tends to increase the amount of char produced. Since the char produced by the CO_2 laser is actually produced above the surface of the tissue by the action of the CO_2 laser beam on the rising laser plume, rapid pulsing of the laser beam does not allow as much time for the plume to be suctioned or to dissipate away between pulses, resulting in increasing amounts of char as the repetition rate increases.

A more recent variation in pulsing the CO_2 laser is commonly known as *ultrapulsing* (other terms used are *char-free pulse* and *enhanced superpulse*). Ultrapulsing (23) represents a more advanced pulsing technology that allows the laser to produce high-peak-power pulses similar to those in the superpulsed mode, but with more variable and longer pulse widths (typically up to 950 μsec in duration). Because of these longer pulse widths, higher average powers can be produced at much lower repetition rates, and the average power delivered to tissue typically can equal the maximum power output of the laser when operating in its continuous mode (Fig. 9). Therefore, the operating speed of the laser is not hindered as much in this pulse mode and less oozing of the incision is noted compared to that of superpulsed lasers. Since the repetition rate is less for a given average power, more time is available for the plume to be evacuated between pulses, resulting in less char. Thus, ultrapulsed CO_2 lasers provide the capability to tailor the pulsing of the laser to provide a near optimal trade-off between vaporization and coagulation for a given tissue type without sacrificing speed and while minimizing adjacent thermal necrosis and char.

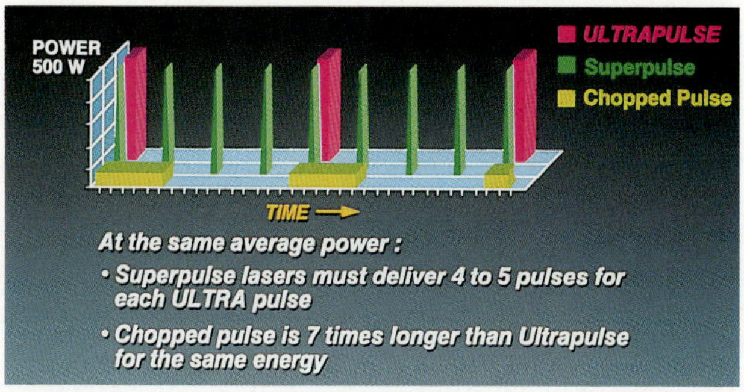

FIG. 9. The relative pulsing characteristics of pulsed, superpulsed, and ultrapulsed CO_2 lasers.

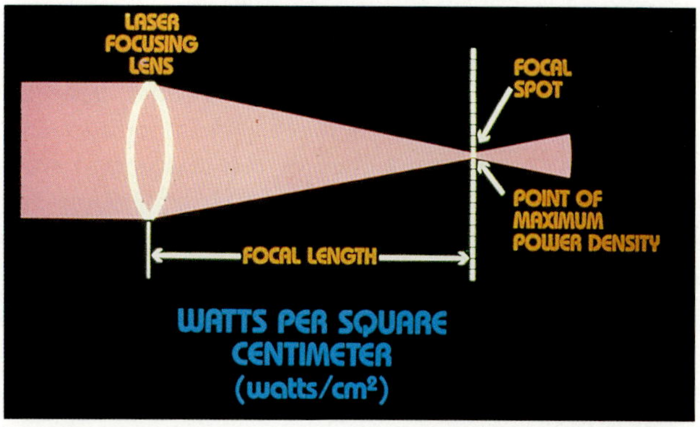

FIG. 10. The delivery of laser energy by means of a focusing lens.

Even shorter pulses are possible by means of a process known as Q switching. Q switching is a technique often applied to the Nd:YAG laser that produces extremely short pulses of laser energy lasting only 10–20 nsec. These high-power, extremely short pulses produce primarily a photoacoustic rather than thermal effect on biological tissues, causing miniexplosions with minimal thermal effect. However, a great deal of concern exists regarding the use of this type of energy on any potentially cancerous tissue. Early investigative work showed evidence for the scattering of potentially viable, malignant cells by surface explosions when Q-switched Nd:YAG energy was used experimentally on tumor tissue (24). Therefore, laser pulses of this type are restricted to applications on nonmalignant tissues only.

BEAM DELIVERY DEVICES

Laser surgical delivery devices deliver the laser energy to the surgical site either through contact or by noncontact means. Noncontact laser beam delivery devices can be further roughly divided between the two categories of lens-focusing and fiberoptic/waveguide devices (25).

Lens-focusing devices cause a collimated, Gaussian-type laser beam to converge to a minimum spot size at a distance equivalent to the focal length of that lens and to diverge again beyond that point. The minimum spot size with its high power density is most useful for incisional-type procedures, whereas the divergent, larger spot with its lower power density is more useful for coagulative or ablative procedures.

For a given laser, the minimum spot size is directly proportional to the focal length of the lens. Smallest minimum spot sizes and highest power densities are obtainable only with the shorter focal length lenses used for surface-type procedures. Focusing the beam through the operating channel of a laparoscope requires 300- to 400-mm focal length lenses, which produce a typical minimum spot size of only approximately 0.8 mm, severely limiting the range of power densities available (Fig. 10).

In addition, the long distance necessary to reach convergence dictates that an equally long distance is necessary to achieve divergence. Laser beams delivered through laparoscopic couplers are very difficult to defocus within the tight confines of the abdominal space without the aid of specially designed defocusing couplers, limiting their application to primarily incisional rather than coagulative procedures. Therefore, many laser laparoscopists advocate the use of laser in conjunction with bipolar electrosurgery in order to best perform both incisional and coagulative procedures through the laparoscope.

Because the laser beam from lens-focused delivery devices does not diverge readily, the use of backstops is strongly encouraged to prevent the beam from damaging tissues that may be exposed once overlying pathologic tissues are vaporized. Brushed surface, titanium-tipped instruments, such as the hydrodissector, serve as excellent backstops for CO_2 laser energy by diffracting rather than reflecting the incident energy off of the dull, lusterless surface and by evenly distributing any absorbed heat over the entire surface of the instrument. Stainless steel–tipped instruments are not as effective as backstops, as they tend to reflect energy rather than diffract and can develop localized hot spots, which can result in unintentional secondary burns to normal tissues. The best backstop for CO_2 laser energy is a layer of water, which is an excellent absorber of this energy as well as an excellent heat sink and thermal barrier. Hydrodissection, the injection of a thin layer of water or saline to expand virtual spaces and tissue planes, such as the subperitoneal surface, is an excellent ancillary procedure to CO_2 laser surgery. It aids not only in the dissection of tissue planes but also in the surrounding of both pathologic and normal tissues with a protective blanket of water, preventing inadvertent damage of surrounding tissues by the laser energy and increasing the precision of the thermal destruction by limiting secondary conductive spread.

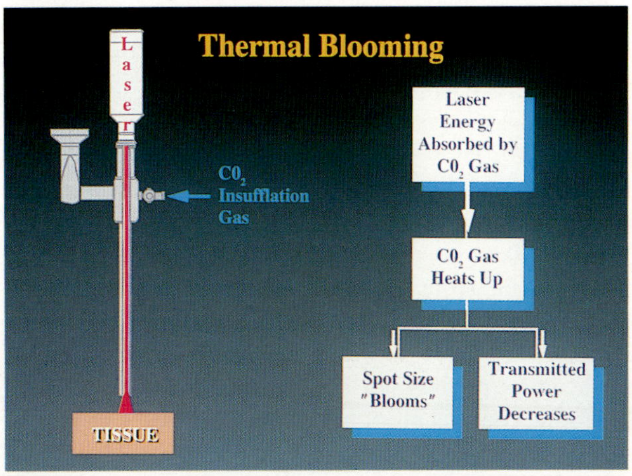

FIG. 11. The mechanisms underlying the problem of thermal blooming of the CO_2 laser beam within a laparoscopic delivery device.

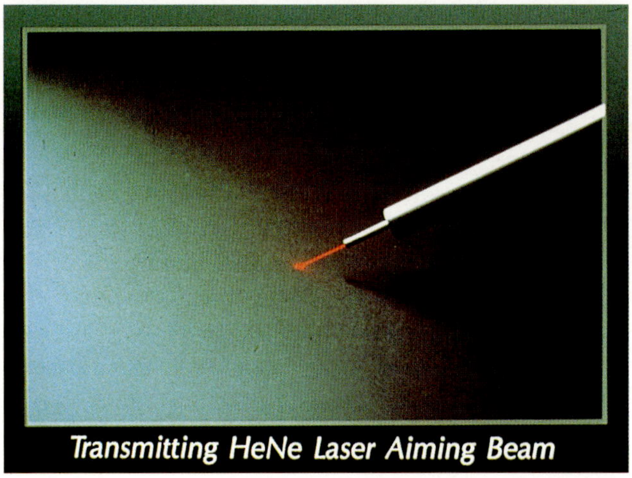

FIG. 12. CO_2 laser fiber.

A recently recognized problem associated with the delivery of CO_2 laser energy by means of long-focal-length, lens-focusing couplers through the laparoscope is the effect of passing the laser beam through a long, narrow operating channel filled with CO_2 insufflation gas (26). Passage of the Gaussian beam through this narrow channel results in some degree of "clipping" of the tails of the Gaussian curve and loss of some of the laser power. Absorption of the laser beam by CO_2 insufflation gas molecules also results in both a loss of power as the beam propagates down the channel and a thermal "lensing" or "blooming" effect as the CO_2 gas expands within the channel, tending to defocus the beam (Fig. 11). Both the absorptive and thermal lensing effects worsen as the CO_2 gas heats, often defeating any attempts to increase laser power during laparoscopic surgery. The recent development of the isotopic $^{13}CO_2$ laser, producing a shifted wavelength of 11.1 μm as opposed to the 10.6-μm wavelength of more conventional $^{12}CO_2$ lasers, has virtually identical tissue effects without the significant absorption and blooming of the laser beam by the CO_2 insufflation gas, allowing the delivery of higher power densities through laparoscopic couplers (23).

Fiberoptic and waveguide laser delivery devices are very similar to each other with regard to the physics and optics underlying their operation (25,27). These devices are composed of a clear inner core (composed of plastic, glass, or quartz materials in the case of fiberoptics or air in the case of waveguides) and an opaque or reflective outer cladding. In the case of infrared energy waveguides, a specially designed ceramic coating is often applied to the inner aspect of the reflective metal shell to enhance reflectivity and minimize power losses. A laser beam, tightly focused to enter the clear inner core, is repetitively bounced within the confines of the outer cladding along the length of the fiberoptic or waveguide until it emerges at the opposite end (Fig. 12). These devices have no focusing lenses at the delivery end and hence no true focal point. The emerging beam has a diameter roughly equal to the inner core diameter at the open end and begins to diverge rapidly almost immediately upon exiting. Highest power densities are always at the tip of the device, and the angle of divergence is generally much greater than for lens-focusing devices, allowing very easily obtainable lower power densities and coagulative capability.

For endoscopic and hand-held applications, the addition of a lens to the fiberoptic or waveguide tip would not be of great advantage, since the ability of a lens to focus is limited by the initial laser beam diameter as it emerges from the fiberoptic. Thus, the minimal beam spot size would always be limited by the aperture of the inner core of the fiberoptic and could be achieved only within a few millimeters from the fiberoptic tip. Since these conditions are not very different from those already achieved with the fiberoptic alone, lenses are typically not used with fiberoptic cables. Lenses are useful, however, when enough distance exists for the beam from the fiber to be defocused prior to refocusing using a lens. This defocusing and refocusing principle is used within the optical couplers that adapt fiberoptic systems to slit lamps and operating microscopes.

Although it is necessary to keep the distance between tissue and tip very short in order to obtain highest power densities when using the bare fiberoptic or waveguide during hand-held or endoscopic applications, actual contact with tissue should be avoided. Touching a fiberoptic tip to the tissue while lasing thermally degrades and eventually fuses the tip over time, thus diminishing and blocking transmission of the laser beam. Periodically during use, the fiberoptic must be precisely cleaved (cut) and preferably polished to allow the optimum transmission of laser light. Similarly, repeatedly touching a waveguide tip to the tissue results in the deposition of smoke and plume particles within the hollow bore, resulting in a gradual deterioration of beam transmission with time. Although autoclavable and reusable, the inside bore of a waveguide device cannot be cleaned and these devices have a limited lifetime. Thus, in order to become most efficient with a fiberoptic or waveguide laser and to prolong the lifetime of a fiberoptic or waveguide device, skill must be gained in getting as close as possible to the tissue with the tip of the device without actually touching. With fiberoptics, skill must also be gained in precisely cleaving the end of the fiber so as to reproduce a laser spot as precise and sharp as that produced by a fresh, mechanically cleaved fiber.

Both fiberoptics and waveguides are limited in terms of maximum permissible input powers. Fiberoptics are available with inner core diameters of 1000, 800, 600 μm, and even smaller, permitting similarly small spot sizes. However, the maximum permissible input power also decreases with decreasing inner core diameters. In addition, a certain amount of this laser power will always be lost as the laser beam bounces within the fiberoptic/waveguide, with the percentage lost increasing as the length of the device increases. For this reason, most fiberoptic lasers have a calibration port to compensate for these internal losses through the device. While fiberoptic cables are flexible, waveguide devices generally are not. Although semirigid waveguides are available, waveguides transmit optimally only when perfectly straight. Even when straight, losses of power through these devices range between 10% and 25%. Any deviation from straightness results in some variable loss in delivered power. Typical minimum spot sizes are 0.8 mm, which are identical to those achievable using 400-mm focal length laparoscopic lens-focusing couplers.

Contact laser delivery devices are generally used in conjunction with the fiberoptic lasers. The tips may be composed of crystal (often sapphire), quartz, ceramic, or metal materials that attach to the end of a conventional fiberoptic cable, or may be part of specially fabricated contact fibers with the tip of the fiber extended and sculpted to a desired shape (Fig. 13). The laser beam is primarily used to heat the tip of the delivery device, which then conductively transfers the heat to the tissues in contact with the tip. Even with completely clear contact tip devices, less than 10% of the laser energy actually leaves the tip to interact with the tissues. Therefore, surgery with clear-tipped devices is generally initially slow until after a thin layer of carbonization or pitting forms to accelerate the thermal transfer of energy. Because of the thermal properties of the tip materials, these tips are capable of very rapidly heating and cooling in synchrony with the laser pulses, which help to control the thermal energy conducted into the tissue and to minimize the amount of subsurface thermal necrosis. The zone of thermal necrosis with contact tips can come very close in depth to that obtained using the CO_2 laser. The shape of the tip determines the exact thermal effect on tissue by defining the area of contact.

Thermal surgery with contact devices only occurs when the tip is actually in contact with the tissue and the ability to defocus is virtually nonexistent. Care must be taken in the use of contact laser devices because almost all of the thermal action is concentrated at the very tip of the device, with very little occurring off to the sides. This effect is very different from that obtained with more standard electrosurgical devices in which the entire uninsulated portion of the tip is electrically active. Attempts to

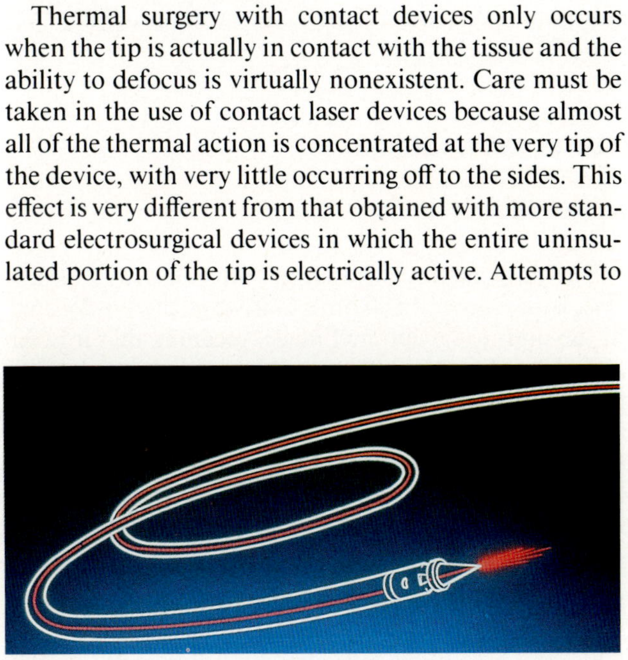

FIG. 13. Contact laser fiber.

use the sides of the tip in a manner similar to that done with electrosurgical devices is very frustrating to the surgeon, since very little thermal effect results to the tissue as desired, other than the overheating and gradual destruction of the contact tip itself.

The thermal destruction associated with contact devices occurs in hemispheric zones about the tip of the device. The depth of penetration is therefore generally equal to the width of destruction, both of which are related to the geometric shape of the contact device. Sharp-tipped devices are better for precise, incisional-type procedures, whereas rounded devices are better suited to coagulative effects. The most advantageous use of these devices is in conjunction with the Nd:YAG laser, since these devices can convert the normally deeply penetrating thermal effect of this laser into a much more precise, less deeply penetrating one. Contact tips are seldom used with other types of lasers because the advantages are not as marked as they are with the Nd:YAG laser.

For precision when using contact tips, the tips must be allowed to cool as rapidly as they heat. Maintaining light contact with the tissue actually serves to keep the tips relatively cool since the heat is rapidly conducted away into the tissue. When these tips are not in actual contact with the tissue, continued administration of the laser beam causes the tips to overheat, shortening the lifetime of the tips and causing even quartz-tipped devices to melt. Burying the tips in tissue also causes the tips to overheat, since the dehydrated and carbonized tissue formed about the tip are not as cooling as moist, soft tissue. Sapphire tips are crystalline, and as such are easily fractured or broken and are extremely expensive. However, these tips are sterilizable and can be reused over many cases if adequate care is taken in handling and storage. Contact fibers are much less expensive, but are much more easily damaged by overheating and are only good for single cases.

TYPES OF LASERS

Carbon Dioxide (CO_2)

The wavelength of photons produced by the CO_2 gas laser is 10.6 μm (10,600 nm). This wavelength is located in the mid- to far-infrared range, meaning that it is far into the infrared spectrum and away from the visible light spectrum. The medium of this laser is typically a mixture of carbon dioxide, nitrogen, and helium to improve the laser's efficiency. Because of the high degree of absorption by most glasses and plastics, CO_2 laser energy cannot be used for medical purposes with conventional fiberoptic cables. The principal means of delivering the laser energy to tissue include the articulated arm coupled to lens-focusing devices, rigid and semirigid waveguides, and directly from the laser tube itself if the laser tube is small enough to be hand-held or easily positionable, as is the case for some of the waveguide lasers. Recently, a new delivery device for the CO_2 laser consisting of a jacketed, flexible laser fiber has become available; however, its length, flexibility, spot size, and power-handling capabilities are all major limitations.

The isotopic $^{13}CO_2$ laser produces a shifted wavelength of 11.1 μm (11,100 nm) as opposed to the 10.6-μm wavelength of more conventional $^{12}CO_2$ lasers. Tissue effects are virtually identical to that of the more conventional $^{12}CO_2$ lasers. However, absorption and attenuation of the laser beam by CO_2 insufflation gas is not as much of a limitation during endoscopic procedures, eliminating the associated problem of spot size blooming and allowing the delivery of higher power densities through laparoscopic couplers.

The CO_2 laser has one of the widest ranges of applications of any of the medical lasers. Since it cuts all soft tissues equally well, regardless of pigment, it can be applied to virtually any surgical operation requiring precise incisions or precise removal of soft tissue or pathology. The field of gynecology has probably applied this laser to the widest range of procedures, including the treatment of endometriosis, tuboplasty, tubal ligation, cervical neoplasia (during colposcopy), condyloma acuminata, and even vulvectomy. Some of the most exciting work with the CO_2 laser has involved its use with the operating laparoscope, making the treatment of many forms of gynecologic pathology by laparotomy nearly obsolete. The combination of video technology with the laser and laparoscope has taken this science one step further, allowing better visualization of the abdominal pathology through magnification and, thus, better treatment of the pathology using minimally invasive surgery (28).

One of the major limitations to any CO_2 laser surgical attachment is that it allows straight line-of-sight propagation of the infrared energy to the tissue from the end of the primary delivery device. The CO_2 laser is adaptable for use with colposcopes, operating microscopes, stiff bronchoscopes, laparoscopes, stiff cystoscopes, arthroscopes, and proctoscopes. The CO_2 laser cannot operate on tissue at a water–tissue or fluid–tissue interface because water absorbs all of the laser energy and allows none to reach the tissue.

Nd:YAG

The neodymium:yttrium-aluminum-garnet, or Nd:YAG, laser produces laser light with a wavelength of 1064 nm, located in the near-infrared portion of the electromagnetic spectrum. The medium within the laser cavity is a crystalline rod composed of rare earth Nd^{3+} ions doped or suspended in a crystalline matrix of YAG. The near-infrared energy, although close to the visible spectrum, is invisible and is often used in conjunction with a coaxial helium-neon aiming beam. As with the visible lasers, the Nd:YAG laser light can be transmitted through conventional fiberoptic cables making it very convenient for delivery of the beam to tissue by hand and through flexible endoscopes. Since the fiberoptic delivery system typically requires the fiberoptic tip to be placed very close to the tissue (the highest power densities will always be at or as close as possible to the tip of the fiber), the Nd:YAG laser is occasionally used without an aiming beam. The Nd:YAG laser beam is effective at both gas–tissue interfaces and water–tissue interfaces. Operation on bleeding or very bloody tissue will not be as hampered as with most other lasers since the hemoglobin pigment and water content of blood do not absorb energy at this wavelength as much as other surgical laser energies. Thus, Nd:YAG laser energy from a bare fiber can penetrate a thin layer of blood somewhat, allowing coagulation of the underlying tissue.

Because of the Nd:YAG laser energy's ability to penetrate deeply into tissue in addition to its relative specificity to absorption by pigmented tissue, a niche was found for it early in the history of medical lasers in the treatment using high power densities on large, bloody lesions and tumors that were relatively untreatable by other techniques. These lesions could, in effect, be "blasted out" by using the Nd:YAG laser before their having a chance to bleed.

More recently, several advances have resulted in a reevaluation of the Nd:YAG laser and expansion of its applications. In gynecology, lower power applications have included the treatment of endometriosis, although the risk of possibly damaging the bowel and sensitive subperitoneal structures is somewhat greater than with other lasers, and hysteroscopic intrauterine endometrial ablation. One of the advantages of using the Nd:YAG laser is the ability of energy of this wavelength to transmit well through water during hysteroscopy and deposit ablative energy to the endometrium. The use of contact tips has vastly expanded the use of the Nd:YAG laser, providing the surgeon with a choice between a more precise ablation of tissue using contact tips or a more blunt and coagulative effect using the bare fiber.

Argon

The argon ion gas laser is an excellent example of a medical laser whose interaction is very dependent on the pigment within the tissue. The argon laser produces visible blue–green laser light with the principal output wavelengths at 488.0 nm (blue) and 514.5 nm (green), although other weaker wavelengths are possible in the green, blue, and even ultraviolet portions of the spectrum. The argon gas atoms are ionized within the specially designed plasma tube to produce the spontaneous and stimulated emission desired. The blue–green photons of this laser are well absorbed by the blood and pigment within tissue in addition to being tightly scattered by the collagen fibers and other opaque constituents of tissue, thus producing its thermal effects. As a result, the thermal effect is mainly coagulative, although high power densities (small beam spot sizes) can heat the tissue pigments and proteins fast enough to transfer heat to the water content of tissue and result in vaporization. The amount of laser plume is not as prominent as with the CO_2 laser, although the amount of charring is more. Early studies showed that the 488.0-nm wavelength performed incisions better than the 514.5-nm wavelength (1). This effect is most likely due to the fact that the blue wavelength does not penetrate as deeply into tissue as the green, thus confining the energy better to a smaller tissue volume at the surface. However, for a given laser, the highest powers and power densities to tissue are always achieved by delivering both wavelengths simultaneously, since both wavelengths are constantly being produced within the laser cavity. The argon laser beam is effective at both gas–tissue and water–tissue interfaces. Operation on bleeding or very bloody tissue is somewhat hampered since the hemoglobin pigment preferentially absorbs the argon laser energy to a very shallow depth, allowing little or none to penetrate to the tissue.

Since argon laser light is visible, an aiming beam is not essential as it is for the CO_2 laser. An attenuated version of the surgical beam is typically sufficient when using a shuttered eye protection system that inserts a protective eye filter into a viewing port to protect the eye while the laser is firing. However, nonshuttered protective glasses and lenses can make the attenuated beam invisible, and an aiming beam of another color light can be very useful. For most hand-held and endoscopic applications, the aiming beam is not necessary because the fiberoptic tip must be almost touching the tissue in order to obtain adequate power densities. In these types of applications, the spatial orientation of the fiberoptic tip can serve the same purpose as the aiming beam. However, an aiming beam is essential when using a slit lamp or operating microscope delivery device because the beam must be focused far from the fiberoptic tip by a focusing lens system. Since it is visible light, the argon laser beam can be transmitted through conventional fiberoptic cables providing a very flexible, lightweight, and convenient system for attaching to slit lamps and operating microscopes using optical couplers, or for delivering the beam directly to tissue either by hand, using either the bare fiber itself or pencil-like handpieces, or through the operating ports of flexible and stiff endoscopes. Because of this flexibility in delivery, the argon laser is extremely easy to adapt to virtually any surgical or endoscopic procedure.

The application of the argon laser in gynecology has had mixed reviews. The fiberoptic delivery system is much easier and less cumbersome to use than the CO_2

articulated arm. The ability of the argon energy to transmit well through water prior to absorption by pigment lends itself to many surgical procedures, whereas CO_2 laser energy cannot transmit through any layer of water. The specific absorption by pigment is very attractive in the treatment of certain pigmented lesions such as endometriosis. However, not all endometriosis-type tissue is deeply pigmented. Additionally, one must be extra careful when using the argon laser intraabdominally since the energy also is specifically absorbed by underlying blood vessels and can cause more extensive deep thermal necrosis to the bowel and to subperitoneal structures, such as the ureter, than the CO_2 laser. The CO_2 laser is confined to surface effects only and can be used (with great care and experience) even on sensitive structures, such as the bowel and the peritoneum overlying blood vessels and ureters.

The argon laser (as well as other fiberoptic lasers, such as the Nd:YAG and the frequency-doubled Nd:YAG or KTP) has also been used in the removal of adhesions during laparoscopy and other endoscopic procedures. However, this application uses the fiberoptic cable primarily as a hot tip or contact tip probe. The argon fiberoptic tip must be touched to the adhesion to remove it effectively. Repeatedly touching the fiberoptic to tissue eventually melts the tip of the fiberoptic, gradually reducing the amount of laser energy actually transmitted. Additionally, adhesions are not typically deeply pigmented, so there is no preferential absorption by the adhesion as compared to normal tissue. Fortunately, the beam rapidly diverges as it leaves the fiberoptic tip, so that damage to tissues behind the adhesion should be minimal as long as the distance between the adhesion and normal tissue is sufficient. This rapid beam divergence also provides an extra margin of safety by reducing somewhat the need for a backstop behind the adhesion. The tip of the fiberoptic should always be recleaved following its use on adhesions and prior to using the laser on any pigmented lesions.

Frequency-Doubled Nd:YAG/KTP

The KTP or frequency-doubled Nd:YAG laser is a relatively new medical laser that produces a visible green energy with a wavelength of 532 nm. The actual lasering part of this laser is a Nd:YAG laser. However, by passing the Nd:YAG energy through a nonlinear crystal composed of KTP, the frequency of the Nd:YAG laser is doubled (corresponding to a halving of the wavelength), thus converting the 1064-nm wavelength energy into 532-nm wavelength energy, which is in the green visible spectrum. The green laser energy is easily transmitted through flexible fiberoptics.

The wavelength of the KTP laser (532 nm) is very close to that of the argon laser (488/514 nm). Therefore, the effects and applications of these two lasers are virtually identical. The green laser energy actually penetrates somewhat deeper in nonpigmented tissue and is somewhat better absorbed by hemoglobin than is the blue–green argon laser energy. However, clinically the difference in effect is almost insignificant. Both lasers penetrate relatively deeply in nonpigmented tissues and have very shallow penetration in pigmented tissues. Generally, the zone of thermal necrosis surrounding and underlying a pigmented lesion is slightly less with the KTP laser than with the argon laser.

Other Lasers

The preceding sections described the lasers most used in gynecology today. Several other new and upcoming lasers bear mentioning. The holmium:yttrium-aluminum-garnet (Ho:YAG) laser is a crystalline laser very similar to the Nd:YAG but doped with rare earth holmium ions instead of neodymium. Its wavelength of 2100 nm is absorbed primarily by the water content of soft tissues and is independent of pigment like the CO_2 laser; however, the depth of penetration and coagulation is more like that of the argon/KTP lasers in pigmented tissue. The energy is produced in precise pulses similar to that of superpulsed and ultrapulsed CO_2 lasers, and can be easily transmitted by means of special, low-water-content fiberoptics. Although absorbed by water, the greater depth of penetration in water allows this laser to be used in an aqueous environment, provided the tip is very close to the tissue surface, with even greater precision than in a gaseous environment since the water prevents carbon formation. Gynecologic applications are still mostly investigational.

The surgical diode laser, typically composed of a gallium-aluminum-arsenide (GaAlAs) medium, has a central output wavelength of 805–810 nm, which is in the very-near-infrared portion of the electromagnetic spectrum. Its interaction with tissue is very similar to that of the Nd:YAG laser for an equivalent amount of power, but with slightly better overall precision and selectivity for blood and other pigments. Because of this similarity, the diode laser has applications almost identical to those of the Nd:YAG laser and is used with both contact and noncontact fiberoptic delivery systems. However, the 25-W power limitation of current diode laser systems restricts their use to primarily contact tip surgical applications. The major advantages of the diode laser are its extremely small size, low electrical power requirements, high-power conversion efficiency, and low cost compared to other surgical lasers. Gynecologic applications are still mostly investigational.

Excimer lasers produce photons with wavelengths in the ultraviolet portion of the spectrum, which are primarily absorbed by water and, at most wavelengths, are better absorbed by water than CO_2 laser photons. Thus excimer lasers are actually more precise than CO_2 lasers but are also slower. Excimer lasers typically produce extremely short, high-energy pulses that enhance their potential surgical precision. Interestingly, the interaction of high-power, ultraviolet laser radiation with tissue results in ionization effects, whereby tissue is instantaneously converted to an ionic gas plasma that then dissipates. Resulting incisions are sharper than those produced by a cold scalpel, with virtually no adjacent thermal effects. Although the delivery devices consist of fiberoptics, current fiberoptics are very limited in terms of power handling capabilities at these wavelengths. Another, more significant problem is that ultraviolet radiation is by nature potentially mutagenic to biological tissues and can result in the development of various types of cancer. Because of the potential for mutagenicity, no surgical procedure has yet received U.S. Food and Drug Administration (FDA) approval, although ophthalmological applications for radial keratotomy are very close to gaining approval.

LASER SAFETY

By its nature, a laser can ignite flammable materials, cause eye injuries, and be reflected. Laser safety revolves about a good understanding and awareness of these three properties, as well as a thorough understanding of all the possible ramifications of these three properties (29).

Anything in the surgical area that is flammable can be potentially ignited by a laser. The liberal use of wetting solutions for gauze squares, lap packs, and drapes in the immediate surgical area prevents the accidental ignition of these materials very effectively with all lasers but is especially effective in absorbing stray CO_2 laser energy. Specifically designed, flame-retardant surgical drapes for laser surgery are also available. During open abdominal procedures, the liberal use of wet packs over the bowel and surrounding the surgical area can be extremely beneficial to a surgeon's peace of mind. During endoscopic procedures, the liberal use of irrigation fluids also confers protection.

Alcohol and ether preps should be avoided during laser surgery. Other prep solutions, such as betadine or hibiclens, are safe as long as they contain no or little alcohol. Anesthesiologists should be aware that no flammable anesthetics should be used during laser surgery. Oxygen is not a flammable gas, and 40% O_2 is commonly used during otolaryngologic laser procedures. However, oxygen does support the combustion of other flammable materials, so that the choice of oxygen concentrations should be made judiciously.

Another potential flammability hazard applies primarily to otolaryngologic procedures but is worthy of note by all medical disciplines that employ the laser. Potentially disastrous complications can result (and have resulted in the past) from the ignition of plastic endotracheal tubes, particularly those composed of polyvinylchloride, while a patient is intubated. Special endotracheal tubes and endotracheal tube wraps are available specifically for endotracheal laser surgery. Although this problem is not of concern in gynecologic procedures, attention should be given to the presence of any plastic materials or accessories entering the surgical area. Suction hoses and tips are generally composed of plastics that melt rather than ignite; however, the testing of the results of hitting any plastic accessory with the laser prior to surgery is a worthwhile precaution.

The eye is always the organ of the body most susceptible to serious laser injuries. The need for eye safety during laser surgery cannot be overemphasized. Visible and near-visible laser energy (Nd:YAG, KTP, and argon) can cause burns of the retina, whereas far-infrared energy (CO_2) can cause burns of the cornea and can rapidly penetrate the cornea. The Nd:YAG laser energy is a particularly bad culprit in the generation of eye injuries since the beam is invisible and can cause significant retinal burns without generating a protective blink response. The eye is most sensitive to laser wavelengths in and near the visible spectrum.

Each laser has its own particular set of safety standards and its own required safety eyewear. The tinting of the eyewear is designed to remove maximally the wavelengths of most concern with the specific laser while passing as many of the other wavelengths as possible to allow maximum visibility. Protected wavelength(s) are generally labeled on the frames or temples. Nd:YAG safety eyewear is not protective against argon laser energy, and vice versa. Argon and KTP safety eyewear are generally orange in color, Nd:YAG safety eyewear is generally green, and CO_2 laser safety eyewear is clear.

Since all plastics and glass absorb CO_2 laser energy very well, virtually any plastic or prescription lenses are protective with this laser. When using one's own prescription lenses as eye protection, the use of unvented side shield attachments is recommended to prevent stray laser radiation from entering from the side. Contact lenses, whether glass or plastic, are not considered adequate protection because they can cause secondary burns to the cornea after absorbing the CO_2 laser energy. The optics of an operating microscope and the lenses on operating laparoscopes are completely protective but only to the viewer's eye(s). Lasers other than the CO_2 require special optical filter shutters on the optical lenses that are triggered to swing into place whenever the laser fires to provide protection.

Everyone in the surgical room should wear protective lenses, including the patient. If desired, an anesthetized patient may have laser safety shields taped over the eyes instead of wearing safety goggles. For the CO_2 laser, these safety shields may consist solely of a thick layer of wet eyepads taped over the eyes.

Laser light can be reflected off of any shiny surface. The major surgical safety consideration with this hazard is the risk of reflections off of surgical instruments that enter the laser field, which may result in unintentional burning of the patient or the surgeon. This possibility can be particularly significant intraabdominally, where sensitive structures abound and separation distances are short. Fortunately, most surgical instruments that tend to get in the way of the laser, such as skin hooks, have convexly curved surfaces with small bend radii, so that incident laser light tends to diverge upon reflection. However, even a curved instrument with a bend radius of 2 mm can appear fairly flat to a 0.2-mm laser spot size. Surgical instruments also typically develop localized dents and pits that can potentially refocus incident laser beams onto unintentional neighboring sites.

Many different schemes have been developed to combat this safety hazard. The best and most expensive surgical instruments that minimize the hazards of reflection are those with brushed titanium tips. The titanium metal handles high laser powers and the resultant heat well, while the gray luster and the fine wire brushing of the surface help to scatter the laser light in all directions rather than directly reflecting or refocusing. These instruments are definitely the ones of choice, particularly if backstops are required, as in laser laparoscopy.

Another, less expensive solution is to have one set of laser instruments finely wire-brushed, sand-blasted, or glass-beaded. Although the typical stainless steel does not handle heat as well as titanium and breakdown of the metal may occur with time, especially when it is used as backstop, the roughened surface still helps in scattering the incident laser light rather than directly reflecting it. However, localized heating with these instruments may occur, resulting in the additional hazard of secondary thermal burns upon contact with tissue.

A third solution has been the use of ebonized coatings on instruments. Ebonized coatings eliminate the hazard of reflections, not by scattering but by the absorption of any stray, incident laser energy. Unfortunately, many of the ebonized coatings tend to degrade with time and laser impact and flake. In addition, by absorbing all of the laser energy, the instrument heats much more quickly with each laser impact and can cause secondary burns to tissue. Newer ebonization techniques are more durable and last longer. However, it is still wise to avoid laser impact on the surface of ebonized instruments and never to use an ebonized instrument as a laser backstop.

The hazards associated with the production of biological smoke during either laser surgery or electrosurgery are often ignored. There is no such entity as safe biological smoke. Although studies have repeatedly documented the absence of significant hazards due to viable cancerous cells, bacteria, or fungal particles (30), recent studies have documented potential hazards associated with the survival and possible transmission of viral particles in both laser surgical and electrosurgical smoke (31,32). Laser surgery produces a high percentage of smoke particles with diameters comparable to those of lung-damaging dust particles, easily capable of penetrating deeply into the terminal bronchioles and alveoli and among the most difficult particles to filter adequately. Particles of this size are also large enough to enclose many types of viral particles, potentially insulating them from thermal damage. In addition to the hazards associated with viruses and particle size, both laser and electrosurgical smoke have also been shown to contain potentially hazardous chemicals and to be potentially as mutagenic as cigarette smoke (33). No smoke-producing surgical procedure, whether laser or electrosurgical, should ever be performed without the assistance of adequate suctioning and filtration of the smoke.

HIGHLIGHTS

Lasers now play a significant role in gynecology and particularly in laparoscopic surgery. This chapter briefly reviews the physics of laser energy as well as the interactions between laser energy and tissue that result in the thermal destruction of tissue. These physical principles provide a logical basis for the subsequent discussion of the various surgical laser operating parameters, with particular emphasis on the importance of time and pulsing parameters and the selection of appropriate laser beam delivery devices. Individual sections discuss in greater depth the surgical principles and utilization of four of the major laser types with applications in gynecologic surgery (the CO_2, Nd:YAG, argon, and KTP lasers), as well as some of the newer lasers that may soon find applications in this field. The chapter concludes with a section discussing laser safety.

REFERENCES

1. Goldman L, Rockwell RJ Jr. *Lasers in medicine.* New York: Gordon and Breach; 1971.
2. Bruhat MA, Mage G, Manhes M. Use of CO_2 laser via laparoscopy. In: Kaplan I, ed. *Proceedings of the third international congress for laser surgery,* Jerusalem: Academic Press; 1979:275-276.
3. Bellina JH, Bandieramonte G. *Principles and practice of gynecologic laser surgery.* New York: Plenum Press; 1984.
4. Nezhat C, Nezhat FR. Safe laser endoscopic excision or vaporization of peritoneal endometriosis. *Fertil Steril* 1989;52(1):149–151.
5. O'Shea DC, Callen WR, Rhodes WT. *Introduction to lasers and their applications.* Reading, MA: Addison-Wesley, 1978.
6. Mihashi S, Jako GJ, Incze J, Strong MS, Vaughan CW. Laser surgery in otolaryngology: interaction of CO_2 laser and soft tissue. *Ann NY Acad Sci,* 1976;263–294.
7. Anderson RR, Parrish JA. The optics of human skin. *J Invest Dermatol* 1981;77(1):13–19.
8. Walsh J, Morelli J, Parrish JA. Laser–tissue interactions and their clinical applications. *Curr Prob Dermatol* 1986;15:94–110.
9. McKenzie AL, Carruth JAS. Lasers in surgery and medicine. *Phys Med Biol* 1984;29(6):619–641.
10. Landry RJ, Sliney D, Scott R. *Optical and laser technology in medicine,* vol. 605. Proceedings of SPIE—The International Society for Optical Engineering, Bellingham: Washington, 1986.
11. Henriques FC, Moritz AR. Studies of thermal injury. I. The conduction of heat to and through skin and the temperatures attained

therein. A theoretical and an experimental investigation. *Am J Pathol* 1947;23(4):531–549.
12. Moritz AR, Henriques FC. Studies of thermal injury. II. The relative importance of time and surface temperature in the causation of cutaneous burns. *Am J Pathol* 1947;23(5):695–720.
13. Moritz AR. Studies of thermal injury. III. The pathology and pathogenesis of cutaneous burns. *Am J Pathol* 1947;23(6):915–943.
14. Henriques FC. Studies of thermal injury. V. The predictability and the significance of thermally induced rate processes leading to irreversible epidermal injury. *Arch Pathol* 1947;43:489–502.
15. Hall RR, Beach AD, Baker E, Morison PCA. Incision of tissue by carbon dioxide laser. *Nature* 1971;232:131–132.
16. McKenzie AL. A three zone model of soft tissue damage by a CO_2 laser. *Phys Med Biol* 1986;31:967–983.
17. Simpson GT, Shapshay SM. Symposium on the use of lasers in otolaryngologic surgery. *Otolaryngol Clin North Am* 1983;16(4):739–827.
18. Symposium on laser surgery. *Surg Clin North Am* 1984;64(5):839–859.
19. Unger M. Symposium on laser techniques. *Clin Chest Med* 1985;6(2):179–217.
20. Baggish MS, ElBakry MM. Comparison of electronically superpulsed and continuous-wave CO_2 laser on the rat uterine horn. *Fertil Steril* 1986;45(1):120–127.
21. Walsh JT Jr, MacGregor TS, Anderson RR, Deutsch TF. Pulsed CO_2 laser tissue ablation: effect of tissue type and pulse duration on thermal damage. *Lasers Surg Med* 1989;8:108–118.
22. Green HA, Domankevitz T, Nishioka NS. Pulsed carbon dioxide laser ablation of burned skin: in vitro and in vivo analysis. *Lasers Surg Med* 1990;10:476–484.
23. Adamson GD, Reich H, Trost D. $^{13}CO_2$ isotopic laser used through the operating channel of laser laparoscopes: a comparative study of power and energy density losses. *Obstet Gynecol* May 1994;83(5):717–724.
24. Oosterhuis JW, Verschueren RCJ, Eibergen R, Oldhoff J. The viability of cells in the waste products of CO_2-laser evaporation of Cloudman mouse melanomas. *Cancer* 1982;49:61–67.
25. Meyer-Arendt JR. *Introduction to classical and modern optics.* Englewood Cliffs, NJ: Prentice-Hall; 1984.
26. Reich H, MacGregor TS III, Vancaillie TG. CO_2 laser used through the operating channel of laser laparoscopes: in vitro study of power and power density losses. *Obstet Gynecol* 1991;77(1):40–47.
27. Katzir A. *Optical fibers in medicine II,* vol. 713. Proceedings of SPIE—The International Society for Optical Engineering, Bellingham: Washington, 1986.
28. Nezhat C, Crowgey SR, Nezhat F. Videolaseroscopy for the treatment of endometriosis associated with infertility. *Fertil Steril* 1989;51:237.
29. *Laser hazards and safety in the military environment.* AGARD Lecture Series No. 79, North Atlantic Treaty Organization Advisory Group for Aerospace Research and Development, Technical Editing and Reproduction Ltd., London, 1975.
30. Voorhies RM, Lavyne MC, Strait TA, Shapiro WR. Does the CO_2 laser spread viable brain-tumor cells outside the surgical field? *J Neurosurgery* 1984;60:819–820.
31. Bellina JH, Stjernholm RL, Kurpel JE. Analysis of plume emissions after papovirus irradiation with the carbon dioxide laser. *J Reprod Med* 1982;27(5):268–270.
32. Matthews J, Newsom SWB, Walker NPJ. Aerobiology of irradiation with the carbon dioxide laser. *Journal of Hospital Infection* 1985, 230–233.
33. Tomita Y, Mihashi S, Nagata K, et al. "Mutagenicity of smoke condensates induced by CO_2-laser irradiation and electrocauterization," *Mutation Research* 1981, 89:145–149.

PART II

Preparation for Operative Laparoscopy

Endoscopic Management of Gynecologic Disease,
edited by G.D. Adamson and D.C. Martin.
Lippincott-Raven Publishers, Philadelphia © 1996.

CHAPTER 5

Indications for Operative Laparoscopy

Andrew S. Cook

The role of operative laparoscopy in the treatment of gynecologic disorders is one of the most controversial subjects in the field of gynecology (1). The most avid proponents are of the opinion that virtually all procedures can and should be performed laparoscopically. At the other end of the spectrum, opponents feel that operative laparoscopy should be restricted to minor procedures, such as tubal ligation and perhaps treatment of minimal endometriosis.

The variety of instruments and the technologic advancements in laparoscopic equipment over the last decade has been dramatic. The current array of instruments and equipment, including high-powered light sources, high-flow insufflators, video cameras, and smoke filtration/recirculation systems, have overcome the vast majority of early technical problems associated with laparoscopy. The length of time to develop sophisticated endoscopic skills may be several years. Therefore there is a lag from the early development of skills by surgical pioneers to the general availability of these skills in the surgical specialty. This dramatic change in laparoscopic equipment and surgical skill over the last decade has contributed to the current state of controversy regarding the role of laparoscopy.

The effect of surgery on tissue and whether this effect is the same or significantly different depending on the surgical approach—laparotomy or laparoscopy—is the real issue. For many procedures, the answer to this question is not clear due to a lack of well-controlled scientific data. The large number of independent variables, including variation in surgical ability, makes arriving at a definitive answer difficult.

Laparotomy offers direct access to the pelvic organs. Direct manipulation of the tissue with the surgeon's hands may be advantageous. If the same tissue effect can be obtained as that at laparotomy, laparoscopy is superior in many ways, including decreased morbidity, decreased recovery time, decreased time lost from work, decreased cost, and potentially decreased adhesion formation and blood loss. The less invasive nature of laparoscopy may actually improve the tissue effect. Laparoscopy provides the surgeon levels of magnification, which can be changed rapidly by varying the distance of the laparoscope from the tissue and visual access to the pelvis unavailable at laparotomy (2).

Advanced laparoscopic surgery requires a level of surgical skill unparalleled in other types of gynecologic surgery. Microsurgery, a surgical technique learned through specialized training and practice, is only once removed from direct surgery through the open abdomen. The surgeon must adapt to the intervening operative microscope. With laparoscopy, not only is the field of view magnified as in microsurgery, but the orientation of the surgical field is different from the view of the surgical field. The view is monocular, which eliminates much of the depth perception; there is continual variation in magnification of the surgical field; movement of the surgeon's hand in one direction results in movement of the tissue in the opposite direction. In addition, the surgeon must have a skilled assistant. All of these factors have a cumulative effect on making laparoscopic surgery one of the most difficult surgical modalities. Not all physicians make good surgeons and even fewer master laparoscopic techniques. Many experienced surgeons who are proficient in laparoscopic techniques feel that equal if not better results are obtained laparoscopically than are obtained by laparotomy.

The objections by gynecologic opponents of advanced operative laparoscopy sound all too similar to the objections of general surgeons to the use of the laparoscope for diagnosis and treatment of such conditions as appendicitis and cholecystitis (3). One is left wondering if the real problem is with the technique, i.e., the laparoscope, or

A. S. Cook: Omega Institute of Health, Metairie, Louisiana 70001-2082.

the ability of the surgeon to develop the necessary skills to use the technique proficiently.

A paucity of prospective randomized studies prevents a definitive answer to which technique, laparoscopy or laparotomy, is superior for which gynecologic procedures. The available studies demonstrate no significant difference in results between laparotomy and laparoscopy for many procedures. Because of the inherent disadvantages of laparotomy, unless the results of a given procedure are clearly superior, laparoscopy must be considered the technique of choice.

SPECIFIC INDICATIONS

Indications for operative laparoscopy are given in Table 1.

Ectopic Pregnancy

The most widely studied indication for laparoscopic surgery is treatment of ectopic pregnancy. The cumulative data are sufficient to support the recommendation of laparoscopic treatment of ectopic pregnancy (4). Vermesh et al., in a prospective randomized trial of 60 patients, compared morbidity, cost, length of hospital stay, and fertility outcome following linear salpingostomy via laparoscopy or laparotomy (5). The laparoscopy group experienced significantly less blood loss, shorter recovery time, and less cost than did the laparotomy group. No significant difference was noted in postoperative patency, pregnancy rates, or complication rates. One patient in each group experienced persistent β-human chorionic gonadotropin (β-hCG) levels. Two patients in the laparotomy group had postoperative wound infections and two patients undergoing laparoscopy required laparotomy to obtain hemostasis. In both cases, the ectopic pregnancy was larger than 5 cm. Detection of significant differences was difficult because of the small sample size.

Bruhat et al. found a 67% intrauterine pregnancy rate with a 12% repeat ectopic pregnancy rate following laparoscopic treatment of ectopic pregnancy (6). These rates compare favorably with intrauterine pregnancy rates reported at laparotomy with salpingectomy (54%), conservative treatment (64%), and microsurgical treatment (53%).

The incidence of persistent trophoblastic tissue after conservative treatment was studied by Lundroff et al. (7). In a nonrandomized fashion, 52 patients underwent linear salpingostomy at laparoscopy and 46 at laparotomy. Overall, 8% of patients experienced persistence of trophoblastic tissue, with no significant difference between the two groups. This study found that a preoperative β-hCG level above 3000 mIU/ml and a level above 1000 mIU/ml on postoperative day 7 was predictive of increased risk for persistent trophoblastic tissue.

The risk of postoperative adhesion formation was addressed by Lundorff et al. (8). One hundred five patients were randomized to either laparotomy or laparoscopic treatment of ectopic pregnancy. Seventy-three patients underwent second-look laparoscopy. Significantly more patients treated at laparotomy experienced adhesion formation on the ipsilateral side. No significant difference was noted in tubal patency between the two groups.

Based on the current literature, there is fair evidence to recommend that operative laparoscopy be used for removal of an ectopic pregnancy (4). The intrauterine pregnancy rate, recurrent ectopic rate, persistence of trophoblastic tissue, and complication rate all seem to be comparable between the surgical techniques. Thus laparoscopy offers the same results with deceased morbidity and cost.

Ovarian Cysts

Laparoscopic treatment of ovarian cysts is the third most common application of operative laparoscopy, yet its use remains controversial (9). The primary concern is failure or delay in diagnosis of ovarian cancer and/or dissemination following rupture of the capsule (10). Systematic preoperative evaluation and counseling is imperative. Some have advocated routine preoperative sonography and CA-125 assay to help exclude malignancy (11). If cancer is suspected preoperatively, laparotomy should be considered. The possibility of ovarian cancer and its ramifications should be discussed with the patient preoperatively. For example, should laparotomy and staging be performed at the initial procedure or

TABLE 1. *Indications for operative laparoscopy in gynecologic surgery*

Laparoscopic treatment usually indicated	Laparoscopic treatment possibly indicated	Laparoscopic treatment rarely indicated
Ectopic pregnancy	Salpingitis	Myomectomy
Ovarian cysts	Uterosacral nerve ablation	Polycystic ovarian syndrome
Endometriosis	Presacral neurectomy	
Salpingoovariolysis	Laparoscopic-assisted vaginal hysterectomy	
Neosalpingostomy		
Fimbrioplasty		

would the patient prefer to return for a second procedure after full consideration?

The visual appearance of the ovarian cyst at laparoscopy further helps the surgeon to differentiate between functional and organic cysts. In a series by Bruhat et al., all ovarian malignancies were recognized: seven by their external appearance and two by the appearance of the cyst wall (intracystic growths) (12). A survey by the Society of Gynecologic Oncologists "concerning the laparoscopic management of ovarian neoplasms subsequently found to be malignant" is noteworthy (13). One in five surgeons responded to the questionnaire reporting a total of 42 cases of ovarian cancer. Only 17% of cases underwent laparotomy at the time of laparoscopy, and 12% never had a laparotomy. For the remaining 71% of cases, laparotomy was performed an average of 5 weeks following laparoscopy. Less than half of the cases were stage I. The frequent delay in treatment reported in this questionnaire study has been criticized by many proponents and opponents of laparoscopic surgery.

Incidental rupture of an unrecognized stage I ovarian malignancy during laparoscopic cystectomy would change the classification from stage Ia or Ib to stage Ic. The potential for a worse prognosis with this change in classification is a prime consideration in the argument against laparoscopic treatment of ovarian cysts. Dembo et al. analyzed data on 519 patients with stage I invasive epithelial ovarian cancer to determine which factors were predictive of relapse (14). Grade, dense adherence, and large-volume ascites were predictive of recurrence, whereas cyst rupture, capsular penetration, tumor size, and bilaterality were not predictive of relapse. These data suggest that cyst rupture does not disseminate disease or adversely affect prognosis.

Several reports have documented the low complication rate of laparoscopic treatment of ovarian cysts. However, simple aspiration is not sufficient; the cyst capsule must be removed or completely ablated.

Endometriosis

Resection and vaporization of endometriosis is the most common indication for operative laparoscopy (9). All stages of endometriosis are probably best treated at laparoscopy (15). The laparoscope is an ideal instrument for diagnosis and, in conjunction with the CO_2 laser, is ideal for treatment of endometriosis. Laparoscopic treatment of minimal and mild endometriosis is as effective or more effective than medical treatment and does not require a 6-month period in which the fecundity is zero (16). Laparoscopic treatment of moderate and severe endometriosis yields results as good as and potentially better than those obtained with macrosurgical or microsurgical techniques (17,18). Treatment of severe endometriosis may involve lysis and/or resection of dense adhesions, resection of deep fibrotic endometriosis, and sometimes vaporization of a portion of the bowel wall involved with endometriosis. These situations are ideally suited for treatment with the CO_2 laser.

Some have argued that results at laparoscopy are not significantly better than those following laparotomy and, therefore, laparoscopy cannot be recommended over laparotomy (19). I submit that the opposite is true. Unless laparotomy is demonstrated to be significantly better, it cannot be recommended over laparoscopy.

Salpingoovariolysis

Several studies have demonstrated the benefit of laparoscopic adhesiolysis. De novo adhesion formation is significantly less and adhesion reformation tends to be less extensive and less dense with laparoscopic treatment (20). An overview of the literature demonstrated an improved but not statistically significant increase in the viable pregnancy rate following laparoscopic salpingo-ovariolysis compared to results at laparotomy (19). Decreased morbidity, decreased risk of adhesion formation, and the potential increase in pregnancy rates together make laparoscopic salpingoovariolysis the technique of choice.

Neosalpingostomy and Fimbrioplasty

The results of laparoscopic treatment of distal tubal obstruction are comparable to those obtained with microsurgery, both with and without laser. Studies by the same group have demonstrated intrauterine pregnancy rates of 34.5% with laparoscopic tuboplasty and 30.8% with microsurgical techniques (6). The intrauterine pregnancy rate, despite the surgical technique, correlates directly with the degree of tubal damage. A review of the literature demonstrates a not statistically significant higher viable pregnancy rate (19). Patients with tubal damage and/or distal tubal occlusion disease should be treated laparoscopically or with in vitro fertilization, depending on the severity of disease.

Salpingitis

Although laparoscopy often is an integral component in the diagnosis of salpingitis, studies describing the use of operative laparoscopy to drain pelvic abscesses or to remove pus loculations have been limited. The few studies that do describe laparoscopic treatment of salpingitis failed to demonstrate complications (21). Laparoscopic treatment of pelvic abscesses carries the theoretical possibility of increasing the efficiency of antibiotic treatment and, thus, decreasing long-term sequelae of salpingitis (22).

Treatment of Polycystic Ovary Syndrome

Ovarian cautery, laser vaporization, and administration of human menopausal gonadotropins are equally effective approaches to inducing ovulation in women with polycystic ovary syndrome (23). Surgical treatment results in a decrease in androstenedione, testosterone, and luteinizing hormone levels (24). Concern arises over potential adhesion formation resulting from surgical trauma to the ovary. The true frequency of postoperative parovarian adhesion formation is uncertain. Some authors have noted low adhesion rates (<5%), whereas others have observed a high incidence (6 of 6 patients) (25). Laparoscopic treatment is effective in patients who are resistant to treatment with clomiphene citrate.

Laparoscopic Uterosacral Nerve Ablation

Laparoscopic uterosacral nerve ablation (LUNA) is a commonly performed procedure for the treatment of dysmenorrhea. There is a lack of well-designed studies demonstrating the efficacy of LUNA. One study claimed that 71% of patients experienced little or no dysmenorrhea one year after treatment (26).

Presacral Neurectomy

Complete resection of the hypogastric nerve plexus at laparotomy provides relief of midline dysmenorrhea in patients with stage III and stage IV endometriosis (27). Presacral neurectomy is not effective in the treatment of dyspareunia, lateral pelvic pain, or back pain. Inappropriate patient selection and incomplete resection of the hypogastric nerve plexus may account for variation in reported results. The efficacy of laparoscopic presacral neurectomy has not been demonstrated in appropriate studies.

Laparoscopic-Assisted Vaginal Hysterectomy

Laparoscopic-assisted vaginal hysterectomy (LAVH) is a new procedure whose appropriate role in gynecology has yet to be determined. Approximately two thirds of the 650,000 hysterectomies performed annually in the United States are currently performed at laparotomy. The role of laparoscopic-assisted vaginal hysterectomy may be to convert abdominal hysterectomies to vaginal cases. This may result in decreased morbidity, shorter hospital stay, and reduced time off work.

Myomectomy

Myomectomy is a procedure that remains in the domain of laparotomy, with occasional exception. Laparoscopic excision of myomas is technically possible. However, issues of hemostasis, closure of the defect, and removal of the myoma currently usually preclude laparoscopic myomectomy as a sensible procedure, especially for women desiring subsequent pregnancies. Indications for laparoscopic myomectomy may include excision of a pedunculated myoma with removal through a colpotomy incision or by morcellation, or removal of small myomas as a secondary procedure during operative laparoscopy.

HIGHLIGHTS

The paucity of well-controlled, prospective, randomized studies to provide irrefutable data has resulted in lack of agreement as to the role of operative laparoscopy. Recommendations regarding which procedures should be performed laparoscopically because of improved outcome must be based on a substantial number of cohort studies, case-control studies, case series, case reports, and expert opinions. These procedures include removal of an ectopic pregnancy, treatment of ovarian cysts, treatment of all stages of endometriosis, adhesiolysis, and treatment of polycystic ovarian syndrome resistant to clomiphene citrate therapy. Fimbrioplasty, neosalpingostomy, and treatment of salpingitis will probably yield better results at laparoscopy, but this is open to debate. Laparoscopic-assisted vaginal hysterectomy may be beneficial if an increased number of hysterectomies can be converted from abdominal to vaginal procedures with a resulting decrease in morbidity. The role of laparoscopic uterosacral nerve ablation and its efficacy is controversial. Laparoscopic myomectomy is rarely favored over removal at laparotomy.

REFERENCES

1. Candiani GB, Vercellini P, Fedele L, Bianchi S, Vendola N, Candiani M. Conservative surgical treatment for severe endometriosis in infertile women: are we making progress? *Obstet Gynecol Surv* 1991;46:490.
2. Nezhat CR, Nezhat FR, Silfen SL. Videolaseroscopy. *Obstet Gynecol Clin North Am* 1991;18:585.
3. Hunter JG. Laser use in laparoscopic surgery. *Surg Clin North Am* 1992;72:655.
4. Grimes DA. Frontiers of operative laparoscopy: a review and critique of the evidence. *Am J Obstet Gynecol* 1992;166:1062.
5. Vermesh M, Lilva PD, Rosen GF, Stein AL, Fossum GT, Sauer MV. Management of unruptured ectopic gestation by linear salpingostomy: a prospective randomized clinical trial of laparoscopy versus laparotomy. *Obstet Gynecol* 1988;73:889.
6. Bruhat MA, Mage G, Chapron C, Pouly JL, Canis M, Wattiez A. Present day endoscopic surgery in gynecology. *European J Obstet Gynecol Reprod Biol* 1991;41:4.
7. Lundroff P, Hahlin M, Sjoblom P, Lindblom B. Persistent trophoblast after conservative treatment of tubal pregnancy: prediction and detection. *Obstet Gynecol* 1991;77:129.
8. Lundorff P, Thorburm J, Hahlin M, Lindblom B, Kallfelt B. Ad-

hesion formation after laparoscopic surgery in tubal pregnancy: a randomized trial versus laparotomy. *Fertil Steril* 1991;55:911.

9. Peterson HB, Hulka JF, Phillips JM. American Association of Gynecologic Laparoscopists' 1988 membership survey on operative laparoscopy. *J Reprod Med* 1990;35:587.
10. Larsen JF, Pedersen OD, Grgersen E. Ovarian cyst fenestration via the laparoscope. *Acta Obstet Gynecol Scand* 1986;65:539.
11. Levine RC. Pelviscopic survey in women over 40. *J Reprod Med* 1990;35:597.
12. Mage G, Canis M, Manhes H, Pouly JL, Wattiez A, Bruhat MA. Laparoscopic management of adnexal cystic masses. *J Gynecol Surg* 1990;6:71.
13. Maiman M, Seltzer V, Boyce J. Laparoscopic excision of ovarian neoplasms subsequently found to be malignant. *Obstet Gynecol* 1991;77:563.
14. Dembo AJ, Davy M, Stenwig AE, Berle E, Bush RS, Kjorstad K. Prognostic factors in patients with stage I epithelial ovarian cancer. *Obstet Gynecol* 1990;75:263.
15. Adamson GD, Hurd SJ, Pasta DJ, Rodriguez BD. Laparoscopic endometriosis treatment: is it better? *Fertil Steril* 1993;59:35–44.
16. Fayez JA, Collazo LM, Vernon C. Comparison of different modalities of treatment for minimal and mild endometriosis. *Am J Obstet Gynecol* 1988;159:927.
17. Olive DL, Lee KL. Analysis of sequential treatment protocols for endometriosis associated infertility. *Am J Obstet Gynecol* 1986;154:613.
18. Rock JA, Guzick DS, Sengos C, Schweditsch M, Sapp KC, Jones HW Jr. The conservative surgical treatment of endometriosis: evaluation of pregnancy success with respect to the extent of disease as categorized using contemporary classification systems. *Fertil Steril* 1981;35:131.
19. Grant NF. Infertility and endometriosis: comparison of pregnancy outcomes with laparotomy versus laparoscopic techniques. *Am J Obstet Gynecol* 1992;166:1072.
20. Operative Laparoscopy Study Group. Postoperative adhesion development after operative laparoscopy: evaluation at early second-look procedures. *Fertil Steril* 1991;55:700.
21. Reich H, McGlynn F: Laparoscopic treatment of tubo-ovarian and pelvic abscess. *J Reprod Med* 1987;32:747.
22. Reich H, McGlynn F. Laparoscopic treatment of tuboovarian and pelvic abscess. *J Reprod Med* 1987;32(10):747–752.
23. Abdel Gadir A, Mowafi RS, Alnaser HMI, Alrashid AH, Alonezi OM, Shaw RW: Ovarian electrocautery versus human menopausal gonadotropins and pure follicle stimulating hormone therapy in the treatment of patients with polycystic ovarian disease, *Clin Endocrinol* 1990;33:585.
24. Greenblatt E, Casper RF: Endocrine changes after laparoscopic ovarian cautery in polycystic ovarian syndrome. *Am J Obstet Gynecol* 1987;156:279.
25. Dabirashrafi H, Mohamad K, Behjatnia Y, Moghodami-Tabrizi N: Adhesion formation after ovarian electrocauterization on patients with polycystic ovarian syndrome. *Fertil Steril* 1991;55: 1200.
26. Feste JR: Laser laparoscopy: a new modality. *J Reprod Med* 1985;30:413.
27. Tjaden B, Schlaff WD, Kimball A, Rock JA: The efficacy of presacral neurectomy for the relief of midline dysmenorrhea. *Obstet Gynecol* 1990;76:89.

Endoscopic Management of Gynecologic Disease,
edited by G.D. Adamson and D.C. Martin.
Lippincott-Raven Publishers, Philadelphia © 1996.

CHAPTER 6

Operating Room Setup

Joseph S. Sanfilippo and G. David Adamson

With the advent of new surgical techniques, expertise in minimally invasive surgery has truly revolutionized gynecologic surgical care. It is of paramount importance that an operating room team be well versed with respect to communication, preparation, and intraoperative as well as postoperative activities. Preoperatively the patient should be appropriately informed by means of a thorough discussion regarding the risks/benefits of the particular procedure; this hopefully should allay anxiety for the patient as she prepares for surgery. The necessary preparation by the surgical team should provide for an uneventful surgical procedure. Knowledge of instrumentation as well as the ability to troubleshoot on the part of the surgeon, surgical technologist, and circulating nurse is of the utmost importance. This concerted effort should create the circumstance on the part of the surgical team for optimal results with respect to patient care.

CAPABILITIES AND FACILITIES

An operative laparoscopic surgeon must have an objective evaluation of his or her own skill level and experience and be knowledgeable regarding the appropriateness of a proposed surgical procedure for the specific clinical situation. Technical competence is assumed in that operative laparoscopic procedures are almost always more complex and difficult than similar procedures performed via laparotomy.

The most common scenario is that initially a diagnostic laparoscopy is performed with the facilities available for proceeding immediately with operative endoscopic surgery when necessary. Therefore, having a well-coordinated surgical team with evaluated and properly functioning equipment with backup equipment available as needed sets the stage for an efficient surgical procedure.

Appropriate anesthesia conducted by a well-trained anesthesiologist and perhaps anesthetist who is knowledgeable of the specific potential problems intrinsic to endoscopic surgery is another prerequisite for operative laparoscopy (1). Depending on the specific circumstance, a nasogastric tube may be indicated to deflate the stomach and thus avoid injury during placement of the Veress needle and trocars. Monitoring of pulse oximetry, electrocardiogram, and end-tidal CO_2 volume are imperative for patient safety (see the chapter by Collins and Jackson, "Anesthesia in Hysteroscopic and Laparoscopic Infertility Procedures").

Operating Room Setup and Initial Procedures

The operating room setup includes proper positioning of the patient and of operative laparoscopic and video equipment (Fig. 1). The use of Allen's universal stirrups (Fig. 2) facilitates proper patient positioning and avoids neurologic damage (2).

The initial incision is usually made at the umbilicus. A vertical incision within the Langer lines of turgor provides an excellent cosmetic result. A Veress needle is then inserted to create a pneumoperitoneum. Most recently, this needle has been further developed to provide pressure monitoring and facilitate intraperitoneal placement of the needle (3) (Fig. 3). Alternative placement of the Veress needle, especially in obese patients, in large part depends on the planned procedure. Transvaginal (cul-de-sac) placement has been advocated with the patient in the Trendelenburg position, thus permitting creation of a pneumoperitoneum (Fig. 4).

An open laparoscopic approach may be more feasible than direct insertion of a Veress needle or trocar for the

J. S. Sanfilippo: Department of Obstetrics and Gynecology, University of Louisville School of Medicine, Louisville, Kentucky 40292.

G. D. Adamson: Fertility Physicians of Northern California, Palo Alto, California 94301.

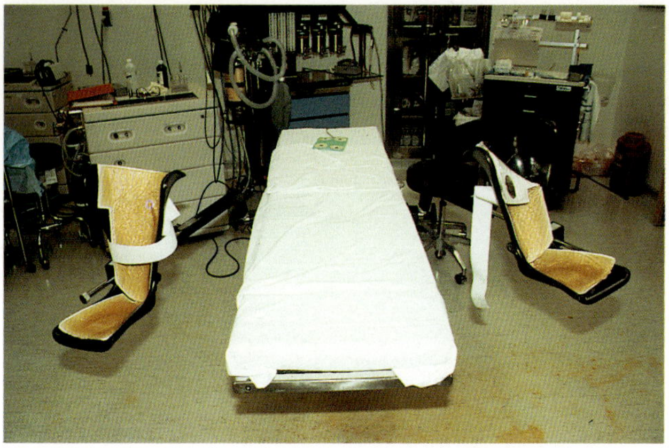

FIG. 1. Patient positioning for operative laparoscopy.

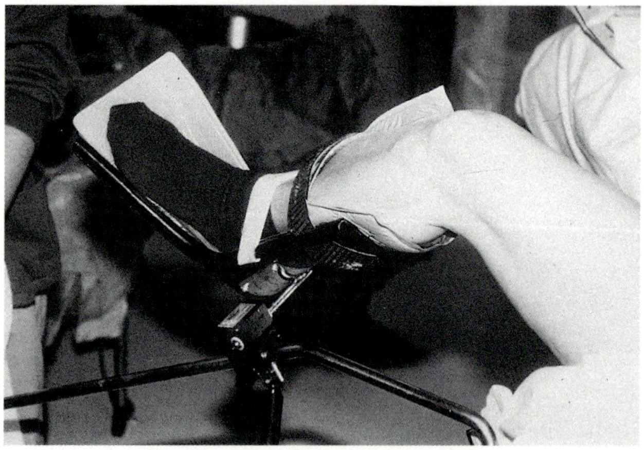

FIG. 2. Allen universal stirrups.

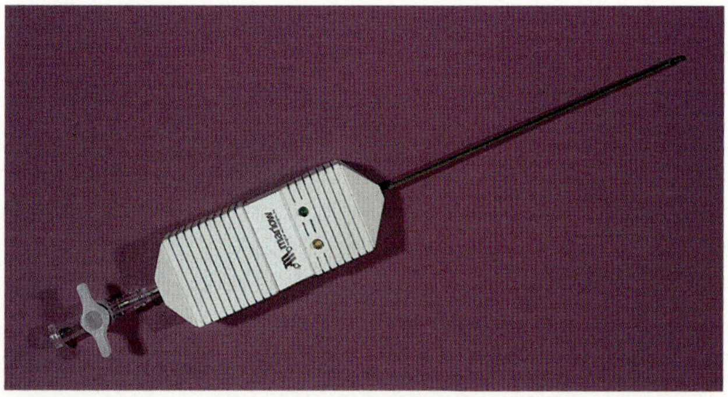

FIG. 3. Marlow pressure needle.

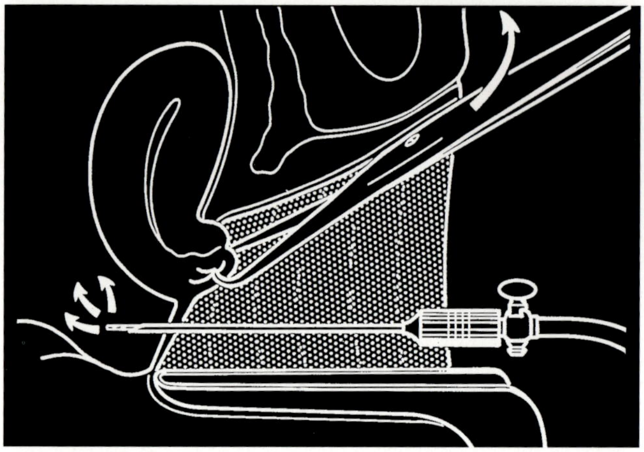

FIG. 4. Cul-de-sac placement of Veress needle for intraabdominal insufflation.

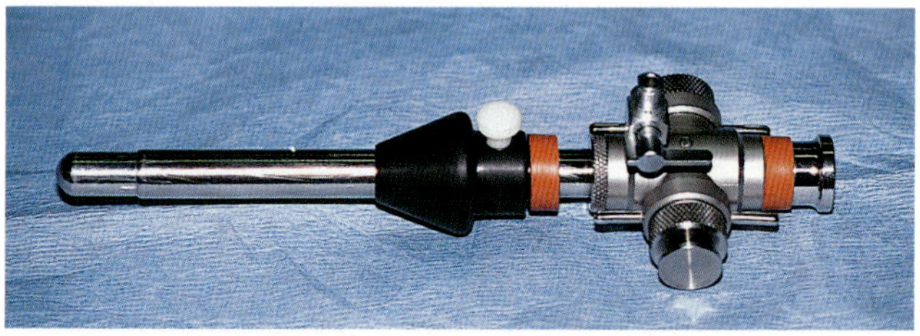

FIG. 5. Hasson cannula for open laparoscopy.

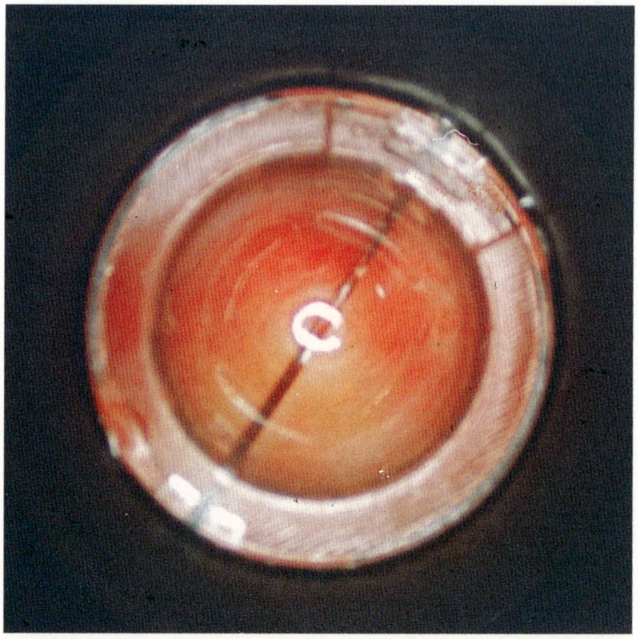

FIG. 6. U.S. Surgical transparent trocar with knife blade.

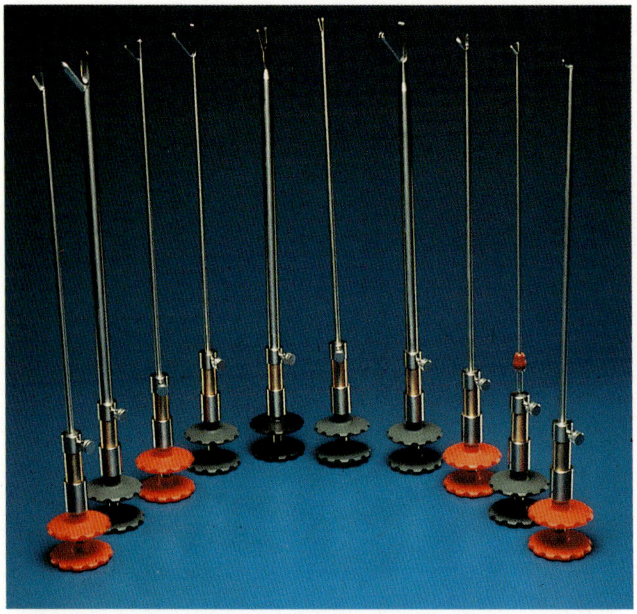

FIG. 7. Instrumentation designed without scissors-type handle. (Courtesy WISAP, Tomball, Texas.)

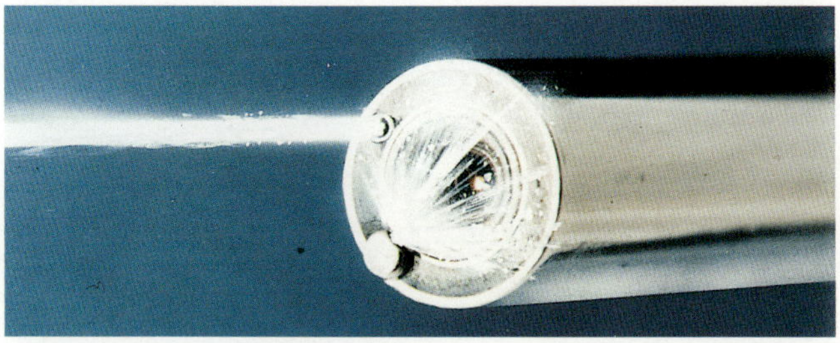

FIG. 8. Laparoscope with irrigation system. (Courtesy Circon/ACMI, Stamford, Connecticut).

TABLE 1. *Basic instrumentation*

Grasping forceps
Laparoscopic scissors
Suction irrigator
Instrumentation associated with electrosurgical systems
Bipolar
Monopolar

patient who has had prior abdominal surgical procedures, especially in the area immediately beneath the incision. Introduction of a Veress needle into the left upper quadrant is an alternative. (A nasogastric tube should first be placed.) Nondisposable and disposable cannulas are designed specifically for open laparoscopy (Fig. 5). Another recent development is a transparent trocar with a knife blade which can be fired multiple times to cut through the abdominal wall under direct vision (Fig. 6). An array of new instrumentation designed without scissors-type handles are available (Fig. 7). Further advancement in laparoscope development includes a model that enables irrigation of the laparoscope lens while the scope is in the abdomen (Fig. 8).

Insufflators

A number of insufflators are available. It is important that the endoscopic surgeon have fundamental knowledge of the mechanics of high-flow insufflators. In general, the operative laparoscopic insufflator delivers insufflation at a rate of 1–6 L/min. Specific gauges indicating intraabdominal pressure as well as the total volume of gas delivered are monitored throughout the surgical procedure. The endpoint of abdominal pressure,

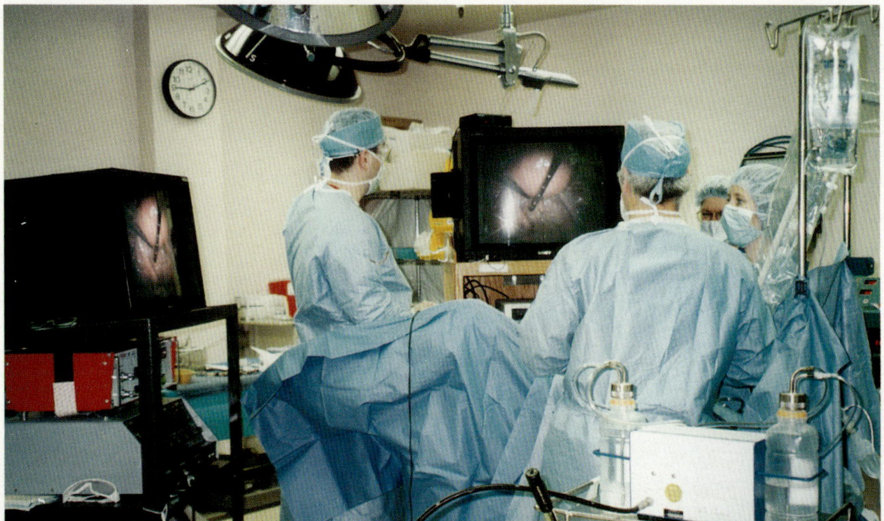

FIG. 9. Video setup with use of separate monitor for surgeon and assistant.

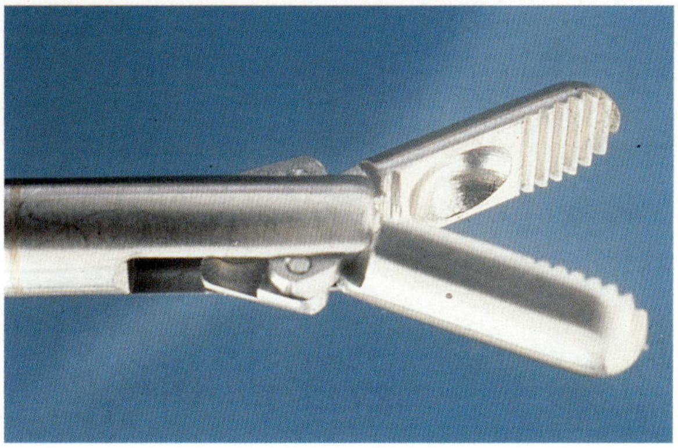
A

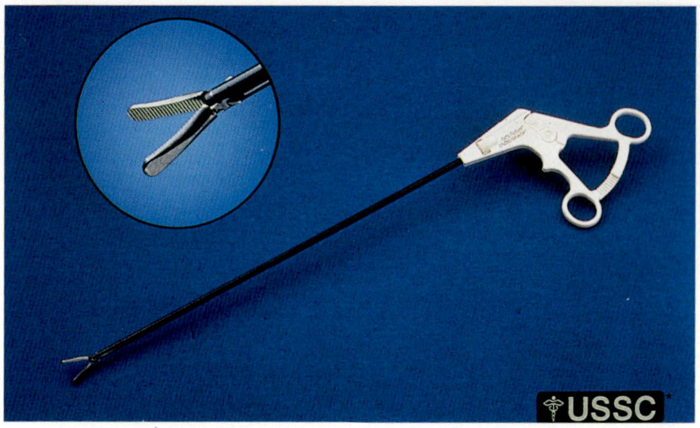

B

FIG. 10. A, B: Forceps.

i.e., 8–14 mm Hg, can be appropriately selected. This setting is of particular importance in prevention of compromise in venous return. Lower pressures should be used in the young adolescent as well as the pediatric patient (e.g., 8 mm Hg). Intraoperative monitoring of oxygen saturation, end-tidal pCO_2, CO_2 partial pressure, along with cardiac status, is mandatory. Use of an esophageal stethoscope facilitates detection of any abnormal murmurs that can be associated with problems, such as CO_2 emboli (characteristic mill wheel murmur). The insufflator should be positioned in such a way that the surgeon can easily read the pressure gauges.

Laparoscopes, Light Sources, Video Equipment

In general, 10-mm laparoscopes are used with a visual angle of 0°. This allows a head-on or more normal perspective for visualization of intraabdominal organs. The endoscope provides low-power magnification in direct proportion to its distance from the object. A video monitor is highly recommended. Ideally, two monitors are positioned for ready access by the surgical team (Fig. 9). The television monitor should be placed at eye level.

An instrument cart is positioned on the side of the table opposite the surgeon. This facilitates access to the electrical devices, insufflator, and suction irrigator apparatus. Ideally a separate unit for the light source, video monitor, and any video recording or photographic equipment is situated as one unit to prevent cluttering and thus provide a more compact placement of equipment (Fig. 9).

Fogging of the laparoscope can be prevented with use of UltraStop (Richard Wolf, Vernon Hills, IL) or similar fluid medium. A number of surgeons use warm water or saline, sometimes kept in a thermos to warm the laparo-

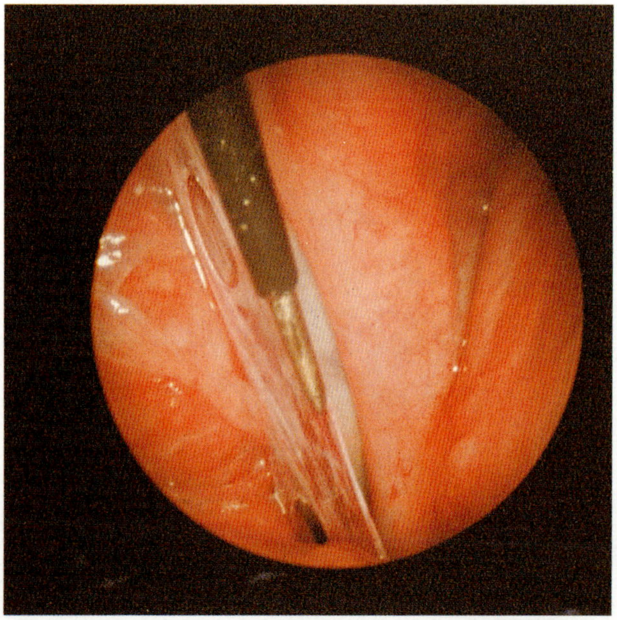

FIG. 11. Unipolar electrode for electrosurgical dissection.

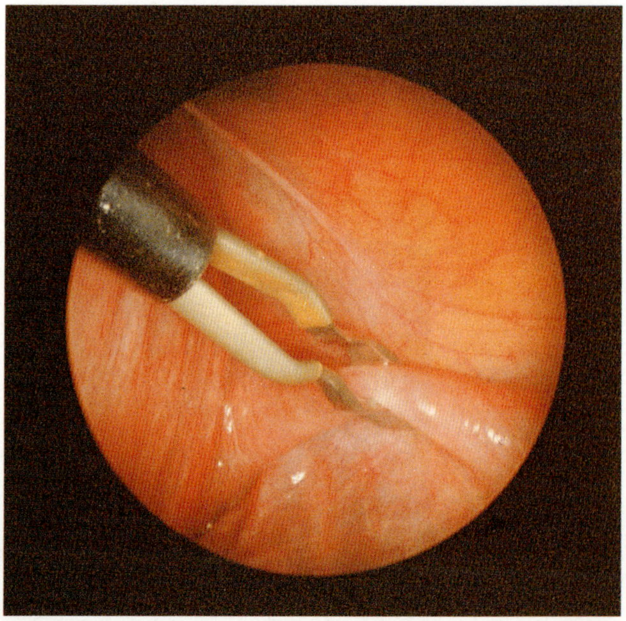

FIG. 12. Bipolar electrode for electrosurgical coagulation.

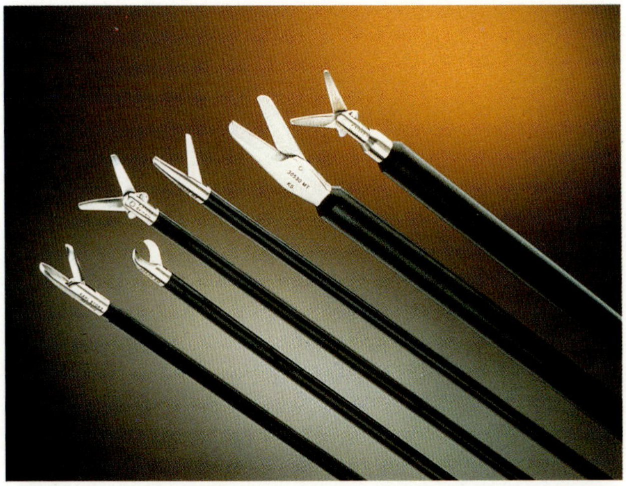

FIG. 13. Scissors (Courtesy Marlow, Willoughby, Ohio.)

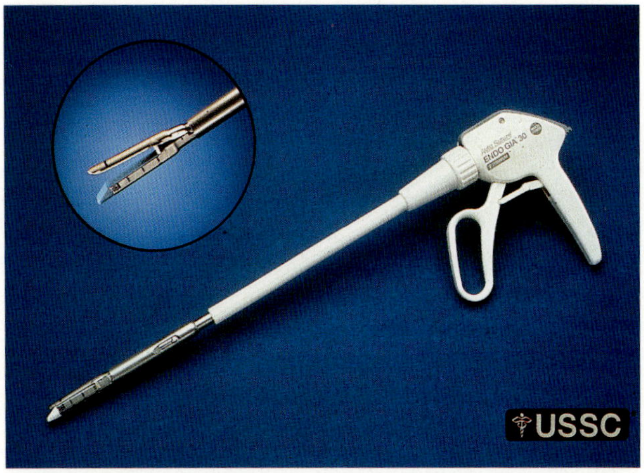

FIG. 15. EndoGIA stapler. (Courtesy Ethicon Endo-Surgery, Cincinnati, Ohio.)

scope to body temperature, thus minimizing lens fogging.

The subject of light sources and photographic equipment is indeed an entity within its own and is discussed in depth elsewhere (see the chapter by Sanfilippo and Leventhal, "Visual Documentation in Endoscopy"). Appropriate methods of visual documentation cannot be overemphasized. This would include documentation in the form of a videotape and/or still photographs for medical documentation and patient education.

Suction Irrigation Systems

A number of systems are available, including the AquaPurator (WISAP, Germany), the Cabot system (Karl Storz Endoscopy, Culver City, CA), and the Nezhat Dorsey equipment (American Hydro-Surgical Instruments, Delray Beach, FL). This instrumentation permits irrigation fluid to be instilled at a pressure of up to 200 mm Hg and also can be used for aspiration of serosanguinous fluid. The irrigation solution usually used is lactated Ringer's, which is ideally warmed to body temperature. These systems also can be used for separation of adhesions or for dissection.

Basic Instrumentation

Appropriate instrumentation, suitable for the planned surgical procedure, should be readily available (Table 1).

Forceps

There are many types of forceps or graspers. They are available in 3-, 5- and 10-mm sizes (Fig. 10A,B). An atraumatic grasping forceps provides little risk of damage to tissue while allowing appropriate traction.

Bipolar coagulation forceps are used for control of bleeding. The instrument can be placed through the op-

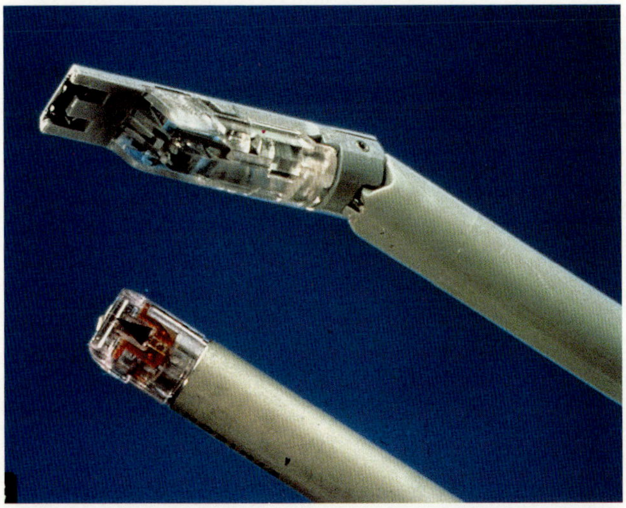

FIG. 14. Hernia stapler with articulating head. (Courtesy United States Surgical Corp., Norwalk, Connecticut.)

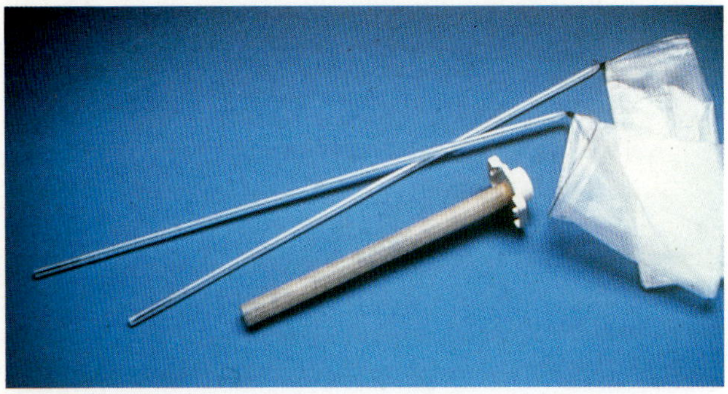

FIG. 16. Endopouch. (Courtesy Ethicon Endo-Surgery, Cincinnati, Ohio.)

erating channel (5 mm) of the laparoscope or through a second puncture site. Instrumentation for electrodissection includes a host of different types and application tips (Figs. 11 and 12).

Scissors

Many types of scissors, ranging in size from 3 to 10 mm, are available (Fig. 13).

Staplers

Staplers are used primarily to achieve hemostasis. Both those with and without an articulated head permit suitable staple placement (Fig. 14). Delivery of rows of staplers with scissors/incising capabilities are available, such as the GIA stapler (Figs. 14 and 15).

Endopouches or Sacs

Endopouches facilitate tissue removal. The device shown in Fig. 16 prevents spillage of tissue contents.

LASERS

The CO_2 laser is the most commonly used laser in laparoscopy (see the chapter by Crowgey and Adamson, "Endoscopic Energy: Laser"). A wide range of suitable models is available. It is important that the laser one chooses has appropriate power with a minimum of 20 W, preferably 40–60 W. It is important that the device have a configuration and a long enough arm that the laser beam can be delivered to the laparoscope without difficulty. General anesthesia is required and endotracheal intubation is essential. Gastric suctioning is recommended. During long laser laparoscopic procedures with the patient in Trendelenburg position, and large volumes of carbon dioxide gas being transferred in and out of the abdominal cavity, the patient should be monitored with state-of-the-art anesthetic equipment. She should be placed in a modified lithotomy position with significant padding around the legs. Ideally, at least every 2 hr the patient's legs should be elevated for several minutes to allow recirculation. Operating room personnel should follow the usual laser safety precautions even though only a diagnostic laparoscopy is being performed.

Equipment for laser laparoscopy includes a laser laparoscope (see Fig. 17). These usually are ~11 mm in size and can be purchased from different vendors. The laparoscope is attached to the laser via a coupler. Direct couplers are available for most instruments and are much easier to use than the joystick-type couplers. Newer waveguides allow delivery of the laser energy directly to the tissue and have certain advantages; these

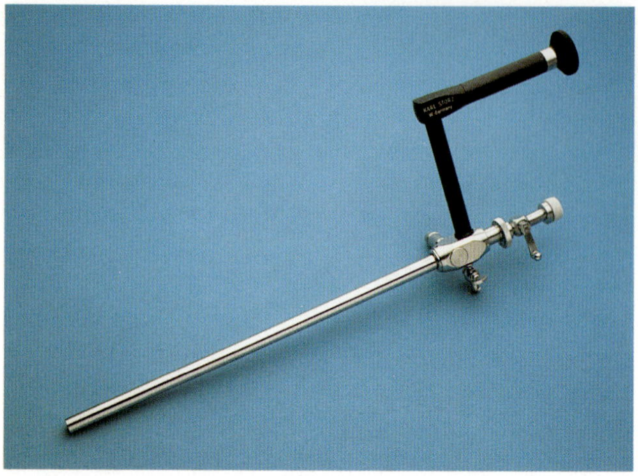

FIG. 17. Stortz right-angle operative laparascope, which can be used with or without coupling to laser.

may include high power density, variable spot size, and ability to compensate for beam misalignment. A full array of operative laparoscopic equipment is necessary and should be readily available in advance of the surgery; this includes bipolar and unipolar electrosurgery equipment. A high stand containing all of the necessary equipment should be available on the medial aspect of the patient's right leg beside the scrub tech. The high stand should contain all of the operating instruments, including aspirators, irrigators, backstops, scissors, grasping instruments, and coagulator. The irrigation and aspiration equipment with appropriate intravenous adapters should also be on the high stand, as should four-by-four sponges and Q-tips for cleaning of the scope and lenses.

Once the decision is made to proceed to laser laparoscopy, the surgeon can introduce the laser laparoscopic trocar subumbilically and can make a third incision in the left lower quadrant for the vacuum aspirator and irrigator. After the arm of the laser has been draped, the laser laparoscope can be attached to the laser. The gas line is attached at the upper end of the laser laparoscope (not to the sheath of the trocar) and the helium-neon (HeNe) beam is checked for alignment against a moistened tongue blade with moistened sponge behind it. The laser beam should be checked by being fired to determine the spot size as well as the beam alignment. Laparoscopy is generally performed from the left side of the table, with the laparoscope held in the right hand and with the left hand used for manipulation of the lower abdominal instruments.

The advent of advanced video technology has allowed small cameras to be attached to the laser laparoscope. This permits more challenging surgical procedures to be completed more easily and comfortably and enhances interest and assistance from the surgical team. The cameras require powerful light sources, the most recent of which is the xenon light source. The operating room setup usually involves the surgeon's standing at the left side of the patient viewing the video over the patient. Both of the patient's arms should be at her side. The nurse stands between the patient's legs with the patient in a modified lithotomy position. In this way the nurse can manipulate the cervical uterine cannula as necessary. A pair of weights is placed on the cannula to hold the uterus in position. A vacuum aspirator with plunger or some other type of apparatus to control evacuation of the plume is necessary. This can be attached either to the middle or left lower quadrant instrument site. Some surgeons prefer to aspirate the plume when their foot is on the laser pedal whereas others prefer to have the nurse perform this function. Automatic gas recirculators (Sun Medical, Arlington, TX) can be very useful in improving plume evacuation (Fig. 18). A high-flow insufflator is necessary to produce a flow of 6–10 L of CO_2/min. It is imperative that one of the operating room assistants monitor the CO_2 pressures at times and keep pressures below 20 mm Hg. Recent high-flow machines have automatic popoff valves. A wide array of lower quadrant instruments can be utilized. Maximum instrumentalization is achieved by use of three 5-mm puncture sites, so that all of the instruments can be transferred to alternative sites. When extensive operative laparoscopy is performed, a single 10-mm site also is required.

Surgical Principles

Careful systematic initial evaluation of the pelvis, as with diagnostic laparoscopy, is mandatory prior to proceeding with operative laparoscopy. This enables the surgeon to diagnose any pathology in the pelvis as well as the upper abdominal area. The type and degree of disease can then be determined and a decision made on optimal treatment approach.

Having an adequate number of puncture sites for instruments is critical to the success of the endoscopic procedure. Several principles of operative laparoscopy are important to remember to assist in the efficacious use of equipment. Visualization of the pelvis under direct vision without the camera may facilitate diagnosis of subtle disease such as the various types of endometriotic lesions.

The laparoscope magnifies tissue, so that when this instrument is about 1 cm from the tissue the magnification is approximately six times, at 2 cm four times, 3 cm two times, and 4 cm no magnification. At a distance greater than 4 cm demagnification or the appearance of a smaller structure appears through the laparoscope. The effects of laser or electrical energy on tissue must be understood by all operative laparoscopists.

Laser safety is also important. This involves prevention of fires, avoidance of inhalation of the plume, electrical injury or application of the laser beam in unintended areas, and numerous other laser safety standards. These standards should be understood and followed at all times.

SURGICAL TECHNIQUES

Surgical techniques utilized at operative laparoscopy attempt to maximize exposure, minimize trauma, and produce the desired result in minimal time. Hemostasis must be carefully maintained at all times and the appropriate instruments freely used in any port as necessary. Irrigation and aspiration can significantly assist in good visualization and in the maintenance of a clean surgical field.

A most important principle in operative laparoscopy is that of control of the surgical field. This requires good visualization of all pelvic organs, awareness of anatomic structures and normal tissue, as well as knowledge of the location and extent of diseased tissue. For increased risk procedures, it is necessary to evaluate whether the benefit of the procedure outweighs the risk. For some surgeons this may occur relatively frequently. Alternative methods of treatment should be carried out in such situations. It is important to recognize that at operative laparoscopy the surgeon is working without binocular vision but with a video monitor/camera placed at a distance from the surgical field. In addition, instruments rather than hands are being used for grasping tissue. Laser energy effects have to be appreciated in advance on a theoretical basis

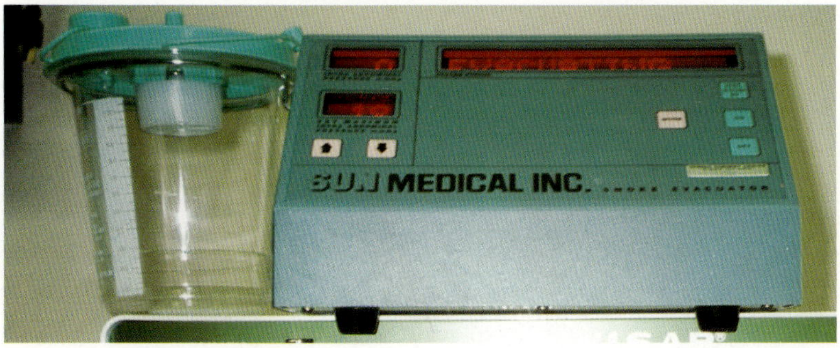

FIG. 18. Gas recirculator. (Courtesy of Sun Medical Inc.)

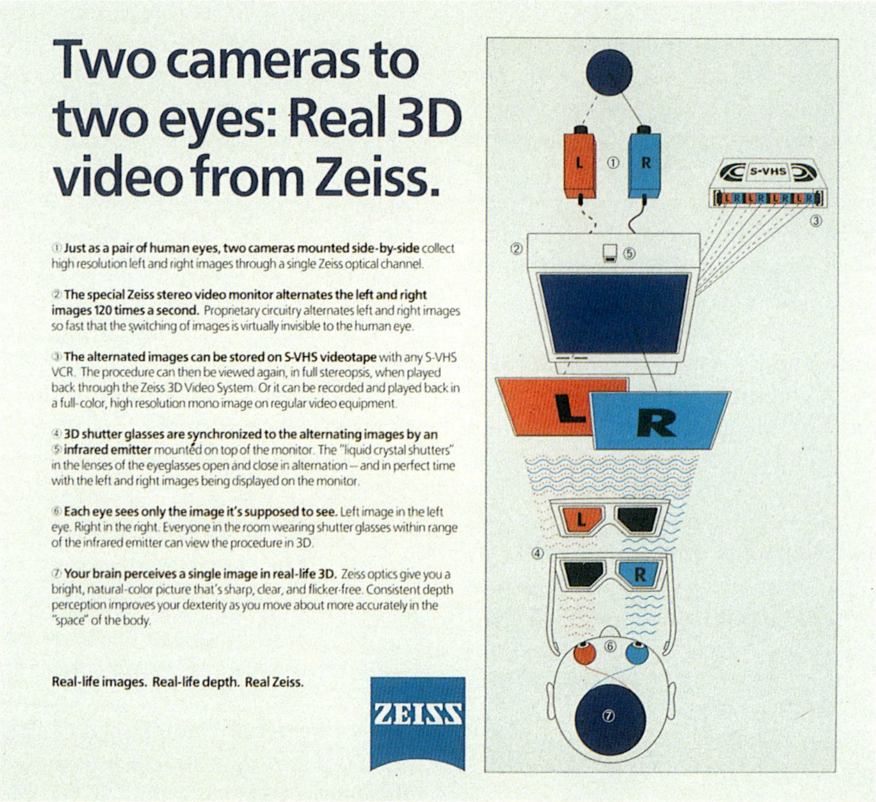

A

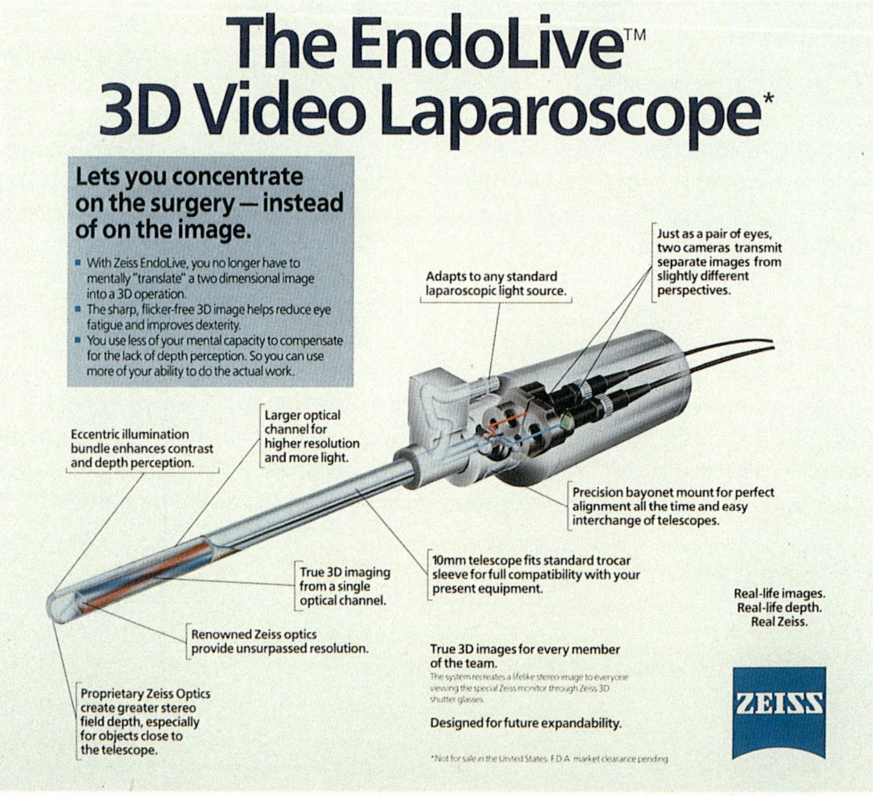

B

FIG. 19. A, B: Three-dimensional laparoscopic equipment. (Courtesy Zeiss, Thornwood, NY.)

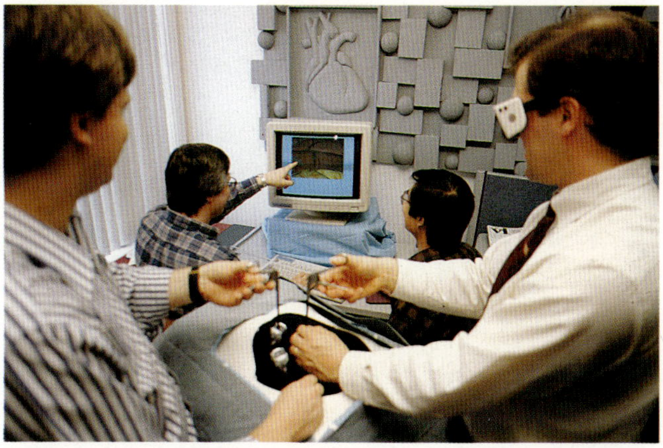

FIG. 20. Virtual Clinic Surgical Skills Simulator. (Courtesy Cine-Med, Woodbury, Connecticut.)

and are not directly related to usual surgical senses. Therefore, the apparent control of the surgical field is less than one has at laparotomy, although the actual degree of control can be significantly maximized with surgical experience.

FUTURE PERSPECTIVES

A number of technical advances are occurring rapidly in the field of minimally invasive surgery. These include use of three-dimensional laparoscopic equipment (Fig. 19A,B) as well as progress in teaching endoscopic surgery with equipment such as Virtual Reality (Fig. 20). Clearly an increasing array of gynecologic surgical procedures are rapidly becoming amenable to an endoscopic approach.

HIGHLIGHTS

Operative laparoscopy can only be performed with skill and safety when an adequate operative room setup is available and equipment is used properly. Much of the equipment is complex and sophisticated, and it is constantly being improved. Surgeons are responsible for assisting in acquisition of equipment, understanding its use, and educating their staff about operating room setup.

REFERENCES

1. Matthew K. Pelviscopy, an endoscopic alternative to laparotomy. *AORN J* 1988;47:1218–1229.
2. Hershlag A, Loy RA, Lavy G, DeCherney AH. Femoral neuropathy after laparoscopy. A case report. *J. Reprod Med* 1990;35(5):575.
3. Janicki T. The new sensor-equipped Veress needle. *J Am Assoc Gynecol Laparosc* 1994;1(2):154.

Endoscopic Management of Gynecologic Disease,
edited by G.D. Adamson and D.C. Martin.
Lippincott-Raven Publishers, Philadelphia © 1996.

CHAPTER 7

Preoperative Patient Preparation

Carmelo S. Sgarlata

In the past 10 years, the rapid advancement and improvement of endoscopic equipment has allowed the surgeon to perform a wide variety of procedures previously considered impossible without laparotomy. With the change from diagnostic to therapeutic procedures, the preoperative patient evaluation and preparation differs significantly from prior routines. It is critical to consider both the physical aspects of patient preparation and the patient's psychological concerns and expectations. As always, the clinical indications for surgery and the preliminary investigations prior to operative procedures allow the best possible preparation and outcome for the patient. A flow chart diagramming considerations and steps from presenting complaints to surgery is given in Fig. 1.

The prospective patient must be completely familiarized with the proposed procedures and their respective risks and side effects, complications, potential benefits and alternatives, expense, and the chance of successful treatment.

CLINICAL INVESTIGATION

Operative laparoscopy is used primarily for the confirmation of pathologic conditions and their surgical repair and/or extirpation. Patient evaluation should include a complete medical and gynecologic history, a comprehensive physical exam, and appropriate diagnostic studies to further define the condition for which surgery is proposed. The preliminary or initial consultation should allow enough time for a thorough review of prior records, detailed descriptions of the patient's symptoms, and an appropriate physical examination. The objectives of this visit are twofold: to provide a clear and concise outline of the proposed surgical procedures and to formulate any preoperative testing or preparation necessary for a successful outcome.

Depending on the clinical situation, preliminary imaging studies may be indicated. These would include ultrasound; magnetic resonance imaging (MRI); or conventional radiographic studies, such as hysterosalpingogram, kidney-ureter-bladder (KUB), intravenous pyelogram (IVP), or barium enema. In patients with bowel symptoms or a fixed cul-de-sac, sigmoidoscopy should be strongly considered as part of the presurgical evaluation. Consultations with gastroenterologists or urologists are occasionally indicated.

With the development of endovaginal ultrasound, precise and detailed imaging in the pelvis is now available. Endovaginal ultrasound is most helpful in the evaluation of pelvic masses contained within the true pelvis or of <10 cm in size. Clinically, ultrasound can determine the size and location of pelvic structures and/or masses, determine the internal consistency (whether they are cystic, solid, papillary, or calcified), and detect associated findings such as ascites. The endovaginal approach may be especially valuable in the identification and localization of early pregnancy. It is advisable that any patient undergoing pelviscopy—particularly those patients with pelvic mass—undergo an ultrasonographic study prior to surgery. In addition, at the time of the patient's preoperative visit, an endovaginal study can be easily and quickly performed to provide valuable information for both the surgeon and the patient. The use of transvaginal color Doppler flow studies may be useful in postmenopausal patients or in those having complex adnexal masses, as the tests show significant neovascularization. Also, preliminary data indicate that Doppler flow studies are helpful in the early detection and localization of tubal ectopic pregnancy (1).

C. S. Sgarlata: Private Practice, San Jose, California 95124; and Stanford University School of Medicine, Stanford, California 94305.

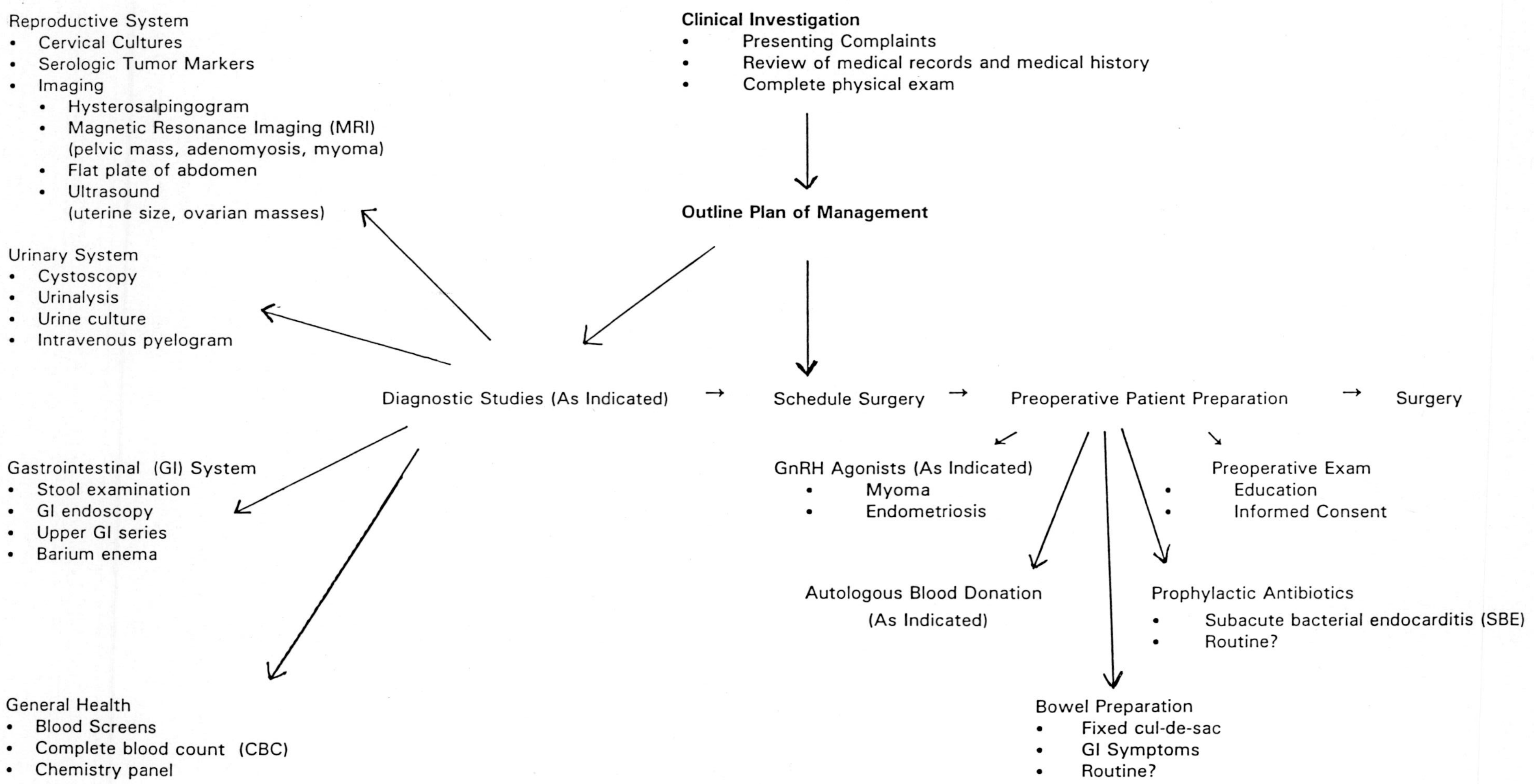

FIG. 1. Flow chart of the surgeon's considerations and the steps that should be taken from the time of presenting complaints to that of surgery.

Preoperatively, the patient should undergo screening laboratory studies including complete blood count (CBC) and chemistry panel. For patients with a complex adnexal mass, the surgeon should consider obtaining a CA-125 assay.

Although the available circulating serologic tumor markers are insufficiently sensitive for routine screening, they may be helpful in the assessment of a patient with a pelvic mass. Whereas markers for germ cell tumors are highly specific, the markers for epithelial tumors are limited. Approximately 80% of patients with epithelial ovarian carcinoma exhibit elevated levels of CA-125. A number of benign pelvic conditions, including endometriosis, pelvic inflammatory disease, or uterine leiomyoma, may cause elevated levels in the perimenopausal patient. Because of the limitations of the specificity and sensitivity of the CA-125 assay, other preoperative tests should be obtained prior to surgery to further evaluate a complex pelvic mass. Other serologic markers, such as α-fetoprotein, human chorionic gonadotropin (hCG), or carcinoembryonic antigen (CEA), may be useful in selected cases. In patients with hirsutism and/or rapid onset virilization or in the postmenopausal patient with marked hyperestrogenism, appropriate endocrine studies should be obtained.

PATIENT PREPARATION

The patient must be informed that operative laparoscopy may require three to five lower abdominal (mini) incisions for the introduction of appropriate instruments. The possibility of operative laparoscopy followed by immediate laparotomy should be fully discussed with the patient. Informing the patient about and preparing her for the possibility of laparotomy, including obtaining the proper informed consent, increases the patient's understanding of the limitations and risks associated with operative laparoscopy. It also allows the surgeon to proceed immediately to laparotomy if it is clinically indicated.

In our offices, all patients receive a comprehensive preoperative information packet when surgery is contemplated. In this packet we include written pre- and postoperative instructions, including diet and bowel preparation, information concerning specific types of surgery proposed, and a copy of the written consents that the patient signs prior to any surgical procedure. In patients undergoing either sterilization or possible hysterectomy, appropriate consents must be obtained.

In patients with leiomyoma or with advanced stages of endometriosis, especially if associated with endometriomas, preoperative medical suppressive therapy may be indicated. Currently, the gonadotropin-releasing hormone (GnRH) agonists, danazol and, less frequently, progestins, have been used to inhibit ovulation and suppress menses. Treatment typically is administered for 3–6 months prior to the planned procedure. In cases where myomas are present, the uterus and myomas may shrink by 30–50% within 3 months, thereby reducing the vascularity of the uterus and potentially decreasing intraoperative blood loss. Reduction in uterine and myoma size may also reduce operative time and aid in the successful laparoscopic removal of the myomas. In advanced endometriosis, preoperative suppressive therapy may reduce the vascularity of the pelvis and stabilize the size of the endometriomas. Suppressive therapy also controls uterine bleeding, allowing restoration of the normal hematocrit in the anemic patient. Once the anemia is resolved, the patient may consider autologous blood donation prior to surgery.

In California, it is required that all patients undergoing elective surgery be informed of the potential risks associated with blood transfusion at the time of surgery and of alternatives, including autologous and/or directed blood donation. This information should be provided to the patient several weeks in advance of the proposed surgical procedure so that the patient may make an informed decision and decide whether she would choose to donate autologous blood or have directed blood available.

PREOPERATIVE EVALUATION

Within 7–10 days of surgery, the patient should be seen for a preoperative review, examination, and appropriate laboratory testing as indicated. All patients should have recent negative cultures for *Chlamydia* and gonorrhea, a current Pap smear, and CBC. Any patient who has an ongoing medical condition or who is taking prescription medications should obtain clearance from her primary care physician as indicated. This consultation ensures that no recent medical problems or issues have occurred since the patient's last office visit. In addition, this visit also allows review of any consultations or laboratory studies performed as part of the patient's preoperative evaluation and gives the patient the opportunity to ask any questions immediately prior to her surgery.

A preoperative bowel preparation should be obtained for all patients undergoing endoscopic procedures. Community standards and the protocols used by local general surgeons/colorectal surgeons may be instrumental as guidelines to determine which are the best preparations. For diagnostic-only procedures, a cleansing enema or oral Dulcolax (Ciba Geigy, Woodbridge, NJ) given the evening before or on the morning of surgery is sufficient. In any patient for whom operative procedures are contemplated, we use a mechanical bowel preparation in addition to a liquid diet beginning 2 days prior to surgery. On the day prior to surgery, we administer 4 L of Colyte (Reed and Carnrick, A Division of Block Drug Company, Jersey City, NJ) or similar preparation. A formal 3-day bowel preparation is indicated for those patients with known bowel involvement or previous bowel surgery. In addition, a general surgeon or colorectal surgeon should see the patient in consultation and should be available to assist at the time of operative laparoscopy if clinically indicated either by examination or by sigmoidoscopy.

Prophylactic antibiotics may be administered, especially in cases involving extensive dissection or colpotomy. Patients with known mitral valve prolapse or valvular heart disease should receive systemic bacterial endocarditis (SBE) prophylaxis, as indicated in the American Heart Association Guidelines.

HIGHLIGHTS

With the recent advances in operative laparoscopy, nearly all gynecologic surgery performed abdominally can be performed through the laparoscope. With the recent interest in laparoscopic-assisted vaginal hysterectomy, an increasing number of patients undergo laparoscopic surgery followed by vaginal hysterectomy, further reducing the likelihood of laparotomy. With this rapid advent in operative laparoscopy, appropriate patient evaluation and preparation is more critical to successful outcome than ever.

REFERENCE

1. Jurkovic D, Bourne TH, Jauniaux E, Campbell S, Collins WP. Transvaginal color Doppler study of blood flow in ectopic pregnancies. *Fertil Steril* 1992;57:68–73.

PART III

Surgical Technique: Laparoscopy

Endoscopic Management of Gynecologic Disease,
edited by G.D. Adamson and D.C. Martin.
Lippincott-Raven Publishers, Philadelphia © 1996.

CHAPTER 8

Laparoscopy

Anthony A. Luciano and Deborah A. Metzger

Since the first recorded optical inspection of the abdominal cavity by culdotomy incision in 1901 (1), the concept of visualization of the pelvic cavity for both diagnosis and operative procedures has expanded and, over the past decade, endoscopic surgery has practically exploded. The modern era of laparoscopic technique began in 1954 when Palmer (2) reported 250 patients in whom gynecologic celioscopy was performed without a serious accident. His procedure included the production of a pneumoperitoneum at a rate of 300–500 cm^3 of gas per minute, and he warned that the intraabdominal pressure should not exceed 25 mm Hg. He readily recognized that laparoscopy had advantages over culdoscopy because the former was associated with lower rates of infection and it provided better visualization and access to the pelvic organs and cul-de-sac.

Laparoscopy creates a picture window in the abdomen, through which the intraperitoneal organs can be closely inspected. It provides a far better view than what is possible through an incision a few centimeters long and stuffed with instruments, sponges, and lap sheets. The basic principles of laparoscopy today do not differ significantly from those described by Palmer in 1954 (2). Adequate pneumoperitoneum is essential to introduce the instruments safely and to visualize the abdomen. What has changed significantly over the past 40 years is the sophistication of the instruments and the complexity of the procedures that can be performed.

A. A. Luciano: Department of Obstetrics and Gynecology, University of Connecticut School of Medicine, Farmington, Connecticut 06030; and Center for Fertility and Reproductive Endocrinology, New Britain General Hospital, New Britain, Connecticut 06050.

D. A. Metzger: Department of Obstetrics and Gynecology, University of Connecticut Health Center, Farmington, Connecticut 06030.

PATIENT POSITIONING AND PREPARATION

Preoperatively, the patient is appropriately informed by the surgeon and the anesthesiologist of the potential therapeutic effects of the contemplated endoscopic procedure, the potential complications associated with the surgery and anesthesia, and the therapeutic alternatives—both surgical and medical—for her condition. A mini-mons preparation is performed prior to surgery by the operating room team or by the patient at home the night before. If extensive cul-de-sac dissection is anticipated, the bowel should be prepared using liquid diet, enemas, or hyperosmolar fluids as appropriate. The bowel preparation that we frequently use involves fleet phosphosoda 45 ml orally on the night before surgery, metroniadizole (Flagyl) 1.0 mg BID on the day before surgery, and a fleet enema on the morning of surgery. Cefoxitin sodium MSD (Mefoxin) 2.0 mg intravenously is administered on call to the operating room.

The anesthesia team, along with the circulating nurses, help coordinate patient transfer onto the operating table. The table must be of a design that can provide steep Trendelenburg positioning. After the induction of anesthesia and placement of the endotracheal tube, the patient's legs are placed in padded stirrups and positioned in such a way as to provide good support and normal anatomic position. Particular attention is paid to padding in the vicinity of the peroneal nerve. No joint in the legs is extended over 60° thus avoiding nerve compression. The patient's sacrum must rest on the table to avoid compression of the vertebral spine, and the buttocks must protrude a few centimeters off the table to permit uterine manipulation. The arms of the patient may be placed at her side, padded with foam troughs, and secured by a sheet, thus allowing the surgeon and the surgical assistants to stand adjacent to the patient unencumbered. Alternatively, one or both arms can be secured on arm boards, which give the anesthesiology team access

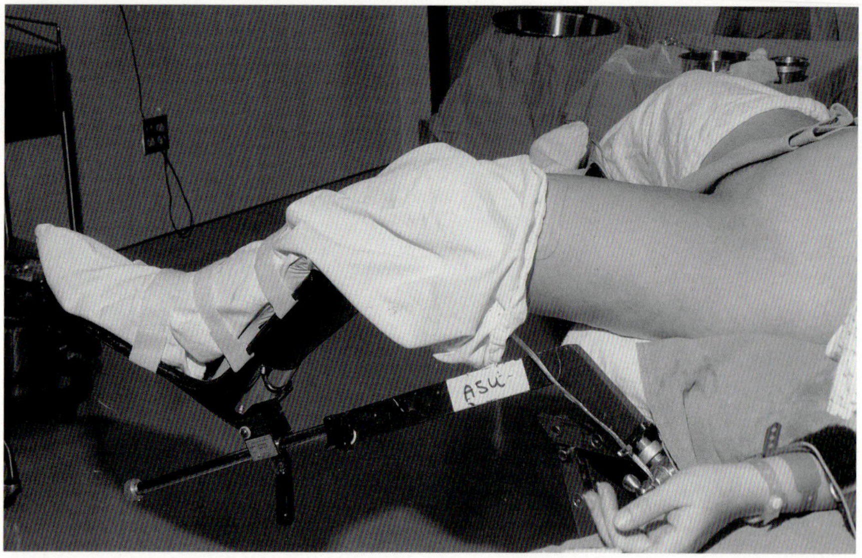

FIG. 1. Positioning of patient for operative laparoscopy. The patient is in a dorsolithotomy position but the thighs are not flexed so that the suprapubic trocars can be properly maneuvered.

to veins and other monitors without compromising the ability of the surgeon to access the abdomen, as shown in Fig. 1.

Once the patient is positioned, a circulating nurse or assistant prepares the patient's abdomen, perineum, and vagina with Betadine or other suitable bactericidal solution and places a Foley catheter to empty the bladder and to monitor urine output during the surgical procedure. The patient then is draped with either reuseable cloth or disposable drapes, exposing only the lower abdomen and the perineum. After pelvic examination, a uterine manipulator is applied to the cervix to mobilize the uterus and for chromopertubation through an injection port.

For better definition of the tissue planes of the cul-de-sac, rectal and/or vaginal probes may be used to manipulate and separate these structures, as shown in Fig. 2. We use ring forceps in the vaginal fornix and push posteriorly to outline the pouch of Douglas or anteriorly to identify the vesicouterine space. Similarly, ring forceps may be inserted into the anus as a rectal probe to outline the rectum and sigmoid colon and to separate the rectum from the uterosacral ligaments and lower posterior uterine segment. The Hume uterine manipulator or a large curette may be placed at the fundus of the uterus to stretch out the cul-de-sac and identify the tissue planes between the rectosigmoid and posterior uterus.

PLACEMENT OF THE VERESS NEEDLE

The purpose of the Veress needle is to establish the pneumoperitoneum, which is a critical step for a successful laparoscopic procedure. The needle consists of a

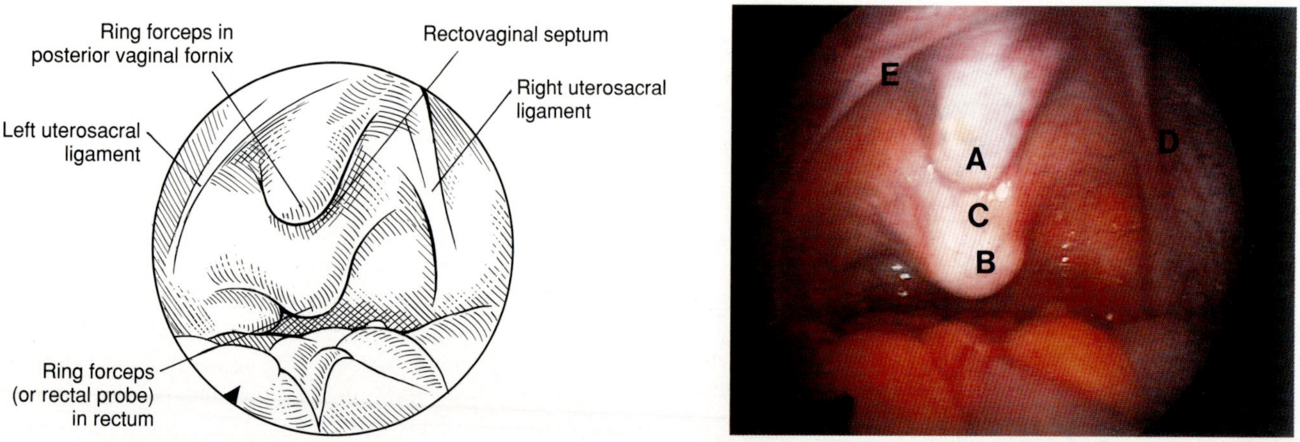

FIG. 2. Use of rectovaginal probes. Ring forceps are placed in the posterior fornix (**A**) and in the rectum (**B**) to define their location and the rectovaginal septum (**C**). The right and left uterosacral ligaments (**D** and **E**) define the boundaries of the posterior cul-de-sac.

blunt-tipped, spring-loaded inner stylet and a sharp outer needle. As pressure is applied to the needle as it passes through the abdominal layers, the stylet retracts to allow penetration. Once the peritoneum is entered, the lack of tissue resistance allows the blunt stylet to protrude, preventing perforation of abdominal structures. A lateral hole on the blunt stylet allows gas to be delivered intraabdominally. Veress needles are available in both disposable and reusable systems, both of which have advantages and disadvantages.

The umbilicus provides the best location for insertion of the Veress needle and the primary trocar. At the level of the umbilicus, the skin of the anterior wall is attached to the fascial layer and anterior parietal peritoneum without any intervening subcutaneous fat or muscle. Therefore, the intraumbilical approach offers the shortest distance between the skin and the peritoneal cavity and can be successfully used even in very obese patients. A cutaneous (not through-and-through) incision is made prior to needle insertion for easier access. The incision should be superficial enough to avoid the deeper rectus muscle layers. Most surgeons make the incision large enough to accommodate the primary trocar, which is inserted after the pneumoperitoneum is established. Either a transverse or vertical incision may be made in the umbilicus. However, patients prefer the vertical incision deep in the umbilicus since it provides the best cosmetic result (3). An Allis clamp can be used to grasp the base of the umbilicus and evert it to incise it more easily and to raise it away from the abdominal structures beneath, as shown in Fig. 3A. These instruments can remain in place to allow application of countertraction while the Veress needle is inserted, as shown in Fig. 3B. It is important to note that when the Veress needle is received by the surgeon from the scrub nurse, it is inspected for proper alignment and checked to make sure that its outer sheath is screwed snugly against the hub so that the cannula aperture is completely visible. The needle should be examined for sharpness and the tip of the inner sleeve should be intact. The integrity of its spring action and unimpeded gas flow must be ascertained before it is introduced into the abdomen.

It is important that the angle of insertion be approximately 45° from the vertical or surface of the skin. It is also imperative that the patient be in a completely horizontal position since premature Trendelenburg positioning may alter the usual landmarks and allow the bowel to move out of the pelvis to a location closer to the peritoneal site of needle penetration. Palpation of the abdominal aorta and the sacral promontory aids in determining the angle of insertion for the needle and later for the trocar. The Veress needle should be grasped by the hub and directed to the hollow of the sacrum. Countertraction should be applied by grasping the skin and fat of the lower abdomen or by pulling on the Allis clamp holding the base of the umbilicus (Fig. 3). In very obese patients, a more vertical initial orientation of the needle may be necessary in order to enter the peritoneal cavity

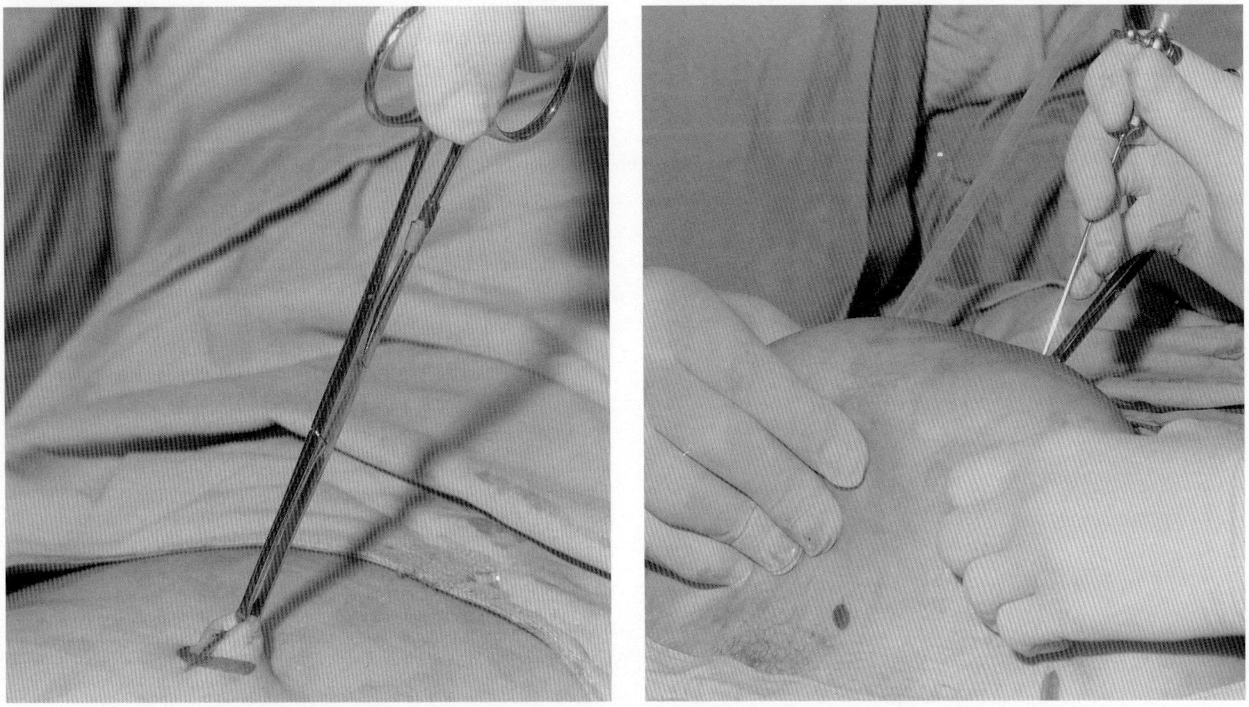

A B

FIG. 3. Intraumbilical placement of Veress needle. The base of the umbilicus is grasped and pulled upward to evert and expose it for either a vertical or horizontal incision (**A**). The Veress needle is grasped by the hub and directed toward the hollow of the sacrum (**B**).

(4,5). Once the peritoneum is traversed, however, the needle should be positioned at a 45° angle. When placing a Veress needle in very thin individuals, the vital structures i.e., major vessels and intestines, are much closer to the abdominal wall thus leaving much less margin for error.

VERIFICATION OF INTRAPERITONEAL PLACEMENT OF THE VERESS NEEDLE

Failure to achieve and maintain a suitable pneumoperitoneum is the most common source of procedural failure. It results in an inordinate number of complications. Most laparoscopic injuries occur at the time of needle insertion for establishing a pneumoperitoneum. Correct placement of the Veress needle can be verified by various means, including the hanging-drop technique whereby a drop of saline is placed on the Veress needle after it is inserted into the abdominal wall. Lifting the abdominal wall establishes negative pressure within the abdomen that sucks the drop of fluid into the Veress needle. Lack of this sign indicates improper placement of the Veress needle. Alternatively, a 10-cm^3 syringe with 5 cm^3 of normal saline is attached to the Veress needle and aspiration is performed to verify that there are no gas bubbles, bowel contents, or blood (Fig. 4). The saline is then injected into the peritoneal cavity, with particular attention paid to the presence of resistance. If placement of the Veress needle is correct, the injected normal saline cannot be reaspirated because it is dispersed intraperitoneally. If placed within a small space, i.e., adhesions or preperitoneal space, it forms a sequestered fluid that can be recovered by applying negative pressure with the syringe. If the needle has been placed intravascularly, blood is aspirated; if the needle is placed within the intestine, intestinal fluid or fecal material is recovered; if the needle is in the bladder, urine is obtained. Likewise, if the needle is within adhesions, fluid is aspirated. The several methods of determining proper placement of the Veress needle are summarized in Table 1.

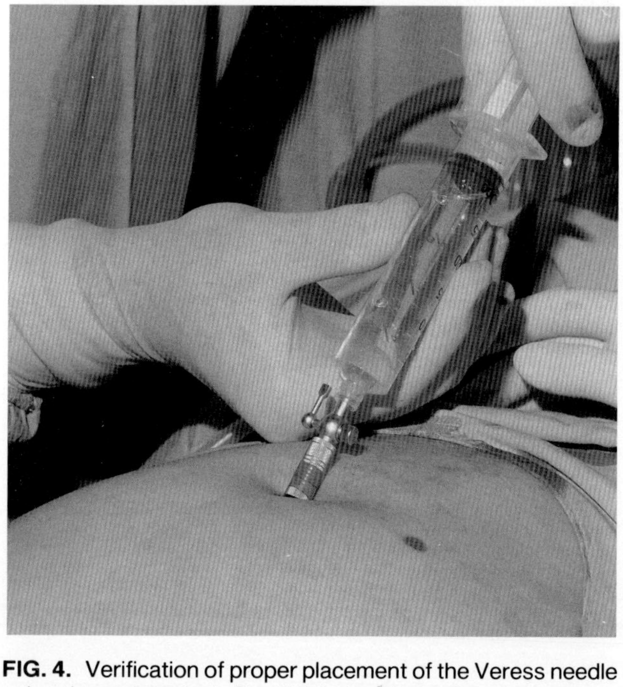

FIG. 4. Verification of proper placement of the Veress needle using the syringe test. See Table 1 and text for other options and narrative description.

TABLE 1. *Tests to confirm the proper position of the Veress needle*

Hanging drop test
Injection and aspiration of fluid through the Veress needle
An unimpeded arc of rotation of the needle to detect anterior abdominal wall adhesions
Loss of liver dullness early in insufflation
Sound of air entering Veress needle with elevation of the abdominal wall (29)
Free flow of gas through the Veress needle
Observation of the fluctuation of pressure gauge needle with inspiratory and expiratory diaphragmatic motions

None of these tests is entirely adequate except for the saline instillation-aspiration method, and each method has shortcomings. A single drop of saline placed on the distal end of the needle can be aspirated by the negative pressure created by the expansion of any space, including preperitoneal space. A low initial insufflation pressure can be obtained if the tip of the Veress needle is located in any distensible organ, such as the bowel or bladder. Tympany can be obtained by percussing any gas-filled chamber including subcutaneous emphysema or a distended stomach. The loss of liver dullness on percussion is a late sign elicited after about 500 cm^3 of gas has been administered via insufflation. An overdistended stomach can be similarly misleading.

ALTERNATIVE SITES FOR VERESS NEEDLE INSERTION

On occasion, it is not possible to place the Veress needle in the appropriate space within the abdomen when using the umbilicus. Alternative sites for insertion are shown in Fig. 5. If the umbilical area is deemed unsuitable for insertion or if the patient is extremely obese, other sites and techniques may still allow safe establishment of a pneumoperitoneum. The site that is used most often other than the umbilicus is the left costal margin. This site is located 3–4 cm below the left costal margin in the midclavicular line. It is important to palpate and percuss this area first to rule out splenomegaly or an insufflated stomach. Insertion of a nasogastric tube preoperatively can prevent the latter. Other sites should be used with extreme caution, since they deviate signifi-

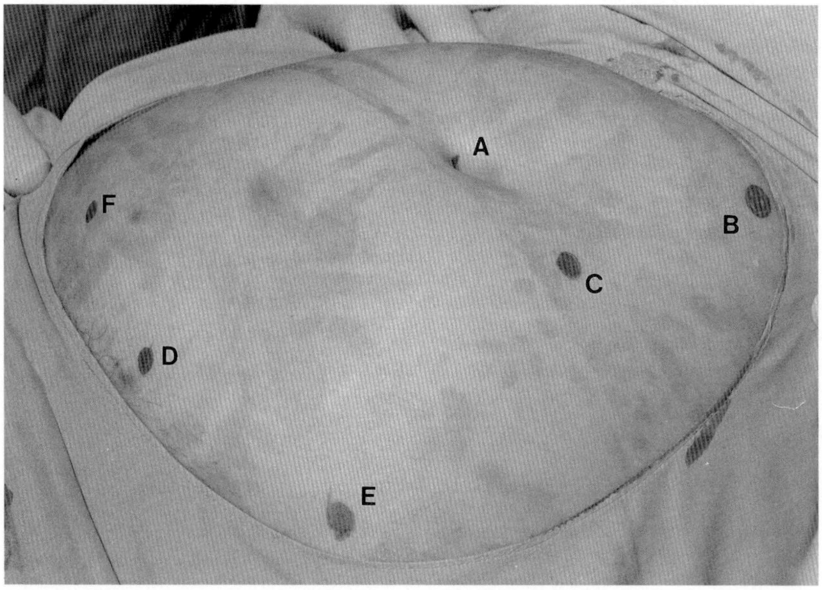

FIG. 5. Puncture sites for operative laparoscopy. Alternative sites for Veress needle placement, in decreasing order of preference. Umbilicus (**A**), left infracostal midclavicular line (**B**), and left periumbilical midclavicular line (**C**). Entry sites for accessory trocars include suprapubic midline (**D**), left and right lower quadrants (**E** and **F**).

cantly from the usual practice of an individual surgeon and thus the risk of injury is much greater.

It is also possible to use a transvaginal approach by inserting the needle through the posterior cul-de-sac (6), provided that there is no evidence of pelvic thickening, the uterus is mobile, and there is no evidence of masses in the cul-de-sac. This technique can be used in the patient who has already developed preperitoneal emphysema from several attempts at inserting the needle through the umbilicus or other abdominal sites.

Another technique for insertion, which is mentioned here only to condemn it, is the use of the uterine fundus, either transcervically or transabdominally (7,8). With the latter approach, the fundus of the uterus is pushed up against the abdominal wall by means of the uterine manipulator. The needle is then passed through all layers of the abdomen and into the fundus of the uterus. The uterus is then pulled away from the tip of the needle. With this technique, the needle then theoretically achieves an intraabdominal placement. There are several concerns about the general use of transuterine insertion of the Veress needle. Puncture of the uterus by this technique can result in persistent low-grade bleeding throughout the procedure. It is possible that inadvertent anterior perforation of the bladder may occur, and if the uterus is deviated to one side because of disease, broad ligament perforation and hemorrhage may result. The Veress needle may slip back to an intrauterine or intramyometrial position during insufflation, risking gas embolism. Furthermore, the technique is undesirable when fundal adhesions are anticipated or in cases where chromopertubation is necessary (9). For cases in which the surgeon anticipates difficulty inserting the Veress needle, direct trocar insertion may be a much simpler and less hazardous procedure, as described below.

Proper placement of the Veress needle is probably the most difficult obstacle to overcome in the obese patient. If it is placed below instead of within the umbilicus at the traditional 45° angle to the abdominal wall, it frequently dissects into the preperitoneal space. In the obese patient it is preferable to insert the needle and the trocar at the base of the umbilicus (Fig. 3)—not at its margin—and at a 90° angle using towel clips for traction and elevation of the abdominal wall (5).

ESTABLISHMENT OF PNEUMOPERITONEUM

The establishment of a pneumoperitoneum is essential for proper visualization and adequate room to perform the intraperitoneal manipulations of endoscopic surgery. If all of the above steps in establishing proper placement of the Veress needle have been taken, then the automatic insufflator can be switched to fill. It is important that high flow not be used at this point, since improper placement of the Veress needle will be further complicated by insufflation of CO_2 at high pressures, which can only lead to additional complications. The maximum flow rate should be 1 L/min.

In a well-anesthetized patient, the difference between the operating pressure of the insufflator outside and within the abdomen should be no greater than 5 mm Hg. If higher pressures are recorded, then the surgeon should suspect improper placement of the needle. Occasionally this is due to placement of the needle tip in the omentum. The needle can easily be dislodged by gently elevating the lower abdominal wall and shaking it. If this fails, the needle hub should be manipulated in a different direction since the distal hole may be impinging against the anterior abdominal wall. If neither of these maneuvers relieves the increased pressure, the Veress needle should be removed and a second attempt made. Occasionally, on passing through the different layers of the abdomen, some tissue may get lodged in the tip thus obstructing its opening. If the Veress needle needs to be withdrawn because of high pressures, it is prudent to examine the tip carefully for tissue.

Once the peritoneum has been insufflated with 1 L of gas, the surgeon should percuss the right costal margin to demonstrate loss of liver dullness. Sometimes tympany occurs with only several hundred cubic centimeters of CO_2 gas insufflation. This is one of the most convincing demonstrations of correct placement of the Veress needle, although not foolproof. If there is no loss of liver dullness, then it is quite likely that the Veress needle is within the preperitoneal space or in a viscus. The needle should be withdrawn and repositioned. If insufflation is allowed to proceed, sufficient gas will accumulate either in a hollow viscus or in the preperitoneal space so that liver dullness is lost and the surgeon gains a false sense of security.

Most insufflators have gauges that indicate the volume of gas insufflated. However, this volume should not be an indicator of whether or not there is sufficient pneumoperitoneum. Rather, the surgeon should use the palpable distention of the abdomen as a gauge rather than the volume, which varies considerably from patient to patient depending on the depth of anesthesia and the size and parity of the patient.

INTRODUCTION OF THE LAPAROSCOPIC TROCAR

The entry of the trocar into the abdomen is the moment of truth during a laparoscopic procedure. As such, it represents the point in the procedure when an instrument capable of producing considerable injury to an organ is inserted blindly into the abdomen. Because of the potential for injury, it is important that this procedure be accomplished with controlled entry and with the trocar aimed toward the hollow of the sacrum.

The principal trocar is designed for initial entry into the peritoneum and therefore as a port through which to operate the laparoscope. Trocars are constructed of metal, plastic, or a combination of both. A feature common to all cannulas is a valve that prevents gas leakage when the laparoscope or other instrument is removed from the abdomen. This mechanism may be either a trumpet or a flapper-type valve. Unfortunately, the valve mechanism also creates a significant amount of friction on the laparoscope and it is not uncommon after a long procedure for the trocar to move in concert with the laparoscope, often resulting in removal of the trocar from the abdominal cavity and subsequent loss of pneumoperitoneum. This problem can be avoided in several ways. On the reusable trocars, the spring can be removed from the valve so that there is significantly less resistance to the necessary movement of the laparoscope. A feature on disposable cannulas is a retention mechanism that may screw in (Ethicon, Inc., Somerville, NJ; United States Surgical Corp., Norwalk, CT), or expand under the abdominal wall like either an umbrella (Dexide Inc, Fort Worth, TX) or an inflatable balloon (Marlow Surgical Technologies, Willoughby, OH). In addition to anchoring the trocar sleeve, this mechanism may also tamponade any abdominal wall bleeding that may obscure the operating field.

DISPOSABLE VS. REUSABLE TROCARS

Much attention has been given to the disposable trocar because of its sharp tip and spring-loaded safety shield. The advantages and disadvantages of reusable and disposable trocars are summarized in Table 2. Dullness of trocars may result in the need for increased force, multiple insertions, and excessive instrumental manipulation; all are associated with increased risk of laparoscopic complications. Insertion of a disposable, shielded trocar in the presence of a pneumoperitoneum has been shown to require half the force needed for a reusable trocar that was professionally sharpened on a regular basis (10). Theoretically, a permanently sharp trocar that provides controlled entry should decrease the risk of injury

TABLE 2. *Advantages and disadvantages of disposable and reusable instruments*

	Reusable	Disposable
Advantages	Familiarity Single expenditure Less wasteful	Consistent sharpness No need for maintenance Minimizes spread of disease Transfer safety shield Retention mechanism to the abdominal wall
Disadvantages	Dullness Bends or breaks Lacks safety shield Lacks retention mechanism to the abdominal wall	Expensive Environmental concerns Adds to medical waste

to intraabdominal structures (10). No studies address the issue of whether this reduction in force is associated with a lower incidence of trocar-related injuries, but it may lessen the proximity of the abdominal wall to the spine and the subsequent compression of bowel and vessels (11). There have been no large-scale clinical trials to establish this as an advantage of single-use trocars; in fact, a surgeon using these new devices may risk injury because of the unexpected ease of insertion. At our institution, the first use of a disposable trocar was associated with laceration of a mesenteric vessel, which was not discovered until several hours postsurgery. This experience underscores the importance of consistency of technique and instruments as well as the potential hazards of alterations in procedure.

There are several types of safety tips for disposable trocars. Some have a spring-loaded safety shield that is retracted into the cannula as the trocar is depressed into the abdomen. This action exposes the sharp trocar for entry but once it is inside the peritoneal cavity the plastic shield automatically releases to cover the sharp tip of the trocar and protect the intraabdominal organs. Another trocar is like the Veress needle in that the sharp trocar tip has a hollow core with a blunt stylet that is spring-loaded. After penetration, the blunt stylet moves beyond the tip, thus preventing puncture of viscera.

Under normal circumstances and with a well-inflated abdomen, these safety features are adequate. However, with excessive force or with an insufficiently inflated abdomen, the shield may not deploy quickly enough to prevent injury. Finally, in the presence of adhesions to the anterior abdominal wall, these devices offer no advantage.

HIGH-RISK SITUATIONS

Special considerations are required for patients at the extremes of body weight. In the obese patient, the trocar may need to be angled close to the vertical, which means that the distance between the sacral promontory and trocar is small, leaving little room for error. The very thin patient may be at even greater risk, as the distance between the anterior abdominal wall and sacral promontory is often very small. Furthermore, the force required to introduce the trocar is often less than anticipated because the fascia is thin and offers little resistance (12). In these patients, it may be safer to overdistend the abdominal wall with additional gas prior to trocar insertion.

Bowel distention secondary to obstruction is a relative contraindication to laparoscopy unless there are compelling reasons for the procedure such that the benefits outweigh the risks. However, bowel distention may be iatrogenic, resulting from the placement of the Veress needle within the bowel lumen. The surgeon may be unaware of this problem because of a lack of difference in filling pressures between the abdominal cavity and the bowel due to the large capacity of the small bowel. Once an apparent pneumoperitoneum is created and the Veress needle removed, the distended bowel is an easy target for significant laceration with the trocar.

The presence of small bowel adhesions to the anterior abdominal wall is associated with a high risk of trocar injury. Patients with previous, uncomplicated abdominal surgery are generally not at increased risk and do not require special considerations. In contrast, those who have had a bowel resection or exploratory laparotomy for trauma probably have an increased risk. Similarly, women who undergo a second-look laparoscopy for carcinoma of the ovary not only have risks of adhesions from previous abdominal surgery but generally have had an omentectomy and a disease process associated with adhesion formation (4).

Patients at high risk for bowel adhesions, i.e., those with previous bowel surgery, may be more appropriately managed by open laparoscopy rather than closed laparoscopy. In spite of this precaution, bowel lacerations still can occur upon entering the peritoneum (13). Moreover, it is difficult to determine which patients who have had pelvic surgery should have an open laparoscopy.

Several procedures have been described to assess the anterior abdominal wall for the presence of bowel adhesions. DeCherney (14) advocates the use of a small-gauge laparoscope called a needle scope which is an endoscope 2-3 mm in diameter. This instrument can be advanced, instead of the Veress needle, under direct visualization on the umbilical, preperitoneal, and immediately subperitoneal structures. Thus the needle can be placed intraabdominally and insufflation can proceed under direct visualization. Exploration of the periumbilical area with an 18-gauge needle attached to a syringe after the establishment of pneumoperitoneum, as shown in Fig. 6, also has been very useful (15).

Should the presence of adhesions be detected by these relatively atraumatic techniques, the options for surgical approach include switching to open laparoscopy (described below) or choosing alternative sites of entry, as previously described and illustrated in Fig. 5. The main trocar can be inserted at any point in the midline between the xyphoid and the pubic symphysis, provided care is taken to remain at least 5 cm below the xyphoid and 5 cm above the pubic symphysis (12).

When managing a patient at risk for bowel adhesions, it is prudent to administer a mechanical and antibiotic bowel preparation preoperatively. This effectively eliminates bowel contents, decompresses the bowel, and serves as a prophylaxis against infection should perforation occur.

INSERTION TECHNIQUES

Successful insertion of the laparoscopic trocar depends on (a) an adequate skin incision, (b) an instrument

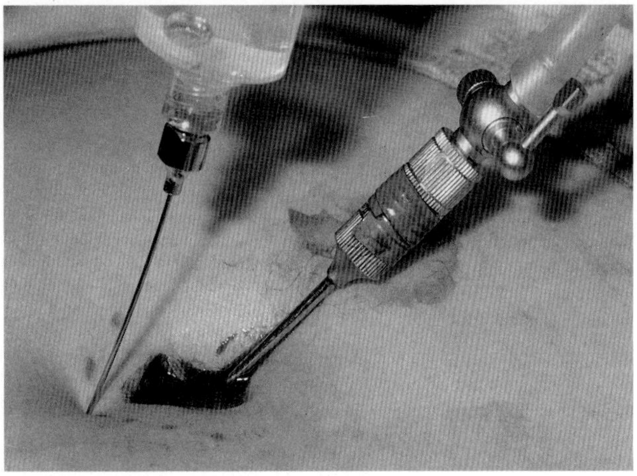

FIG. 6. Syringe test to ascertain that bowel and/or blood vessels are not adherent under the umbilicus prior to trocar insertion. A 10-cm^3 syringe with a 20-gauge needle is inserted under negative pressure at the four cardinal points of a 20-mm circle around the umbilicus. If blood or bowel content is aspirated instead of CO_2 gas at any of these points, it indicates vascular or intestinal infraumbilical adhesions and alternate sites for trocar insertion should be chosen.

in good working condition, (c) proper orientation of the trocar, (d) appropriate insertion force, and (e) control over the depth of insertion of the instrument. As the trocar penetrates each layer of the anterior abdominal wall, there are associated sensations which the experienced operator learns to anticipate and interpret. Each step in the laparoscopic approach should not deviate from the surgeon's standard procedure without good cause. This is especially true for the trocar insertion technique. Soderstrom and Butler (16) demonstrated in a program for laparoscopic sterilization that the complication rate could be reduced tenfold with the adoption of a consistent operating format.

Regardless of the technique used, the trocar should be inserted with the patient in a completely horizontal position. Premature Trendelenberg positioning does nothing to avoid injuries to the abdominal viscera, particularly if bowel adhesions are present. It may alter the surgeon's perspective of important landmarks, such as the sacral promontory and sacral hollow, toward which the trocar is advanced to avoid the major blood vessels and to provide the greatest distance between the sharp point of the trocar and the unyielding, solid tissue. When the patient is horizontal, viscera such as the bowel almost invariably easily slides out of the way of the advancing trocar.

To comprehend fully the importance of the direction for insertion, the major anatomic landmarks and their relationships must be known. The umbilicus is located at the level of L3 and L4. The abdominal aorta usually bifurcates between L4 and L5. Proper direction of insertion of the trocar should be at approximately a 45°–60° angle with respect to the abdominal wall plane, which should place it toward the hollow of the sacrum.

The trocar and its sleeve are grasped by the operator with the index finger extended to the point of maximal planned penetration. The extended finger helps prevent the sharp trocar tip from thrusting too deeply and causing intraabdominal injury. It is important that the surgeon use the dominant hand for this procedure since there is little room for error. The remainder of the fingers grasp the trumpet valve or the insufflation valve. The trocar itself is held in the palm of the hand. The trocar is rotated in a semicircular fashion along its long axis while controlled, firm, downward pressure is applied. As the trocar is advanced, the operator senses when the fascia has been traversed, at which point the force is relaxed as the trocar is slowly advanced to enter the peritoneum. The correct placement of the trocar is confirmed by the free escape of gas when the sharp trocar is removed from its sleeve.

TECHNIQUES REQUIRING A PNEUMOPERITONEUM

Establishment of a large pneumoperitoneum before trocar insertion and elevation of the abdominal wall to increase the distance between the abdominal wall and viscera help decrease the chance of viscous injury. The following two methods of trocar insertion require that pneumoperitoneum be established first. In the first procedure, shown in Fig. 7A, the operator places upward traction on the lower abdomen in the midline, thus providing countertraction for insertion of the trocar through the umbilicus. Alternatively, an assistant can also apply traction to the lower abdomen, but it is important that the operator and assistant apply traction symmetrically. Difficulties may occur with this technique if trocar insertion is difficult, or if the patient has a large panniculus, or if the operator does not have adequate strength. In such cases, several attempts may be necessary and significant abdominal bruising may result. To avoid this, the operator can use his or her nondominant hand to apply upper abdominal pressure, thus increasing transiently the lower abdominal pressure, and insert the trocar without applying countertraction (see Fig. 7B). Controlled entry of the trocar is very important with either technique.

DIRECT TROCAR INSERTION

Laparoscopy involves entering the peritoneal cavity via three blind steps: Veress needle insertion, induction of pneumoperitoneum, and trocar insertion. Direct insertion of the laparoscopic trocar without a pneumoperitoneum reduces the number of blind steps to one;

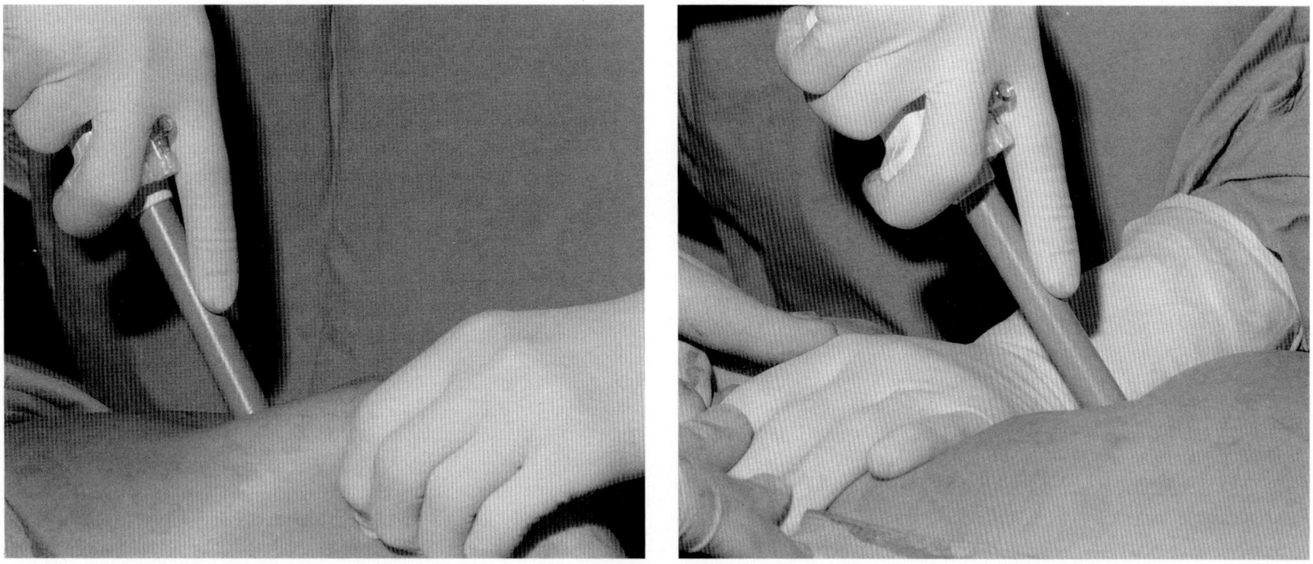

FIG. 7. Insertion of trocar. Elevation of lower abdominal wall (A); application of pressure on the upper abdomen to further distend the lower abdominal wall (B).

this provides savings in operating time and potential complications (17). Direct insertion of the laparoscopic trocar, without previous pneumoperitoneum, has been reported to be a safe alternative to Veress needle insertion (17–23), although only one study prospectively compared the two methods. A disposable, shielded trocar has been introduced and provides two advantages: a safety shield which snaps into position after the peritoneum is entered and a freshly sharpened instrument for each surgical case. This instrument also has been investigated for direct abdominal insertion (21). Nezhat et al. recently conducted a randomized, prospectively controlled study to compare the ease of use and safety of (a) Veress needle insertion and establishment of a pneumoperitoneum vs. (b) direct insertion of the conventional reusable trocar vs. (c) direct insertion of the disposable shielded trocar. Minor complication rates of 22%, 6%, and 0% were observed, respectively (see Table 5) (17). None of these methods resulted in major complications in a series of 200 patients. Although the study demonstrated fewer complications with direct insertion of the trocar, it did not confirm fewer or easier insertions

TABLE 3. *Comparison of Veress needle or direct trocar insertion*

Factor	Veress needle (n = 100)	Direct trocar insertion (n = 100)
Complications	22	3*
Two insertions required	20	20
Failed insertions	3	6

* $P < 0.05$.

(see Table 3). In addition, this study was performed only in low-risk patients who had not undergone prior laparotomy.

Direct trocar insertion is accomplished by elevating the abdominal wall either manually or with towel clips inserted close to the umbilicus. The trocar is then inserted into the peritoneal cavity, aiming toward the hollow of the sacrum. The laparoscope is immediately introduced in order to verify correct intraperitoneal placement. The pneumoperitoneum then is created. Since proper placement of the trocar has been verified, high-flow insufflation can be utilized from the beginning.

OPEN LAPAROSCOPY

In 1971, Hasson introduced the concept of open laparoscopy to eliminate risks associated with blind introduction of the Veress needle and laparoscopic trocar (24). The technique involves direct trocar insertion without prior pneumoperitoneum using specially designed equipment. The equipment consists of a laparoscope cannula with a trumpet valve fitted with a cone-shaped stainless steel sleeve and a blunt obturator; the obturator protrudes 1 cm from the tip of the cannula. The cone sleeve acts like a cork to seal the peritoneal and fascial gap.

The procedure involves making either a small, transverse, curved incision or a vertical incision at the level of the umbilicus. Instruments for open laparoscopy are listed in Table 4. After the initial skin incision is made either within or around the umbilicus, the surgeon uses Allis clamps to grasp the edges of the incision to provide better visualization and to elevate the abdominal

TABLE 4. *Instruments used in open laparoscopy*

Two Allis clamps
One knife handle with small blade
One straight scissors
One tissue forceps with teeth
One right-angle skin hook
Four S-shaped retractors
One needle holder
Two curved Kocher clamps
Four small curved hemostats
Two sutures of 0-PDS
Hasson blunt trocar and obturator

wall. S-shaped retractors may also be used to expose the surgical incision. Once the fascia is incised, the exposed peritoneum is incised vertically for a distance of 1 cm. It is important to keep upward traction on the skin and the fascia to elevate the abdominal wall away from the intraabdominal organs and to minimize the risk of bowel injury. Extreme caution is exercised in incising the peritoneum to avoid possible injury to the bowel wall. Two sutures of 0-PDS are passed, one through each peritoneal edge and fascia, and are subsequently tagged. The cork-like cannula with the blunt obturator is inserted through the opening into the peritoneal cavity. The obturator is withdrawn and gas is insufflated through the cannula to effect a pneumoperitoneum. To prevent the escape of gas, the surgeon inserts the cannula further as required to block the incisional gap. The previously placed sutures are used to tie down the trocar sleeve so that no gas escapes and the laparoscope can move freely within the abdominal cavity. At the end of the procedure, the abdominal wall is closed using the previously placed sutures of 0-PDS.

This method was designed to eliminate certain flaws of the blind trocar insertion method: (a) The Veress needle and sharp laparoscopic trocar, which are placed blindly and forcibly, are not used. (b) Gas consistently insufflates the peritoneal cavity. (c) Anatomic repair of the fascia and peritoneum is possible, thus avoiding the complications of an umbilical hernia.

Open laparoscopy usually takes about 5–10 min more than does closed laparoscopy and requires operators of comparable expertise. The recovery time is identical. Open laparoscopy is contraindicated only in patients with conditions in which the creation of a pneumoperitoneum may be harmful, such as diseases associated with acute respiratory distress and significant chronic disability. Abdominal hernia is not a contraindication because the maximum intraabdominal pressure obtained at laparoscopy is less than that associated with coughing or sneezing.

The complications of open laparoscopy are those of an umbilical minilaparotomy, i.e., wound infection and small bowel injury. In more than 1000 consecutive cases performed by Hasson and his colleagues, the frequency of minor wound infection was 0.6% and that of small bowel injury was 0.1% (25). A review of the complications associated with open and closed laparoscopy indicates that the former procedure reduces the risks and complications of failed attempts, inappropriate gas insufflation, gas embolism, bladder or pelvic kidney puncture, major vessel injury, and postoperative herniations (25). With experience and proper technique, surgeons seldom encounter difficulties with either the closed or the open method.

Penfield conducted a survey that suggested that bowel laceration is the most serious complication of laparoscopy (13). Interestingly, most of the complications with open laparoscopy occurred early in the use of this technique. In a series of 10,840 open laparoscopies performed by 18 board-certified obstetrician/gynecologists, six bowel lacerations occurred. Four were recognized instantly and repaired. Two of the bowel lacerations, however, were not suspected until several days after surgery. The following measures have been suggested to minimize the risk of bowel laceration:

1. Utilize a focused spotlight when operating through the small incision.
2. Use an experienced assistant.
3. Make a vertical, not transverse, incision as it greatly facilitates exposure.
4. Grasp and elevate the fascia with small Kocher clamps, then incise slowly between the clamps.

Infraumbilical minilaparotomy, as a substitute for needle and trocar puncture, continues to be attractive to gynecologists for safety reasons. Unfortunately, the gynecologist who performs open laparoscopy only in special situations, such as for patients with suspected intraperitoneal adhesions, will find the procedure slow and cumbersome and may have difficulty exposing and identifying each layer of the abdominal wall.

ACCESSORY TROCAR INSERTION

To perform diagnostic laparoscopy, it is necessary to insert accessory trocars through which various instruments can be introduced into the abdomen for manipulation and operative procedures. The site of accessory trocar placement depends on the patient's anatomy, the contemplated procedure, and the surgeon's preference. For diagnostic purposes, the incision is generally made

TABLE 5. *Comparison of conventional and disposable trocars*

	Conventional (n = 50)	Disposable (n = 50)
Complications	3	0
Two insertions required	10	10
Failed insertions	4	2

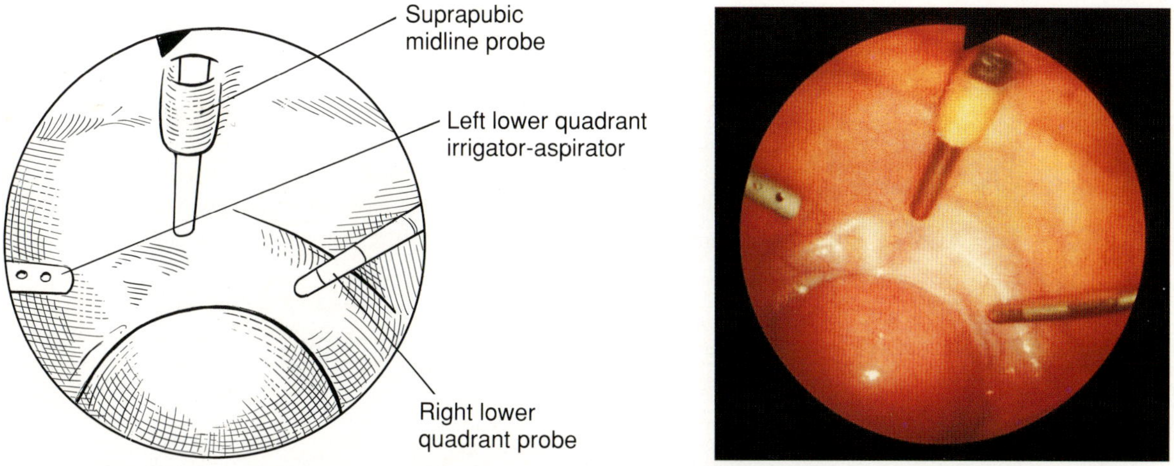

FIG. 8. Insertion of accessory trocars. The trocars are placed high enough to clear the fundus of the uterus to gain free access to the posterior cul-de-sac. It is important to insert the accessory trocars under direct visualization to minimize injury to intraabdominal organs and to inferior epigastric vessels.

6–8 cm above the symphysis pubis in the midline. This area, which is delineated by the two umbilical ligaments and the dome of the bladder, is safe and usually avascular. For operative laparoscopy, two 5-mm accessory trocar sleeves are generally placed 6–8 cm above the symphysis pubis at the outer border of the rectus muscle (Fig. 8).

It is important to insert the accessory trocars under direct visualization from the laparoscope to minimize the risk of injury to intraabdominal organs and epigastric vessels (Fig. 9). Also they must be placed high enough to clear the fundus of the uterus to gain free access to the posterior cul-de-sac. The inferior epigastric vessels may be difficult to identify by transillumination of the abdominal wall, particularly in obese patients. However, they invariably run lateral to the umbilical ligaments, which are easily identified laparoscopically on either side of the bladder, and medial to the internal inguinal ring where the round ligament runs into the anterior abdominal wall (Fig. 10). In order to avoid these vessels, the surgeon may insert the accessory trocar medial to the umbilical ligaments or lateral to the internal inguinal ring, under direct visualization of the underside of the abdomen using the laparoscope. The area between the umbilical ligament and the inguinal ring should be avoided, since that is where the inferior hypogastric vessels are most commonly located.

In cases where the location of the vessels may be anomalous, they may be seen protruding in front of the advancing trocars. In these instances, last minute corrections can be made with the accessory trocar to avoid them. In order to avoid trauma to the abdominal structures, the site of secondary puncture should be indented by applying abdominal pressure with the index finger and should be observed with the laparoscope, as shown in Fig. 10. This maneuver is particularly important in a patient who has evidence of anterior abdominal wall adhesions. The site of the indentation is inspected to ensure that it provides the necessary access.

The trocar is held with the index finger extended on

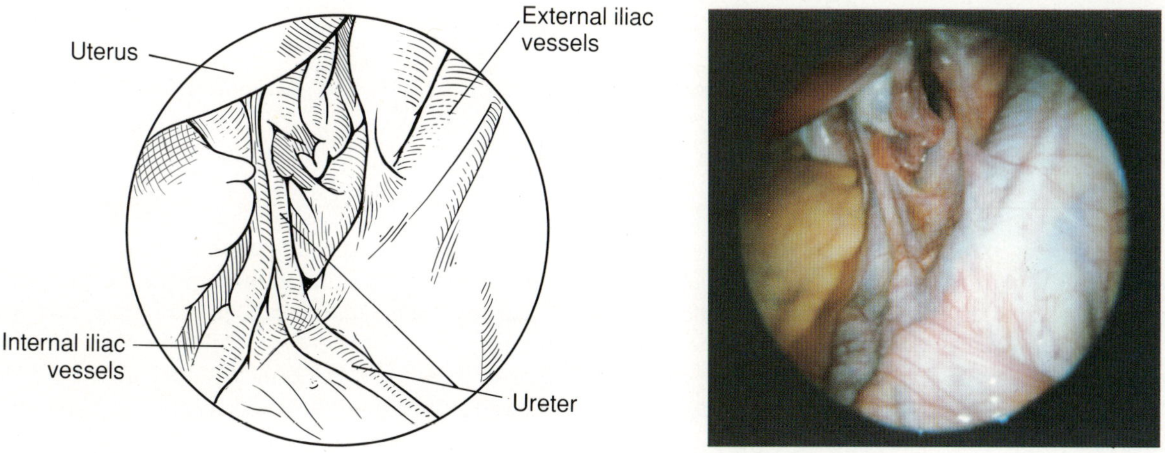

FIG. 9. Major vascular structures at risk of injury during laparoscope and accessory trocar insertion.

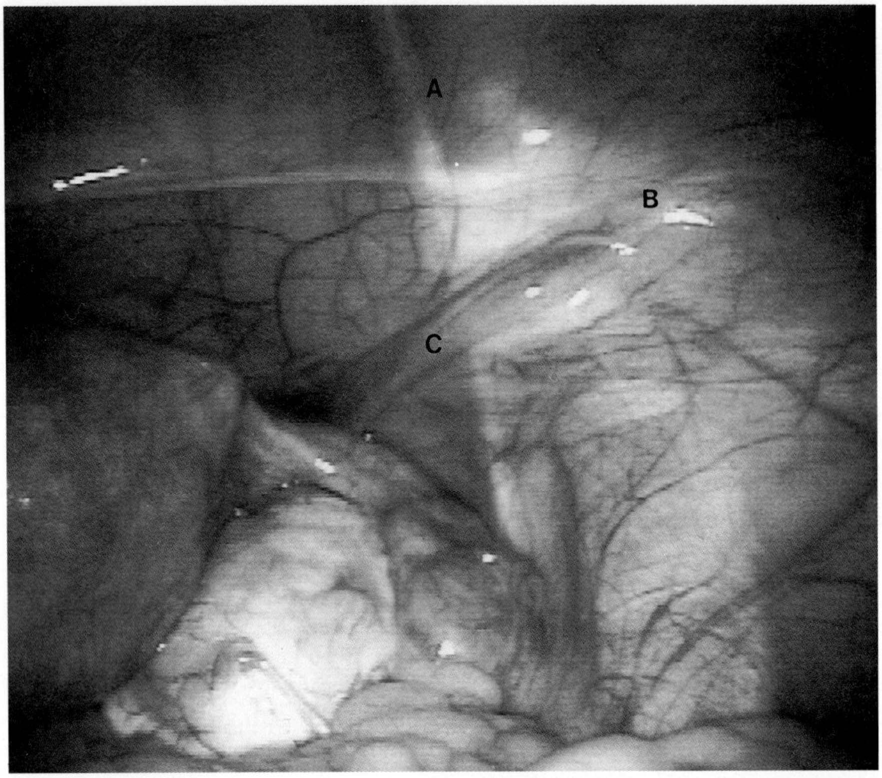

FIG. 10. The inferior epigastric vessels are invariably located lateral to the umbilical ligaments (**A**) and medial to the internal inguinal ring (**B**), where the round ligament (**C**) inserts into the anterior abdominal wall. To avoid these vessels, the accessory trocars may be safely inserted either medial to the umbilical ligament or lateral to the inguinal ring.

the sheath to control the depth of penetration, as shown in Fig. 7. The trocar and sheath are inserted through the skin, fat, and fascia, and further advancement is controlled under direct laparoscopic visualization. It is important that the trocar be aimed toward the hollow of the sacrum just as other instruments are inserted. If the trocar is aimed laterally instead of medially, it is possible that the trocar can go down the pelvic side wall without being visualized through the laparoscope. This obviously can result in significant injury to the iliac vessels. The accessory trocar must never be inserted without clear laparoscopic visualization of its indentation on the lower aspect of the abdominal wall.

In general, most laparoscopic procedures do not require more than two accessory trocars. On occasion third and rarely fourth ancillary instruments can be introduced. Other sites of introduction include the midpoint between the symphysis and the umbilicus and 6–8 cm above the symphysis pubis, as shown in Fig. 5.

Many of the early trocar sleeves present problems for the laparoscopic surgeon; these problems may be overcome with some of the newer models (26). The lower quadrant sleeves are often too long for free access to the pelvic structures and may slip out of the peritoneal cavity, unnecessarily prolonging the operative time. In addition, trap valves interfere with efficient instrument exchange and prohibit the introduction and removal of suture material and evacuation of tissue. As with the main trocars mentioned earlier, several new accessory trocar sleeves either screw in or have an umbrella to secure them to the abdominal wall at a fixed location so that these problems do not occur and there is more room for intraabdominal manipulation.

Currently trocars come in sizes of 5–12 mm. It is wise to minimize the use of 12-mm trocars, since they require separate closure of the fascia to prevent hernia formation.

EVALUATION OF THE ABDOMEN

The initial phase of laparoscopy is exploration of the pelvic anatomy to assess and map out the extent of disease. Preferably this is done with photographs or video recordings, and the surgeon must identify anatomic landmarks and become familiar with the patient's pelvic anatomy. Each laparoscopic procedure offers a lesson in anatomy and a wondrous sight of the abdominal organs, whose anatomic relationship and integrity may be viewed from a panoramic perspective or close up for microscopic inspection.

A thorough diagnostic evaluation and documentation

of the initial findings at the time of laparoscopy is important for many reasons. First, a complete survey of the pelvis helps the operator to plan the surgical procedures to be performed. Second, careful documentation of the operative record allows the surgeon to refer back to the procedure, particularly if a second laparoscopic procedure is performed. Third, the documentation serves as a reference for determining future treatment of the patient. Finally, both evaluation and documentation are excellent tools with which to educate oneself, residents, and patients.

It is important that the exam be conducted in a standardized and thorough manner. The procedure that is presented here has served us well and we describe it only as an example. The initial examination should be completed soon after the laparoscope and accessory trocar(s) have been inserted. The omentum and bowel directly beneath the trocar should be inspected first, since this is where Veress needle and trocar injuries are more likely to occur and become evident either as bleeding or as spillage of bowel content.

Initially, a general survey of the pelvis is undertaken from a distance so that all the pelvic structures are within sight of the laparoscope, providing a panoramic view. The upper abdominal organs, abdominal walls, liver, gall bladder and diaphragm should be examined for the presence of endometriosis or other pathology that may contribute to the patient's symptoms. Forceps or blunt probes may be used to manipulate gently the organs of interest. The laparoscope then is moved closer to the left adnexa, which is lifted if possible, and the pelvic side wall is carefully inspected. The left ovary is examined at all sides and then released and the scope is placed over the anterior cul-de-sac and swept over the right adnexa. The right ovary is examined and elevated and the pelvic side wall is carefully inspected. The cul-de-sac is then carefully evaluated. The appendix is inspected as is the upper abdomen.

In the presence of extensive adhesions, this technique must be modified. It is important that the surgeon ascertain approximately where the normal structures are and assess the type of adhesions that will be encountered so that the procedure can be planned. It is also important at this point that the surgeon make a very clear assessment of whether the procedure should be performed by laparotomy or laparoscopy. This decision will take into account the anatomic distortions that are present, the amount of time involved, and the surgeon's experience.

CONCLUSION OF THE PROCEDURE

Following the operative procedure, chromotubation is performed, when indicated. Although some surgeons may prefer performing chromotubation at the beginning rather than at the end of the operative procedure, we prefer the latter when, after all adhesions have been lysed, we can clearly see the fimbria and distal tubal ostium for a final inspection of fimbrial adhesions. Moreover, on occasions the tubes may be kinked by adhesions showing initial obstruction, which is relieved after adhesiolysis.

At the end of the procedure, the entire peritoneal cavity is irrigated copiously with isotonic fluid, usually Ringer's lactate, and thoroughly inspected for further pathology, debris (such as blood clots, pieces of adhesions, cyst wall, endometriosis implants), or bleeding (Fig. 11). At this point, any bleeders should be identified and coagulated with bipolar forceps. Because the pressure created by the pneumoperitoneum may tamponade bleeding from small venules or capillaries, the surgeon should temporarily evacuate the gas and inspect again for bleeding while reinsufflating the abdominal cavity. The presence of clear irrigating fluid confirms adequate hemostasis. At this point the procedure can be terminated by evacuating the abdomen of the CO_2 gas.

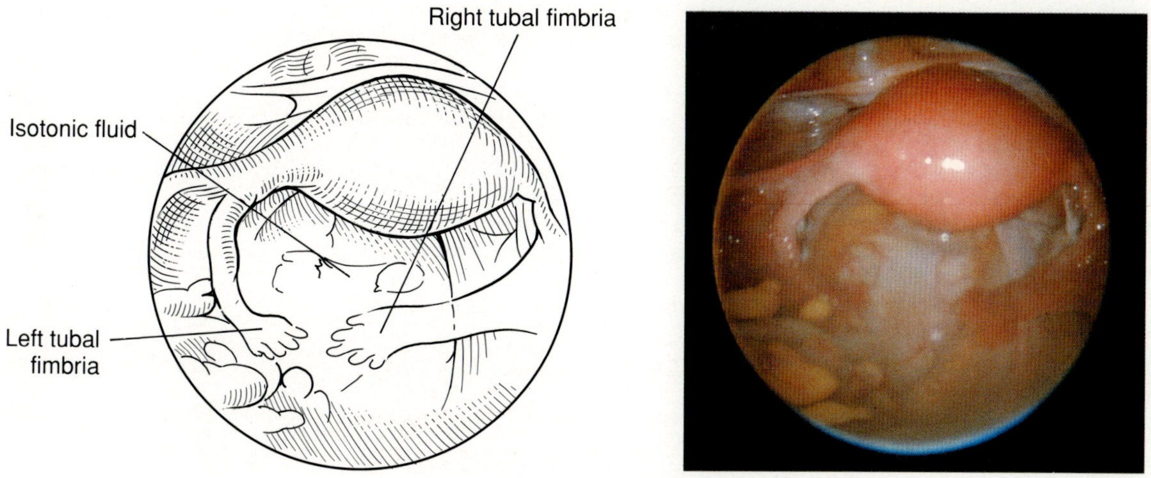

FIG. 11. Pelvis filled with isotonic fluid.

RELEASE OF PERITONEUM

The CO_2 gas must be completely evacuated to avoid postoperative pain. Of all of the common postoperative problems, patients complain most vehemently about the referred shoulder pain from gas trapped under the diaphragm. Therefore, it is important that the surgeon attempt to remove as much of the trapped gas as possible. A procedure that is quite successful involves keeping the patient in Trendelenberg position as the instruments are removed from the trocar sleeves. The gas source is disconnected and as much of the pneumoperitoneum as possible is allowed to escape from the umbilical and the two suprapubic trocars. Since the patient is in a Trendelenberg position, most of the gas is trapped in the suprapubic area. Therefore the umbilical trocar can be removed at this point and the remainder of the gas is milked out of the trocar sleeves by applying moderate upper abdominal pressure.

Except in cases where Interceed (Tc-7, Johnson and Johnson Medical, Inc., Arlington, TX) is applied, the surgeon usually leaves within the abdominal cavity 500–1000 cm^3 of Ringer's lactate solution; this may serve two important purposes. The large fluid volume displaces the gas, further promoting its full evacuation from the abdominal cavity, thereby decreasing postoperative shoulder pain. The second purpose, which is more tenuous but may be even more important, is the potential for decreased formation of postoperative adhesions associated with the use of large volumes of isotonic solution (27). The prevalence of shoulder pain has decreased dramatically in our institution since the procedure has been implemented.

The 5-mm incisions used for the accessory trocars can be closed with Steri-Strips (3M Co., St. Paul, MN). Alternatively, the surgeon may apply an inverted subcutaneous suture of 4-0 Dexon or Vicryl. A similar sort of closure can be used for vertical umbilical incisions. Incisions for trocars larger than 10 mm need to be closed in layers with particular attention paid to closure of the fascia.

POSTOPERATIVE CARE AND INSTRUCTIONS

We routinely provide our patients with postoperative instructions prior to the day of surgery so that they are maximally prepared for their postoperative experience. The surgeon ordinarily sees the patient in the outpatient surgery recovery room to explain the operative findings and the surgical procedure performed. The patient's questions are answered and the expected postoperative course explained. Prior to discharge, she is given a prescription for pain medication as indicated, and routine postoperative instructions, as shown in Table 6. It is rou-

TABLE 6. *Same day surgery laparoscopy/hysteroscopy discharge instructions*

1. You will have one small incision in your navel and possibly other small incisions further down on your abdomen and to the side. You may notice a small amount of bleeding on the bandages covering these incisions. When all bleeding has stopped, the bandages may be removed for showering or bathing. At this time it is all right to leave the dressings off completely. If irritation occurs with tight clothing, you may want to apply a dressing for comfort. It is a good idea to leave the incision open to the air. You will feel numbness and hardness around your incision—this is normal. Some women may notice bruising on their lower abdomen—this is normal and will resolve in several days.
2. You had gas (CO_2) put into your abdomen during surgery in order to enable the physician to see inside the abdominal cavity. Your physician removed as much air as possible when he or she finished with the laparoscopy and before he or she put your stitches in. However, if some of the gas remains in the abdomen, it may cause some shoulder pain or chest discomfort. This generally resolves in a day or two. You will probably feel more comfortable if you lie on your abdomen with a pillow under your hips. In addition, you may notice leakage of variable amounts of pinkish fluid from your incision(s). This is normal and resolves in 1–2 days.
3. Resume normal activities as you feel up to them. Working may generally resume within 3 days. Recovery from laparoscopic surgery varies greatly depending on the length of time you were under anesthesia, the surgical procedure performed, the nature of your job, and your constitution.
4. If only a laparoscopy was performed, sexual activity may resume as soon as you are comfortable and vaginal bleeding has stopped. If a hysteroscopy has been performed, do not put anything in your vagina for one (1) week (i.e., no tampons, douching, or intercourse).
5. Menses should occur as expected or earlier. Tampons may be used. Do not douche unless you are instructed to do so.
6. Unrestricted bathing or showering is allowed. No swimming for 48 hr.
7. Please follow your physician's instructions if you are given prescriptions for a vaginal cream, douche, or an antibiotic.
8. Contact your physician if you notice any of the following:
   a. Chills or fever over 101°
   b. Heavy or prolonged vaginal bleeding, soaking pads
   c. Heavy incisional bleeding
   d. Heat, swelling, or pus from the incisions
   e. Frequency or burning on urination
   f. Severe pelvic pain
   g. Vaginal discharge that itches, burns, or has an odor
   h. Fainting, dizziness, persistent nausea or vomiting, constipation, or diarrhea
   i. Inability to urinate

tine in our hospital for the outpatient surgery nurses to contact the patient 1 or 2 days after surgery to ensure that there are no problems and to answer whatever questions they may have.

It is important that the patient's progress be one of improvement each day. A patient's developing significant pain, fever, or bowel or bladder symptoms indicates that something out of the ordinary has interfered with the normal recovery process and the patient needs to be evaluated. Generally patients are seen in a routine postoperative visit 1–2 weeks following their surgery. Most women return to work 3–10 days following their procedure. This period depends on a number of factors, such as the length of time under anesthesia, the surgical procedure performed, the nature of the patient's job, and the individual patient's constitution.

COMMON POSTOPERATIVE PROBLEMS

There are several postoperative problems that are exceedingly common and can be handled with standard measures. Nausea and vomiting are common and are most likely related to intraabdominal CO_2 gas and to narcotics that are frequently used perioperatively. Most of the time nausea and vomiting respond to parenteral antiemetic medications, but on occasion the patient needs to be admitted overnight for continued care.

Referred shoulder pain is a frequent complaint of the patient and generally takes 1–2 days to resolve. If a patient develops this pain, she can be instructed to rest on her abdomen with a pillow under the lower part of her abdomen to elevate the lower pelvis where the gas collects in preference to the diaphragm. This should alleviate this severe type of pain.

Subcutaneous crepitation may be palpable over the abdomen and occasionally extends superiorly to the chest and neck or inferiorly to the buttocks and thighs. This is caused by the escape of carbon dioxide gas from the peritoneal cavity into the subcutaneous tissues, where it dissects superiorly and inferiorly resulting in crepitation and subcutaneous swelling of the chest, face, abdomen, buttocks, and thighs. Although worrisome to the patient and family, this is a minor complication and usually resolves spontaneously without sequelae. Subcutaneous crepitation occurs more frequently in obese patients having undergone prolonged operative procedures or in cases where multiple punctures are made to reinsert trocars that have slipped out of the abdominal wall. On occasion a patient develops profound hypotension, which apparently is idiosyncratic in its appearance and unrelated to blood loss. Often these patients do quite well after being administered a bolus of intravenous fluid.

Postoperative pain from incision sites usually is mild and can be managed using a heating pad and nonnarcotic analgesics. In contrast, many patients who undergo extensive intraabdominal procedures may have significant visceral pain from these procedures. Ordinarily this pain requires either narcotics or nonsteroidal antiinflammatory agents. A heating pad applied to the abdomen does much to help relax the abdomen and provide significant analgesia.

When large amounts of isotonic fluid is left in situ, it may drain as pinkish fluid through the abdominal puncture wounds, which may be very worrisome to the patient. The drainage usually resolves within 24–48 hr, and simple reassurance is all that is required.

CONCLUDING REMARKS

In this chapter we have provided guidelines, recommendations, and suggestions that may be useful in the perioperative preparation of the patient and in updating the surgeon with the more current laparoscopic instruments and techniques. It is hoped that this material will facilitate these operative procedures and increase the safety of the laparoscopic approach to pelvic surgery.

Operative laparoscopy allows the surgeon to perform very complex, extensive, and delicate surgery through small puncture wounds, thus minimizing patient discomfort, morbidity, expense, and duration of convalescence (28). However, laparoscopy is not a method of treatment but rather a way of accessing the patient's diseased organs. The ability to remove disease and reconstruct damaged organs depends on the surgeon's training, experience, and talent. Only those surgeons who are well trained to treat a certain disease by laparotomy should attempt treatment of the same disease by laparoscopy.

The transition from microsurgery by laparotomy to microsurgery by laparoscopy is a slow but rewarding process, and it cannot be accomplished after a 2- to 3-day postgraduate course or from reading the literature. The learning curve should be progressive—but not too rapid, and should not be accelerated at the expense of the patient. Occasionally the laparoscopic attempt may be converted to laparotomy, if in the opinion of the surgeon the latter approach would result in a more complete surgical procedure and yield better outcome. Thus the debate of laparoscopy vs. laparotomy is moot. The goal is the complete and best possible treatment of the disease. Only when it can be achieved as well by laparoscopy should the economic and social benefits of the laparoscopic approach be considered. The savings in hospital cost and recovery periods obtained with the laparoscopic approach do not compensate for its failure to achieve the best treatment for the disease.

REFERENCES

1. Ott DO. Die beleuchtung der bauchhohle (ventroskopie) als methode bei vaginaler coeliotomie. *Abl Gynakol* 1902;231:817.
2. Palmer R. La coelioscopie gynecologique, ses possibilities et ses indications actuelles. *Sem Hop Paris* 1954;30:4441.

3. East MC, Steele PRM. Laparoscopic incisions at the lower umbilical verge. *Br Med J* 1988;296:753.
4. Loffer FD. Endoscopy in high risk patients. In: Martin DC, ed. *Manual of endoscopy.* Santa Fe Springs, CA: American Association of Gynecologic Laparoscopists; 1990:43.
5. Loffer FD, Pent D. Laparoscopy in the obese patient. *Am J Obstet Gynecol* 1976;125:104.
6. Neely MR, McWilliams R, Makhlouf HA. Laparoscopy: routine pneumoperitoneum via the posterior fornix. *Obstet Gynecol* 1975;45:459.
7. Morgan HR. Laparoscopy: induction of pneumoperitoneum via transfundal puncture. *Obstet Gynecol* 1979;54:260.
8. Wolfe WM, Pasic R. Transuterine insertion of Veress needle in laparoscopy. *Obstet Gynecol* 1990;75:456.
9. Awadalla SG. Letter to the editor. *Obstet Gynecol* 1990;76:314.
10. Corson SL, Batzer FR, Gocial B, Maislin G. Measurement of the force necessary for laparoscopic entry. *J Reprod Med* 1989;34:282.
11. Phillips JM. *Laparoscopy.* Baltimore: Williams & Wilkins; 1977: 220.
12. Gomel V, Taylor PJ, Yuzpe AA, Rioux JE. The technique of endoscopy. In: *Laparoscopy and hysteroscopy in gynecologic practice.* Chicago: Year Book; 1986:32.
13. Penfield AJ. How to prevent complications of open laparoscopy. *J Reprod Med* 1985;30:660.
14. DeCherney AH. Laparoscopy with unexpected viscus penetration. In: Nichols DH, ed. *Clinical problems, injuries and complications of gynecologic surgery.* Baltimore: Williams & Wilkins; 1988.
15. Semm K. *Operative manual for endoscopic abdominal surgery.* Chicago: Year Book; 1987:130.
16. Soderstrom RM, Butler JC. A critical evaluation of complications in laparoscopy. *J Reprod Med* 1973;10:245.
17. Nezhat FR, Silfen SL, Evans D, Nezhat C. Comparison of direct insertion of disposable and standard reusable laparoscopic trocars and previous pneumoperitoneum with Veress needle. *Obstet Gynecol* 1991;78:148.
18. Borgatta L, Gruss L, Barad D, Kaali SG. Direct trocar insertion vs. Veress needle use for laparoscopic sterilization. *J Reprod Med* 1990;35:891.
19. Copeland C, Wing R, Hulka JF. Direct trocar insertion at laparoscopy: an evaluation. *Obstet Gynecol* 1983;62:655.
20. Dingfelder JR. Direct laparoscopic trocar insertion without prior pneumoperitoneum. *J Reprod Med* 1978;21:45.
21. Jarrett JC. Laparoscopy: direct trocar insertion without pneumoperitoneum. *Obstet Gynecol* 1990;75:725.
22. Kaali SG, Bartfai G. Direct insertion of the laparoscopic trocar after an earlier laparotomy. *J Reprod Med* 1988;33:739.
23. Saidi MH. Direct laparoscopy without prior pneumoperitoneum. *J Reprod Med* 1986;31:684.
24. Hasson HM. Open laparoscopy: a modified instrument and method for laparoscopy. *Am J Obstet Gynecol* 1971;110:886.
25. Hasson HM. Open laparoscopy vs closed laparoscopy: a comparison of complication rates. *Adv Plann Parent* 1978;13:41.
26. Reich H, McGlynn F. Short self-retaining trocar sleeves for laparoscopic surgery. *Am J Obstet Gynecol* 1990;162:453.
27. Pagidas K, Tulandi T. Effects of Ringer's lactate, Interceed (TC7) and Gore-Tex surgical membrane on Post-surgical adhesion formation. *Fertil Steril* 1992;57(1):199–201.
28. Luciano AA, Lowney J, Jacobs SL. Endoscopic treatment of endometriosis-associated infertility: therapeutic, economic and social benefits. *J Reprod Med* 1992;37:573.
29. Lacey CG. Laparoscopy: a clinical sign for intraperitoneal needle placement. *Obstet Gynecol* 1976;47:625.

Endoscopic Management of Gynecologic Disease,
edited by G.D. Adamson and D.C. Martin.
Lippincott-Raven Publishers, Philadelphia © 1996.

CHAPTER 9

Postoperative Adhesion Development After Operative Laparoscopy

Evaluation at Early Second-Look Procedures

Fayek N. Shamma and Michael P. Diamond

Adhesions tend to develop after most reproductive surgical procedures and present as either de novo formation or adhesion reformation. In addition to decreased fertility of the female patient, which is presumably secondary to a hindrance in ovum pickup, the impact of adhesions is manifested by development of acute and chronic pelvic pain and by gastrointestinal dysfunction. Thus, concern for the development of postoperative adhesions is a pervasive issue. The following is a discussion of the etiology of the development of these pelvic adhesions and addresses the role of various therapies in their prevention.

PREVALENCE

Despite the use of elaborate surgical techniques and various adjuvants, adhesions tend to develop after most types of reconstructive operative surgeries. The use of second-look laparoscopy allows the surgeon to assess the extent of these adhesions. Most studies show that after reproductive pelvic surgery, adhesions redevelop in ~55–100% of the cases with an average of 85–90% (1). In addition, de novo adhesion formation is also a concern. De novo adhesion formation is the development of adhesions identified at the time of a second-look procedure at sites where there were no adhesions at the time of the initial procedure. This would include sites that were operated on at the time of the initial procedure or other sites in the pelvis. Such adhesions are noted in approximately 50% of patients, and in these patients such adhesions are noted on approximately a third of the available sites (2).

PATHOGENESIS

The etiology of pelvic adhesions is not well established. The peritoneal lining consists of a continuous layer of mesothelial cells overlying loose connective tissue. This loose tissue is made up of collagen and elastin fibers, fibroblasts, other mononuclear cells, adipocytes, and blood vessels. In response to injury and in normal healing, the peritoneum repairs itself by metaplasia of the underlying connective tissue rather than from the defect margins.

Generally, adhesions are believed to occur secondarily to abnormalities in the normal healing processes. When peritoneal injury occurs, there is exudation of a proteinaceous, serosanguinous fluid. In normal healing, this fluid is resorbed as a result of peritoneal fibrinolytic activity. The mesothelium is restored and healing occurs without scarring. This fibrinolytic activity is mostly secondary to the intrinsic peritoneal plasminogen activator activity. However, in situations accompanied by devascularization, such as tissue ischemia or where suture materials are present, there is a decrease in the natural endogenous plasminogen activator activity. Consequently, the serosanguinous coagulum persists, and fibroblasts migrate into the fibrin matrix consisting of the coagulum and cellular debris and commence proliferating with

F. N. Shamma: Department of Obstetrics and Gynecology, Michigan State University; and Ann Arbor Reproductive Medicine Associates, Ypsilanti, Michigan 48197.

M. P. Diamond: Division of Reproductive Endocrinology and Infertility, Wayne State University, Detroit, Michigan 48201.

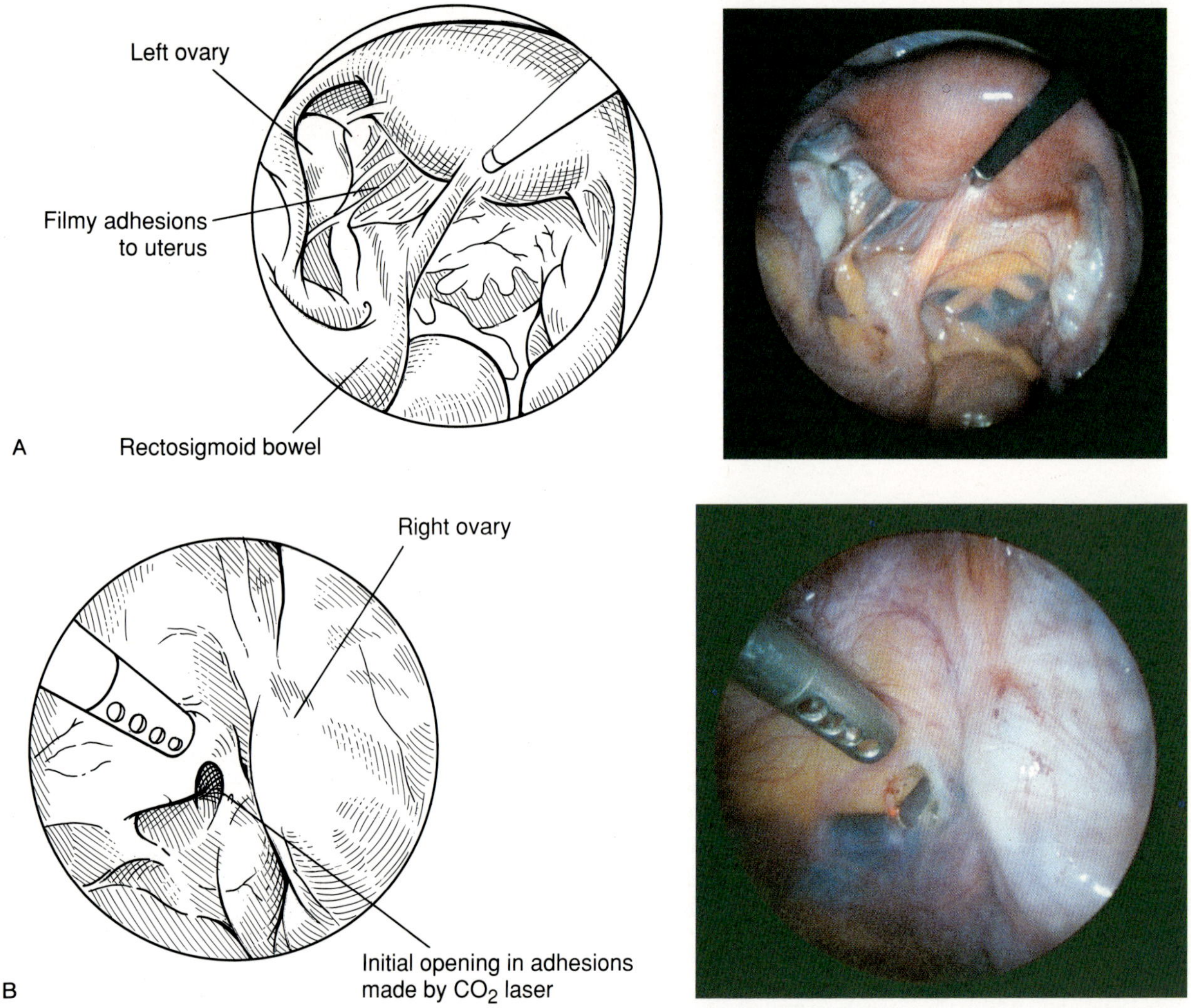

FIG. 1. Filmy pelvic adhesions. **A:** Overview of pelvis. **B:** At higher magnification. (Courtesy of G. David Adamson, M.D.)

subsequent collagen deposition and resultant scar formation (3).

SURGICAL APPROACHES IN PELVIC ADHESION PREVENTION

The clinical impact of adhesions on fertility depends on the extent and location of the adhesions. Jessen first described an improved pregnancy rate in the presence of low-grade (64%) vs. high-grade (22%) adhesions (4). Hulka then showed that pregnancy is more likely to occur when less than 50% of the ovary is covered with adhesions and when these adhesions are filmy and avascular (Figs. 1–3) rather than dense and vascular (Fig. 4) (5). Similarly, Caspi demonstrated that pregnancy rates are higher in association with fine, avascular adhesions than with fibrous, dense adhesions (6).

The role of adhesions and adhesiolysis is clouded by the degree and the extent of tubal disease. Rock and associates developed a classification system of distal tubal disease based on hydrosalpinx diameter, rugal pattern, and the extent of fimbrial damage and of coexistent pelvic adhesions; they demonstrated a worsening outcome with progression of the disease from mild to moderate to severe (7). Boer-Meisel and colleagues added two other parameters: hydrosalpinx tubal wall thickness and macroscopic assessment of the condition of the endosalpinx. They also noted a worsening pregnancy outcome with worsening disease (8). The American Fertility Society developed and proposed a standard classification system to describe the extent of pelvic disease. The system scores adhesions, based on whether they are filmy or dense, whether the cul-de-sac is partially or completely obliterated, and on the extent of ovarian and tubal enclosure by the adhesions (9). However, validation of this scoring system for prediction of pregnancy outcome remains to be performed.

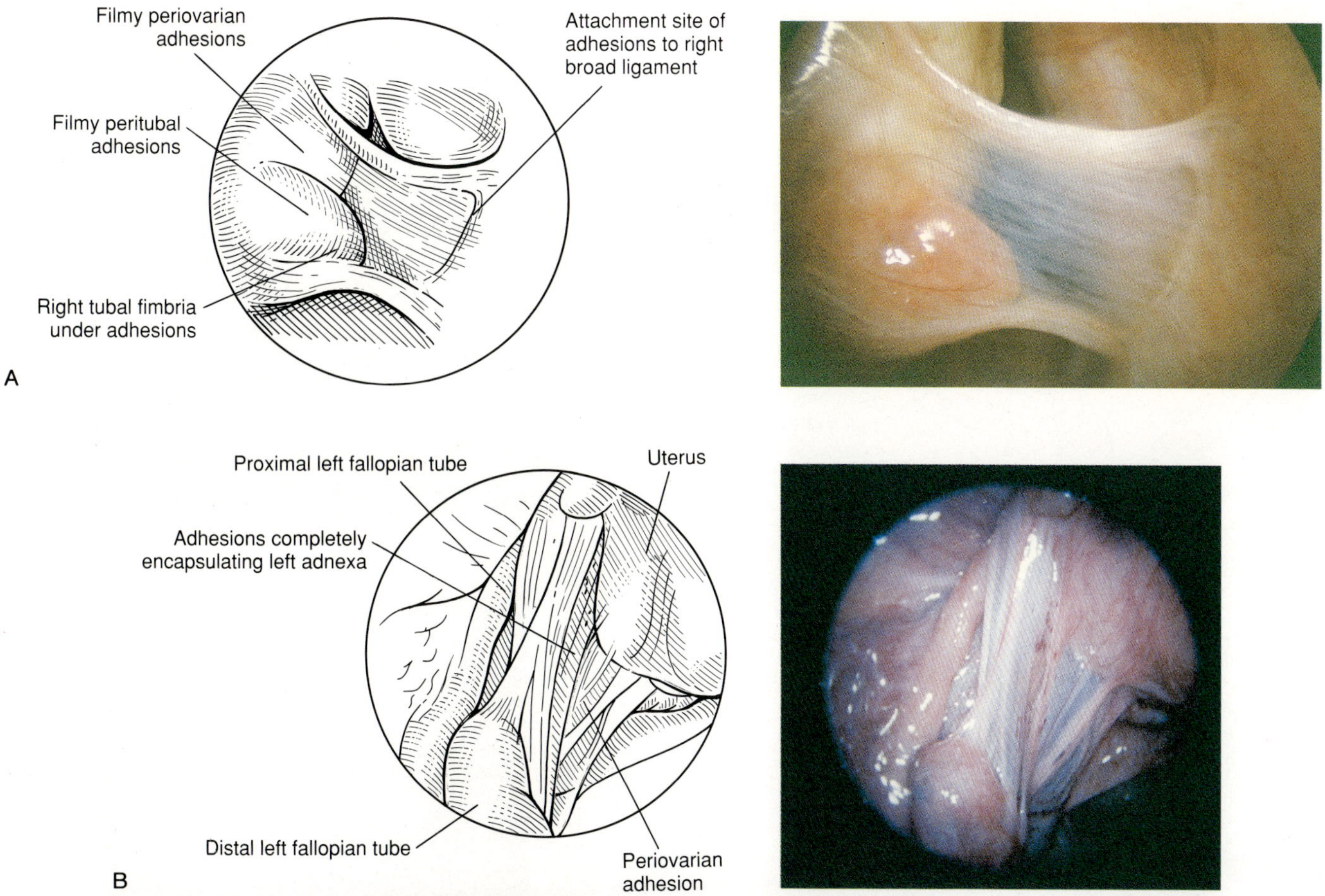

FIG. 2. Filmy periovarian and peritubal adhesions. **A:** Partial encapsulation. **B:** Complete encapsulation.

In the face of the deleterious reproductive effect of adhesions, various techniques exist and can be used in their prevention. During laparotomy, the use of microsurgical technique has been shown in various studies to improve the pregnancy rate and result in fewer adhesions as assessed by second-look laparoscopy (1,10,11). The microsurgical principles do not include only tissue magnification but also gentler tissue handling, meticulous hemostasis, precise approximation of tissue planes, and careful attention to sterile techniques. Magnification is important as it allows the use of smaller caliber suture material with resultant less foreign body reaction, closer inspection and differentiation between normal and abnormal tissue, and precise microcoagulation of bleeding points. All of this results in a decrease in tissue ischemia with less secondary adhesion formation. Adequate irrigation is important as it keeps the tissues moist and helps prevent ischemia. Certainly irrigation is better than sponging as the latter is associated with persistence of foreign materials and abrasion of peritoneal surfaces and, hence, an increased possibility of adhesion formation. However, the value of precise approximation of tissue planes has now been called into question with some investigators thinking that tissue approximation may actually cause rather than prevent postoperative adhesion development. This adverse outcome may be hypothesized to be due to tissue ischemia created by the sutures or clips used in tissue approximation (12).

Operative laparoscopy has replaced laparotomy in some patients not only in the diagnosis of pelvic adhesions but also in their management. Operative laparoscopy is hypothesized to be associated with less patient morbidity, hospital time, and hospital expense and with a shortened time for the patient to return to full activity.

The microsurgical principle of operative laparoscopy is similar to that described above with laparotomy. The Trendelenburg position and adequate pneumoperitoneum help displace the bowel from the operating field and enhance visualization. A multiple puncture technique is encouraged in order to manipulate pelvic structures properly and improve access to areas of pathology. Appropriate instrumentation is mandatory as is surgical assistance. As in laparotomy, the laparoscopic surgical technique should be as atraumatic as possible, with emphasis on hemostasis, gentle handling of tissue, avoidance of foreign substances, and continuous irrigation. In

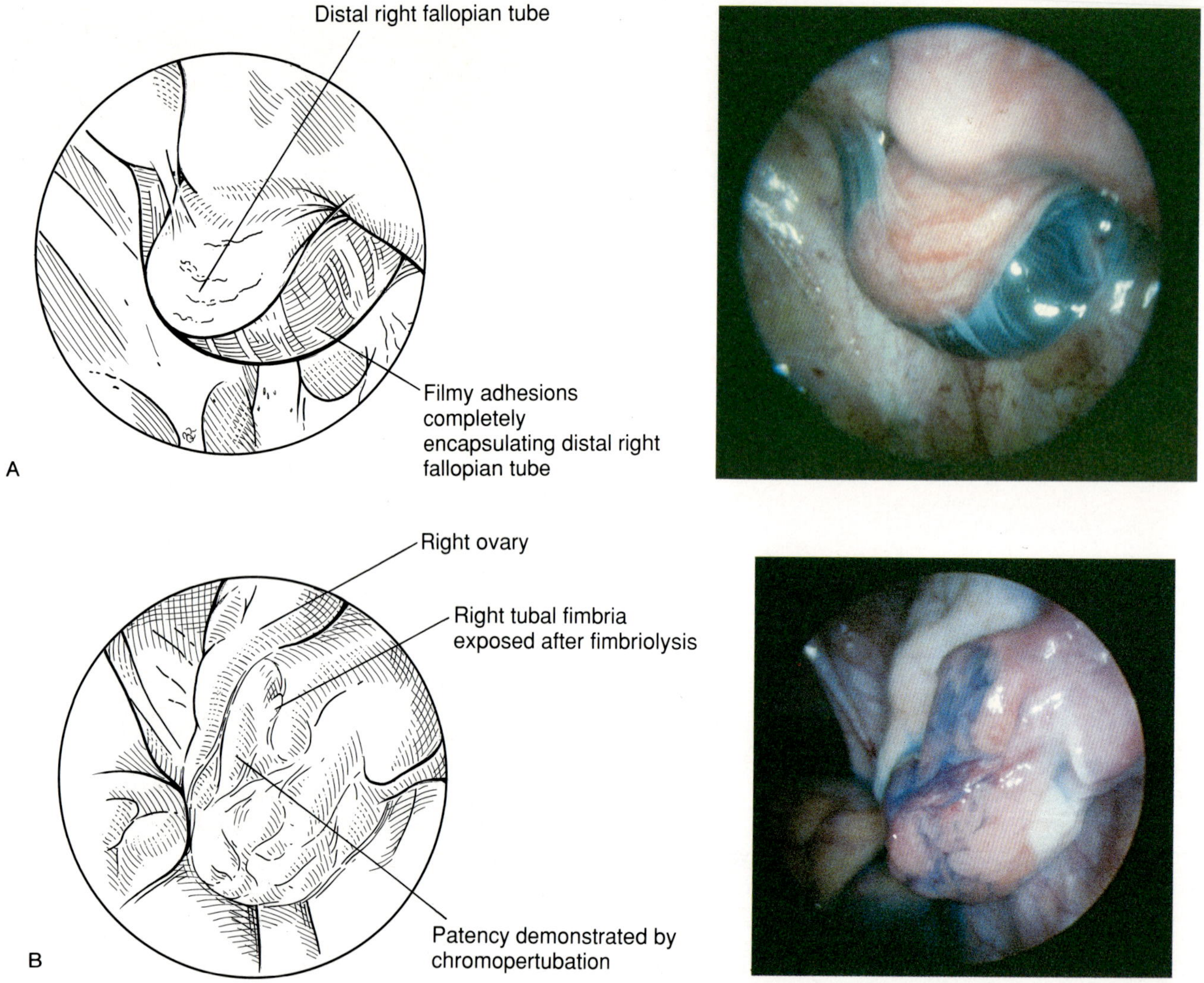

FIG. 3. Filmy, avascular perifimbrial adhesions. **A:** Before treatment. **B:** After treatment.

addition, as in laparotomy, the use of adjuvants for adhesion prevention might be helpful. Finally, the laparoscopic expertise of the surgeon is likely to play a role in the successful outcome of operative laparoscopy. This has been demonstrated to be the case at laparotomy in both the animal model and clinical experience (3).

Randomized clinical trials to assess the advantages of laparoscopy over laparotomy are lacking. Fayez and his colleagues have suggested that operative laparoscopy may be more advantageous when salpingolysis, ovariolysis, or salpingoovariolysis is performed, whereas laparotomy with the use of microsurgical techniques may be beneficial when fimbrioplasty or neosalpingostomy are performed (11,13). This is based on lower pregnancy rates—35% and 10%, respectively—when the latter two procedures were performed laparoscopically. These rates are lower than what have been traditionally reported with laparotomy (13).

Operative laparoscopy seems to offer some advantages over laparotomy in de novo adhesion formation. In contrast to adhesion reformation, which occurred in 97% of patients following adhesiolysis, de novo adhesion formation tended to occur in only 12% of patients in a recent study by the Operative Laparoscopy Study Group (14). This rate of de novo adhesion formation is considerably lower than what has been reported following laparotomy. However the potential perils of direct comparisons of different study groups make definitive conclusions difficult.

The laser has been utilized in the past decade for reconstructive surgery. Its ability to make precise incisions with little adjacent tissue injury has been suggested as possibly preventing adhesion formation. Animal model studies suggest that use of high power density laser seems to result in fewer adhesions when compared with microelectrosurgery (15,16). However, results from a pro-

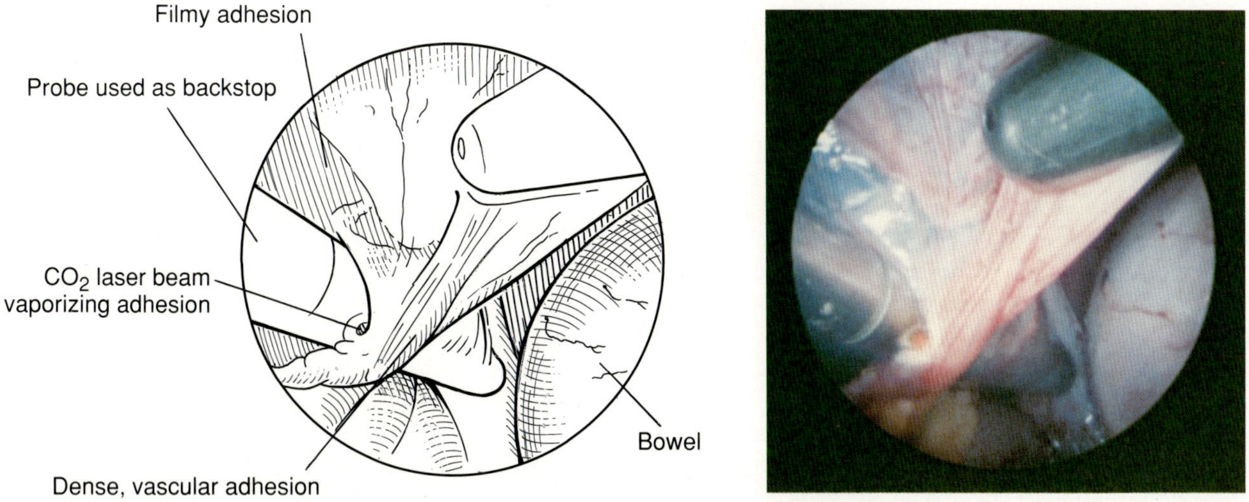

FIG. 4. Dense, vascular adhesion being treated with CO_2 laser.

spective randomized clinical trial comparing the CO_2 laser and microdiathermy for salpingoovariolysis failed to show improved pregnancy rates (17). Currently the general consensus is that use of a laser per se does not offer advantages over other techniques with regard to either postoperative adhesion development or subsequent pregnancy outcome.

The use of second-look laparoscopy has been utilized not only diagnostically but therapeutically to lyse the reformed and newly formed adhesions (18). Trimbos-Kemper, using third-look laparoscopy to evaluate the effectiveness of the adhesiolysis performed during second-look laparoscopy, concluded that second-look laparoscopy significantly reduced the occurrence of pelvic adhesions (19). However, Tulandi in a small prospective randomized study, in which intrauterine pregnancy was an endpoint after operative second-look laparoscopy was performed a year after reproductive surgery, found no significant difference in pregnancy rates (20). Thus, the role of second-look laparoscopy awaits further, larger randomized prospective studies.

ADJUVANTS AND MATERIALS UTILIZED IN ADHESION PREVENTION

Various agents have been used in an attempt to curb the development of adhesions following reproductive surgery. These include antiinflammatory agents, antico-

TABLE 1. *Classes of adhesion reduction adjuvants*

Fibrinolytic agents	Mechanical separation
Fibrinolysin	Dextran
Papain	Mineral oil
Streptokinase	Silicone
Urokinase	Povidine
Hyaluronidase	Vaseline
Chymotrysin	Crystalloid solutions
Trypsin	Carboxymethylcellulose
Pepsin	Barriers
Plasminogen activators	Endogenous tissue
Anticoagulants	Omental grafts
Heparin	Peritoneal grafts
Citrates	Bladder strips
Oxalates	Fetal membranes
Antiinflammatory agents	Exogenous material
Corticosteroids	Oxidized cellulose
Nonsteroidal antiinflammatory agents	Oxidized regenerated cellulose
Antihistamines	Polytetrafluoroethylene (PTFE)
Progesterone	Gelatin
Calcium channel blockers	Rubber sheets
Antibiotics	Metal foils
Tetracyclines	Plastic hoods
Cephalosporins	

agulants, antibiotics, fibrinolytic agents, agents that promote plasminogen activator activity, intraabdominal instillates, and endogenous or exogenous barriers (see Table 1).

Corticosteroids—with their ability to decrease vascular permeability, mitigate the inflammatory tissue response to injury, and stabilize lysosomal membranes thus inhibiting the release of various humoral factors—have been utilized perioperatively for adhesion prevention. They have been commonly used in conjunction with promethazine, an antihistamine. However, most studies in large animals or humans have failed to show an improvement in adhesion prevention. Other antiinflammatory agents, such as ibuprofen, have also been utilized perioperatively. Again, most studies have failed to show ibuprofen to be effective in adhesion prevention (21–23).

Anticoagulants, including low-dose heparin (5 IU/ml), have been used as intraabdominal irrigants. However, Jansen, Rock, and colleagues found anticoagulants not to be more effective than use of lactated Ringer's solution alone (24,25). The systemic use of heparin is not recommended in view of the high incidence of associated bleeding complications. Similar potential complications after use of intraperitoneal urokinase make it unpopular for adhesion prevention. Various new adjuvants were recently investigated in animal models (26). These include calcium channel blockers, recombinant tissue plasminogen activator, and pentoxifylline, a methylxanthine derivative. Although effective in certain animal models, human clinical studies are lacking (27,28).

Mechanical separation has been used in adhesion prevention and involves either intraabdominal instillates or barriers. The most commonly used instillate is 32% dextran 70 (Hyskon; Pharmacia, Piscataway, NJ). Its mechanism of action is probably related to its ability to induce hydroflotation of pelvic organs and to its siliconizing properties. The instillation of dextran 70 was noted to prevent adhesion formation in various animal models. However, the results of human clinical trials have been mixed (3). Its use has been associated with certain complications including leakage from the incision, labial

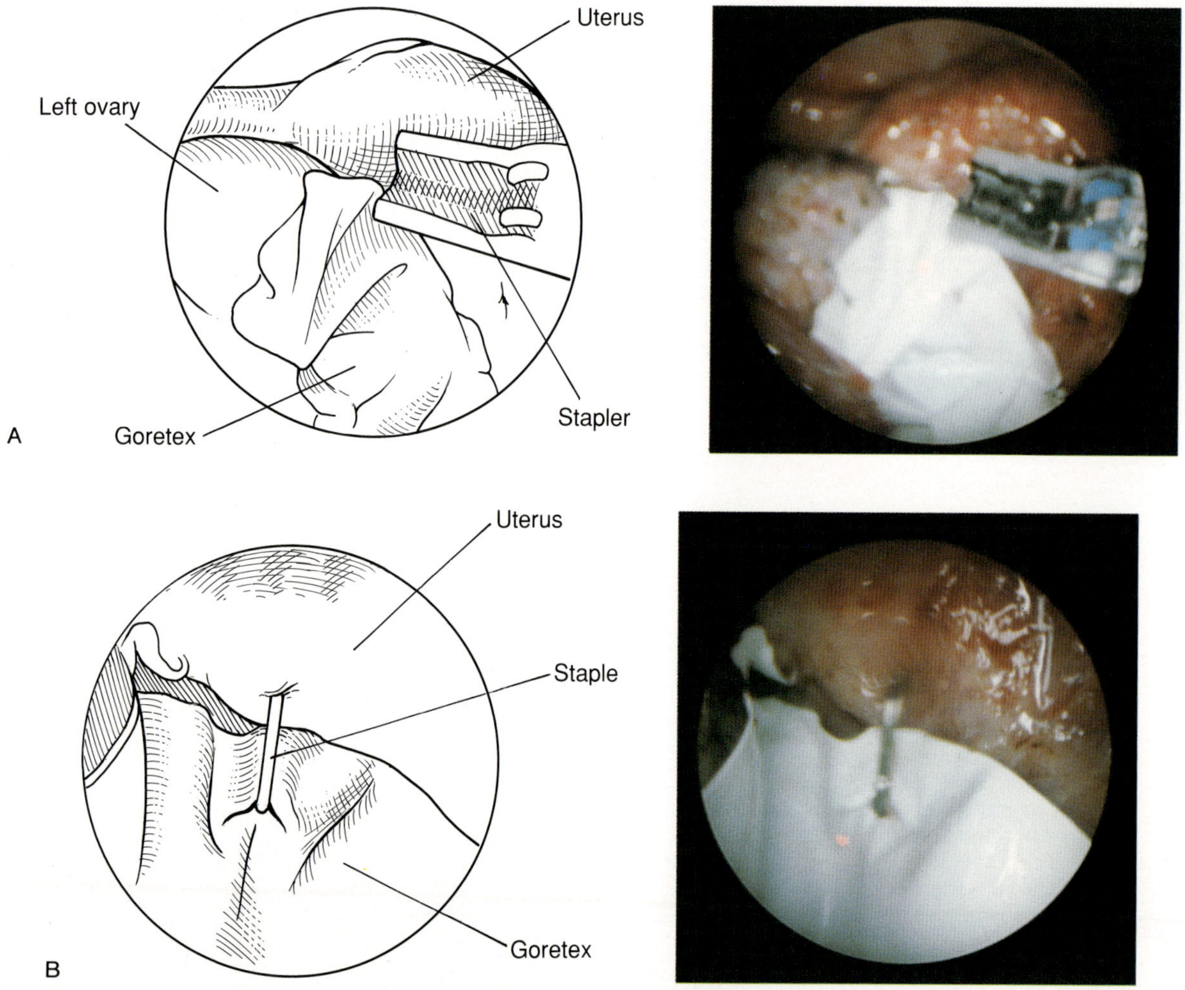

FIG. 5. A: Endoscopic stapling of Gore-Tex. **B:** Gore-Tex stapled in place.

swelling, abdominal bloating, and transient increases in liver function tests.

Mechanical barriers of endogenous materials, such as omental and peritoneal grafts, are not recommended as their use has resulted in increased adhesion formation. However, two exogenous materials have been used in an attempt to decrease adhesion reformation and de novo adhesion formation. These are Interceed (Tc-7; Johnson & Johnson Medical, Inc., Arlington, TX), a fabric made up of oxidized regenerated cellulose similar to Surgicel (Ethicon, Inc., Somerville, NJ), and Gore-Tex surgical membrane (W. L. Gore, Flagstaff, AZ), a material of nonreactive expanded polytetrafluoroethylene (PTFE). Tc-7 has been noted to reduce the incidence and severity of postsurgical pelvic side wall adhesions in a multicenter clinical trial (29). The Gore-Tex surgical membrane has been shown to be an effective barrier in the rabbit model. Although it requires suturing to hold it in place and subsequent removal (unless it is to be left in place chronically) (30), it can be used endoscopically (Fig. 5).

Polaxamers, which are biocompatible and bioabsorbable materials, have been successfully utilized as barriers for adhesion prevention in animal models (31). They have the property of reverse thermal gelation: they change from a viscous fluid at low temperature (e.g., between 4°C and room temperature) to a firm gel at body temperature. This property offers significant promise for clinical use.

HIGHLIGHTS

Prevention of pelvic adhesions continues to be of paramount importance after reconstructive pelvic surgery. It should be emphasized that the use of adjuvants, materials, and new surgical techniques cannot replace and should complement the pivotal role of the pelvic surgeon in adhering to sound microsurgical techniques during laparoscopy and laparotomy.

REFERENCES

1. Diamond MP. Surgical aspects of infertility. In: Sciarra JJ, ed. *Gynecology and obstetrics*. Vol 5. Philadelphia: Harper and Row; 1988:1–23.
2. Diamond MP, Daniell JF, Teste J, et al. Adhesion reformation and de novo adhesion formation following reproductive pelvic surgery. *Fertil Steril* 1987;47:864–866.
3. Diamond MP, DeCherney AH. Pathogenesis of adhesion formation/reformation: application to reproductive pelvic surgery. *Microsurgery* 1987;8:103–107.
4. Jessen H. Forty-five operations for sterility. *Acta Obstet Gynecol Scand* 1971;50:105.
5. Hulka JF. Adnexal adhesions: a prognostic staging and classification system based on a five-year survey of fertility surgery results at Chapel Hill, North Carolina. *Am J Obstet Gynecol* 1982;144:141.
6. Caspi E, Halperin Y, Bukovsky I. The importance of periadnexal adhesions in tubal reconstructive surgery for infertility. *Fertil Steril* 1979;31:296.
7. Rock JA, Katayama KP, Martin EF. Factors influencing the success of salpingostomy techniques for distal fimbrial obstruction. *Obstet Gynecol* 1978;52:591.
8. Boer-Meisel ME, te Velde ER, Habbema JDF, et al. Predicting the pregnancy outcome in patients treated for hydrosalpinx: A prospective study. *Fertil Steril* 1986;45:23.
9. American Fertility Society. Classifications of adnexal adhesions, distal tubal occlusion, tubal occlusion secondary to tubal ligation, tubal pregnancies, Mullerian anomalies and intrauterine adhesions. *Fertil Steril* 1988;49:944.
10. Gomel V. The impact of microsurgery in gynecology. *Clin Obstet Gynecol* 1980;23:1031–1310.
11. Fayez JA, Suliman SO. Infertility surgery of the oviduct: comparison between macrosurgery and microsurgery. *Fertil Steril* 1982;37:73.
12. Meyer WR, Grainger DA, DeCherney AH, Lachs MS, Diamond MP. Ovarian surgery in the rabbit: Effect of cortex closure on adhesion formation and ovarian function. *J Reprod Med.* 1981;36:639.
13. Fayez JA. An assessment of the role of operative laparoscopy in tuboplasty. *Fertil Steril* 1983;39:476.
14. Operative Laparoscopy Study Group. Postoperative adhesion development after operative laparoscopy: evaluation at early second-look procedure. *Fertil Steril* 1991;55:770.
15. Filmar S, Gomel V, McComb P. The effectiveness of CO_2 laser and electromicrosurgery in adhesiolysis: a comparative study. *Fertil Steril* 1986;45:407.
16. Bellina JF, Hemmings R, Voros JI, et al. Carbon dioxide laser and electrosurgical wound study with an animal model: a comparison of tissue damage and healing patterns in peritoneal tissue. *Am J Obstet Gynecol* 1984;148:327.
17. Tulandi T. Salpingo-ovariolysis: a comparison between laser surgery and electrosurgery. *Fertil Steril* 1986;45:489.
18. Jansen RP. Early laparoscopy after pelvic operations to prevent adhesions: safety, efficacy. *Fertil Steril* 1988;49:26–31.
19. Trimbos-Kemper TCM, Trimbos JF, Van Hall EV. Adhesion formation after tubal surgery: results of the eighth day laparoscopy in 188 patients. *Fertil Steril* 1985;43:395.
20. Tulandi T, Falcone T, Kafka I. Second-look operative laparoscopy 1 year following reproductive surgery. *Fertil Steril* 1989;52:421.
21. Granat M, Schenken JC, Mor-Yosef S, et al. Effects of dexamethasone on proliferation of autologous fibroblasts and on the immune profile in women undergoing pelvic surgery for infertility. *Fertil Steril* 1983;39:180.
22. Jansen RPS. Failure of intraperitoneal irrigation with heparin during pelvic operations upon young women to reduce adhesions. *Surg Gynecol Obstet* 1988;166:154.
23. Holtz G. Failure of a nonsteroidal anti-inflammatory agent (ibuprofen) to inhibit peritoneal adhesion reformation after lysis. *Fertil Steril* 1982;37:582.
24. Jansen RPS. Failure of intraperitoneal irrigation with heparin during pelvic operations upon young women to reduce adhesions. *Surg Gynecol Obstet* 1988;166:154.
25. Rock JA, Cohen SM, Franklin RR, et al. Clinical evaluation of Interceed (TC7) absorbable adhesion barrier: role of adhesiolysis techniques and heparin irrigation on adhesion formation. Presented at the 45th Annual Meeting of the American Fertility Society, San Francisco, CA, November 1989.
26. Drollette CM, Badawy SZA. Pathophysiology of pelvic adhesions. *J Reprod Med* 1992;37:107.
27. Montz FJ, Fowler JM, Wolff AJ, Lacey SM, Mohler M. The ability of recombinant tissue plasminogen activator to inhibit post-radical pelvic surgery adhesions in the dog model. *Am J Obstet Gynecol* 1991;165:1539.
28. Steinleitner A, Lambert H, Kazensky C, Danks P, Roy S. Pentoxifylline, a methylxanthine derivative, prevents postsurgical adhesion reformation in rabbits. *Obstet Gynecol* 1990;75:926.
29. Interceed (TC7) Adhesion Barrier Study Group. Prevention of postsurgical adhesions by Interceed (TC7), an absorbable adhesion barrier: a prospective randomized multicenter clinical study. *Fertil Steril* 1989;51:933.
30. Boyers SP, Diamond MP, DeCherney AH. Reduction of postoperative adhesions in the rabbit with Gore-Tex surgical membrane. *Fertil Steril* 1988;49:1066.
31. Steinleitner A, Lopez G, Suarez M, Lambert H. An evaluation of Flowgel as an intraperitoneal barrier for prevention of postsurgical adhesion reformation. *Fertil Steril* 1992;57:305.

Endoscopic Management of Gynecologic Disease,
edited by G.D. Adamson and D.C. Martin.
Lippincott-Raven Publishers, Philadelphia © 1996.

CHAPTER 10

Salpingoplasty and Neosalpingostomy

Joseph R. Feste

The fimbriated end of the fallopian tube is crucial to fertility. Without patency and reasonably normal fimbria, pregnancy rarely occurs without the aid of assisted reproductive technology, i.e., in vitro fertilization, regardless of other pelvic pathology. Therefore, how one approaches fimbrial disease is extremely important, since the first attempt at surgical repair is the most critical one.

PATHOPHYSIOLOGY

Salpingoplasty, in contrast to salpingostomy, is the repair of only partial rather than complete obstruction of the fimbria. Other terms used to describe these procedures are *fimbrioplasty* and *neosalpingostomy,* respectively. The long-term sequelae of salpingitis includes chronic pelvic pain, ectopic pregnancy, and infertility (1). Forty percent of infertility in women has been reported to result from tubal damage due to salpingitis (2). Westrom reported bilateral tubal occlusion in 13% of patients after one episode of salpingitis, in 35% after two episodes, and in 75% after three or more episodes (3). The majority of cases of complete hydrosalpinx have been found secondary to tubal infection with either *Neisseria gonorrhea* or *Chlamydia trachomatis* or both. It is presumed that infection associated with either one of these organisms, if treated early and aggressively, may lead to only minimal damage. In these cases, the mucosal folds are less severely damaged and pregnancy rates are better. With respect to endometriosis, partial or complete obstruction of the fimbria is most often due to extensive adhesion formation. The fimbria become trapped within adhesions, sparing destruction of the mucosal folds.

J. R. Feste: Department of Obstetrics and Gynecology, Baylor College of Medicine, University Health Science Center, Houston, Texas 77054.

Other gram-negative bacteria have been described as major infecting organisms in pelvic inflammatory disease. The predominant facilitative aerobic pathogen found in the tuboperitoneal fluid obtained from women with salpingitis is *Escherichia coli,* whereas the prominent anaerobic pathogens are in the *Bacteroides* species. It is thought that the major damaging effect on tubal mucosa is mediated through endotoxin liberated from the bacterial cell wall. Close observation in those cases of partial obstruction reveals mostly normal infundibulum, with its concentric folds leading to the ostium. Normal folds contain a multitude of ciliated cells covering approximately 50% of the surface of the infundibulum. However, in the case of a total hydrosalpinx, there is marked damage of the cilia. When total obstruction is present, the pressure within the tube eventually flattens out the mucosal folds and the ciliated epithelium is completely destroyed. This lack of ciliated epithelium greatly contributes to low pregnancy rates, even after neosalpingostomy is performed and tubal patency is achieved.

DIAGNOSIS

Many patients with distal tubal disease present with a history of salpingitis manifested by fever, pelvic pain, foul vaginal discharge, and extreme tenderness on pelvic examination. For years, the most common cause of salpingitis was *Neisseria gonorrhea.* However, over the last several years, the presence of *Chlamydia trachomatis* has become more prevalent. The latter has been coined the silent infection because in many instances it causes no clinically demonstrable symptoms. Only at the time of a hysterosalpingogram or diagnostic laparoscopy is the hydrosalpinx recognized (Figs. 1 and 2). In such cases, it is extremely important for patients to be treated with prophylactic antibiotics during and after the procedure to prevent recurrent infection in the susceptible endosalpinx.

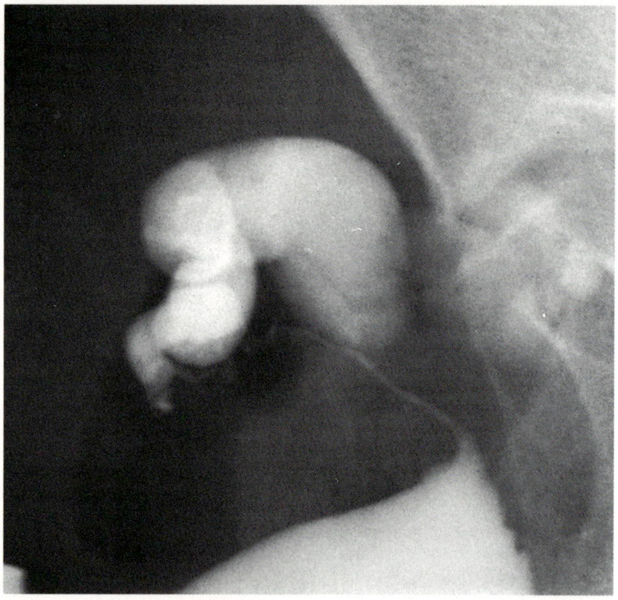

FIG. 1. Hysterosalpingogram revealing unilateral hydrosalpinx.

PATIENT SELECTION

The next important issue is proper selection of patients. This decision often is made only at the time of the diagnostic laparoscopy. If the patient has had prior surgery, an operative record from a referring physician helps on occasion in the counseling of the patient on what to expect and may alter the approach taken at the time of surgery. However, even with a very good description of the pelvic structures, only the exterior surface of the fallopian tube is evaluated on routine laparoscopy. On the other hand, tuboscopy performed at the time of a diagnostic laparoscopy is an excellent technique for evaluation of endosalpingeal architecture and, hence, the extent of inner tubal damage (4,5). Usually, a small hole is drilled in the area of puckering, and a small flexible tuboscope is inserted. Three different conditions may exist that would help in deciding which surgical approach would be best (see Table 1). A patient with a very thin-walled, markedly dilated hydrosalpinx and with no interstitial adhesions is an ideal candidate for laparoscopic neosalpingostomy. However, tubes of this type usually are associated with a poor prognosis for pregnancy, i.e., 20–25% term pregnancy rates. This type of anatomic defect comprises more than 80% of the hydrosalpinges seen. If the wall is of normal thickness and there are no interstitial adhesions, it becomes difficult to keep the fimbriated end open when the Bruhat technique is used or the edges are sutured back (6). These tubes probably would be best treated by laparotomy in which proper placement of fine sutures would allow a greater likelihood for the tube to stay open. This type of anatomic defect is certainly not the one most likely to occur but probably has the best prognosis for pregnancy, usually a 45 to 50% pregnancy rate. In those cases where the tuboplasty reveals extensive intratubal adhesions, repair should not be attempted because of dismal postoperative pregnancy rates and the high incidence of ectopic pregnancies. These latter patients should undergo in vitro fertilization.

TABLE 1. *Neosalpingostomy: selection of procedure based on tuboscopy*

Finding	Procedural approach
>1–3 cm dilated fimbria; no interstitial adhesions; thin wall	Laparoscopy
Undilated fimbria; no interstitial adhesions; wall of normal thickness	Laparotomy
Interstitial adhesions; thick or thin wall; dilated/undilated fimbria	In vitro fertilization

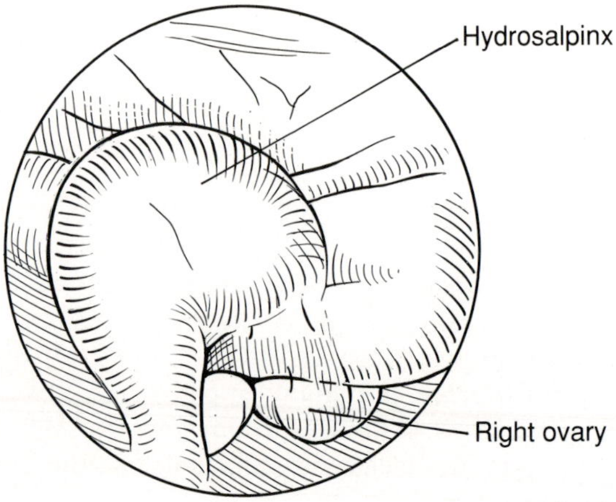

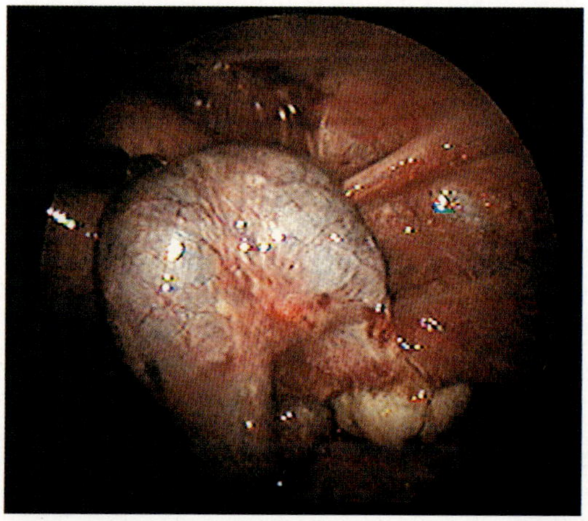

FIG. 2. Dilated and "clubbed" end of a hydrosalpinx.

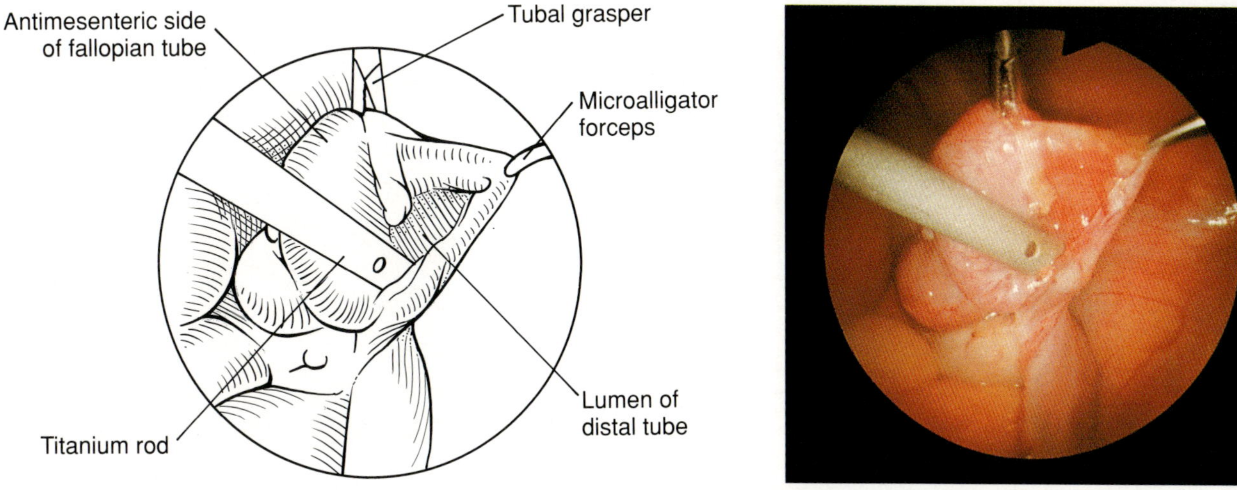

FIG. 3. Antimesenteric ampullary tube is stabilized with grasper, serosal edge is exposed with microalligator forceps, and titanium rod is used as a backstop for CO_2 laser beam.

PREPARATION FOR SURGERY

Before a salpingoplasty or neosalpingostomy is attempted, the tube and ovary must be freed of external adhesions. Unless the fimbria is freely movable, ovum pickup will be limited. Needless to say, if the ovary is covered with adhesions, ovum release will also be obstructed. Following adhesiolysis, there is the unfortunate possibility that adhesions will reform. Every effort should be made to reduce the recurrence of adhesions. Among the more common adjunctive measures used are irrigating solutions containing heparin, Interceed (7) or Gortex (8) barrier grafts, and administration of various intraoperative and postoperative medications. These alternative methods are described in other chapters.

Of note is the importance of a proper bowel preparation prior to surgery in cases of known hydrosalpinx. Although the likelihood of injury to the bowel may be remote, on occasion the rectosigmoid or small bowel may be densely adherent to the tubes and/or ovaries, and inadvertent entry could lead to disastrous consequences.

TECHNIQUES OF TREATMENT

Salpingoplasty

If adequate evaluation of the fallopian tube by tuboscopy shows only minimal adhesions of varying degrees around the end of the fimbria and less than total hydrosalpinx, it may be possible to remove the adhesions with scissors. For more vascular adhesions, laser or electrosurgical energy can be used. However, the choice of the laser wavelength is important as is the amount of

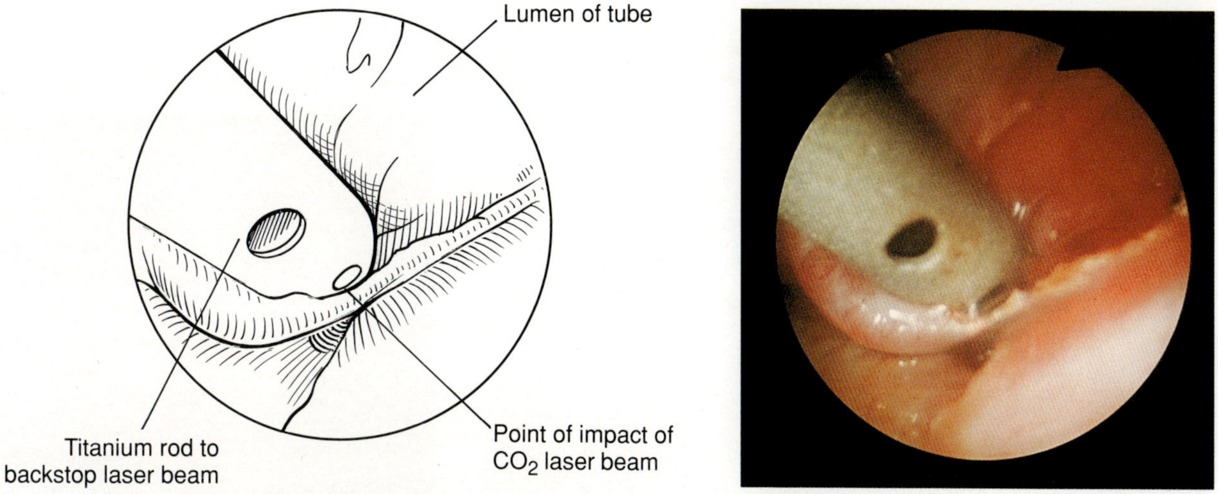

FIG. 4. Laparoscope is placed close to the distal fallopian tube, thereby providing magnification for creation of neosalpingostomy with titanium rod as backstop for CO_2 laser beam.

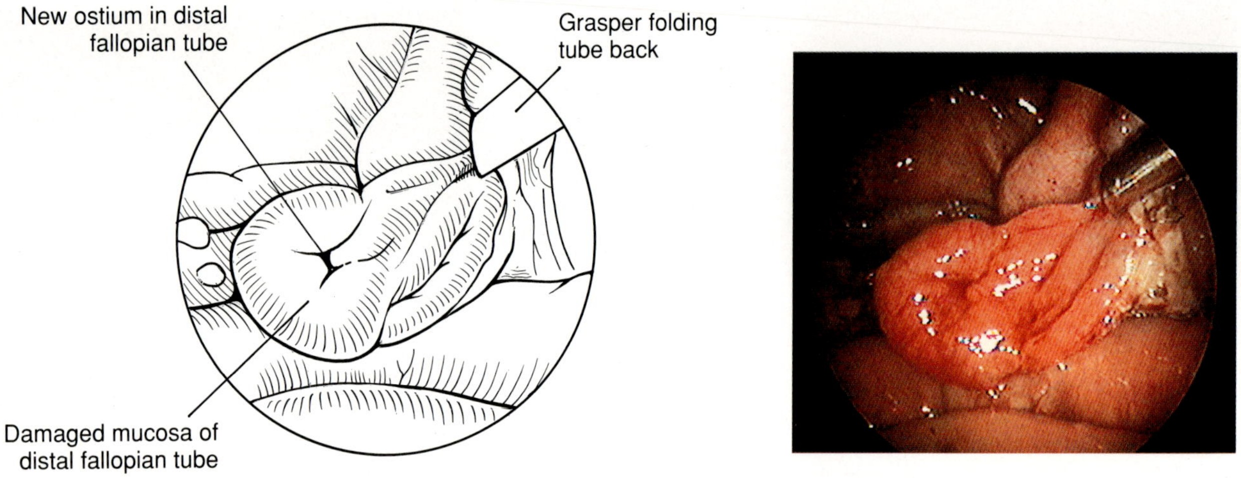

FIG. 5. Following the completion of the incisions to create the neosalpingostomy, the tube is folded back mechanically to ensure absence of tension on tissues. The Bruhat technique then is used to maintain the distal flaps in place.

exposure time of each burst of energy. In general, a focused CO_2 superpulse or a green wavelength with a 300-μm fiber can vaporize the adhesions precisely without significantly damaging the mucosa. It is important to use a titanium rod backstop within the tube to prevent damage to the normal mucosa. With careful dissection, the results can greatly improve the chances for pregnancy.

Neosalpingostomy

Using a transcervical insufflator, the surgeon distends the tube with indigo-carmine dye (Fig. 2). The end of the tube is superficially marked with an "X" so the lines of dissection are visible after the fluid within the tube is released and the tube collapses. In tubes with hydrosalpinges having obvious, discrete scarred areas, the incision line should be modified to follow and to remove scarred tissue. The linear incisions are etched on the distal end of the tube with a finely focused, high-wattage (35 W) CO_2 laser beam. The incision can be made with a quartz fiber from a YAG, argon, or potassium-trideuterium-phosphate (KTP) laser or with a pair of scissors after the markings are made. The first incision is made for a distance of at least 2–3 cm or along obvious scar lines, as modified by the nature and extent of the tubal scarring. A second incision in the tube is then extended with the same high-power-density laser beam 90° to the first linear incision in the end of the hydrosalpinx. When the blue dye begins to spill through the open tube, there is a complete collapse of the tube. At this time all references to the proper locations of the incisions are lost unless one has properly marked the tube as described. The incised ends of the tube are carefully grasped with two accessory forceps (Fig. 3 and 4). Atraumatic forceps are passed through second and third puncture sites for

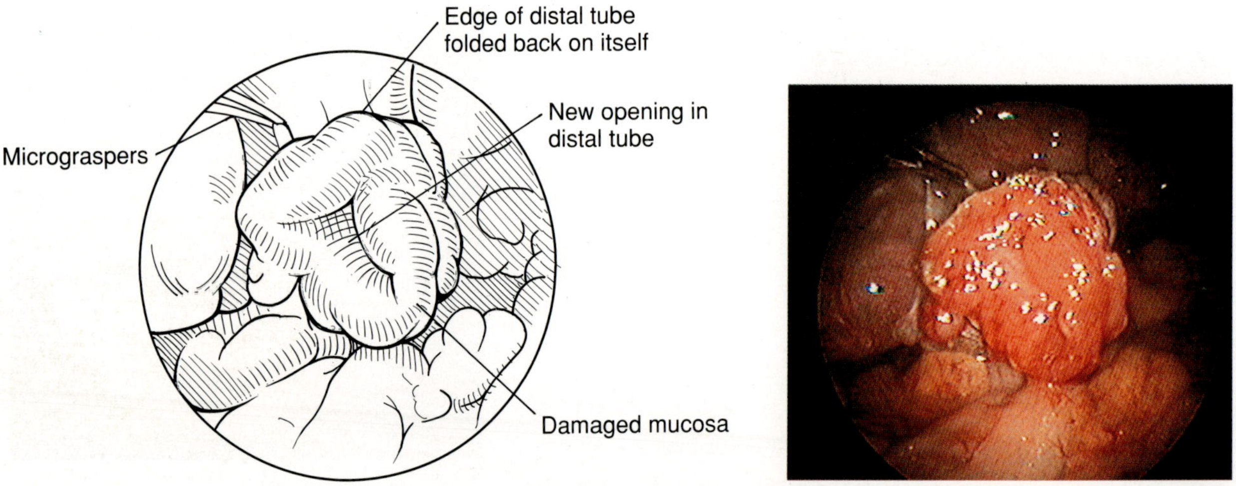

FIG. 6. Completed neosalpingostomy.

gentle countertraction on the tubal opening. When all four flaps are completely developed, the laser power is reduced to 5 W for the CO_2 laser, or is defocused in the case of the shorter wave lasers, 1–2 cm from the peritoneal surface of the newly developed flaps (Fig. 5). Next the beam is aimed at the peritoneum of the hydrosalpinx a few millimeters proximal to the apex of each flap. With the firing of this defocused, lower power density beam, the peritoneum contracts slowly and everts the edges of the hydrosalpinx. This procedure, described by Bruhat and known as the Bruhat maneuver, causes the newly constructed distal opening of the tube to flower back. As long as the developed flaps are long enough, this maneuver will adequately roll back each flap, and the peritoneum on the serosal surface of the tube will eventually agglutinate to help keep the new ostium open (Fig. 6).

Another technique may be a little simpler to develop but a little more difficult to complete. A single incision is made over the area of puckering. With two alligator forceps, the serosa proximal to the opening is pushed through the opening created in the tube. The tube is everted on itself for a distance of at least 2–3 cm to prevent the edges from retracting and the opening from returning to its original position. Neither this technique nor the Bruhat technique generally requires suturing open the tube unless it appears that the ostium created will not stay open. However, I prefer to suture all the flaps to maintain tubal patency. If a suture is used, size 4-0 or smaller is preferred under the shelving edge of each flap.

In severe cases, it may be necessary to incise along scar lines to obtain a more natural opening of the tube. In all cases, the surgical objective is to obtain the most functional distal fallopian tube.

RESULTS

In most instances, results of salpingoplasty or neosalpingostomy are based on the condition of the mucosal folds and the number of remaining ciliated cells. Tuboscopy probably is the best visual method to evaluate the prognosis for pregnancy. It is obvious that if the fimbria can be restored to normal with a simple fimbrioplasty the pregnancy rates will be excellent. Tubes that are partially blocked certainly are expected to provide a better chance of pregnancy than those that are completely blocked.

In the literature there are numerous reports of neosalpingostomies by laser techniques and conventional methods (9–16). Most studies cite pregnancy rates of 20–40%. The maximum full-term pregnancy rates are 18–32%, with an ectopic pregnancy rate of 2–14%. It is important to educate patients as to their prognosis for pregnancy after laparoscopic repair of tubal disease. The success rates for in vitro fertilization in some centers is now comparable to results obtained following distal tubal surgery. In vitro fertilization is less invasive, has a lower rate of ectopic pregnancies, but is more expensive. The patient who presents with distal tubal obstruction should be properly counseled with regard to the best approach.

HIGHLIGHTS

Laparoscopic neosalpingostomy offers less patient discomfort and is more economical than tubal surgery performed via laparotomy. The pregnancy rates have been equal to those achieved by laparotomy. However, these procedures must be performed by a skilled laparoscopist. With proper selection of patients, operative laparoscopy is often a desirable alternative to microsurgery by laparotomy for management of distal tube disease.

REFERENCES

1. Adler MW, Belsey EH, O'Conner BH. Morbidity associated with pelvic inflammatory disease. *Br J Vener Dis* 1982;58:151.
2. Weinstein L. Effect of pelvic inflammatory disease on infertility. *Am J Obstet Gynecol* 1980;1212:707.
3. Westrom L. Incidence, prevalence and trends of acute pelvic inflammation disease and its consequences in industrialized countries. *Am J Obstet Gynecol* 1980;138:880.
4. De Bruyne F, Puttemans P, Boeck W, Brosens I. The clinical value of salpingoscopy in tube infertility. *Fertil Steril* 1989;51(2):339–340.
5. Brosens IA, Puttemans PJ. Double-optic laparoscopy. Salpingoscopy, ovarian cystoscopy and endo-ovarian surgery with the argon laser. *Baillieres Clin Obstet Gynaecol* 1989;3(31):595–608.
6. Bruhat MA, Mage G, Manhes H, Soualhat C, Robert JF, Pouly JL. Laparoscopic procedures to promote fertility: ovariolysis and salpingolysis results of 93 selected cases. *Acta Eur Fertil* 1983;14:113.
7. Interceed (TC7) Adhesion Barrier Study Group, Johnson & Johnson Patient Care, Inc., New Brunswick, New Jersey. Prevention of postsurgical adhesions by INTERCEED (TC7), an absorbable adhesion barrier: a prospective, randomized multicenter clinical study. *Fertil Steril* 1989;51:933–938.
8. Boyers SP, Diamond MP, DeCherney AH. Reduction of postoperative pelvic adhesions in the rabbit with Gore-Tex surgical membrane. *Fertil Steril* 1988;49:1066–1070.
9. Donnez J, Nisolle M. CO_2 laser laparoscopic surgery. Adhesiolysis, salpingostomy, laser uterine nerve ablation and tubal pregnancy. *Baillieres Clin Obstet Gynaecol* 1989;3(3):525–543.
10. Daniell JF, Herbert CM. Laparoscopic salpingostomy utilizing the CO_2 laser. *Fertil Steril* 1984;41:558.
11. Reich H. Laparoscopic treatment of extended pelvis adhesions including hydrosalpinx. *J Reprod Med* 1987;32:736.
12. Dubuisson JB, Aubriot FX, Foulot H, Henrion R. Place de la coelioscopie operatoire dans le traitement des sterilites tubaries distales. *Contr. Fert. Sex* 1988;16:13.
13. Mage G, Pouly JL, Bouquet de Joliniere J, Chabrand S, Ridouallan A, Bruhat MA. A preoperative classification to predict the intrauterine and ectopic pregnancy rates after distal tubal microsurgery. *Fertil Steril* 1986;46:807.
14. Fayez JA. An assessment of the role of operative laparoscopy in tuboplasty. *Fertil Steril* 1983;39:476.
15. Bruhat MA, Dubuisson JB, Pouly JL, et al. La coeliochirurgie. In: *Encycl. med. chir., techniques chirurgicales, urologie-gynecologie.* vol 6. Paris: Editions Techniques: 1989:38.
16. Mage G, Bruhat MA. Pregnancy following salpingostomy: comparison between CO_2 laser and electrosurgery procedures. *Fertil Steril* 1983;40:472.

Endoscopic Management of Gynecologic Disease,
edited by G.D. Adamson and D.C. Martin.
Lippincott-Raven Publishers, Philadelphia © 1996.

CHAPTER 11

Ectopic Pregnancy

Steven J. Ory

Ectopic pregnancy, the occurrence of a pregnancy outside the uterine cavity, has been recognized as a complication of pregnancy for over 1000 years. The incidence of ectopic pregnancy appears to be increasing; from 1970 through 1987 the number of ectopic pregnancies reported to the U.S. Centers for Disease Control increased every year except in two (1). In 1987, 88,000 women were hospitalized in the United States with diagnoses of ectopic pregnancy; this represents a 19% increase over the previous year. The rate of ectopic pregnancies in 1987 was 16.8 per 1000 reported pregnancies, 23.1 per 1000 live births, and 15.3 per 10,000 women ages 15–44. The risk of ectopic pregnancy is greatest in women over 30, in nonwhite populations, and in the southern United States. The death rate during the same interval declined by 90%. In 1987 there were 30 deaths from ruptured ectopic pregnancies, or 3.4 deaths per 10,000 ectopic pregnancies.

Embryologic development of the fallopian tube is generally normal in patients with ectopic pregnancies, although some patients with Mullerian anomalies, such as rudimentary horns or tubes or partial tubal atresia, may be at higher risk for ectopic pregnancy. A fertilized embryo may implant along the normal route of migration through the fallopian tube or some distance from it (Fig. 1) (2). Approximately 97% of ectopic pregnancies are tubal and the ampullary portion of the tube is most often affected. Isthmic followed by true fimbrial ectopics are the next most commonly noted sites. Cornual and interstitial pregnancies are less common, and cervical and ovarian ectopic pregnancies are relatively rare, as are abdominal implantations.

Ectopic implantation proceeds developmentally in a similar fashion to nidation within the uterine cavity. The embryo implants approximately 6.5 days following fertilization with deep penetration of the developing trophoblast into adjacent tissues. Successful nidation is influenced by the vitality of the trophoblast, the adjacent vascularity, the ability of the implantation site to sustain the trophoblast, and the ability of the penetrating trophoblast to weaken the underlying tissues (3). Penetration of the muscularis by chorionic tissue precedes tubal rupture. Decidual tissue is not present at the ectopic implantation site unless there is ectopic endometrium (endometriosis).

S. J. Ory: Division of Reproductive Endocrinology and Infertility, Department of Obstetrics and Gynecology, Mayo Clinic, Rochester, Minnesota 55905.

PATHOPHYSIOLOGY

Several mechanisms have been proposed to account for the development of tubal ectopic pregnancy. Previous tubal damage from infection or prior surgical trauma is the most commonly cited preexisting factor. Resultant abnormalities in the tube might result in impaired embryo transport as a consequence of damaged or absent cilia; intraluminal synechia, which may impede migration and trap the embryo prior to its entry into the uterus; or adhesions on the tubal serosa. However, histologic evidence of previous tubal infections is reported in only 30–50% of cases, suggesting other factors (2,4).

Transmigration of the oocyte from the ovary contralateral to the affected tube has been suggested as a source of delay of ovum or embryo transport, which results in initiation of nidation while the embryo is still in the tube. The presence of a corpus luteum opposite the tubal pregnancy occurs in 24–33% of cases (2). However, the site of implantation is the same whether the corpus luteum is ipsilateral or contralateral to the implantation site. This suggests that the additional delay that is assumed to occur with transmigration is not associated with a difference in the distance migrated through the tube (5). Also, patients who undergo salpingoophorectomy have a subsequent ectopic rate comparable to those treated with

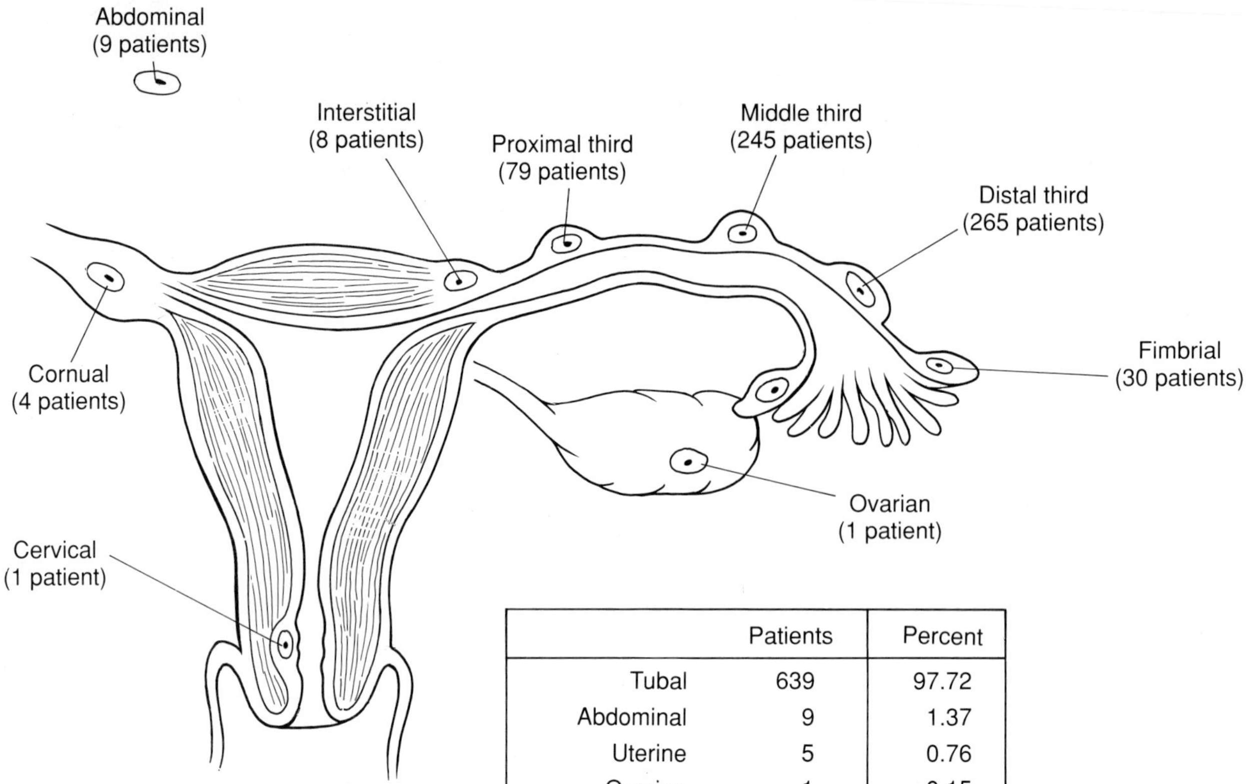

	Patients	Percent
Tubal	639	97.72
Abdominal	9	1.37
Uterine	5	0.76
Ovarian	1	0.15
Total	654	100.00

FIG. 1. Sites of implantation.

salpingectomy alone. These data do not support the notion that transmigration predisposes to ectopic pregnancy.

Salpingitis isthmica nodosa has also been suggested to contribute to ectopic pregnancy. This inflammatory condition of the tubal isthmus may produce partial or complete obstruction of the fallopian tube thereby impeding passage of the embryo. Curiously, many patients with salpingitis isthmica nodosa have ectopic pregnancies in the tubal ampulla, presumably as a consequence of altered tubal transport.

Two additional possible explanations for the pathophysiology of ectopic pregnancy were recently proposed by Pauerstein (4). The oviduct may be unsuccessful in recovering the ovum, and the egg may be released into the cul-de-sac fluid where fertilization occurs. This might occur after ovulation from either ovary, and both oviducts would be equally accessible to the embryo. If blastocyst development begins in this milieu, ultimate pickup of the embryo could be delayed. Tubal implantation could result from the larger cell mass becoming obstructed in the tubal lumen prior to its entry into the uterus, or the stimulus to initiate nidation could begin before the embryo reaches the uterine cavity.

Alternatively, ovulation, ovum pickup, and fertilization could occur in a normal sequence; but there could be tenuous attachment within the tube. The ovum or embryo could be released into the cul-de-sac to be retrieved later by either tube. This might result in a delay of embryo transfer and implantation could occur prematurely.

Previous tubal surgery increases the risk of ectopic pregnancy because of preexisting tubal disease or as a consequence of iatrogenic tubal injury. Following conservative tubal surgery, patients incur a 12–15% risk of future ectopic pregnancies. Ectopic rates as high as 50% have been described in women conceiving after laparoscopic sterilization procedures (6). However, microsurgical tubal anastomosis confers only a 4% risk of ectopic pregnancy, presumably because of minimal tubal alteration.

Several authors have described an increased risk of ectopic pregnancy in two patient groups: those with high serum estradiol levels following ovulation induction therapy with human menopausal gonadotropin and clomiphene citrate therapy and those receiving high doses of estrogen postovulation for contraception (7–9). Tubal motility and cilia activity are modulated by sex steroids.

Abnormal embryonic development also has been postulated as a possible etiology. Although abnormal karyotypes have been described and there appears to be a preponderance of 46 XY over 46 XX karyotypes, genetic abnormalities do not appear to cause ectopic pregnancies and overall they are not more likely to be coincident with abnormal karyotypes (10). No increased familial tendency has been described.

Heterotopic (combined) pregnancies were calculated in 1948 to occur in 1 of 30,000 tubal pregnancies (11). This incidence was computed by multiplying the incidence of ectopic pregnancy by that of dizygotic twinning in 1948. The incidence of ectopic pregnancy has increased dramatically over the past 40 years, as has the incidence of dizygotic twinning resulting from the more prevalent use of ovulation induction agents. The current estimates of heterotopic pregnancy range from 1 in 4000 to 1 in 15,000 (12). In some high-risk populations, such as in vitro fertilization (IVF) patients, the risk of heterotopic pregnancy may exceed 1%.

Currently, there is controversy regarding how trophoblastic tissue spreads following implantation within the tube. Historically, intraluminal spread was suspected. Budowick suggested that the trophoblast invades the lamina propria shortly after attachment and then spreads throughout the muscularis in both a longitudinal and circumferential manner early in the course of disease (13). Hemorrhage tends to be extraluminal until tubal rupture occurs or there is extrusion from the fimbriated end. However, Pauerstein using a slightly different methodology described early invasion of the lamina propria and dissection through the muscularis in only one third of ectopic pregnancies (4). Dissemination of trophoblastic tissue through the muscularis layer may account for difficulty in visualizing ectopic tissue at the time of surgery and persistent ectopic pregnancy following surgery.

CLINICAL PRESENTATION

Classically, patients with ectopic pregnancy present with a triad of abnormal vaginal bleeding, pelvic pain, and an adnexal mass. Over 90% of patients experience abdominal or pelvic pain and 75% of patients have abnormal vaginal bleeding or amenorrhea (14). The diagnosis of ectopic pregnancy should be considered in all women with lower abdominal pain and a positive pregnancy test. Syncope, shoulder pain, and the urge to defecate are reported by 10–15% of patients; and 5–10% pass a decidual cast that is often mistaken for products of conception. In 30–50% of patients, an adnexal mass is palpable. The differential diagnosis includes adnexal torsion, pelvic inflammatory disease, uterine leiomyoma degeneration, threatened or incomplete abortion, ruptured corpus luteum, endometriosis, appendicitis, and other gastrointestinal disorders.

More recently, a second type of presentation was described. These patients are often diagnosed earlier, prior to developing symptoms, and have a more insidious presentation. Generally, these are patients who are at increased risk for ectopic pregnancy by virtue of a history of prior ectopic pregnancy, tubal surgery, or tubal infection. They are followed prospectively with sonograms and laboratory tests from the time that pregnancy is confirmed. The diagnosis can usually be reliably established early on, and a broader array of therapeutic options are available to this group.

DIAGNOSIS

Signs associated with ectopic pregnancy are quite variable. For many patients with early ectopic pregnancy there are no demonstrable findings. Assessment of vital signs is important in the initial evaluation. Many young, otherwise healthy individuals can tolerate a large reduction of intravascular volume without exhibiting signs of cardiovascular collapse; and tachycardia and orthostatic changes may be the first clue. Other potential causes of shock, such as sepsis, must be excluded. Occasionally, patients with intraabdominal hemorrhage demonstrate temperature elevation secondary to a nonspecific reaction to peritoneal irritation. Deep tenderness on palpation, often with rebound, may be present on abdominal examination. This is usually localized to the lower abdomen but may be more diffuse with significant hematoperitoneum. The abdomen may be distended, and the umbilicus may develop a bluish hue (Cullen's sign) if there is massive intraabdominal bleeding. Nonspecific signs of pregnancy, such as vaginal and cervical cyanosis, may be present on vaginal examination. Cervical motion tenderness usually is present and the posterior cervix may be particularly tender. Tender adnexal enlargement is palpable in 30–50% of cases. The uterus may enlarge to 8-week size. Palpable surface irregularities of the cornu may suggest interstitial pregnancy. One quarter of patients have hematocrits less than 30% after tubal rupture. Approximately 50% of patients have associated mild leukocytosis.

Quantitative Human Chorionic Gonadotropin

The development of highly sensitive serum radioimmunoassays for human chorionic gonadotropin (hCG) and its subunits has been a major advance in the diagnosis of ectopic pregnancy. Currently available radioimmunoassays (RIAs), enzyme-linked immunoabsorbent assays (ELISAs), and immunoradiometric assays (IRMAs) identify the presence of hCG in over 99% of ectopic pregnancies; this is in contrast to the previously used urinary hCG determinations, which were positive in 50% of ectopic pregnancies (15). Of greater significance, the hCG levels reflect the status of the pregnancy; hCG concentrations arc roughly correlated with the amount of trophoblastic tissue present, which is influenced in part by the duration of the gestation. Normally developing intrauterine pregnancies have a characteristic doubling rate of hCG of 1.98 days (16). Pregnancies not characterized by a normal rate of hCG increase are most often abnormal; hCG increases of less than 66% within 48 hr are associated with ectopic pregnancies and intrauterine pregnancies that abort in 87% of cases. Fifteen percent of normal pregnancies may have abnormal doubling times. Determining serial hCG levels at 48-h intervals is helpful in following a pregnant patient in whom the site of implantation has not yet been determined, but diagnosis may be delayed. The rate of hCG increase appears to be consistent through the first 6 weeks following the last menstrual period (17). The usefulness of tracking hCG doubling times in a population of asymptomatic patients was not confirmed in a recent prospective study, but most investigators find it to be helpful clinically (18).

Human chorionic gonadotropin (hCG) appears to be eliminated in two phases following term pregnancy and therapeutic abortion. During the initial, major phase of elimination hCG has a half-life of 5–9 hr. There is a second phase with a half-life of 22–32 hr (19). Following salpingectomy and conservative surgery for ectopic pregnancy, similar rates have been described (20).

Progesterone

A single serum progesterone determination within the first 6 weeks of pregnancy can be used to predict pregnancy viability (21–23). Serum progesterone values less than 10 ng/ml are associated most often with ectopic pregnancies and pregnancies destined to abort; higher values are more likely to be associated with normally developing intrauterine pregnancies. Neither serum progesterone determinations nor serial hCG testing permit the physician to distinguish ectopic pregnancy from spontaneous abortion.

Ultrasound

Ultrasound has been an essential component of diagnostic testing for ectopic pregnancy for over 10 years. Initially, transabdominal ultrasound was used to exclude the presence of intrauterine pregnancy in clinically suspicious circumstances. However, ectopic pregnancy may be associated with an intrauterine pseudogestational sac in 10–20% of cases (24). Pseudogestational sacs can be distinguished from true gestational sacs by the absence of a second ring around the fluid collection. A true intrauterine gestational sac can be consistently identified when the hCG level exceeds the discriminatory zone. The discriminatory zone is the zone above which the gestational sac is seen with a normal intrauterine pregnancy. This zone occurs at different hCG levels with transabdominal and transvaginal ultrasonography. Kadar et al. initially described a discriminatory zone for transabdominal sonography of 6000–6500 mIU/ml (International Reference Preparation [IRP]) (25). Intrauterine gestational sacs can be visualized in 94% of cases using this discriminatory zone. The absence of a gestational sac when hCG levels exceed the discriminatory zone confirms the presence of ectopic pregnancy in 86% of cases. The major limitation of transabdominal scanning is that diagnosis is usually not possible until 6 weeks following the last menstrual period. Also, only 25–40% of ectopic pregnancies are characterized by hCG concentrations greater than 6500 mIU/ml at initial presentation (26).

Transvaginal ultrasonography permits earlier diagnosis by offering improved resolution and a chance to define the discriminatory zone at a lower level. The actual determination of the discriminatory zone depends on the quality of ultrasound resolution, the skill of the ultrasonographer, the sensitivity of the hCG assay, and the reference standard with which the assay is calibrated. These factors may produce significant variations at the lower end of these ranges and specific discriminatory zones vary among institutions.

It usually is possible to identify an intrauterine gestational sac by transvaginal ultrasonography with a 5.0- or 7.5-mHz transducer when hCG levels are in the 1000- to 1400-mIU/ml (IRP) range (27). The transvaginal approach usually allows confirmation of an intrauterine pregnancy by 35 days gestation or approximately one week earlier than is possible with transabdominal ultrasonography. An ectopic gestational sac occasionally can be identified using transvaginal ultrasonography (Fig. 2).

In addition to identifying the site of the gestational sac, ultrasound may offer other valuable information. The presence of a complex mass in the adnexa predicts ectopic pregnancy in 8% of cases and in 94% of cases if free peritoneal fluid is present with the mass (28). Although these findings are relatively specific for ectopic pregnancy, they are not consistently present in the majority of ectopic pregnancies. New technologies, including pulse and color flow Doppler, may increase the sensitivity of diagnostic tests.

Determination of the discriminatory zone varies depending on which hCG reference standard is used with a particular hCG assay. Currently, there are three reference standards available for quantitating hCG: the Second International Standard (2nd IS); the International Reference Preparation (IRP), now referred to as the 1st IRP; and the Second International Reference Preparation (2nd IRP). The 2nd IS, which paradoxically was the first reference standard introduced, was available as a bioassay for hCG in 1964. It contains heterogeneous material with various amounts of α and β subunits in addition to containing approximately 20% intact hCG molecules. For this reason the 2nd IS is not ideal for use in radioimmunoassays. The 1st IRP was introduced as an hCG standard reference in 1974 and consists of highly purified hCG material (CR 119) with insignificant amounts of the hCG subunits (29). There are separate

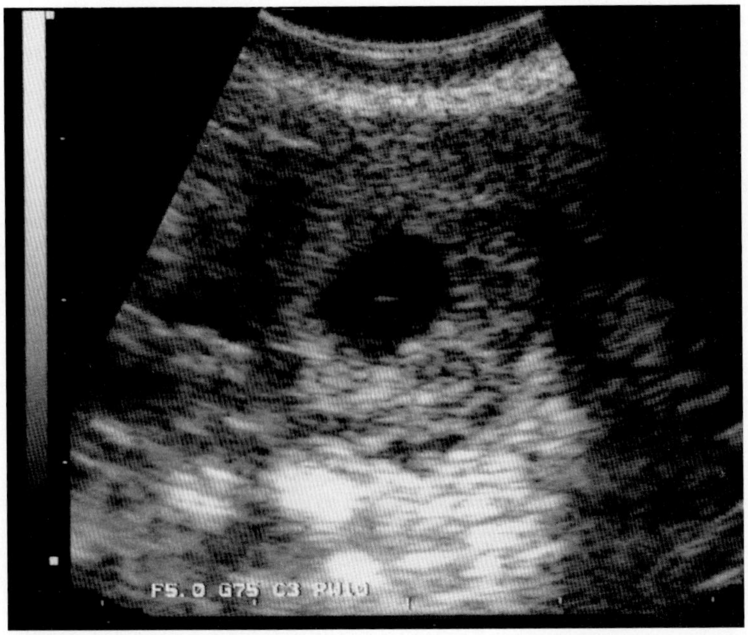

FIG. 2. Transvaginal ultrasound visualization of a gestational sac within the fallopian tube.

IRP reference standards for the subunits. As this stock has been depleted, a second IRP has been introduced which, biologically, is essentially identical to the 1st IRP. The first and second IRP are the preferred reference standards, but references to the 2nd IS and erroneous references to the IRP are in the literature.

The need to perform culdocentesis has decreased with the use of serial hCG determinations and ultrasound, since the presence of fluid in the cul-de-sac can frequently be visualized with ultrasound. However, culdocentesis is very helpful in confirming ectopic pregnancy. A positive culdocentesis, i.e., greater than 5 ml of nonclotting blood, with a positive serum pregnancy test indicates ectopic pregnancy in 99% of cases (30). Positive culdocentesis occurs in 62% of unruptured ectopic pregnancies; 45% of patients with positive culdocentesis have no peritoneal signs at initial evaluation. The principal reason for culdocentesis is to determine whether immediate surgery is indicated in patients with otherwise equivocal findings when ultrasound is not readily available.

Dilatation and Curettage

Dilatation and curettage may be helpful in the evaluation of patients with possible incomplete abortion in which the gestational age is greater than 5 weeks and conclusive sonographic evidence of an intrauterine gestation is absent. The curettings can be histologically examined by frozen section and laparoscopy should be performed if chorionic villae are not identified. Occasionally chorionic villae can be grossly identified by floating the tissue in saline. A variety of types of endometrial histology have been described with ectopic pregnancy, including proliferative endometrium, secretory endometrium, decidua, and Arias–Stella reaction. None of these findings conclusively establishes the diagnosis of ectopic pregnancy.

LAPAROSCOPY

Laparoscopy usually is required to establish definitively the diagnosis of ectopic pregnancy, although diagnosis occasionally can be done with ultrasound alone if an ectopic gestational sac can be identified. False-negative and false-positive rates for laparoscopy are 2–5% (31). Laparoscopic surgery is the principal treatment method for ectopic pregnancy.

Indications

Patients suspected of having an ectopic pregnancy should be evaluated as expeditiously as possible. Those evidencing intraabdominal hemorrhage or significant pelvic pain require immediate surgery. If the diagnosis is less apparent and the patient is not acutely ill, ultrasound, serial hCG determinations, and serum progesterone levels are useful. Prior to surgery, all reasonable therapeutic options and the risks and benefits of each should be reviewed with the patient. An in-depth knowledge of the patient's fertility expectations, previous tubal surgery, and concerns about future ectopic pregnancy should be established before surgery. The general risks of abdominal surgery and those unique to laparoscopy also should be reviewed.

Alternative Treatment

Observation without surgical intervention, systemic methotrexate therapy, and salpingocentesis with a variety of agents have been reported to be successful alternatives to surgery. Many tubal pregnancies spontaneously resolve by tubal abortion without evident clinical sequelae if surgery is not performed. At surgery for ectopic pregnancy, spontaneous complete or evolving tubal abortion is often apparent. Tubal abortion often is evidenced clinically by declining hCG levels. Several studies have confirmed that early ectopic pregnancies associated with falling hCG levels can be safely and reliably followed (32–34). This management option should be limited to the occasional asymptomatic patient in whom ectopic pregnancy is suspected but not confirmed but whose hCG levels are declining. In general, patients with hCG concentrations of less than 1000 mIU/ml experience the most rapid and uneventful clinical course (26).

Systemic methotrexate therapy has been confirmed to be safe and effective treatment for ectopic pregnancy (35–41). Regimens of intramuscular or intravenous methotrexate 1 mg/kg/day every other day for four doses with administration of leucovorin on alternating days are successful in effecting the resolution of the pregnancy in 95% of cases. A single-dose regimen of methotrexate 50 mg/m^2 without leucovorin has become popular and appears to have comparable efficacy (39). Treatment with all regimens generally is well tolerated and side effects are mild and infrequent. Additional variations in the regimen include outpatient administration, shorter courses of therapy, and treatment without laparoscopic confirmation (39,40). Fertility following treatment has been evaluated in a preliminary fashion and is encouraging (41). Clinical response usually is more rapid and less complicated when hCG levels are below 5000 mIU/ml IRP. However, in most centers, laparoscopy is still required for diagnosis. Methotrexate administration offers no distinct advantage if laparoscopy must be performed and definitive treatment can be accomplished.

Salpingocentesis—the injection of methotrexate, potassium chloride, prostaglandin $F_2\alpha$, or hypertonic glucose into the gestational sac at the time of laparoscopy or by transvaginal ultrasound-directed needle—has been attempted to minimize effects of systemic agents such as methotrexate. The treatment can be accomplished by transvaginal ultrasound and does not necessitate a general anesthetic or hospitalization. Although salpingocentesis has been successful in small series, more recent larger series describe success rates significantly lower than those achieved with systemic methotrexate or surgery (42–46). As of this writing, salpingocentesis cannot be endorsed as a comparably effective option.

Surgical Technique

Laparoscopy is the initial surgical procedure of choice except when the patient is in obvious shock or there are contraindications to laparoscopy. In all cases the necessary intrumentation for laparotomy should be available in the room at the initiation of the procedure. Laparoscopic treatment has been documented to be associated with shorter operative time, briefer hospitalization, less postoperative pain, decreased cost, earlier return to work, and comparable future fertility potential as compared to patients treated by laparotomy (47–49). Laparoscopic treatment does require additional equipment and surgical training, but it should be offered if appropriately trained personnel are available. All conservative surgical procedures, with the exception of tubal anastomosis after segmental excision, can be performed through the laparoscope.

If a laparoscopic procedure is planned, a technique involving three punctures greatly facilitates surgery. The two ancillary trocars should be in suprapubic sites, at least 4 cm above the pubic symphasis and 5 cm lateral to the midline. Care should be taken to avoid the inferior epigastric vessels. It is desirable to have a 10-mm or larger suprapubic port to facilitate removal of tissue. A laparoscopic approach should not be attempted if the pelvic organs cannot be completely visualized, if the affected tube cannot be completely mobilized, or if there is uncontrolled hemorrhaging. Some clinicians advised against laparoscopic treatment if the affected tube was greater than 4-cm in diameter. However, with additional options for tissue removal, size alone need not be a contraindication to laparoscopic management. If peritubal adhesions are present, the tube should be fully mobilized prior to attempting to remove the ectopic gestation. Necessary equipment includes microtip unipolar and bipolar cautery instruments, a variety of atraumatic grasping forceps, laparoscopic scissors, and a means of removing the tissue. The latter can be accomplished with a laparoscopic morcellator through a 10-mm or larger port or by utilizing a special endoscopic pouch and withdrawing the tissue through the abdomen. A dilute pitressin solution (20 U/50–100 ml of saline) can be injected into the tubal serosa to facilitate hemostasis.

Bipolar cautery, an automatic cutting and stapling device, or appropriate laparoscopic suture should be available for hemostasis, if salpingectomy or segmental excision is planned. A high-quality video system and camera are essential for appropriate surgical assistance.

The choice of procedure depends on several factors. Salpingectomy should be performed on patients with obvious tubal rupture, uncontrolled hemorrhage, or those who have no desire for future pregnancy. In addition, salpingectomy should be considered in patients who have already had two ectopic pregnancies in an affected tube and those who are unwilling to accept increased risk of repeat ectopic pregnancy in the future. However, such patients should understand that they will still have an increased risk of tubal pregnancy in the remaining contralateral tube. In patients desiring future fertility, the choice of procedures is determined by the site and size of the ectopic pregnancy, the condition of the contralateral

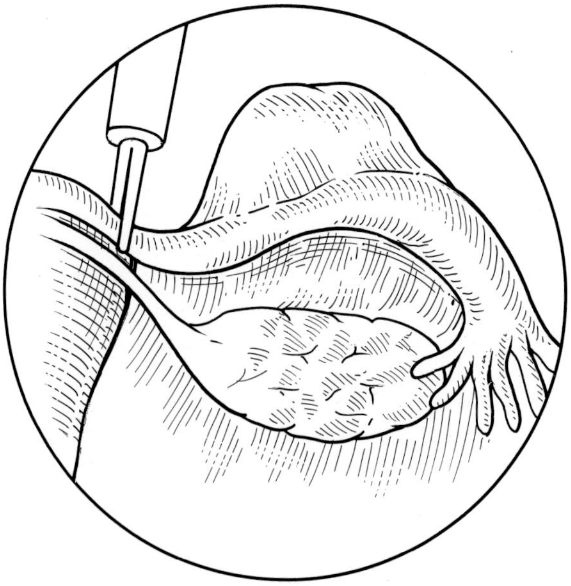

A

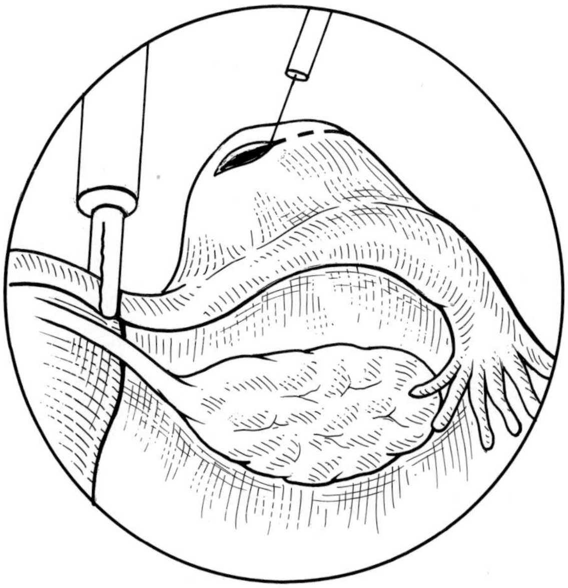

B

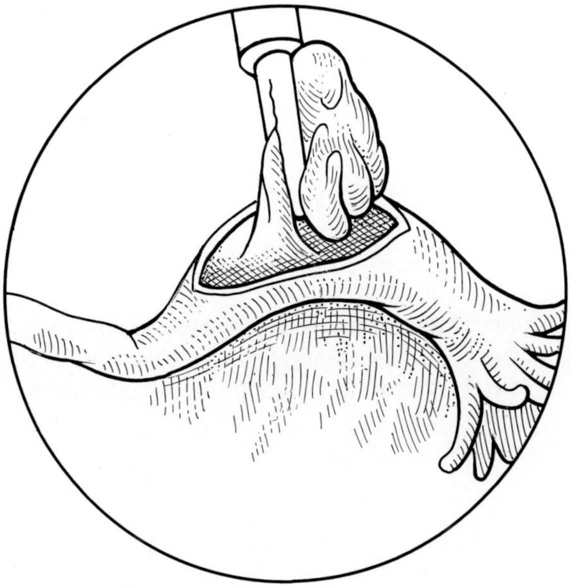

C

FIG. 3. Linear salpingostomy. **A:** An unruptured tubal ectopic pregnancy located in the ampulla is present. The tube is grasped proximally. **B:** An incision is made over the most distended portion of the antimesenteric surface with unipolar microtip cautery. **C:** The tissue is grasped from within the lumen and removed. **D:** Hemostasis is achieved by microtip cautery.

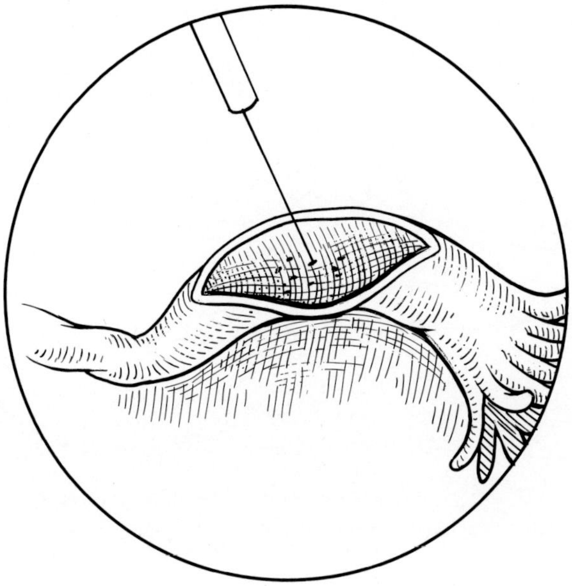

D

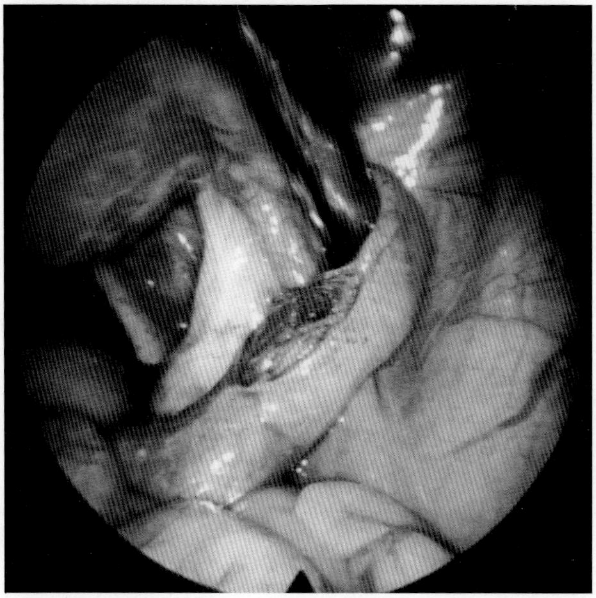

tube, prior history of infertility, previous ectopic pregnancy, and the relative availability of IVF services.

GENERAL SURGICAL PRINCIPLES

Strict adherence to microsurgical principals offers the best potential for future fertility. The laparoscope provides magnification up to three times, thereby permitting careful examination of the exposed endosalpinx and adjacent tissues. Gentle tissue handling, copious irrigation, and meticulous hemostasis are important. The ampullary portion of the fallopian tube is the site of most tubal pregnancies, and linear salpingostomy is the procedure of choice (Fig. 3). The tube is grasped and oriented in a manner to provide the best exposure of the antimesenteric surface of the tube and it is opened at this site. Several techniques have been described including: incision with laser, microtip unipolar cautery tip, or laparoscopic scissors. Most authors inject a dilute Pitressin solution in the tubal serosa before using scissors. Applying Kleppinger forceps in a line over the intended site of the incision also helps ensure hemostasis, but this technique may result in greater thermal damage. After opening of the tube, the products of gestation are grasped and gently extruded from the tube. Bleeding generally occurs over the serosal edges and at the implantation site. This can usually be controlled by unipolar or bipolar cautery or by injection of Pitressin. Compression of the underlying mesosalpinx and coagulation or placing a suture around the vessels in the underlying mesosalpinx may be helpful. As a last resort, salpingectomy or segmental resection may be undertaken to control bleeding. The lumen should be flushed with irrigation fluid, which may dislodge additional tissue. Particular care should be taken to inspect the site proximal to the incision because this may be more commonly associated with retained trophoblastic tissue. Following salpingostomy and once hemostasis is achieved, the tubal incision is left to close by secondary intention. Some authors recommend that salpingotomy be performed in which the tubal defect is closed with fine (5-0 to 7-0), interrupted, nonreactive suture material. Salpingostomy may be associated with earlier conception following conservative surgery than is salpingotomy (50). Also, the sutures used with salpingotomy may lead to more tissue ischemia and additional adhesion formation (51).

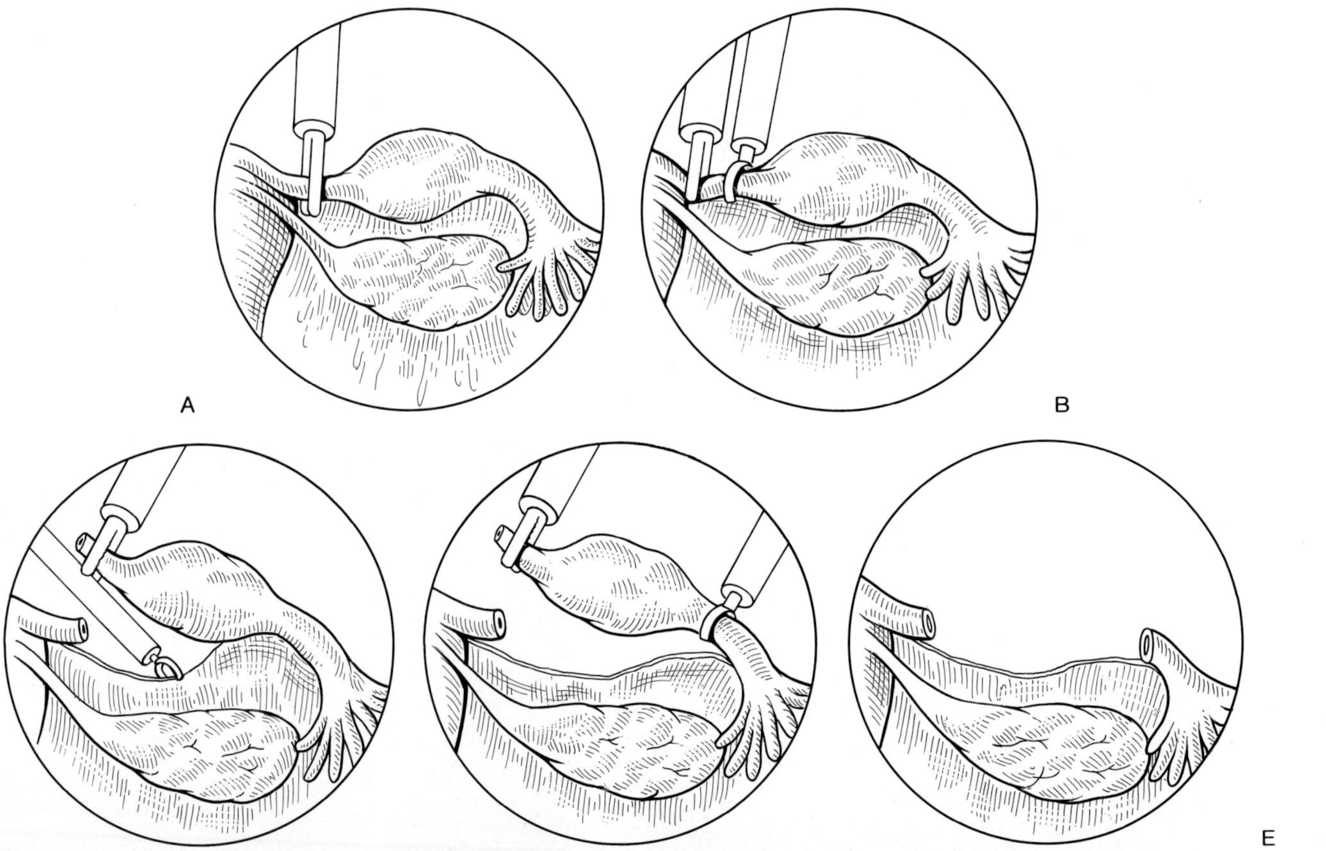

A B

C,D E

FIG. 4. Segmental excision. **A:** A large isthmic ectopic pregnancy is present and the tube is grasped proximal to the site of implantation. **B:** Bipolar cautery is used to coagulate the tube adjacent to the ectopic pregnancy. **C–E:** Tube is divided and the mesosalpinx is progressively coagulated and divided and the affected segment is excised.

Fimbrial expression also is recommended for treatment of ampullary ectopic pregnancy. This technique involves compression of the tube to extrude the conception products from the fimbriated end of the tube. It has limited application for tubal pregnancies in which spontaneous abortion is underway and should generally not be employed for intact tubal pregnancies in which all of the tissue remains within the tube. Otherwise, tubal compression results in greater tissue trauma and potentially more dissection of the trophoblastic tissue through the adventitia. Fimbrial expression is associated with a higher incidence of persistent trophoblastic tissue and recurrent ectopic pregnancy (52). However, if the tissue is already protruding from the tubial ostia, it can be grasped and gently teased away from the fimbria. Encouraging results have been described under these circumstances.

Some authors have reported successful utilization of linear salpingostomy for isthmic tubal pregnancies. This procedure can be attempted for small, unruptured isthmic pregnancies in which bleeding can be easily controlled. However, these pregnancies often present with significant tubal distortion and rupture and are not amenable to linear salpingostomy. Moreover, with significant intraluminal distortion, tubal function will likely be compromised. In this instance, segmental excision is preferable for isthmic ectopic pregnancy (Fig. 4). Segmental excision can be easily performed through the laparoscope using bipolar cautery to coagulate the tube along a tract immediately proximal and distal to the ectopic pregnancy and by resecting the midportion with scissors. Additional cauterization of the mesosalpinx may be necessary for hemostasis. Alternatively, the same procedure can be performed with an automatic stapling and cutting device to achieve hemostasis and divide the tissue simultaneously. An additional alternative involves ligating the affected segment with suture. This can be accomplished either by laparoscopic suturing or by drawing the affected segment into a pretied loop of suture and securing it. Usually two or three loops are placed over the tissue. This technique is less preferable to the use of bipolar cautery and the automatic stapling and cutting devices because of the latter's ease and reliability.

Salpingectomy should be performed in patients who

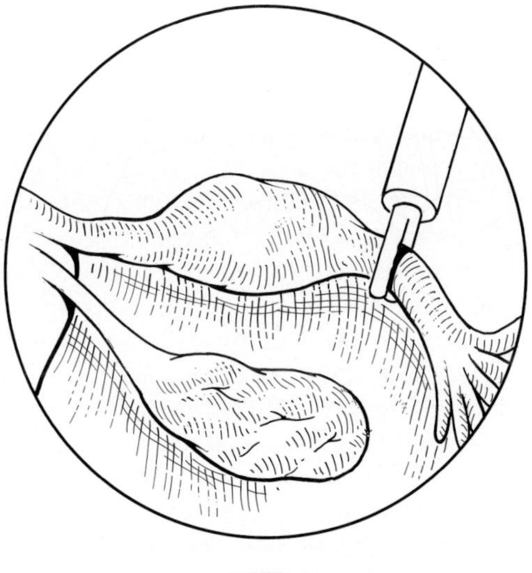

A

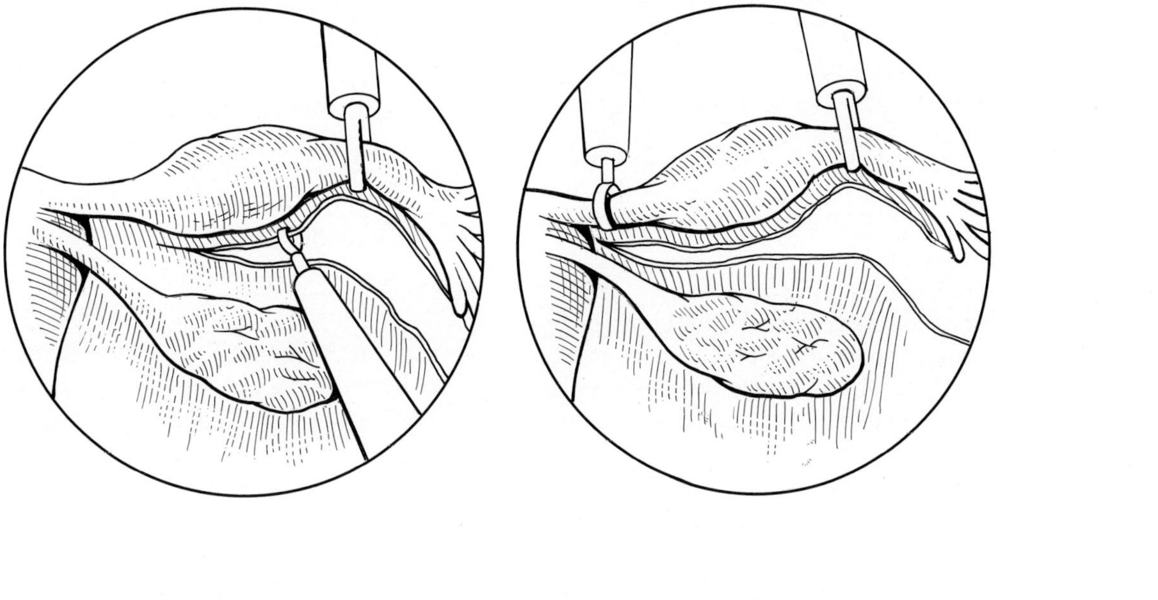

B

FIG. 5. Salpingectomy. **A:** Tubal pregnancy is confirmed and the tube is grasped distally. **B (left):** The mesosalpinx is coagulated with bipolar cautery and divided with scissors progressively to the level of the uterus, or **B (right):** The tube is coagulated with bipolar cautery and divided and the specimen removed.

do not desire future fertility, have tubal rupture or other significant anatomic distortion, or have uncontrolled bleeding. Patients with additional risk factors for poor fertility potential—including a history of a previous ectopic pregnancy, previous tubal surgery, and presence of adhesions involving either adnexa—may be more appropriately managed with salpingectomy and early referral for IVF. They have a very poor prognosis for future fertility in the affected tube. Salpingectomy can be accomplished easily during laparoscopy by extending the dissection described for segmental resection (Fig. 5). The tube is grasped and elevated and the mesosalpinx is coagulated and divided with bipolar cautery and scissors, respectively. The tube is then removed at the site of its uterine attachment. Tubal closure can be ensured with laparoscopically placed sutures or bipolar coagulation. The dissection can proceed from either the proximal or the distal end of the tube, but it is usually easier for right-handed surgeons to work from right to left. The dissection should be as close to the fallopian tube as possible to prevent compromise of the ovarian vascular supply. Following excision, the tissue can be removed through a 10-mm or larger operating channel with a claw or with spoon forceps. Occasionally, morcellation of the tissue in the pelvis is necessary prior to its removal. Alternatively, the specimen can be placed inside a special pouch which passes through an operating channel and is drawn out through the abdominal incision as the whole sleeve is withdrawn. Following removal in this manner, the surgeon loses the pneumoperitoneum and the sleeve either must be reintroduced or the incision must be closed if the procedure is not completed.

Previously, cornual wedge resection and oophorectomy were recommended as integral parts of surgical treatment for ectopic pregnancy. There does not appear to be any basis for continuing to perform either of these procedures.

INTERSTITIAL PREGNANCY

Pregnancy in the tubal interstitia poses unique surgical challenges. These pregnancies are generally more advanced than tubal pregnancies and patients typically present at 12 weeks gestation or later. The advanced gestation, proximity to large uterine vessels, and uterine distention make laparoscopic management potentially hazardous. A laparoscopic approach has been performed successfully in several instances, but this procedure should be undertaken only by an experienced surgeon. The fallopian tube is transected distal to the ectopic pregnancy and dissection of the mesosalpinx is developed toward the uterus and into the myometrium. Cautery and/or laser is useful for the myometrial dissection. The uterine serosa and myometrium should be injected with a dilute Pitressin solution prior to the dissection. Additional options include wedge resection of the involved area at laparotomy, administration of systemic methotrexate, or salpingocentesis—all of which have been successfully employed (42,53). Occasionally, hysterectomy may be necessary for an advanced, ruptured, interstitial pregnancy. Cesarean section in subsequent pregnancies may be advisable to reduce the risk of uterine rupture.

OVARIAN PREGNANCY

Ovarian pregnancies are rare but can usually be treated laparoscopically. The diagnosis may be difficult to make and can be facilitated by ultrasound. Both ovaries should be inspected very carefully in patients in whom an implantation site is not obvious. The ectopic pregnancy can be dissected from the ovary using microtip unipolar cautery or laser. All trophoblastic tissue should be carefully removed. The ovarian defect can be either left open to close by secondary intent or closed with interrupted laparoscopic sutures. Larger ovarian pregnancies may necessitate oophorectomy. The ovarian vessels in this situation may be significantly enlarged and the decision to proceed with a laparoscopic approach should be undertaken by an experienced surgeon.

OUTCOME

Several authors have confirmed that surgical treatment of ectopic pregnancy laparoscopically is comparable to that achieved through laparotomy (47–49,54). Approximately 95% of patients treated laparoscopically have successful resolutions of their tubal pregnancies. Laparoscopy has several well-documented advantages over laparotomy: shorter hospitalization and operating time, more rapid convalescence, and less requirement for postoperative analgesia (47).

The primary concern following surgery is future fertility and this too seems comparable to that achieved through laparotomy (48,49). In the largest series described to date, Pouley reported a 57% intrauterine pregnancy rate and a 22% recurrent ectopic rate in 321 patients undergoing laparoscopic surgery for tubal pregnancy (55). However, future fertility is influenced by numerous other factors, including a prior history of infertility, tubal surgery, presence of adhesions, age, and the presence of other infertility factors (56). An accurate appraisal of future fertility following laparoscopic treatment for ectopic pregnancy requires additional prospective studies with appropriate stratification.

COMPLICATIONS

All of the previously described laparoscopic operative complications exist for laparoscopic treatment of ectopic pregnancy. The most commonly encountered operative complication is hemorrhage. Management of intraoperative hemorrhage was reviewed earlier; hemorrhage following surgery is rare.

The primary, short-term, nonoperative complication of conservative treatment of ectopic pregnancy is persistent ectopic pregnancy. The continued proliferation of trophoblasts after surgery was described in 1979 (57). Detectable hCG levels for over 6 weeks following salpingectomy or conservative surgery for ectopic pregnancy are common. Persistent hCG levels, which indicate remaining viable trophoblastic tissue, should not be of clinical concern unless the tissue begins to proliferate again. The latter event is thought to be consistently depicted by increasing hCG levels. Although hemorrhage does occur with falling hCG levels, it is a rare event (58). Following conservative surgery, patients with increasing hCG levels may re-present with symptoms of ectopic pregnancy and are at additional risk for tubal rupture and hemorrhage. Approximately 5% of patients experience persistent ectopic pregnancy following conservative surgery, but rates as high as 20% have been described and the rate appears to increase after a laparoscopic approach (59,60). A patient's hCG levels should be determined weekly following conservative surgical procedures until nonpregnant levels are attained. Persistent ectopic pregnancy may be observed as long as the hCG levels do not increase. For patients who have two successively increasing values, intervention is necessary. Options include a second conservative surgical procedure, salpingectomy, or systemic methotrexate therapy. As noted earlier, ectopic pregnancy may often be associated with dissection of the trophoblastic tissue through the muscularis layer (4,13). The inability to see this tissue at the time of surgery may be a recurrent problem and should be considered if a second surgical procedure is contemplated. Salpingectomy is effective, but it eliminates any fertility sparing potential of the initial procedure. Systemic methotrexate therapy is effective, well tolerated, and appears to be the best choice for patients with persistent ectopic pregnancy, although treatment efficacy has not been documented in a large series to date.

Recurrent ectopic pregnancy is a long-term complication of laparoscopic surgery for ectopic pregnancy. Risk of recurrent ectopic pregnancy is higher if the affected tube is retained (53,61,62). Risk of recurrent ectopic pregnancy may be as high as 30% in affected tubes. Given the significance of additional risk factors for recurrent ectopic pregnancy, a judicious decision must be made regarding whether to remove or to retain the tube. Recent literature would suggest that patients with additional risk factors would benefit more from salpingectomy and early referral to IVF programs than from conservative procedures.

HIGHLIGHTS

The management of ectopic pregnancy has evolved dramatically over the last 20 years. It is a far more common disease than previously thought, and diagnosis is greatly facilitated by the sensitive diagnostic tests available, including quantitative serum hCG determinations, high-resolution ultrasonography, and advances in laparoscopic equipment and techniques. These diagnostic methods have broadened our appreciation of the natural course of the disease and have led to more treatment options, including observation, systemic methotrexate therapy, and laparoscopic procedures. In most cases, laparoscopy is required to confirm diagnosis; definitive treatment can be performed at the time of laparoscopy in most cases of ectopic pregnancy. As compared to laparotomy, laparoscopic surgery offers the advantages of rapid convalescence, decreased hospitalization and expense, and comparable efficacy and fertility potential. The specific laparoscopic procedure undertaken should be determined by each patient's particular circumstances and needs.

REFERENCES

1. Ectopic Pregnancy—United States, 1987. *MMWR* 1990;39(24):401.
2. Breen JL. A 21-year survey of 654 ectopic pregnancies. *Am J Obstet Gynecol* 1970;106:1004.
3. Philippe E, Bilenki I, Warter A. Pathology of ectopic pregnancy. In: Lager A, Iffy L, eds. *Extrauterine pregnancy*. Littleton, MA: PSG; 1986:107.
4. Pauerstein CJ, Croxatto HB, Eddy CA, Ramzy A, Walters MD. Anatomy and pathology of tubal pregnancy. *Obstet Gynecol* 1986;67:301.
5. Saito M, Koyama T, Yaoi Y, et al. Site of ovulation and ectopic pregnancy. *Acta Obstet Gynecol Scand* 1975;54:227.
6. McCausland A. High rate of ectopic pregnancy following laparoscopic tubal coagulation failures. *Am J Obstet Gynecol* 1980;136:97.
7. McBain JC, Evans JH, Pepperell RJ, et al. An unexpectedly high rate of ectopic pregnancy following the induction of ovulation with human pituitary and chorionic gonadotropin. *Br J Obstet Gynaecol* 1980;87:5.
8. Gemzell CA: Experience with the induction of ovulation. *J Reprod Med* 1978;21(Suppl):205.
9. Morris JM, Van Wagenen G. Interception: the use of postovulatory estrogen to prevent implantation. *Am J Obstet Gynecol* 1973;115:101.
10. Elias, S, LeBeau M, Simpson JL, et al. Chromosome analysis of ectopic human conceptuses. *Am J Obstet Gynecol* 1981;141:698.
11. DeVoe RW, Pratt JH. Simultaneous intrauterine and extrauterine pregnancy. *Am J Obstet Gynecol* 1948;56:1119.
12. Bello G, Schonholz D, Mosirpur J, et al. Combined pregnancy: the Mount Sinai experience. *Obstet Gynecol Surv* 1986;41:603.
13. Budowick M, Johnson TRB, Genardy R, et al. The histopathology of the developing tubal ectopic pregnancy. *Fertil Steril* 1980;34:169.
14. Weckstein LN. Current perspectives on ectopic pregnancy. *Obstet Gynecol Surv* 1985;40:259.
15. Schwartz RD, DiPietro DL. Beta hCG as a diagnostic aid for suspected ectopic pregnancy. *Obstet Gynecol* 1980;56:197.
16. Kadar N, Caldwell B, Romero R. A method of screening for ectopic pregnancy and its indications. *Obstet Gynecol* 1981;58:162.
17. Daya S. Human chorionic gonadotropin increase in normal early pregnancy. *Am J Obstet Gynecol* 1987;156:286.
18. Shepherd RW, Patton PE, Novy MJ, Burry KA. Serial beta hCG measurements in the early detection of ectopic pregnancy. *Obstet Gynecol* 1990;75:417.
19. Midgley A, Jaffe P. Regulation of human gonadotropin II. Disappearance of human chorionic gonadotropin following delivery. *J Clin Endosc* 1968;28:1712.

20. Kamrava M, Taymor M, Berger M, et al. Disappearances of human chorionic gonadotrophin following removal of ectopic pregnancy. *Obstet Gynecol* 1983;62:486.
21. Matthew CP, Coulson PB, Wild RA. Serum progesterone levels as an aid in the diagnosis of ectopic pregnancy. *Obstet Gynecol* 1986;68:390.
22. Gelder MS, Boots LR, Younger JB. Use of a single random serum progesterone value as a diagnostic aid for ectopic pregnancy. *Fertil Steril* 1991;55:497.
23. Cowan BD, Vandermolen DT, Long CA, Whitworth NS. Receiver operator characteristic, efficiency analysis, and predictive value of serum progesterone concentration as a test for abnormal gestations. *Am J Obstet Gynecol* 1992;166:1729.
24. Romero R: The diagnosis of ectopic pregnancy. In: DeCherney AH, ed. *Ectopic pregnancy*. Rockville, MD: Aspen Publishers, 1986:15–33.
25. Kadar N, DeVore G, Romero R. Discriminatory hCG zone: its use in the sonographic evaluation for ectopic pregnancy. *Obstet Gynecol* 1981;58:156.
26. Leach RE, Ory SJ. Modern management of ectopic pregnancy. *J Reprod Med* 1989;34:324.
27. Fossum G, Davajan V, Kletzky O. Early detection of pregnancy with transvaginal ultrasound. *Fertil Steril* 1988;49:788.
28. Romero R, Kadar N, Castro D, Jeanty P, Hobbins J, DeCherney A. The value of adnexal sonographic findings in the diagnosis of ectopic pregnancy. *Am J Obstet Gynecol* 1988;158:52.
29. Bangham DR, Storring PL: Standardization of human chorionic gonadotropin, hCG subunits, and pregnancy test. *Lancet* 1982;1:390.
30. Romero R, Copel J, Kadar N, Jeanty P, DeCherney A, Hobbins J. Value of culdocentesis in the diagnosis of ectopic pregnancy. *Obstet Gynecol* 1985;65:519.
31. Samuellson S, Sjovall A. Laparoscopy in suspected ectopic pregnancy. *Acta Obstet Gynecol Scand* 1972;51:31.
32. Garcia A, Aubert J, Sama J, Josimovich J. Expectant management of presumed ectopic pregnancies. *Fertil Steril* 1987;48:395.
33. Mashiach S, Carp H, Serr D. Nonoperative management of ectopic pregnancy a preliminary report. *J Reprod Med* 1982;27:127.
34. Dericks T, Scholz C, Tauber H. Spontaneous recovery of ectopic pregnancy: a preliminary report. *Eur J Obstet Gynecol Reprod Biol* 1987;25:181.
35. Ory SJ, Villanueva AL, Sand PK, Tamura RK. Conservative treatment of ectopic pregnancy with methotrexate. *Am J Obstet Gynecol* 1986;154:1299.
36. Goldstein DP. Treatment of unruptured ectopic pregnancy with methotrexate with folinic acid rescue (MTX-FA). Presented at the Thirty-Fourth Annual Clinical Meeting of the American College of Obstetricians and Gynecologist in New Orleans, LA, May 1986.
37. Sauer M, Gorrill M, Rodi I, et al. Nonsurgical management of unruptured ectopic pregnancy: an extended clinical trial. *Fertil Steril* 1987;48:752.
38. Ichinoe K, Wake N, Shinkai N, Shiina Y, Miyazaki Y, Tanaka T. Nonsurgical therapy to preserve oviduct function in patients with tubal pregnancies. *Am J Gynecol* 1987;156:484.
39. Stovall TG, Ling FW, Buster JE. Outpatient chemotherapy of unruptured ectopic pregnancy. *Fertil Steril* 1989;51:435.
40. Stovall TG, Ling FW, Carson SA, Buster JE. Nonsurgical diagnosis and treatment of tubal pregnancy. *Fertil Steril* 1990;54:537.
41. Stovall TG, Ling FW, Buster JE: Reproductive performance after methotrexate treatment of ectopic pregnancy. *Am J Obstet Gynecol* 1990;162:1620.
42. Robertson DE, Smith W, Moye MA, et al. Reduction of ectopic pregnancy by injection under ultrasound control. *Lancet* 1987;1:974–975.
43. Lindblom B, Kallfelt B, Hahlin M, Hamberger L. Local prostaglandin F1 and injection for treatment of ectopic pregnancy. *Lancet* 1987;1:776.
44. Feichtinger W, Kemeter P. Conservative treatment of ectopic pregnancy by transvaginal aspiration under sonographic control and injection of methotrexate injection. *Lancet* 1987;1:381.
45. Mottla GL, Rulin MC, Guzick DS: Lack of resolution of ectopic pregnancy by intratubal injection of methotrexate. *Fertil Steril* 1992;57:685–687.
46. Tulandi T, Atri M, Bret P, Falcone T, Khalife S. Transvaginal intratubal treatment of ectopic pregnancy. *Fertil Steril* 1992;58:98–100.
47. Brumsted J, Kessler C, Gibson M. A comparison of laparoscopy and laparotomy for the treatment of ectopic pregnancy. *Obstet Gynecol* 1988;71:889–893.
48. Vermesh M, Silva PD, Rosen GF, Stein AL, Fossum GT, Sauer MV. Management of unruptured ectopic gestation by linear salpingostomy: a prospective randomized clinical trial of laparoscopy vs laparotomy. *Obstet Gynecol* 1989;73:400–408.
49. Vermesh M, Presser SC. Reproductive outcome after linear salpingostomy for ectopic gestation: a prospective three year follow-up. *Fertil Steril* 1992;57:682–684.
50. Tulandi T, Guralnick M. Treatment of tubal ectopic pregnancy by salpingotomy with or without tubal suturing and salpingectomy. *Fertil Steril* 1991;55:53–58.
51. McComb P, Gomel V. Linear ampullary salpingotomy heals better by secondary versus primary closure. *Fertil Steril* 1984;41:454.
52. Timonen S, Nieminen U. Tubal pregnancy, choice of operative method of treatment. *Acta Obstet Gynecol Scand* 1967;46:327.
53. Tanaka T, Hayashi H, Kutsuzawa T, Fujimoto S, Ichinoe K. Treatment of interstitial ectopic pregnancy with methotrexate: report of a successful case. *Fertil Steril* 1982;37:851.
54. Reich H, Johns DA, DeCaprio J, McGlynn F, Reich F. Laparoscopic treatment of 109 consecutive ectopic pregnancies. *J Reprod Med* 1988;33:885–889.
55. Pouly MA, Manhes H, Mage G, Canis M, Bruhat MA. Conservative laparoscopic treatment of 321 ectopic pregnancies. *Fertil Steril* 1988;46:1093–1097.
56. Pouly JL, Chapron C, Manhes H, Canis M, Wattiez A, Bruhat MA. Multifactorial analysis of fertility after conservative laparoscopic treatment of ectopic pregnancy in a series of 223 patients. *Fertil Steril* 1991;56:453–460.
57. Kelly RW, Martin SA, Strickler RC. Delayed hemorrhage in conservative surgery for ectopic pregnancy. *Am J Obstet Gynecol* 1979;133:225.
58. Tulandi T, Hemmings R, Khalifa F. Rupture of ectopic pregnancy in women with low and declining serum beta chorionic gonadotropin concentration. *Fertil Steril* 1991;56:786–787.
59. DiMarchi J, Kosasa T, Kobara T, Hale R. Persistant ectopic pregnancy. *Obstet Gynecol* 1987;70:555.
60. Mecke H, Semm K, Lehmann-Weillenbrock E. Results of operative pelviscopy in 202 cases of ectopic pregnancy. *Int J Fertil* 1988;34:93–100.
61. Makinen JI, Salmi TA, Nikkanen VPJ. Encouraging rates of fertility after ectopic pregnancy. *Int J Fertil* 1989;34(1):46.
62. Querleu D, Boutteville C. Fertility after ectopic. *Fertil Steril* 1989;51:1069.

Endoscopic Management of Gynecologic Disease,
edited by G.D. Adamson and D.C. Martin.
Lippincott-Raven Publishers, Philadelphia © 1996.

CHAPTER 12

Pelvic Inflammatory Disease and Tuboovarian Abscess

Harry Reich

Pelvic inflammatory disease (PID) is an infection of the uterus, fallopian tubes, and pelvic peritoneum. Pelvic abscess, the most severe manifestation of this disease, is a localized collection of a large number of organisms, inflammatory exudate, and necrotic debris separated from surrounding tissue by a fibrous capsule. An adnexal abscess that lacks a classic abscess wall and contains an agglutination of tube and ovary to adjacent pelvic and abdominal structures is termed a tuboovarian complex. True pelvic abscess with a classic abscess wall can occur in the ovary and after rupture of a diverticulum. Whatever the terminology, purulent material exists in a collection within the pelvis. The terms *adnexal abscess, tuboovarian abscess* (TOA), *tuboovarian complex,* and *pelvic abscess* are used interchangeably, with pelvic abscess implying extension of the adnexal abscess to involve most of the true pelvis.

Approximately 1 million women in the United States are diagnosed with PID annually (1). Risk factors include adolescence; multiple sexual partners, especially a new partner within the last two months; failure to use a barrier contraceptive method; use of an intrauterine device, with an increased risk occurring the first 2–3 months after insertion; use of immunosuppression therapy; and frequent douching. Recently, bacterial vaginosis has been implicated as a risk factor (2).

PATHOPHYSIOLOGY

PID is usually an ascending infection. It is estimated that *Chlamydia trachomatis* and/or *Neisseria gonorrhoeae* are the causative organisms in more than half of all cases. Organisms associated with enteric and bacterial vaginosis also have been isolated (2).

Abscess is the end result of an acute or subacute infection beginning with an initial peritonitis stage in which aerobic bacteria predominate, followed by the development of an intraabdominal abscess with emergence of anaerobic bacteria as the predominant flora. Abscesses contain a large number of organisms in high concentration, but they are not in a rapid growth phase; thus, they are less susceptible to antimicrobial agents requiring actively growing organisms for efficacious treatment. The fibrinous capsule may inhibit adequate levels of antimicrobial agents from entering the abscess (3). Also, the anaerobic milieu may hinder host defense mechanisms, thereby reducing the ability of neutrophils to phagocytize and kill bacteria. Consequently, therapy for abscesses must include some technique of adequate drainage along with use of appropriate antimicrobial agents.

CLINICAL PRESENTATION AND DIAGNOSIS

Women with acute or subacute onset of lower abdominal pain and a palpable or ultrasound-suggestive pelvic mass require early laparoscopy for diagnosis and treatment, as even an "obvious TOA" may prove to be an endometrioma, hemorrhagic corpus luteum cyst, or abscess surrounding a ruptured appendix. The routine use of laparoscopy to diagnose acute PID has become widespread in Europe and is accepted by every gynecology department in Sweden (4,5). The worldwide average rate of misdiagnosis of PID is 35% when laparoscopy has been used for confirmation. Conversely, PID can be an unanticipated finding at laparoscopy for pelvic pain.

The diagnosis of an adnexal infection or abscess is suspected in women who have persistent pain and abdom-

H. Reich: Wyoming Valley Health Care System, Wilkes-Barre, Pennsylvania 18704.

inal, adnexal, and/or cervical motion tenderness on examination. "Because of the potential for serious long-term sequelae, even from mild disease, clinicians should have a high index of suspicion and a low threshold for making the diagnosis and initiating treatment" (1).

Temperature, leukocyte concentration, or sedimentation rate may be elevated. Endocervical cultures for gonorrhea and chlamydia may be positive. A recent study indicates that endometrial biopsy has a diagnostic sensitivity of 89% and a specificity of 67% with laparoscopically confirmed disease (6). Serum or urine human chorionic gonadotropin (HCG) must be obtained and a negative result documented. Ultrasound may demonstrate a large hydrosalpinx filled with dense fluid or an adherent adnexal mass. Septations, air fluid levels, internal echoes, and abscess cavity may be identified. Human immunodeficiency virus (HIV) testing should be considered, especially in women with pelvic abscess (7).

More sophisticated diagnostic testing, including gallium 67– and indium 111–labeled white blood cell scans and computed tomographic scans, are rarely necessary, as the diagnosis can be determined at laparoscopy. After a presumptive diagnosis of PID/TOA is made, laparoscopic diagnosis and treatment should be initiated within 24–48 hr. The procedure is explained to the patient/family, and the discussion should include the risk/benefit ratio and treatment alternatives. Informed consent is obtained and documented.

ALTERNATIVE TREATMENTS

Medical Treatment

In recent years, the accepted therapy for PID has been outpatient management with hospitalization and intravenous antibiotics reserved for situations involving an adolescent or when the diagnosis is uncertain, surgical emergencies cannot be excluded, there is suspected pelvic abscess or pregnancy, there is an inability to follow or a failure to respond to outpatient management, or clinical follow-up cannot be obtained otherwise (8). Sexually transmitted diseases treatment guidelines are listed in Table 1 (9). Similarly, an unruptured adnexal abscess is treated with intravenous antibiotics with surgical intervention considered only when the patient does not respond to antibiotics. However, this approach leaves the necrotic and inflammatory tissue in prolonged contact with each other, which is likely to result in the formation of chronic, dense, fibrous adhesions with resultant impaired reproductive potential.

Antibiotic success implies the resolution of symptoms and, often at a much later date, resolution of the pelvic mass as judged by clinical or ultrasound examination; it in no way implies the resolution of pelvic adhesions that could result in future infertility. The literature cited below confirms that when long-term resolution of symp-

TABLE 1. *Regimens for the treatment of pelvic inflammatory disease, as recommended by the CDC*

Type of treatment	Comment
Inpatient	
Regimen 1	
Cefoxitin, 2 g IV every 6 hr, or cefotetan, 2 g IV every 12 hr Doxycycline, 100 mg IV or orally every 12 hr	The cefoxitin regimen is continued for at least 48 hr after the occurrence of substantial clinical improvement after which doxycycline should be given until day 14 of treatment
Regimen 2	
Clindamycin, 900 mg IV every 8 hr Gentamicin, 2 mg/kg of body weight IV or IM (loading dose) followed by 1.5 mg/kg IV or IM every 8 hr (maintenance dose)	The clindamycin regimen is continued for at least 48 hr after the occurrence of substantial clinical improvement, after which doxycycline, 100 mg orally 2 times a day, or clindamycin, 450 mg orally 4 times a day, should be given until day 14 of treatment
Outpatient	
Regimen 1	
Cefoxitin, 2 g IM in a single dose, plus concomitant probenecid, 1 g orally, or ceftriaxone, 250 mg IM, or another third-generation cephalosporin (e.g., ceftizoxime or cefotaxime)	
Doxycycline, 100 mg orally 2 times a day for 14 days	
Regimen 2	
Ofloxacin, 400 mg orally 2 times a day for 14 days	
Clindamycin, 450 mg orally 4 times a day for 14 days, or metronidazole, 500 mg orally 2 times a day for 14 days	

From Ref. 9.

toms and infertility is considered, medical treatment is usually doomed to failure even with modern antibiotics.

Ginsburg and colleagues reviewed 160 patients with tuboovarian abscess (1969–1979) (10). Of these women, 76 (47%) responded to medical therapy with no subsequent surgery, and 84 (53%) required subsequent surgery. Surgery was performed during the acute phase in 50 patients because of failure of the disease to respond to the medical regimen (40 total abdominal hysterectomy/bilateral salpingo-oophorectomy (TAH/BSO), 4 unilateral adnexectomies, and 6 abscess drainage procedures). Thirty-four of the 84 had later surgery for persisting symptomatology related to the abscess. Eighty percent of the women who responded to medical therapy and had no subsequent surgery continued to experience persistent or recurrent disease. Of 120 women in whom reproductive function was preserved, 9 conceived (7.5%); no women with a bilateral tuboovarian abscess conceived.

Hager (1970–1974) also documented poor success with medical therapy alone (11). Of 50 women with the original diagnosis of tuboovarian abscess, only 5 had successful medical treatment.

In 1983, Landers and Sweet reported their results from 175 of 232 women with tuboovarian abscesses treated with antibiotics alone (12). Laparoscopic confirmation was performed in only 15 of these women. Twenty-five percent required surgery as part of their original therapy. Long-term follow-up information was available for 58 women treated with antibiotics alone: 31% required subsequent surgery.

Hemsell and associates reported 41 women with pelvic abscesses treated with cefotaxime during 1980–1981 (13). Chronic pelvic pain and recurrent infection were infrequent during a 31- to 43-month follow-up period, but five women (12%) subsequently required TAH/BSO for persistent adnexal mass, and a sixth underwent unilateral salpingo-oophorectomy for an asymptomatic adnexal mass (hydrosalpinx). Six of thirty (20%) became pregnant.

Diagnoses in these and other studies were based on clinical and sonographic findings without laparoscopy for diagnosis or later evaluation (14). These studies document that antimicrobial treatment of a formed tuboovarian abscess rarely results in complete resolution without adhesion formation. In addition, medical treatment resulted in prolonged initial hospitalization in most cases with a high rate of readmission. Medical treatment has not proved beneficial in ensuring fertility and can be justified only because ovarian preservation results in the possibility of a future in vitro fertilization procedure.

Alternative Surgical Treatment

Primary surgical treatment (laparotomy) for an unruptured tuboovarian abscess within a few days of admission has always been controversial. Early TAH/BSO was advocated by Kaplan and associates who, during 1964–1966, treated 71 women with a presumptive diagnosis of pelvic abscess in this manner (15). Five patients each received more than 2 U of blood. Postoperatively, there were seven superficial wound infections, one subfascial wound infection, and one evisceration. Cuff abscess occurred in three women.

Colpotomy drainage can be performed for those pelvic abscesses dissecting into the upper portion of the rectovaginal septum. Rubenstein and colleagues reported the results of 38 colpotomy procedures for pelvic abscess: 14 (37%) required additional surgery (16). Mean duration of hospitalization was 12.4 days (7.7 days after drainage).

Van Sonnenberg and colleagues reported a 78% success rate with percutaneous drainage of 50 pelvic abscesses (17). Gerzof and colleagues successfully treated six of nine pelvic abscesses (67%) via percutaneous drainage (18). Worthen and Gunning reported percutaneous drainage of 35 pelvic abscesses secondary to pelvic inflammatory salpingitis (19). Nine patients with 11 abscesses were treated by percutaneous catheter placement, with a success rate of 77%; two required surgical procedures. Nineteen women underwent percutaneous aspiration. Among them, there were 23 abscess cavities, 18 (94%) of whom were successfully aspirated; 1 required surgical drainage. Seven women had abscess cavities that could not technically be drained or aspirated. Four of these seven recovered on antibiotic therapy alone, and three required surgical drainage. Long-term follow-up was not part of any of these studies.

LAPAROSCOPIC SURGICAL TECHNIQUE

Laparoscopic treatment of pelvic abscess was first proposed by Dellenbach in 1972 (20). The largest series of laparoscopic treatment of tuboovarian abscess (50 cases) was reported by Henry-Suchet in 1984 and involved lysing of recent friable adhesions with a rod despite the presence of acute infection (21). Success with laparoscopic and laparotomy treatment of TOA by Henry-Suchet et al., Reich, Hudspeth, and Rivlin and Hunt substantiates the laboratory work of Ahrenholz and Simmons (3,21–24). Laparoscopic drainage of a pelvic abscess followed by lysis of peritoneal cavity adhesions and excision of necrotic inflammatory exudate allows host defenses to control the infection effectively.

Preoperative Care

Intravenous antibiotics are initiated on admission to the hospital, usually 2–24 hr prior to laparoscopy. Adequate and sustained blood levels of antibiotics are required to combat transperitoneal absorption of aerobic and anaerobic organisms during the operative procedure. This author prefers cefoxitin, 2 g intravenously, every 4 hr from admission until discharge, usually on postoperative day 2 or 3. Oral doxycycline is started on the first postoperative day and is continued for 10 days. Although clindamycin and metronidazole both have demonstrated greater ability to enter abscess cavities and reduce bacterial counts therein, cefoxitin is used to simplify therapy to a single intravenous agent and assess further the efficacy of the laparoscopic surgical procedure; that is, the intravenous antibiotic alone cannot be considered the reason for successful therapy. Azithromycin is the treatment of choice for *Chlamydia trachomatis* when cost permits.

Operative Technique

Hysteroscopy is done during peritoneal insufflation to inspect the endometrial cavity. Tissue is obtained for histology and chlamydia, gonorrhea, anaerobic, and aerobic bacterial cultures. A uterine manipulator is inserted. A 10-mm laparoscope is used through a vertical intraumbilical incision. Lower quadrant puncture sites are made above the pubic hairline and lateral to the deep epigastric vessels.

The upper abdomen is examined and the patient is placed in 20° Trendelenburg position before the surgeon focuses attention on the pelvis (Fig. 1). A Foley catheter is inserted if the bladder is distended. Either a blunt probe or a grasping forceps is inserted through the right-sided trocar sleeve and is used for traction and retraction. A suction-irrigator-dissector (aquadissector) or a suction probe attached to a 50-cm^3 syringe is inserted through the left-sided trocar sleeve and is used to mobilize omentum, small bowel, rectosigmoid, and tuboovarian adhesions until the abscess cavity is entered. Purulent fluid is aspirated while the operating table is returned to a 10° Trendelenburg position. Cultures should be taken from the aspirated fluid, and inflammatory exudate is excised with biopsy forceps, especially exudate near the tubal ostium.

After the abscess cavity is aspirated, the aquadissector is used to separate the bowel and omentum completely from the reproductive organs and to lyse tuboovarian adhesions (aquadissection) (Figs. 2–4). Aquadissection is performed by placing the tip of the aquadissector against the adhesive interface between bowel–adnexa, tube–ovary, or adnexa–pelvic side wall and by using both the tip and the pressurized fluid gushing from it to develop a dissection plane that is extended either bluntly or with more fluid pressure (Figs. 5, 6). The grasping forceps place the tissue to be dissected on tension so that the surgeon can identify the distorted tissue plane accurately prior to aquadissection (Figs. 7–9). When the dissection is completed, the abscess cavity (necrotic inflammatory exudate) is excised in pieces with 5-mm biopsy forceps (Figs. 10, 11).

It is important to remember that after ovulation purulent material from acute salpingitis may gain entrance into the ovary by inoculation of the corpus luteum, which may then become part of the abscess wall. Consequently, after drainage of the abscess cavity and mobilization of the entire ovary, a gaping hole of varying size may be noted in the ovary that had been intimately involved in the abscess cavity. This area should be well irrigated and should heal spontaneously. Significant bleeding is rare.

The next step is insertion of the grasping forceps into the fimbrial ostia and spreading them to free agglutinating fimbriae. Retrograde irrigation of the tube is performed with the aquadissector to remove infected debris

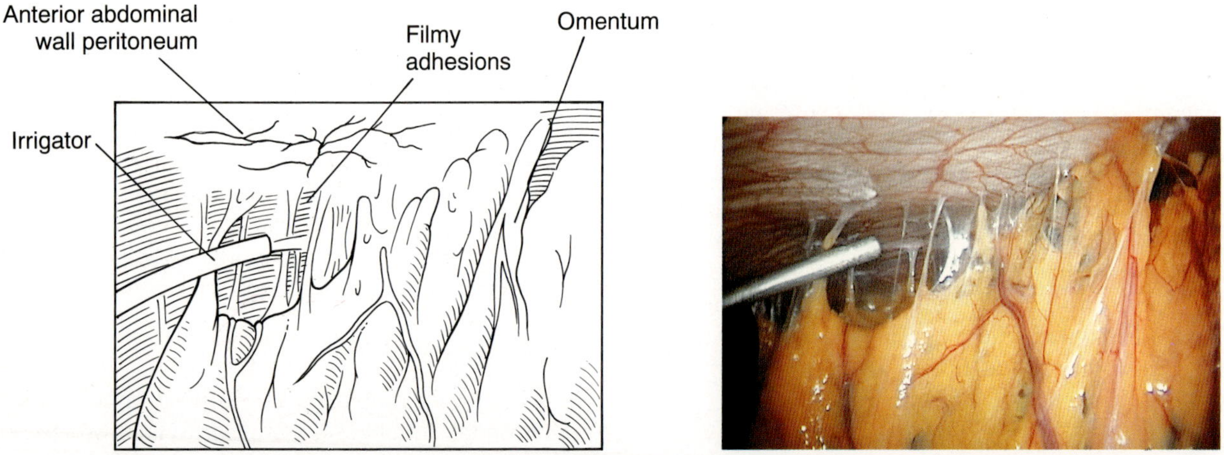

FIG. 1. A 38-year-old woman with large fibroid uterus, stage IV endometriosis with complete cul-de-sac obliteration, and a past history of laparotomy treatment for pelvic abscess. Patient presents with probable recurrent abscess. Slide shows initial view of peritoneal cavity with laparoscope inserted at the left subcostal margin in the midclavicular line.

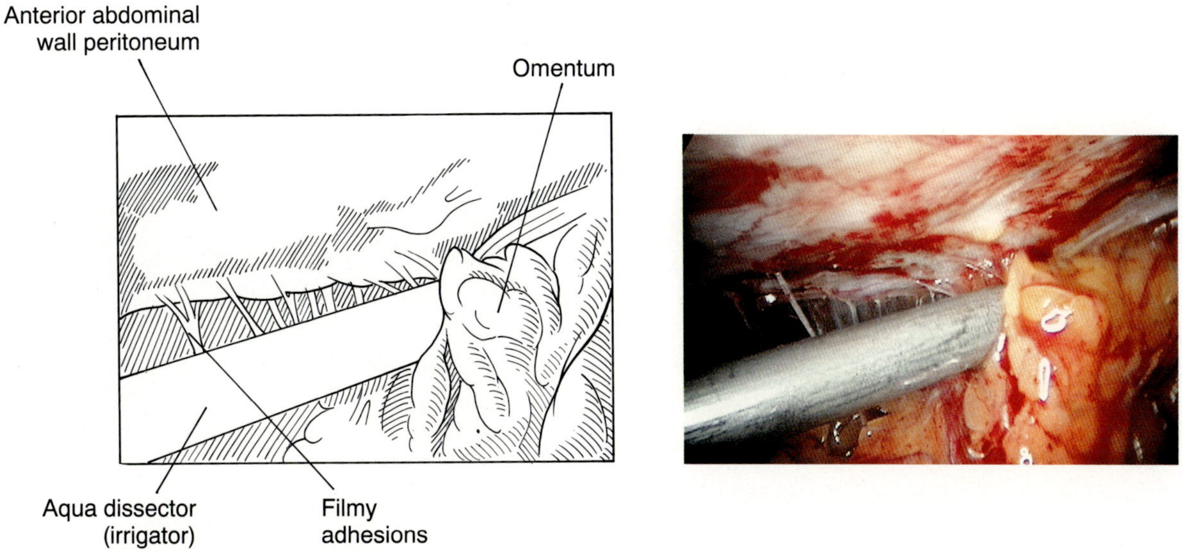

FIG. 2. Aquadissection and blunt dissection is used to separate omental and small bowel adhesions from the anterior abdominal wall.

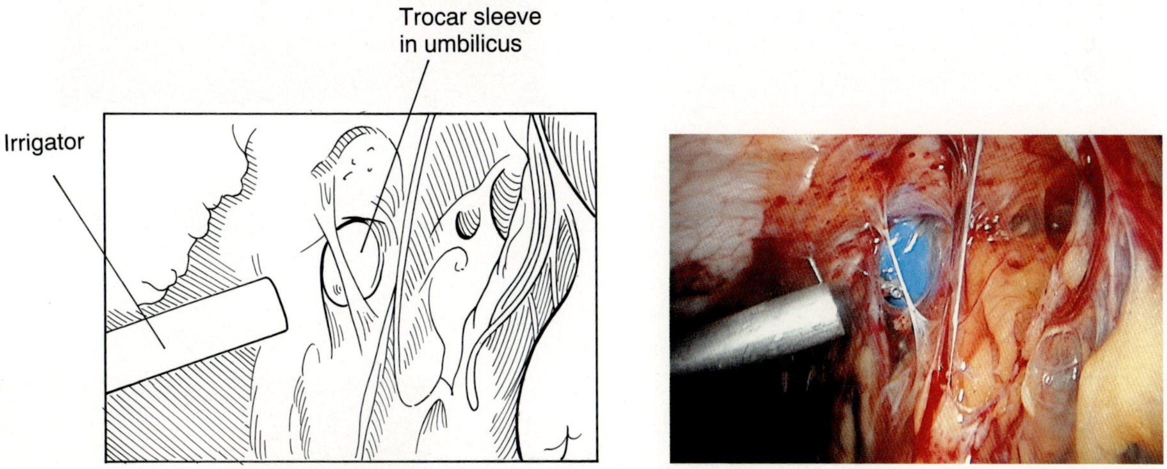

FIG. 3. Previously placed trocar sleeve in umbilicus is uncovered.

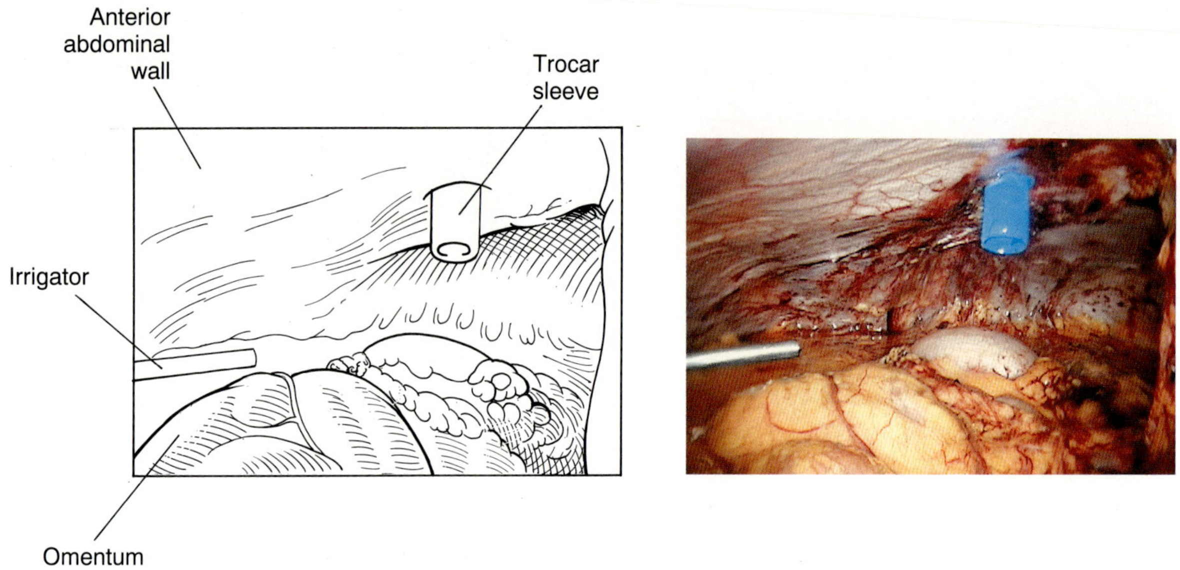

FIG. 4. Anterior abdominal wall adhesions have been divided and umbilical trocar sleeve is free.

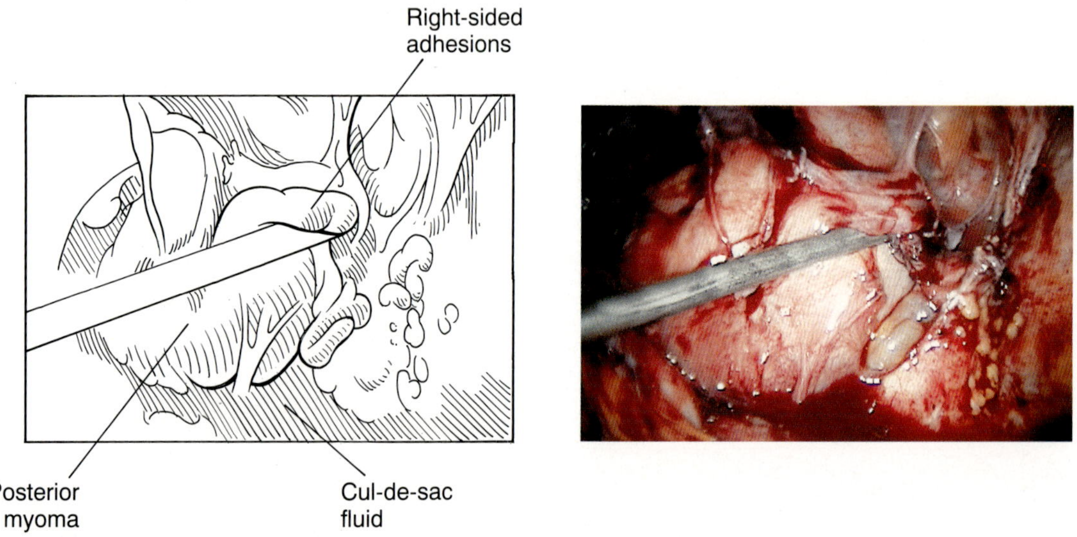

FIG. 5. In deep pelvis, large fibroid uterus is seen with extensive adhesions to it. Right-sided adhesions are divided.

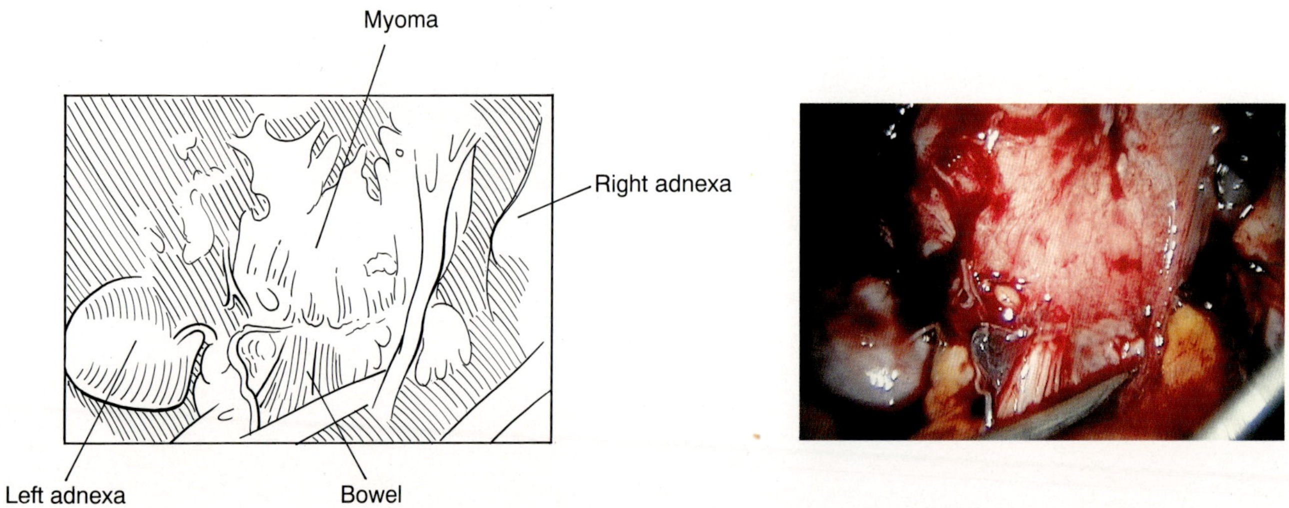

FIG. 6. As the dissection continues, bowel is separated from posterior uterus and cervix on the right.

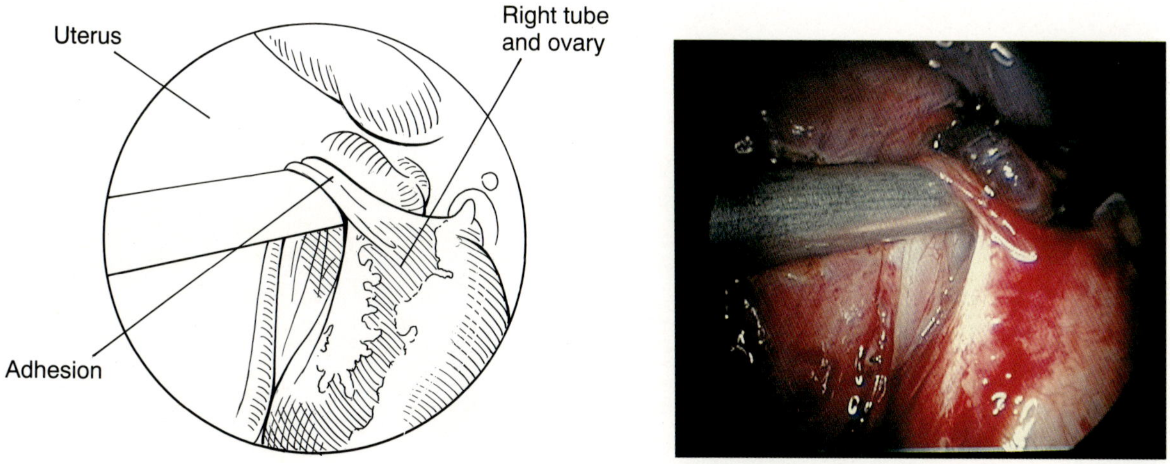

FIG. 7. Right tube and ovary are separated from right side of uterus.

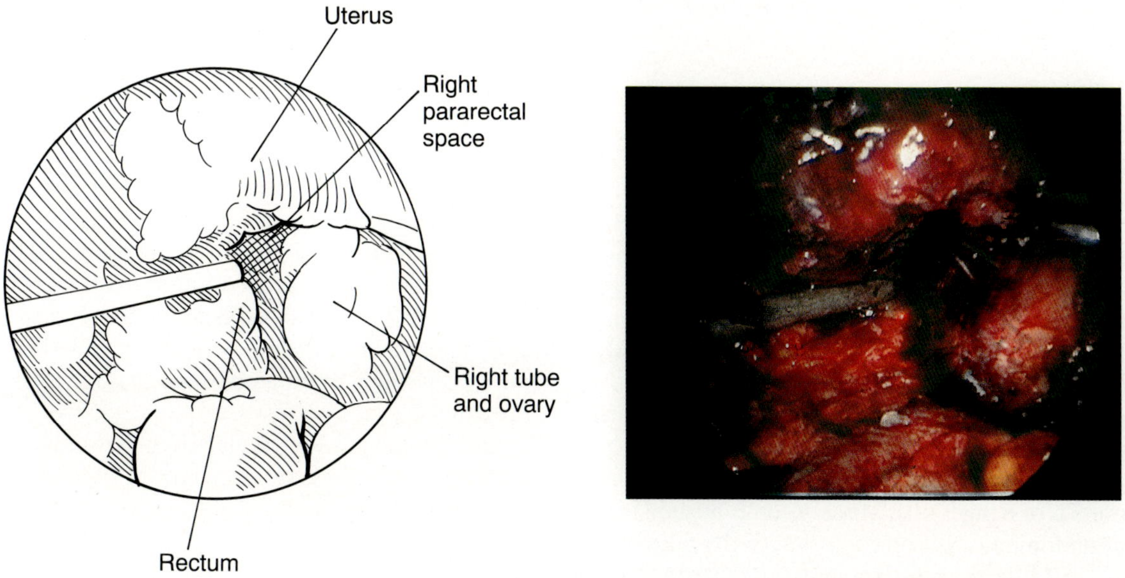

FIG. 8. Right tube and ovary are freed and right pararectal space is entered in search of a chronic abscess.

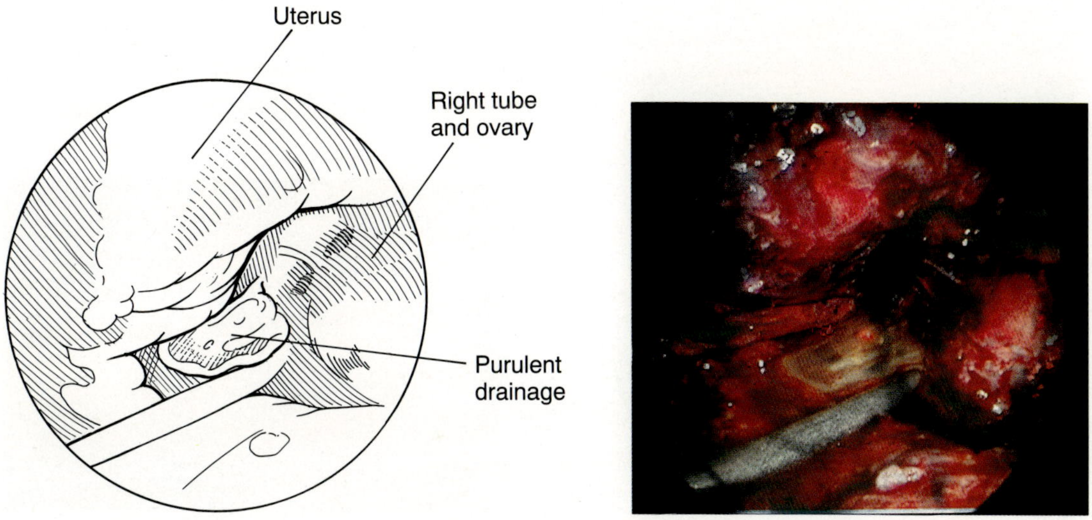

FIG. 9. Purulent drainage is observed from right pararectal space.

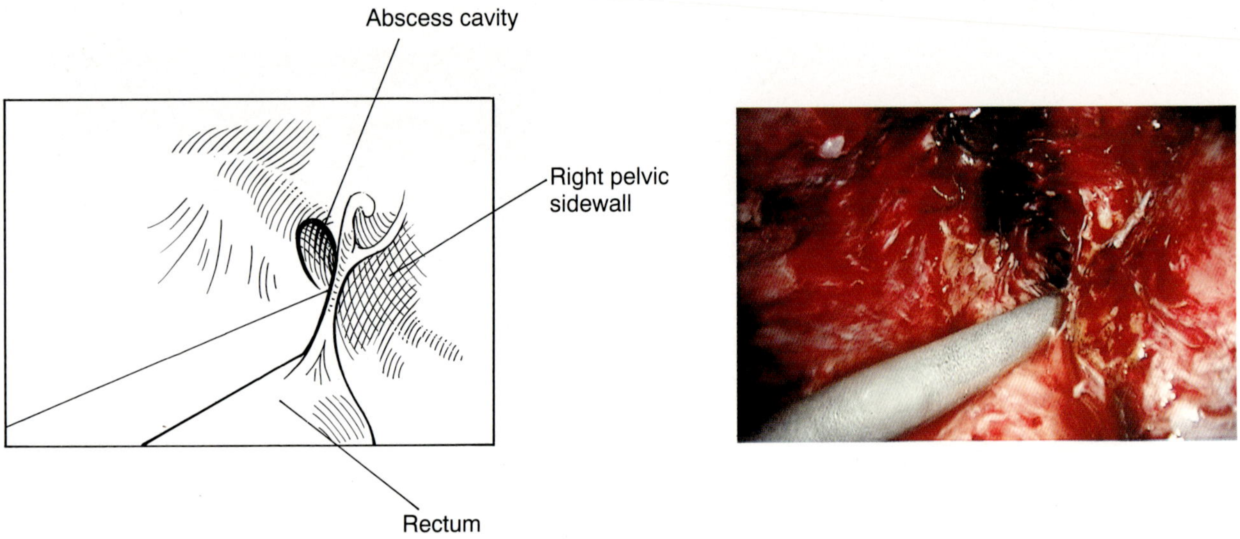

FIG. 10. Purulent drainage is aspirated with aquadissector.

and to diminish the chance of recurrence. The fimbrial endosalpinx is assessed for future prognosis.

Tubal lavage with indigo-carmine dye through a Cohen cannula is attempted. With early acute abscess, the tubes are rarely patent due to interstitial edema. However, when the abscess process has been present for more than a week and/or the patient was previously treated with an antibiotic, lavage frequently documents tubal patency, and inspissated necrotic material can possibly be pushed from the tube.

The peritoneal cavity is irrigated thoroughly with Ringer's lactate solution until the effluent is clear. The total volume of irrigant may exceed 20 L. As part of this procedure, 2 L of Ringer's lactate solution is flushed into the upper abdomen—half on each side of the falciform ligament—to dilute any purulent material that may have gained access to these areas during the 20° Trendelenburg's positioning. The patient is then placed in reverse Trendelenburg position for the underwater exam. The laparoscope and the aquadissector are manipulated into the deep cul-de-sac beneath floating bowel and omentum, and this area is alternately irrigated and suctioned until the effluent is clear. An underwater examination then is performed to observe the completely separated tubes and ovaries and to document complete hemostasis. At the close of each procedure, at least 3 L of Ringer's lactate is left in the peritoneal cavity to prevent fibrin adherences from forming between operated-on surfaces during the early healing phase and to dilute the bacteria present (25).

Blood loss is rarely greater than 100 cm^3. No drains, antibiotic solutions, or heparin are used. Second-look laparoscopy is encouraged.

Postoperative Care

Postoperatively, the patient is ambulatory and on a diet as can be tolerated after recovery from anesthesia.

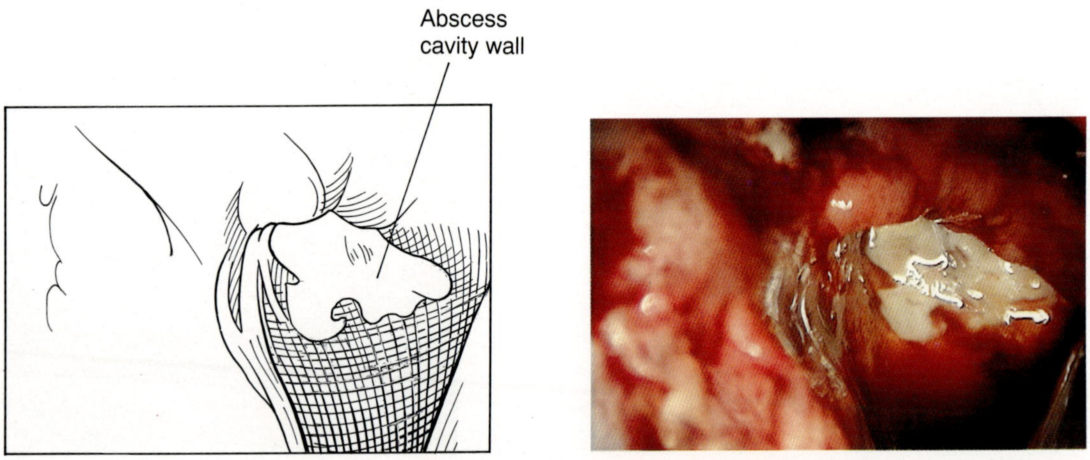

FIG. 11. Abscess cavity is visualized and then removed in many pieces with biopsy forceps.

Leukocytosis and fever rarely persist past the first postoperative day. Discharge is determined by resolution of pain and fever. Intravenous cefoxitin is continued until discharge—usually on the second postoperative day. Oral doxycycline is continued for 10 outpatient days. The patient is examined a week after discharge whereupon all restrictions are removed.

It is critical that the patient's sexual partner undergo medical evaluation and sexually transmitted disease screening. Although frequently asymptomatic, the partner is treated according to the Centers for Disease Control's (CDC) outpatient antibiotic regimen for PID (26).

OUTCOME

In the author's experience from 1976 until 1993, 46 of 48 women with tuboovarian and pelvic abscess were treated with intravenous antibiotics and laparoscopic surgery. One 37-year-old gravida 4, para 4 patient early in the study had laparoscopy for diagnosis alone and underwent total abdominal hysterectomy after no response to antibiotic therapy. One 29-year-old gravida 1, para 1 patient, who underwent laparotomy for a presumed ruptured appendix, was treated for bilateral tuboovarian abscess with preservation of all reproductive organs when the author was consulted during the operative procedure. She has had two subsequent intrauterine pregnancies. Of 46 laparoscopically managed cases, there were 25 unilateral tuboovarian abscesses, 14 bilateral tuboovarian abscesses, 4 diverticular abscesses, 1 vaginal cuff abscess, 1 postappendectomy abscess, and 1 rectal abscess secondary to a delayed bowel perforation. The average age was 28 years (the range was 10–61 years), with a median of 25 years.

Of 46 women treated for abscess, 45 (98%) had complete clinical resolution of the abscess. No laparoscopic complications occurred during the 10 years of the study. The average operating time was 90 min, and the average length of hospital stay postlaparoscopy was 4.1 days. Minimal adhesions were found in the eight women who later underwent second-look laparoscopy.

COMPLICATIONS

In the treatment of PID and abscess, the most serious complications are inaccurate and/or delayed diagnosis and inadequate management. The result to the patient is a lifetime of the sequelae of pelvic adhesive disease. Tubal factor infertility occurs in 8% of women after one episode of PID, in 20% after two episodes, and in 40% after three or more episodes (27).

Complications of laparotomy treatment of pelvic abscess include superficial wound infection, wound dehiscence, bowel injury (including delayed perforation of bowel secondary to unrecognized injury), bowel obstruction, persistent undrained collections, thrombophlebitis, pulmonary embolism, septic shock, and subdiaphragmatic collections with pleural effusion.

At laparoscopy, the subphrenic region can be well visualized and irrigated directly. Delayed bowel perforation secondary to an unrecognized injury is a rare complication of laparoscopy, especially as laser and electrosurgery are infrequently used. Bowel injury, the most common serious operative complication of abscess surgery via laparotomy, occurs only when the bowel is the primary source for abscess formation.

HIGHLIGHTS

The goals in management of acute PID and tuboovarian abscess are prevention of the chronic sequelae of infection, including infertility and pelvic pain; both often lead to further surgical intervention. Laparoscopic treatment in addition to antibiotics is effective and economical. It offers the gynecologist 100% accuracy in diagnosis while simultaneously accomplishing definitive treatment with a low complication rate (21,22).

Authors of most reports on operative technique for treatment of TOA by laparotomy emphasize that the tissues are edematous, congested, friable, and tear easily, and that capillary and venous oozing can be profuse. Blood loss requiring transfusion is common. These reports also suggest that meticulous dissection is virtually impossible and caution that the bowel is particularly vulnerable to injury when it is being separated from the pelvic viscera. The belief that surgical intervention during acute pelvic infection results in greater injury than that after the infection subsides is based on a study published in 1909 suggesting that the technical surgical difficulty is greater in the former case (28).

In contrast, laparoscopic acute adhesiolysis involving aquadissection is rarely bloody. Capillary oozing does occur, but it ceases spontaneously as the procedure progresses. In my experience, blood loss is rarely greater than 100 cm^3. Without question, the more acute the abscess, the easier the dissection. Patient and physician delay often make the laparoscopic procedure more difficult than it need be. However, even chronic abscesses can be successfully treated by careful blunt aquadissection.

It is encouraging that at least one health care plan emphasizes the importance of expedient management of PID [the Oregon health care plan (29)]. We salute the 11 members of the Health Services Commission for their difficult task, but specifically for recognizing that early treatment of PID can prevent significant morbidity and mortality.

Laparoscopy combined with intravenous antibiotic therapy allows for conservation of the tube and ovary with subsequent fertility potential. Additionally, laparoscopy has a high degree of patient acceptance due to minimal incision size, shorter hospital stay, and early return to full activity. The combination of laparoscopic treatment and effective intravenous antibiotics is a reasonable approach to the spectrum of PID from acute salpingitis to ruptured tuboovarian abscess.

REFERENCES

1. McCormack WM. Pelvic inflammatory disease. *N Engl J Med* 1994;330:2:115–119.
2. Eschenbach DA, Hillier S, Critchlow C, Stevens C, DeRouen T, Holmes KK. Diagnosis and clinical manifestations of bacterial vaginosis. *Am J Obstet Gynecol* 1988;155:819–828.
3. Ahrenholz DH, Simmons RL. Fibrin in peritonitis. I. Beneficial and adverse effects of fibrin in experimental *E. coli* peritonitis. *Surgery* 1980;88:41.
4. Jacobson L, Westrom L. Objectivized diagnosis of acute pelvic inflammatory disease. *Am J Obstet Gynecol* 1969;105:1088.
5. Westrom L. Clinical manifestations and diagnosis of pelvic inflammatory disease. *J Reprod Med* 1980;28:703.
6. Paavonen J, Aine R, Teisala K, Heinonen PK, Punnonen R. Comparison of endometrial biopsy and peritoneal fluid cytologic testing with laparoscopy in the diagnosis of acute pelvic inflammatory disease. *Am J Obstet Gynecol* 1985;151:645–650.
7. Hoegsberg B, Abulafia O, Sedlis A, et al. Sexually transmitted diseases and human immunodeficiency virus infection among women with pelvic inflammatory disease. *Am J Obstet Gynecol* 1990;163:1135–1139.
8. Pelvic inflammatory disease: guidelines for prevention and management. MMWR 1991;40(RR-5):1–25.
9. 1993 Sexually transmitted diseases treatment guidelines. MMWR 1993;42(RR-14):75–81.
10. Ginsburg D, Stern J, Hamond R. Tubo-ovarian abscess: a retrospective review. *Am J Obstet Gynecol* 1980;138:1055.
11. Hager WD. Follow-up of patients with tubo-ovarian abscess(es) in association with salpingitis. *Obstet Gynecol* 1983;61:680.
12. Landers DV, Sweet RL. Tubo-ovarian abscess: contemporary approach to management. *Rev Infect Dis* 1983;5:876.
13. Hemsell D, Santos-Ramos R, Cunningham G, et al. Cefotaxime treatment for women with community-acquired pelvic abscesses. *Am J Obstet Gynecol* 1985;151:771.
14. Roberts W, Dockery JL. Operative and conservative treatment of tubo-ovarian abscess due to pelvic inflammatory disease. *South Med J* 1984;77:860.
15. Kaplan A, Jacobs WM, Ehresman JB. Aggressive management of pelvic abscess. *Am J Obstet Gynecol* 1967;98:482.
16. Rubenstein P, Mishell D, Ledger W. Colpotomy drainage of pelvic abscess. *Obstet Gynecol* 1976;48:142.
17. Van Sonnenberg E, Wittich GR, Casola G. Percutaneous drainage of 50 pelvic abscesses; pitfalls and refinements. In ARRS Scientific Program; 1985.
18. Gerzof S, Johnson W, Robbins A, Nabseth D. Expanded criteria for percutaneous abscess drainage. *Arch Surg* 1985;120:227.
19. Worthen N, Gunning J. Percutaneous drainage of pelvic abscesses: management of the tubo-ovarian abscess. *J Ultrasound Med* 1986;5:551.
20. Dellenbach P, Muller P, Philippe E. Infections utero annexielles aigues. *Encycl Med Chir Paris Gynecol* 1972;470:1410.
21. Henry-Suchet J, Soler A, Loffredo V. Laparoscopic treatment of tubo-ovarian abscesses. *J Reprod Med* 1984;29:579.
22. Reich H, McGlynn F. Laparoscopic treatment of tubo-ovarian and pelvic abscess. *J Reprod Med* 1987;32:747.
23. Hudspeth AS. Radical surgical debridement in the treatment of advanced generalized bacterial peritonitis. *Arch Surg* 1975;110:1233.
24. Rivlin M, Hunt J. Surgical management of diffuse peritonitis complicating obstetric/gynecologic infections. *Obstet Gynecol* 1986;67:652.
25. Reich H. Aquadissection. In: Baggish M, ed, *Endoscopic laser surgery*. vol 2. (Clinical Practice of Gynecology series.) New York: Elsevier; 1990:159–185.
26. Gilstrap LC III, Herbert WNP, Cunningham FG, Hauth JC, Van Patten HG. Gonorrhea screening in male consorts of women with pelvic infection. *JAMA* 1977;238:965–966.
27. Westrom L, Joesoef R, Reynolds G, Hagdu A, Thompson SE. Pelvic inflammatory disease and fertility: a cohort study of 1,844 women with laparoscopically verified disease and 657 control women with normal laparoscopic results. *Sex Trans Dis* 1992;19:185–192.
28. Simpson FF. The choice of time for operation for pelvic inflammation of tubal origin. *Surg Gynecol Obstet* 1909;9:45.
29. Huston P. The Oregon Plan: a rational way to "ration" care? *OBG Management* 1991;9:34.

Endoscopic Management of Gynecologic Disease,
edited by G.D. Adamson and D.C. Martin.
Lippincott-Raven Publishers, Philadelphia © 1996.

CHAPTER 13

Laparoscopic Microsurgical Tubal Anastomosis

Charles H. Koh and Grace M. Janik

Although further refinement in instrumentation will ensue, true microsurgery employing 7-0 and 8-0 suturing is possible laparoscopically using the innovations and adaptations described below. This opens a new vista in operative laparoscopy by enabling the incorporation of microsuturing not only for gynecology but for other surgical specialties. For reproductive surgery the additive benefits of operative laparoscopy and true microsurgical technique may now be realized.

The following terms will be used in this chapter:

Microsurgery: Reconstructive surgery using an operating microscope to obtain magnification enabling use of fine instruments and sutures from 7-0 to 10-0. Performed via laparotomy (open).

Microsurgical principles: Surgical style incorporating atraumatic tissue handling, pinpoint accuracy in hemostasis and dissection, and avoidance of tissue desiccation by constant irrigation with the aim of reducing adhesion formation.

Tubal anastomosis: Reversal of sterilization or removal of tubal block due to disease and rejoining of the healthy ends.

Laparoscopic: Procedures performed via laparoscopy or minimally invasive surgery thus replacing the same procedures performed "open" by laparotomy.

CLASSICAL OPEN MICROSURGICAL TUBAL ANASTOMOSIS

Microsurgery through open laparotomy is the established standard today. Swolin (1) in 1967 first proposed the use of magnification and the microsurgical approach for infertility surgery, and Gomel (2) first reported on human microsurgical tubal anastomosis in 1974. In 1977, Gomel (3) and Winston (4) separately reported their results of tubal anastomosis employing microsurgery for reversal of sterilization and soon established microsurgery as the gold standard for reproductive surgery. Microsurgical technique and principles became incorporated in reproductive surgery even where microsuturing was not needed, e.g., endometriosis surgery, myomectomy, and adhesiolysis.

The superiority of the microsurgical vs. macrosurgical approach to tubal anastomosis has been well established in the literature. The former is associated with higher pregnancy rates, lower ectopic rates, and the earlier occurrence of pregnancies (Table 1).

Term delivery rates of 79% have been reported [Gomel, 1983, follow-up more than 18 months (6); Xue Pei et al., 1989, follow-up to 7 years (7)]. An analysis of macrosurgical tubal anastomosis by life table (8) demonstrated a cumulative pregnancy rate of 26% at 12 months and 51% at 66 months. In contrast, Bai et al. (9) in their report on microsurgical tubal anastomosis, achieved a 56% pregnancy rate at 1 year and 70% at 39 months.

LAPAROSCOPIC MICROSURGICAL TUBAL ANASTOMOSIS

Laparoscopic microsurgical tubal anastomosis must be considered experimental until sufficient outcome data are available to compare it favorably with the classical open method. It is important to replicate established principles of classical open microsurgery so as not to compromise its hard-earned gains.

The achievement of true microsurgery at laparoscopy requires four prerequisites:

C. H. Koh and G. M. Janik: Reproductive Specialty Center, Medical College of Wisconsin, Milwaukee, Wisconsin 53211.

TABLE 1. *Macrosurgical vs. microsurgical tubal anastomosis*

Macrosurgical	161 patients	34.8% live births	8.0% ectopics
Microsurgical	486 patients	56.0% live births	2.5% ectopics

By various authors 1979–1980. Modified from ref. 5.

1. Laparoscopic magnification to greater than 20×.
2. Laparoscopic instrumentation capable of handling 7-0 and 8-0 sutures.
3. Advanced laparoscopic skills. The laparoscopist should easily be able to place and tie intracorporeal knots using 4-0 to 6-0 sutures on a curved needle before attempting laparoscopic microsurgical suturing. Extracorporeal and other indirect methods of placing a knot are not suitable for the delicacy of microsuturing. Extensive experience in handling of the adnexa for various tuboplasties and adhesiolysis is essential.
4. Competence in classical microsurgery. Essential prerequisites to classical microsurgery are respect for tissue and gentle handling. It often is necessary for the operator to compensate for unanticipated difficulties of the laparoscopic approach by falling back on his vast open microsurgical experience to complete the operation laparoscopically.

TYPES OF PROCEDURES

Anatomic terminology of the fallopian tube and types of tubal anastomosis are given in Figs. 1 and 2, respectively.

Tubocornual Anastomosis

Tubocornual anastomosis is a very difficult procedure to perform laparoscopically because of the limited mobility of the tubal cornua and its lateral facement, so the laparoscope cannot view the cornual ostium easily. The

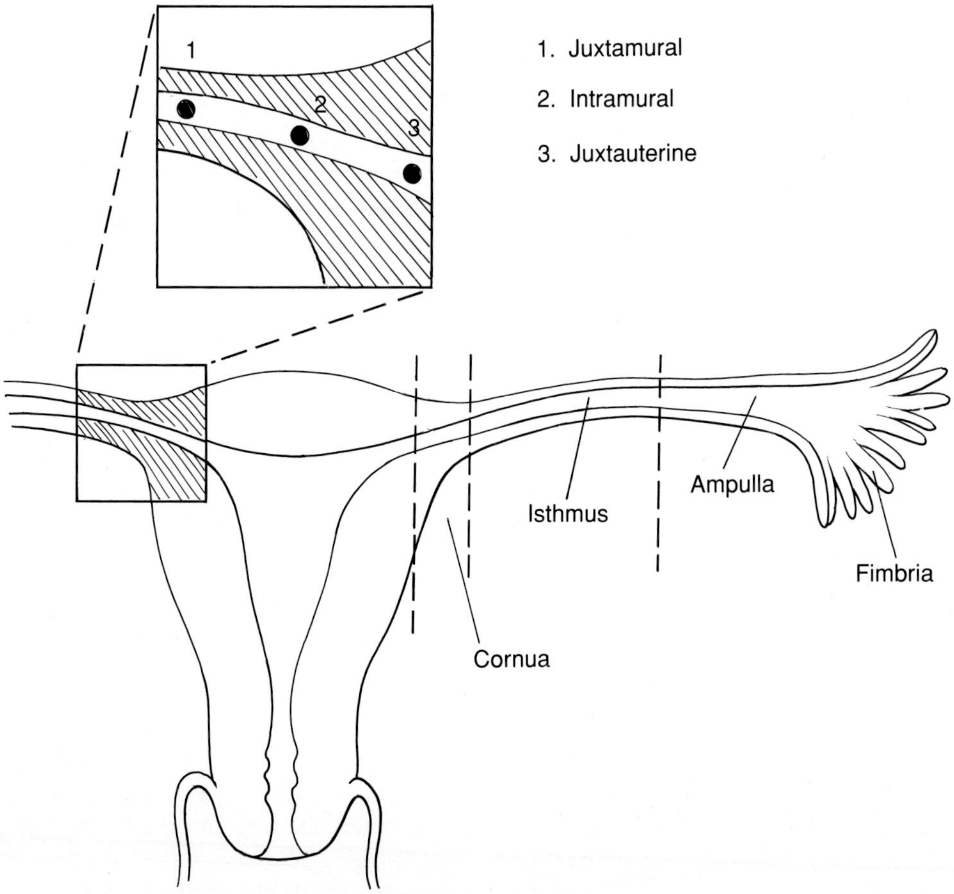

FIG. 1. Terminology of fallopian tube.

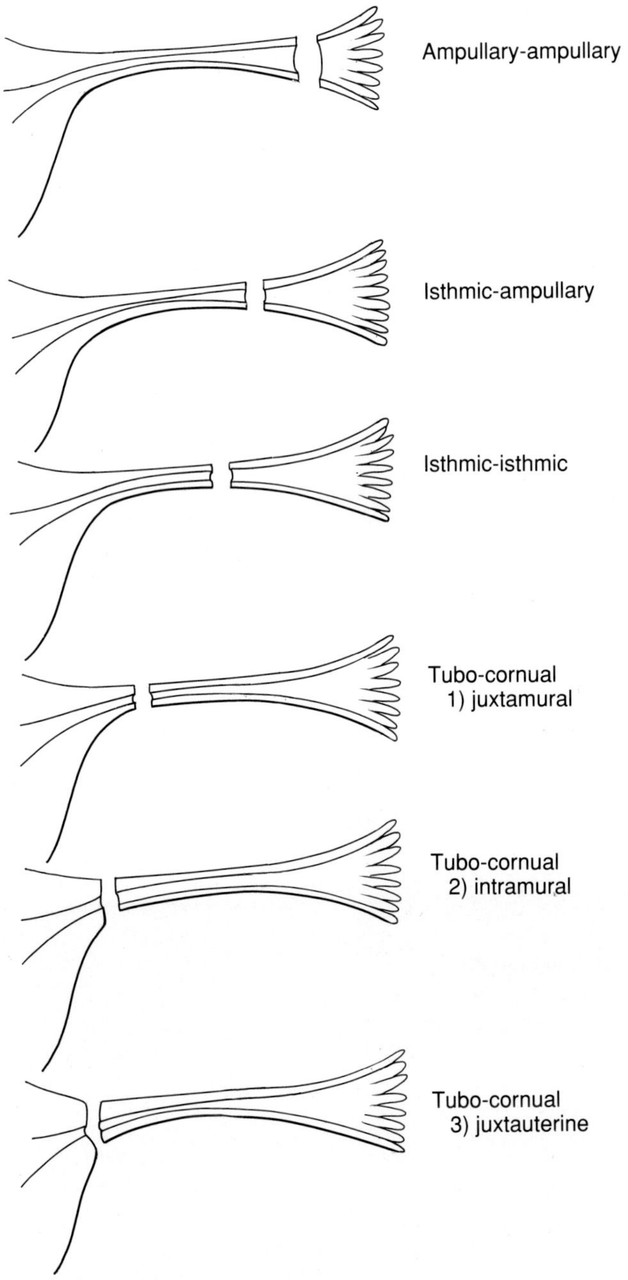

FIG. 2. Types of tubal anastomosis.

difficulty is compounded further if the anastomosis has to be performed deep in the cornua, as in the case of the juxtauterine tubal anastomosis. In order to mobilize the intramural tube, a vertical cut is made into the cornual musculature and the muscle is temporarily sutured back with 5-0 or 6-0 nylon. For the juxtamural anastomosis, the cornua may be mobilized by a contralateral grasper tracting on the muscle medially to turn the tubal lumen toward the laparoscope. We recently performed a juxtauterine anastomosis, which demonstrated tubal patency postoperatively at hysterosalpingogram, while a juxtamural-ampullary anastomosis achieved pregnancy at 3 months postoperatively and the patient recently delivered.

Tubal–Tubal Anastomosis

Isthmic–isthmic

This is the most reproducible procedure as there is good control of the ostial direction, and luminal equality is easily obtained. The muscularis is of similar thickness and this facilitates accurate apposition.

Isthmic–Ampullary

A correct initial ampullary luminal cut is vital as it is very difficult laparoscopically to reduce an overlarge lumen and still perform a good anastomosis. A mini-laparotomy with true microsurgery should be performed to rescue such instances. By initially trimming off the serosa from the ampullary stump we can perform an accurate cut with confidence of matching the proximal tubal luminal diameter.

Ampullary–Ampullary Anastomosis

This is the easiest anastomosis technically because of the larger lumen, but luxuriant mucosa may obscure the already thin muscularis. Gentle irrigation will expose the muscularis for suture placement. One can usually push back the prolapsed mucosa after tying all of the sutures.

INDICATIONS

The following are indications for tubal anastomosis:

Sterilization reversal
Postectopic partial salpingectomy
Salpingitis isthmica nodosa
Failed tubal cannulation for proximal tubal occlusion

SELECTION AND PREOPERATIVE EVALUATION FOR STERILIZATION REVERSAL

Laparoscopic tubal anastomosis should be considered experimental and the patient must be so informed. Alternative treatments, namely, classical microsurgery and in vitro fertilization (IVF), should be fully discussed.

It is advisable that a psychological evaluation be instituted. The most common request for reversal is from patients who have remarried and, interestingly, these women are most likely to be satisfied with surgical reversal whether or not pregnancy is achieved (10). It is important to identify psychosocial reasons for reversal, as some may decide not to conceive after the reversal operation (11).

The prognosis for success following sterilization reversal is inversely correlated with the age of the patient and the interval from sterilization; it also is influenced by the type of sterilization performed. The highest pregnancy rates occur when the reconstructed tube measures more than 4 cm in length. Mechanical occluders, such as a clip or a Falope ring, prognosticate the highest pregnancy rates after reversal, followed by postpartum and all Pomeroy-type procedures. Lower pregnancy rates may be expected from electrosurgical sterilization, whether monopolar or bipolar, because of extensive tubal destruction.

The feasibility of reversal may be inferred from the operative report. In general, all mechanical methods and Pomeroy or postpartum sterilizations are potentially reversible. The length of healthy tube following either monopolar or bipolar electrocautery is unpredictable and cannot be assumed from the operative report.

A preliminary diagnostic laparoscopy is not necessary when dealing with nonelectrical sterilization methods, thereby avoiding two operations. It is advisable for evaluating *all* electrosurgical sterilizations to avoid the inconvenience of a scheduled 3-hr case being aborted because of insufficient tubal length for anastomosis. A hysterosalpingogram is unnecessary preoperatively if one is capable of dealing with a potential tubocornual anastomosis except to evaluate the uterine cavity, if clinically indicated.

The ovulatory status of a patient may be inferred from regular menstrual cycles. Basal body temperature is adequate further confirmatory evidence. If the menstrual cycle is short or there is oligomenorrhea, a timed endometrial biopsy may diagnose luteal phase problems, or a cycle day 3 serum follicle-stimulating hormone (FSH)

TABLE 2. *Equipment for laparoscopic microsurgery*

Instrumentation	Manufacturer	Model no.
Modified needle holder	Jarritt, Chicago, IL	
Director microscissors	Microsurge, Needham, MA	
DaVinci hook cutter (guillotine)	DaVinci Medical, Minneapolis, MN	
Rumi uterine manipulator	Blairden, Lenexa, KS	
Nylon monofilament suture 6-0, 7-0, 8-0	Ethicon, Cincinnati, OH	1696G 1856G 2808G
Prolene 7-0, 8-0 BV 175-6 Ethalloy needle	Ethicon, Cincinnati, OH	M8743
Ureteric catheter (4–6 Fr)	Cook, Bloomington, IL	
Microlaryngeal forceps	Pilling, Ft. Washington, PA	50 − 5420 50 − 6470 (Left) 50 − 6471 (Right)
	Storz, Culver City, CA	8592 A 8593 B (R) 8593 C (L)
	Mueller, Chicago, IL	BE − 2491
Microscissors	Ethicon, Cincinnati, OH	D MS 15
Florestor vessel occluder	BioVascular, Inc., St. Paul, MN	Micro Tip #52005-33
Microneedle electrode (150 μm)	Elmed, Chicago, IL	52205-48
Laparoscope and Camera System		
Three-chip camera; 800-line horizontal resolution; 768 × 494 pixels Laparoscope; 10-mm 0°	Stryker, Kalamazoo, MI	782-050-111
Three-chip camera		Tri-Cam 9070B
Laparoscope 0° Hopkins	Storz, Culver City, CA	26033AP
Monitor: 800 lines horizontal resolution	Sony, Montvale, NJ	PVM1943MD
Generator: Microunipolar and Bipolar		
Force II	Valley Lab, Boulder, CO	1000 Watts 50–60 Hz
MC-MS	Elmed, Chicago, IL	ESU 100E MM-B
Carbon Dioxide Insufflation		
Insufflation tubing with filter	Surgin, California	SU 1101 lot 10642

level may indicate impending ovarian failure. FSH level should be recommended in all women over age 40 who are considering tubal microsurgery.

Semen analysis is mandatory.

EQUIPMENT CONSIDERATIONS AND PREREQUISITES:

Equipment available for laparoscopic microsurgery is listed in Table 2.

MAGNIFICATION

The degree of magnification required for either open or laparoscopic microsurgery should be sufficient to allow differentiation of healthy from diseased tubal mucosa and muscularis, which at the interstitial and isthmic area may involve luminal diameters of 0.5 mm. Although the operating microscope permits magnification of up to 40×, 26× magnification usually is adequate for examination, and 10–15× normally is adequate for suture placement and tying. Laparoscopic microsurgery requires similar magnification. Operating from a television monitor is absolutely essential to reduce fatigue, improve fine control, and enable meaningful assistance from the assistant surgeon. We initially used the single-chip zoom camera system by Storz, which gave reasonable 10–15× magnification. Recently, we have used the three-chip camera, which provides superior resolution at 800 lines. The Stortz 0° Hopkins laparoscope has exceptional depth of field and remains in focus from 4 mm to infinity, thus facilitating magnification. The third component is the Sony 20-in. monitor with 800-line horizontal resolution. With this combination, it is possible to make a 1-cm probe fill the whole screen horizontally giving a magnification of 40:1, with usable resolution rivaling the operating microscope. We think that this is the way to define magnification via the laparoscope, rather than theoretical mathematics, which may not be meaningful in practice. Although stereoscopic vision is absent in videolaparoscopy, it does not pose a problem as one gets used to two-dimensional surgery, particularly with magnification. In fact, current three-dimensional camera systems are inadequate for microsurgery as they introduce a strobe effect to fine movement.

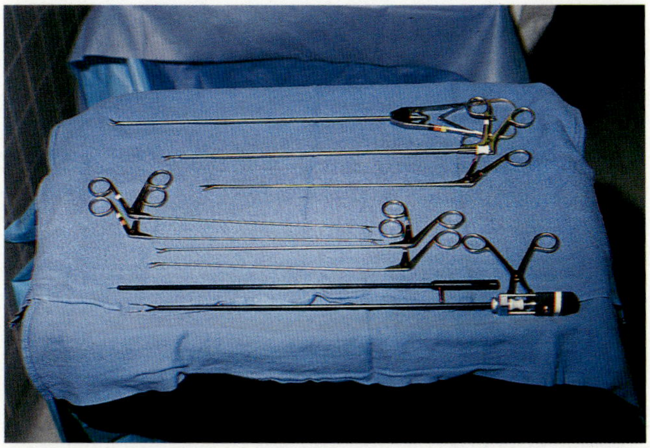

FIG. 3. Laparoscopic microsurgical instruments demonstrated.

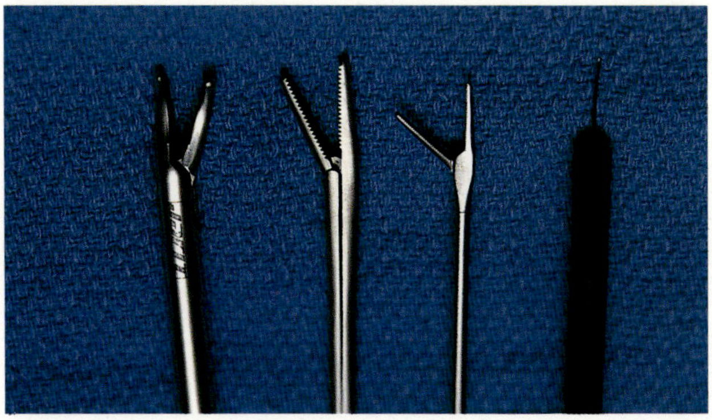

FIG. 4. The fine tips of the instruments are shown. For comparison the needle point is 150 μm and the tips of the instruments range from 1 to 2 mm.

INSTRUMENTATION

There are currently no laparoscopic microsurgical instruments available. Our early attempts at using 8-0 nylon in both the animal and human situation was rewarded with bent needles and suture breakage from grasper trauma. None of the so-called microinstruments available for laparoscopy today are useful, so we are in the process of designing ultramicroinstruments for laparoscopic microsurgery. After considerable experimentation, we found the following currently available instruments to be useful (see Figures 3–10).

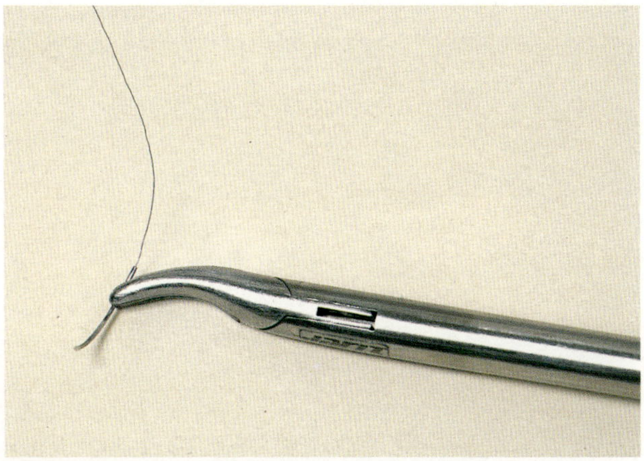

FIG. 5. The position of the needle as grasped by the curved needle holder to facilitate laparoscopic microsurgical suturing.

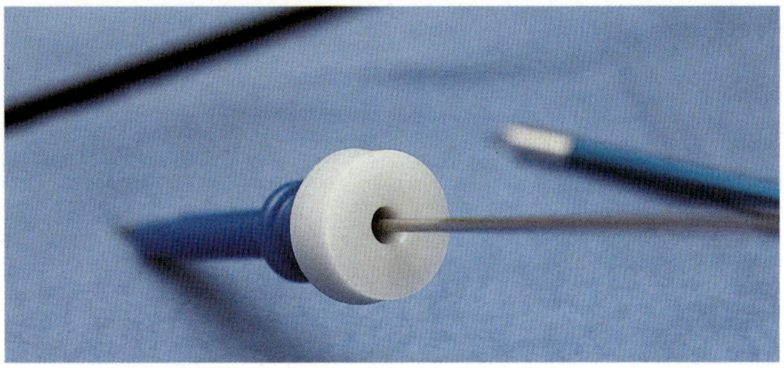

FIG. 6. The Apple trocar reducer admits a 2.5-mm shaft without loss of CO_2.

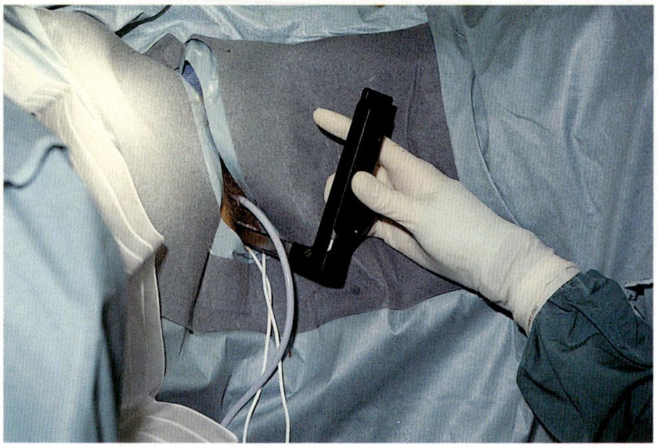

FIG. 8. The Rumi in position.

Needle Driver

We modified the Jarritt needle holder for handling 7-0 and 8-0 sutures by having the tip machined down to 2 mm.

Graspers

Microlaryngoscopic graspers with a tip diameter of 1 mm are useful for handling fallopian tubes and for knot tying. We use the finest emery paper to smooth the jaws from burrs. The frictionless handle mechanism provides a high degree of delicate control without distracting jerkiness. The Mueller microforceps is a strong grasper used for tubal traction to aid the scissor cut, particularly at the cornual tube.

Trocars

We use the Apple 5-mm trocar because its unique cap design allows the introduction of 2.5-mm instruments without the need for distracting adapters to prevent loss of pneumoperitoneum. Suture introduction is also extremely convenient via this cannula.

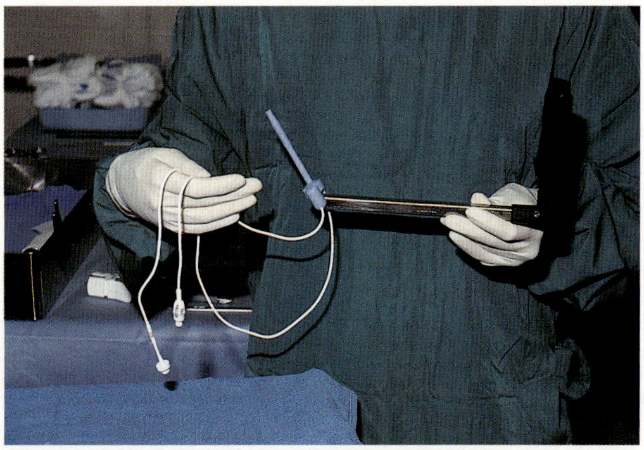

FIG. 7. The Rumi uterine manipulator with lines for methylene blue dye and intrauterine balloon.

Excision of Fallopian Tube

Disposable microscissors from Ethicon are useful for straight cuts.

Director scissors from Microsurge, which allow up to a 75° angulation at the tip, are useful for performing right-angle cuts of the fallopian tube, particularly at the cornua.

In a recent innovation, we use the guillotine (Hook Cutter, DaVinci), which transects both proximal and distal tubes very cleanly, giving a nice ring of muscularis to aid in suturing.

Suction Irrigation

Most disposable probes are roughly machined and cause serosal ecchymosis when used to mobilize the fallopian tube. We use emery paper to smooth nondispos-

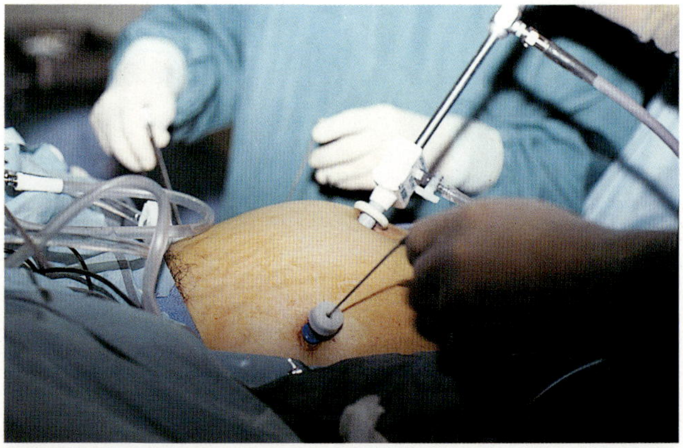

FIG. 9. Demonstration of trocar sites with two on the right side of the patient, one on the left and the laparoscope through the umbilicus. The surgeon, standing on the patient's right, uses both right-sided trocars, while the assistant, standing on the patient's left, handles the camera and left trocar.

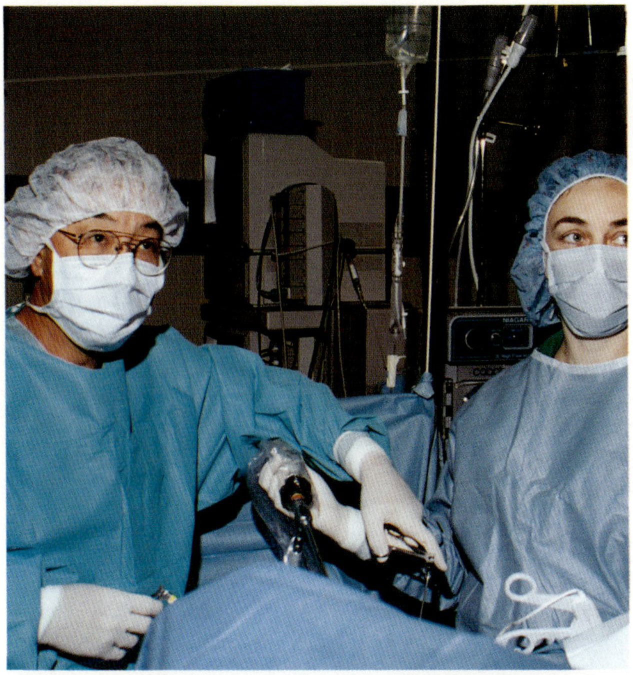

FIG. 10. During intracorporeal suturing, the surgeon's left hand crosses over the patient's abdomen to handle a grasper from the left lower quadrant port.

able probes. For irrigation, 1 L of warm Ringer's lactate with 5000 U of heparin is used.

Particulate Filter

It is important to filter the carbon dioxide used for pneumoperitoneum from particulate impurities and microorganisms. For this purpose, the insufflation tubing with filter from Surgin (Tustin, California) is used.

Stents

With adequate magnification, tubal apposition is more accurately performed without using stents. We occasionally employ the Florestor vessel occluder used for vascular anastomosis as a luminal indicator where there is difficulty seeing the muscularis because of luxuriant mucosa.

Uterine Manipulator/Chromopertubation

We use a Rumi uterine manipulator, which allows the uterus to be anteflexed and deviated to the left or right or pushed upwards into the abdominal cavity. This reduces tension during anastomosis by approximating the proximal to the distal tube. The lateral openings of the tip allow successful retrograde chromopertubation. Other uterine chromopertubators with terminal openings tend to be lodged in the endometrium causing intravasation of dye. The ureteric catheter (Cook, Bloomington, IL), size 4–6 Fr, is introduced through a suction irrigation probe and is used for retrograde chromopertubation of the distal tube after opening its proximal stump.

ENERGY

As an energy source, a 150-μm microneedle is used and powered from a low-voltage generator, like those from Elmed (600 V peak to peak) and ValleyLab (1000 V peak to peak). The power setting is 18 W for cutting and 10 W for coagulation. We can also employ the microlaryngoscopic scissors in place of the needle electrode to dissect the serosa prior to stump excision.

OVERCOMING INHERENT LIMITATIONS OF LAPAROSCOPY

Angle of View

With the operating microscope at laparotomy one is looking perpendicularly down at the uterus and fallopian

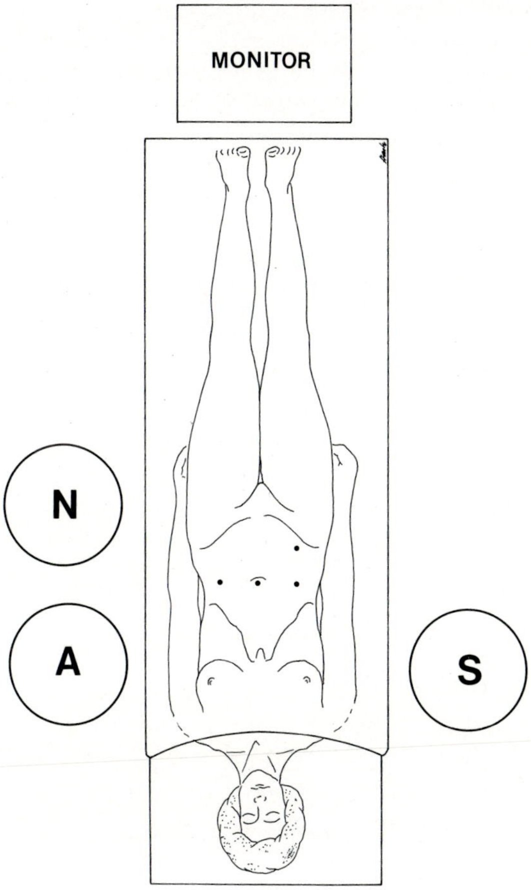

FIG. 11. Portals for microsurgery.

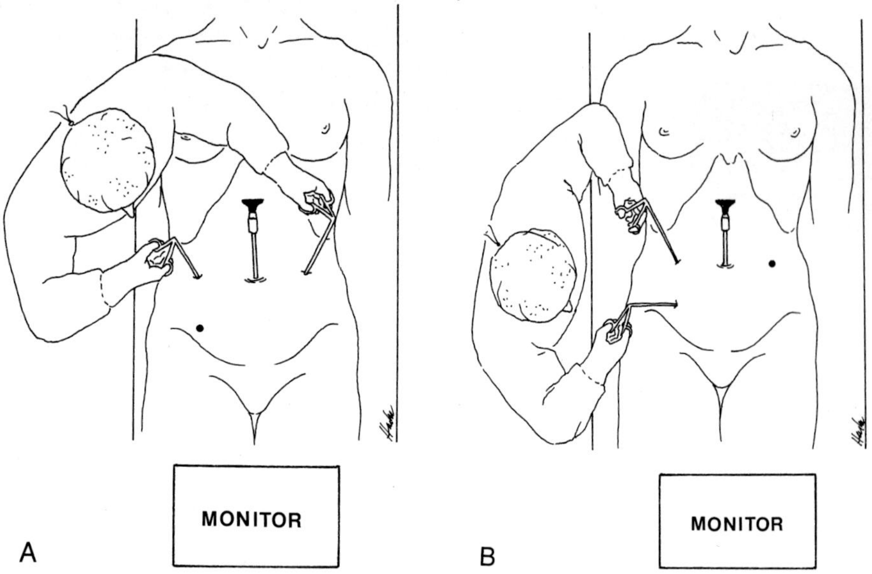

FIG. 12. Intracorporeal suturing. A: Contralateral method. B: Ipsilateral method.

tubes while the instruments come in at a near-horizontal angle. There is also good lateral mobility of the operating microscope for cornual visualization. With laparoscopy, the angle of view is caudad with the scope angled at 20–45° from the horizontal. (The use of other than 0° scopes reduces coordination and is not recommended.) This requires modifications in technique. For example, holding the needle on the convex of the needle holder, which is the technique at open microsurgery, will result in poor visualization of the needle, as it is obscured by the convexity of the needle holder jaws. Hence, the needle is held in the direction of the concavity.

Portals for Instrumentation

At laparotomy there is an unlimited approach angle of the instruments, which allows precise and accurate placement of cuts and sutures. In contrast, at laparoscopy the angle of approach of accessory instrumentation is limited by the three or four portals employed (Fig. 11). The use of curved and articulating instruments (e.g., Director scissors) provides increased versatility, but one is very dependent on good uterine manipulation to achieve the desired angle of approach to the proximal tubes and in approximating the ends.

Transmission of Fine Delicate Movements

This is possible first by appropriate trocar placement at an angle facing the pelvis, so that one is not overcoming abdominal wall resistance. Second, the shorter microlaryngoscopic instruments, together with their fine delicate design, allow the transmission of tactile information sensitively, so that it is possible to tie even 8-0 sutures with

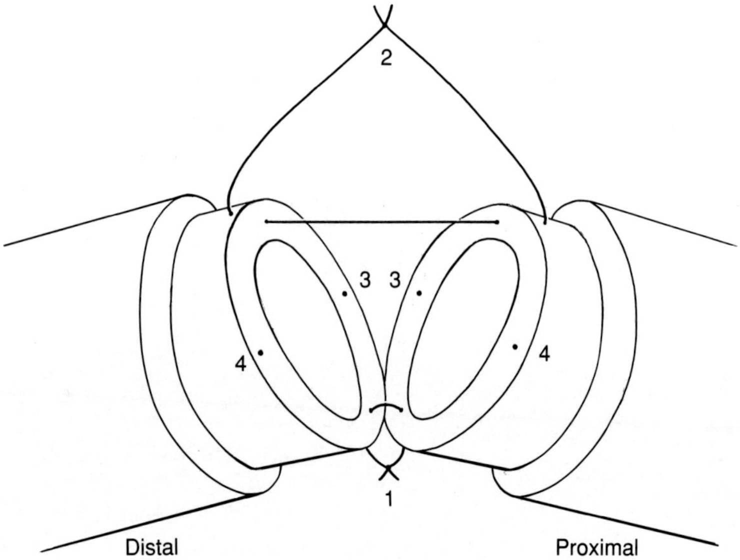

FIG. 13. Microsuturing using 7-0 or 8-0 nylon, proline, or vicryl. (1) 6 o'clock is tied first. (2) 12 o'clock is held to orient other sutures. (3) 9 o'clock placed and tied. (4) 3 o'clock placed and tied. The 12 o'clock suture is tied last.

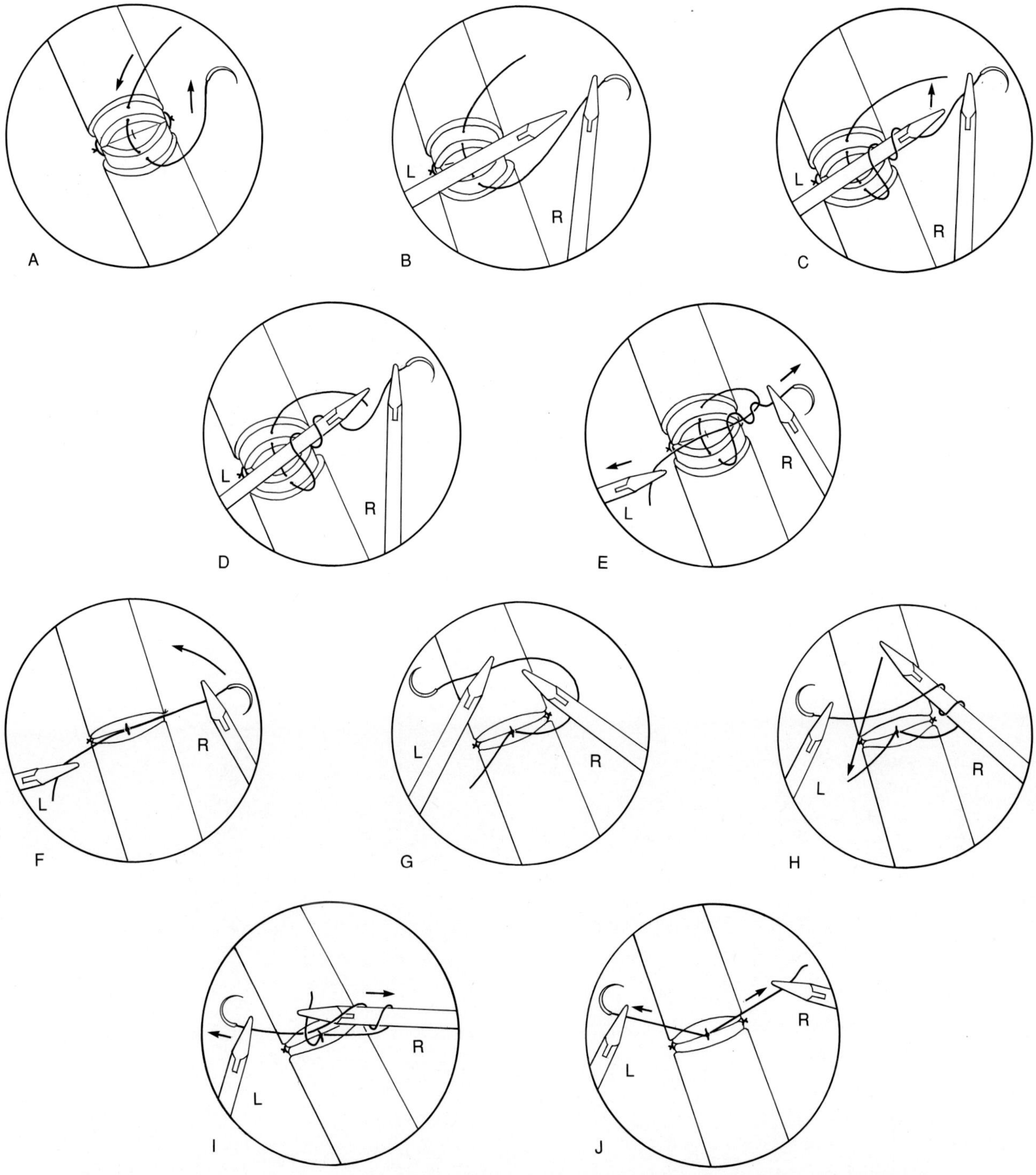

FIG. 14. Contralateral method. **A:** The most important aspect is a proper initial grasper positioning similar to the address in golfing. The address for intracorporeal suturing is the U position as illustrated. Failure to adopt the address position as depicted will result in frustration and often failure. The 6, 3, and 9 o'clock sutures have been tied. The suturing technique is being demonstrated for the 12 o'clock suture. **B:** The contralateral left grasper (L) is positioned at the base of the U parallel to the long (needle) arm of the U. **C:** The needle end of the suture is held with the right-hand grasper (R), which proceeds to throw a clockwise double loop over the left grasper. **D:** The left (contralateral) grasper picks up the short end. **E:** Pull is exerted in opposite directions (*note arrows*) to cinch the knot squarely. **F:** The first knot has been tightened. Arrow shows movement of right grasper to pass the long end of the suture to the left contralateral grasper. **G:** After the left grasper picks up the long end, the address now becomes an inverted U or inverted C. **H:** The second knot is counter clockwise single loop over the right grasper. **I:** The short end has been picked up by the right grasper and cinching begins. **J:** The completed surgeon's square knot is shown.

just the right amount of tension without breaking the suture.

To avoid tremors and maintain more delicate control, it is a good idea to have the upper arm rest against the side of one's body and to have the table elevated enough, such that it is possible to rest the palm on the patient's body while employing the microneedle electrode.

INTRACORPOREAL MICROSUTURING

The left and right paraumbilical portals are used for the left and right hands of the surgeon, while the assistant holds the camera and the remaining portal to assist. Steep Trendelenburg positioning minimizes arm fatigue.

Figures 12–15 demonstrate our technique of laparoscopic microsuturing.

APPLICATION OF TECHNIQUE

Slides depicting three procedures are presented. Steps illustrating in detail bilateral ampullary–ampullary tubal anastomosis are provided in Figs. 16–39. The patient had undergone previous sterilization with nonabsorbable sutures by the Pomeroy technique. The next set

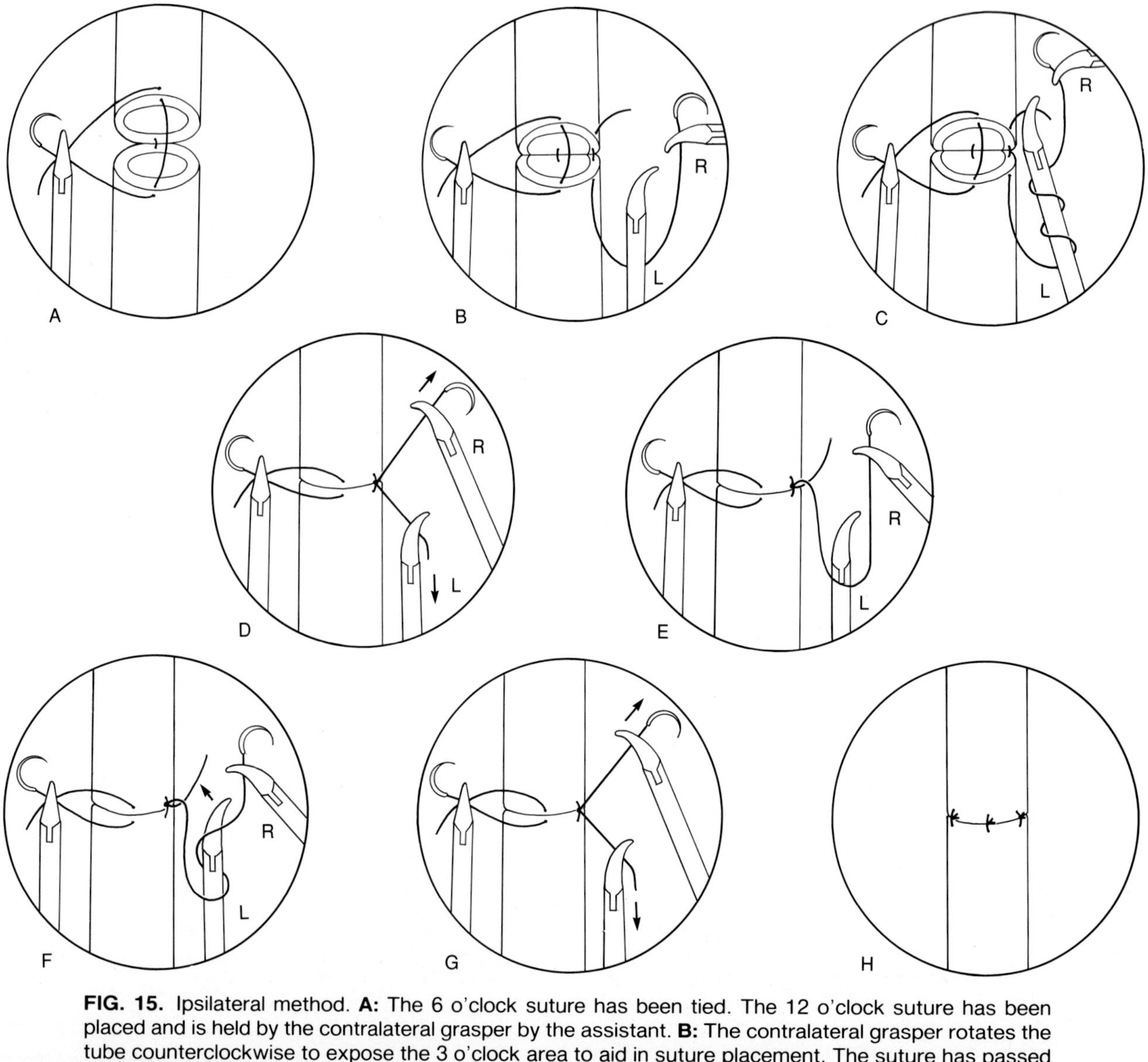

FIG. 15. Ipsilateral method. **A:** The 6 o'clock suture has been tied. The 12 o'clock suture has been placed and is held by the contralateral grasper by the assistant. **B:** The contralateral grasper rotates the tube counterclockwise to expose the 3 o'clock area to aid in suture placement. The suture has passed from proximal to distal tube, and pulled through. The U address is now prepared by the right grasper (R) holding the needle end. **C:** A double clockwise loop has been thrown over the left (L) ultramicrograsper, which then picks the short end of the suture. **D:** The knot is cinched by pulling in the direction of the arrows. **E:** The U address is again formed. **F:** A single counterclockwise loop is thrown over the left grasper (L) held by the left hand of the operator which then picks up the short end. **G:** After pulled in opposite directions the knot is completed. **H:** 7-0 interrupted serosa sutures complete the anastomosis.

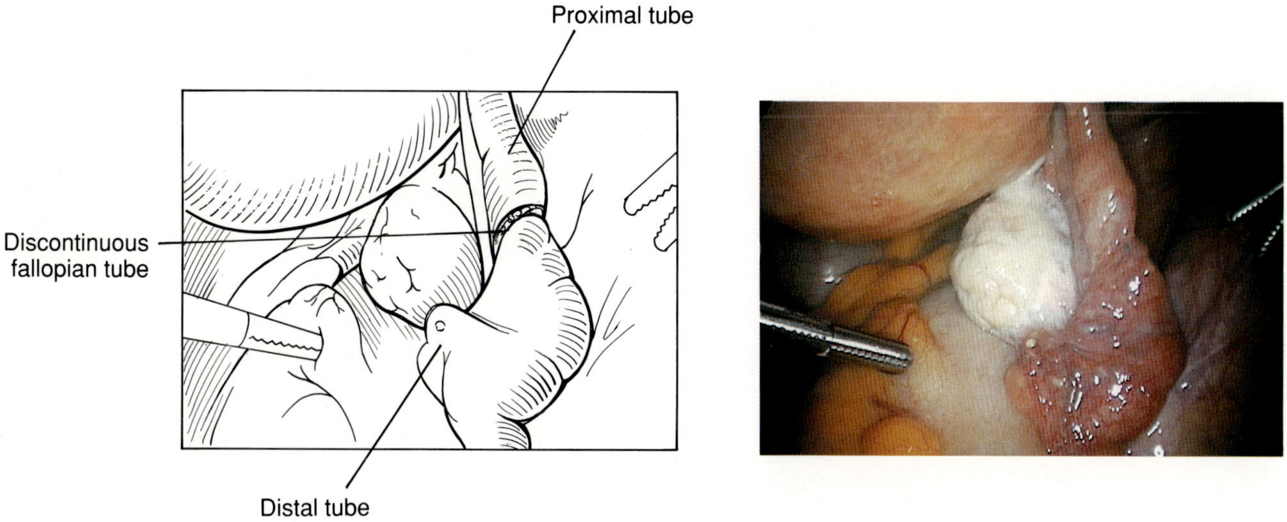

FIG. 16. Right fallopian tube with previous midampullary ligation with nonabsorbable suture.

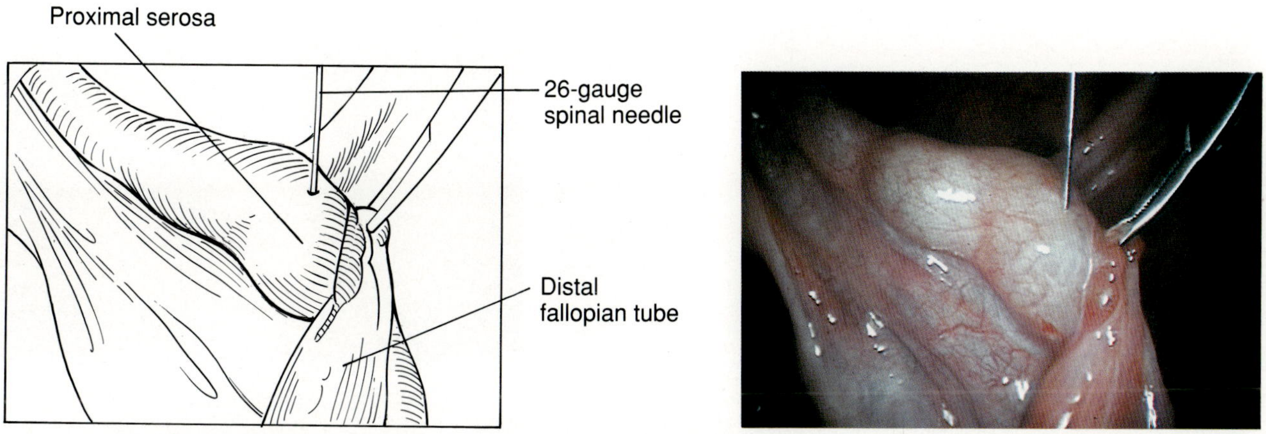

FIG. 17. Pitressin 1:50 dilution is injected into proximal tubal serosa with a 26-gauge spinal needle through the abdominal wall.

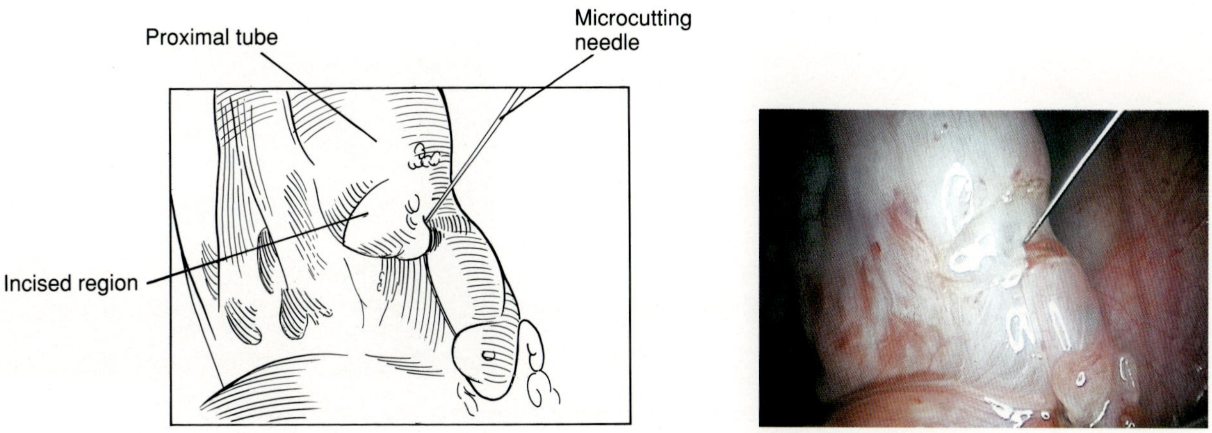

FIG. 18. Serosa of proximal tube is incised circumferentially up to muscularis with a 150-μm microneedle at 18 W unipolar cutting. This facilitates later scissors cut by reducing tissue volume.

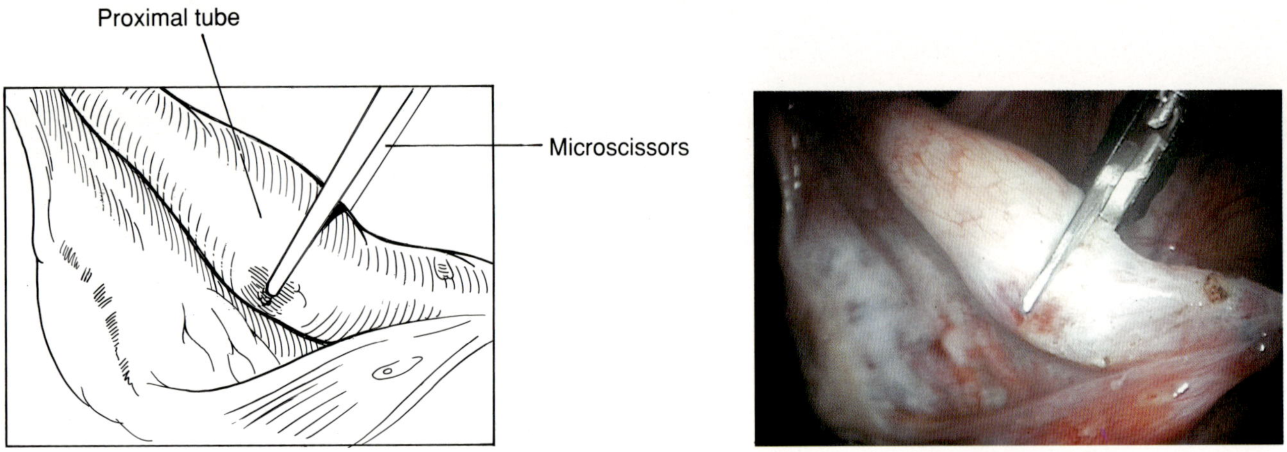

FIG. 19. Proximal tube is cut using disposable Ethicon microscissors.

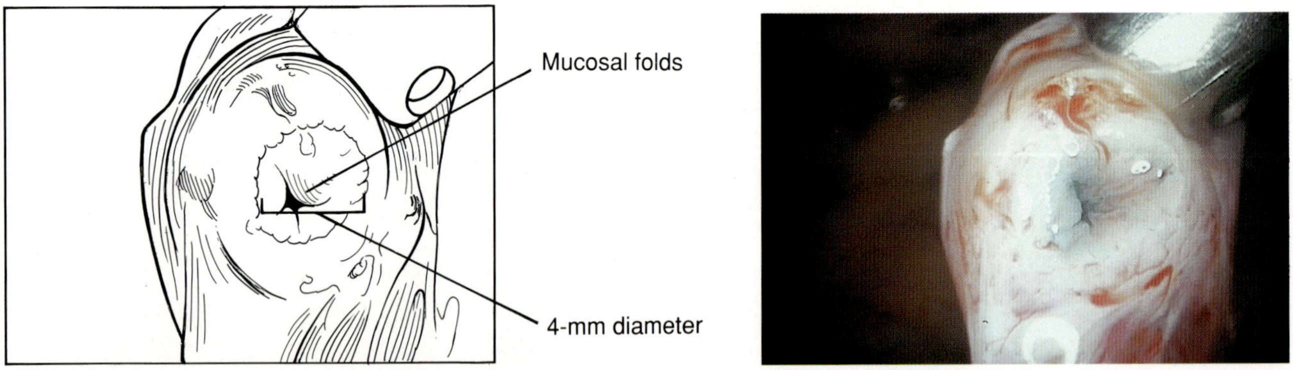

FIG. 20. Cut end of proximal tube shows healthy muscosal folds and a luminal diameter of 4 mm. The magnification is 27× as measured on a 20-in. diagonal TV monitor.

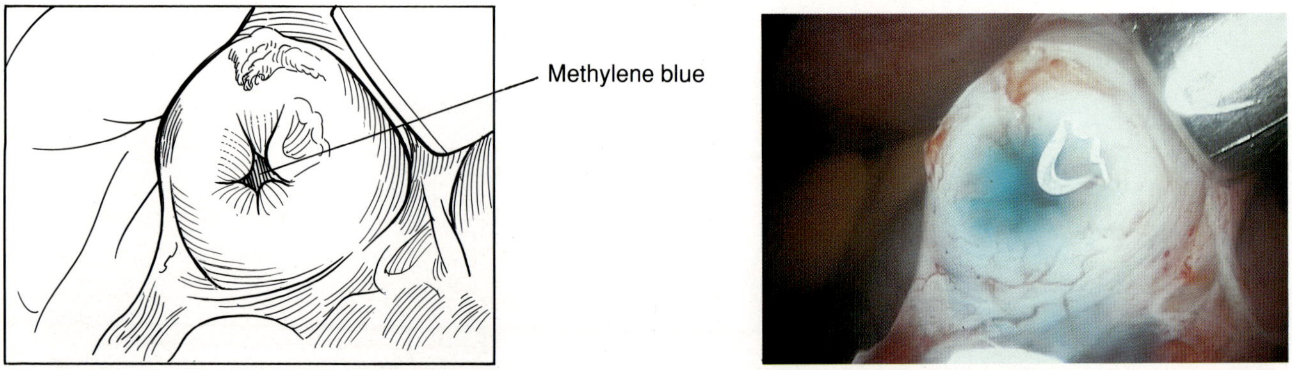

FIG. 21. Methylene blue emerges from the proximal tube. Magnification is 36×.

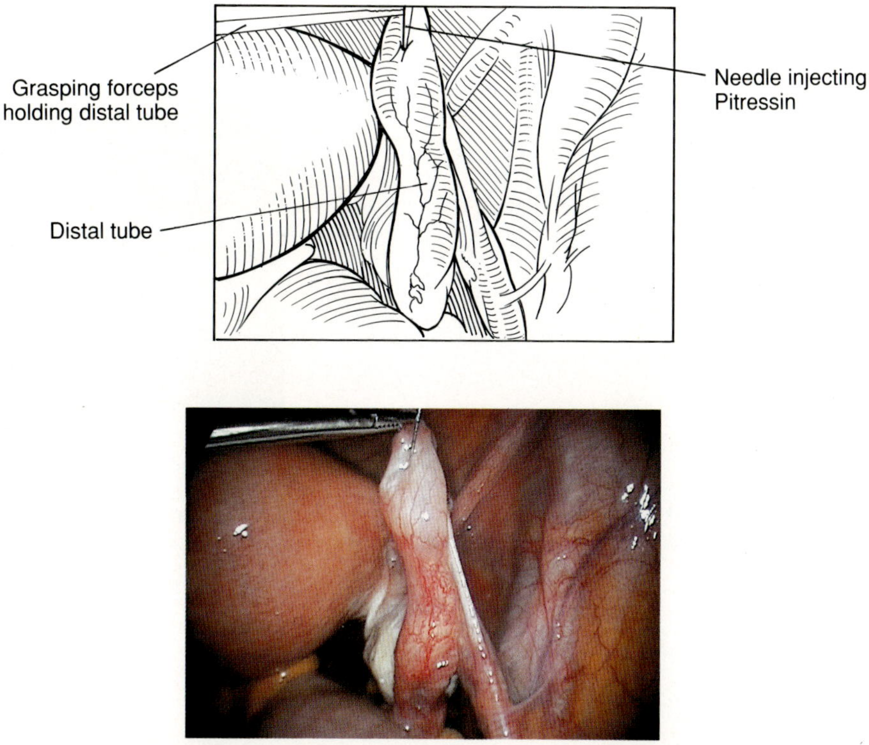

FIG. 22. Pitressin 1:50 is injected into distal stump.

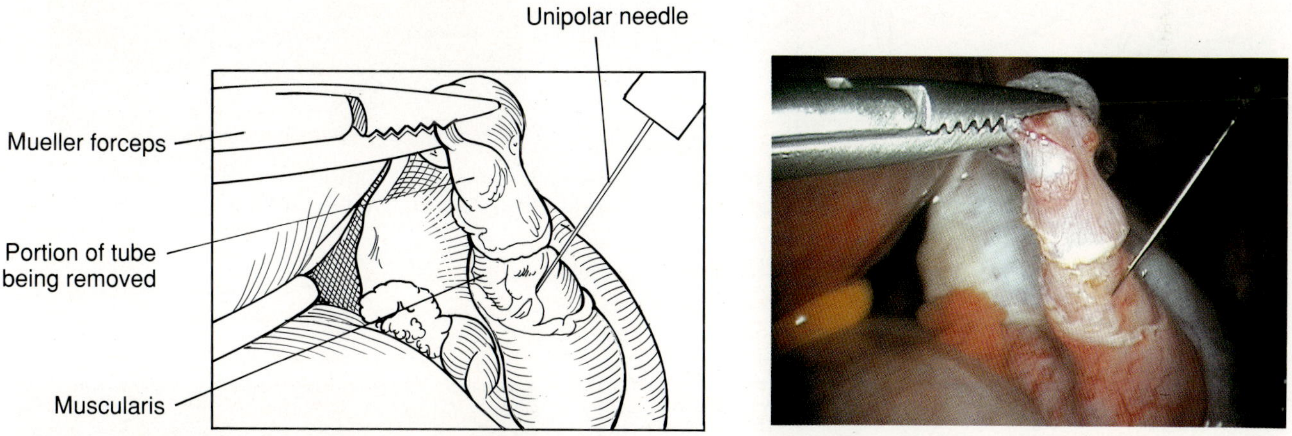

FIG. 23. Circumscription of serosa with a 150-μm unipolar needle. Muscularis is exposed to assess potential luminal size prior to being cut with microscissors. Mueller forceps are used for forceful grasping of tissue. These forceps should only be used on tissue which eventually will be removed because of the tissue trauma created by the graspers.

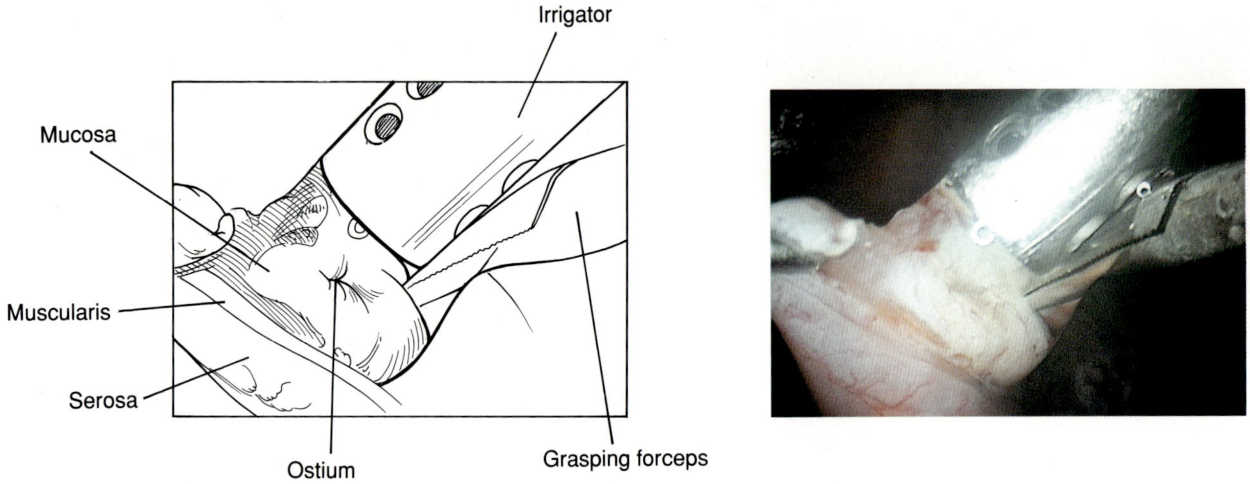

FIG. 24. Distal stump has been excised revealing a 5-mm luminal diameter. The normal mucosal folds exhibit delicate movement when irrigated with Ringer's lactate.

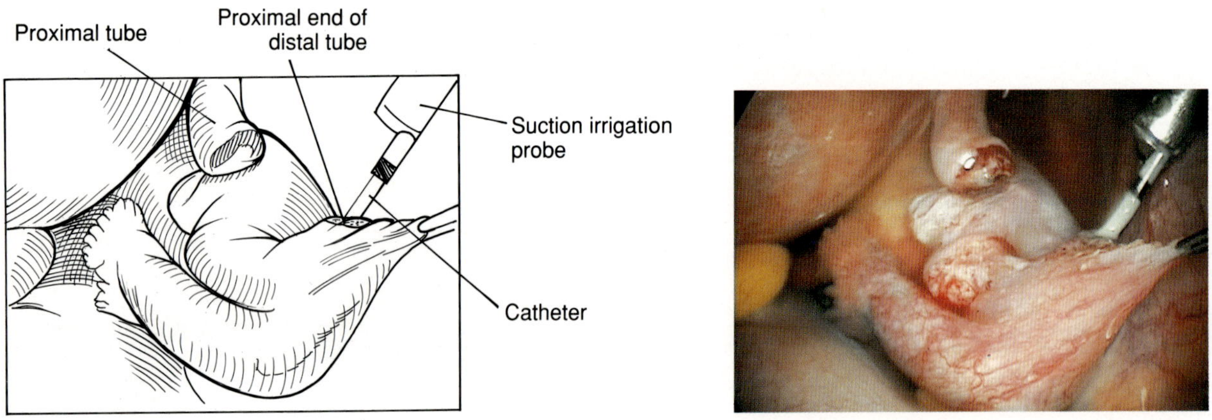

FIG. 25. A no. 4 Fr ureteric catheter is introduced via the suction irrigation probe into the proximal end of the distal tube. Methylene blue emerges at the fimbria indicating patency of the distal tube.

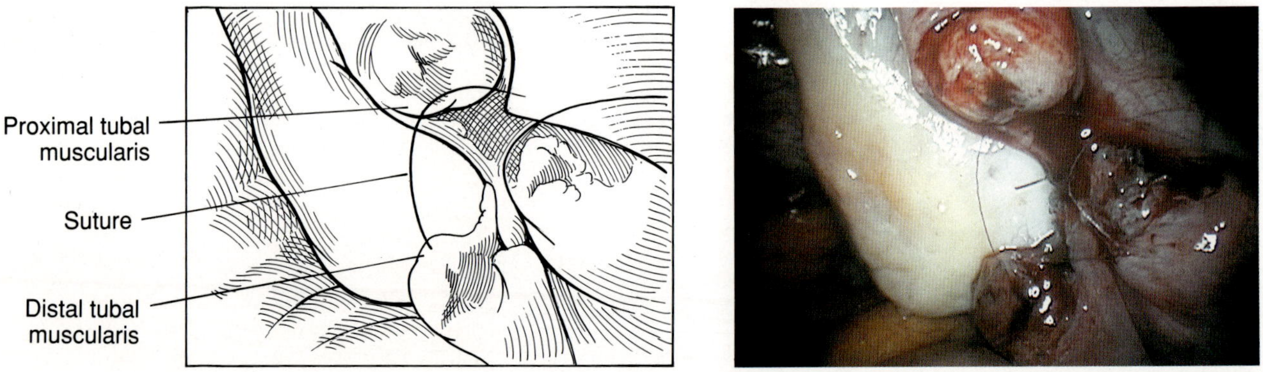

FIG. 26. 8-0 vicryl has been inserted at the 6 o'clock position into the muscularis of both stumps; care is taken to avoid the muscosa.

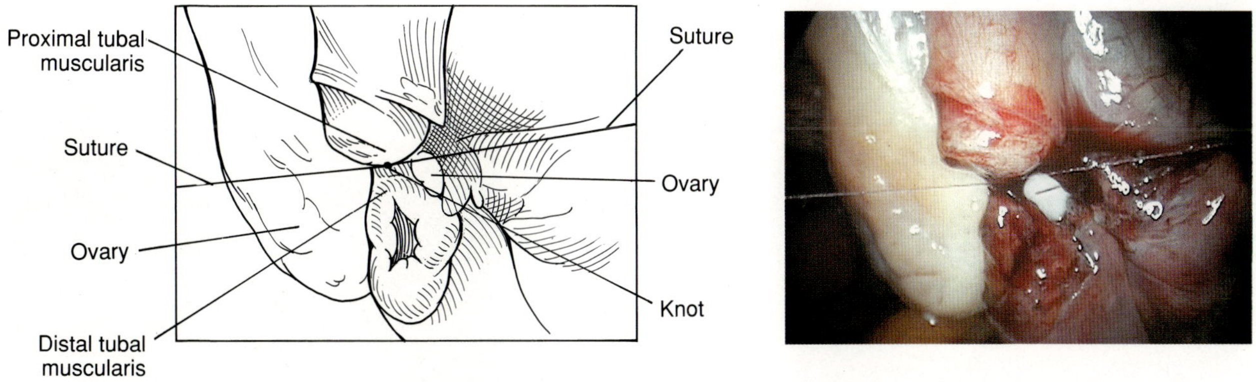

FIG. 27. The 6 o'clock suture completed after second throw of surgeon's knot.

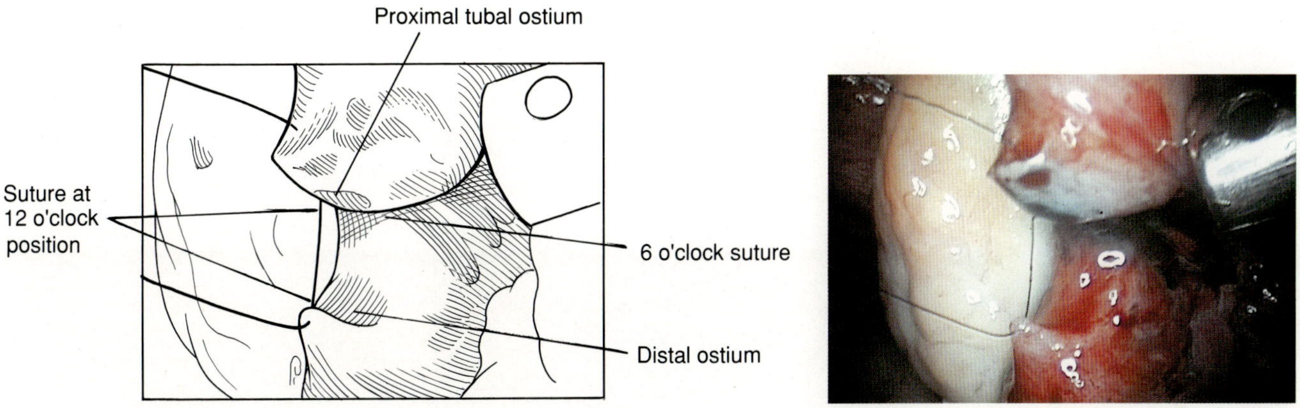

FIG. 28. 7-0 nylon at the 12 o'clock position through the muscularis. The suture is held by a grasper and is pulled to facilitate placement of the 3 and 9 o'clock sutures.

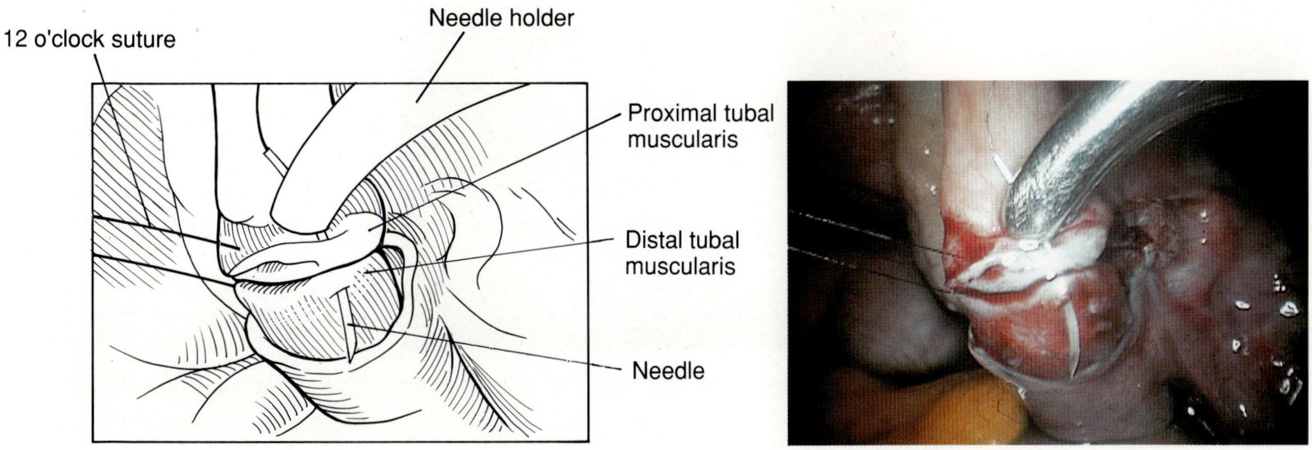

FIG. 29. With the 12 o'clock suture pulled to the left, the 3 o'clock muscularis stitch is placed, using 7/0 nylon.

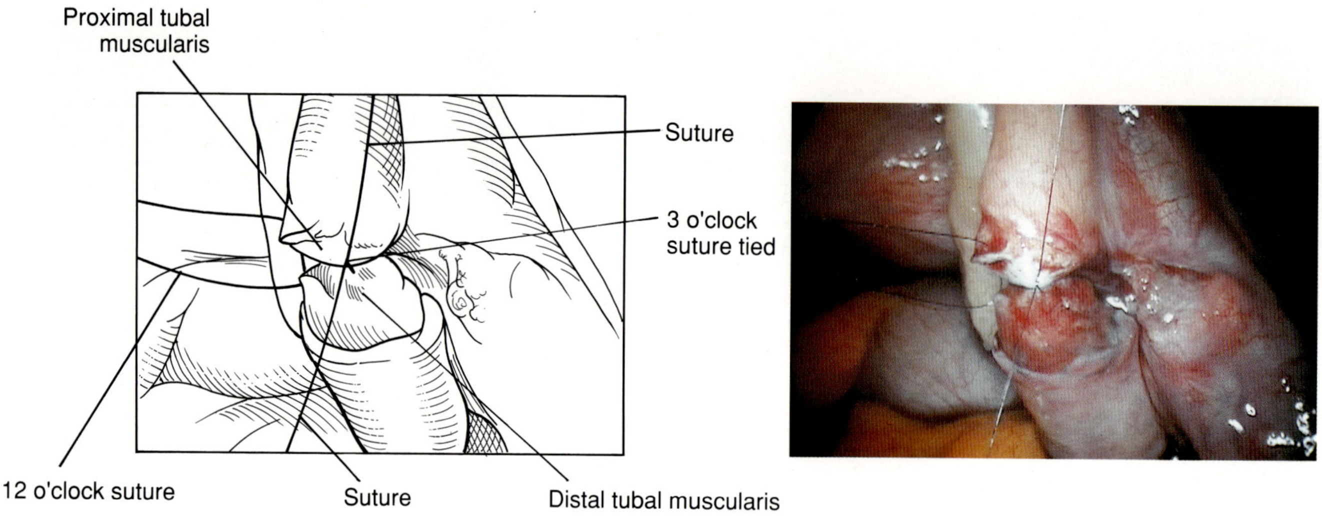

FIG. 30. The 3 o'clock suture is tied.

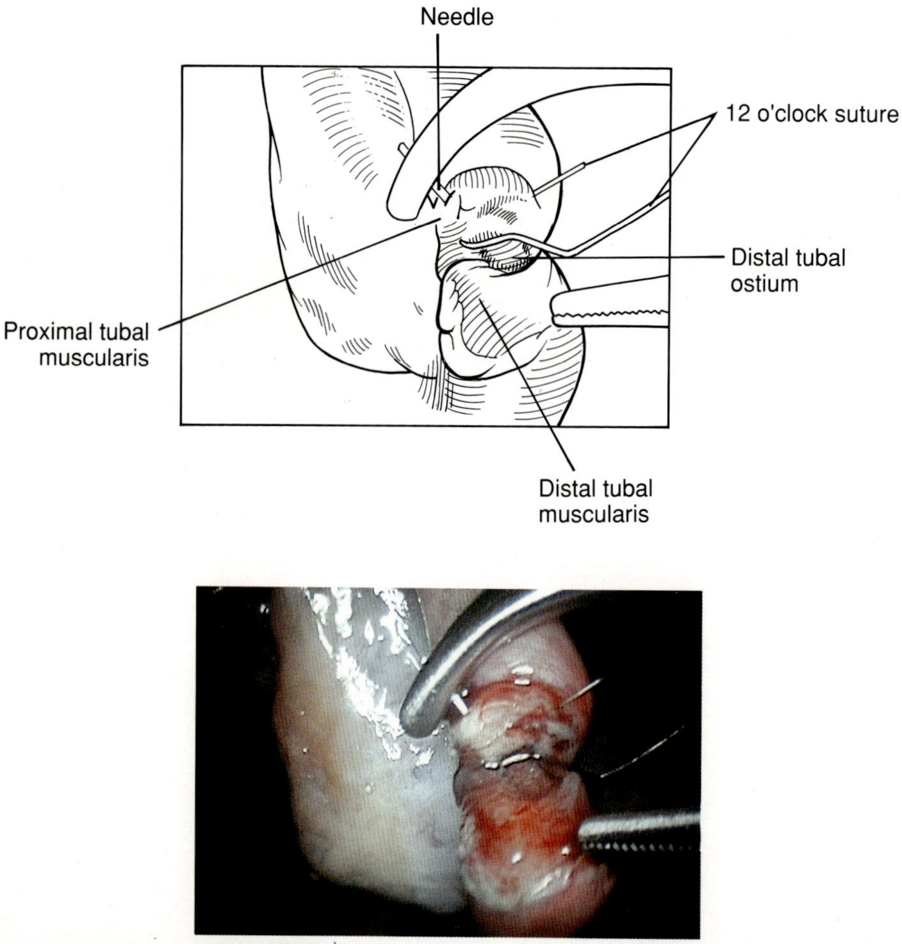

FIG. 31. The 12 o'clock suture is pulled to the right and the 7-0 muscularis stitch is placed at the 9 o'clock position on the proximal tube.

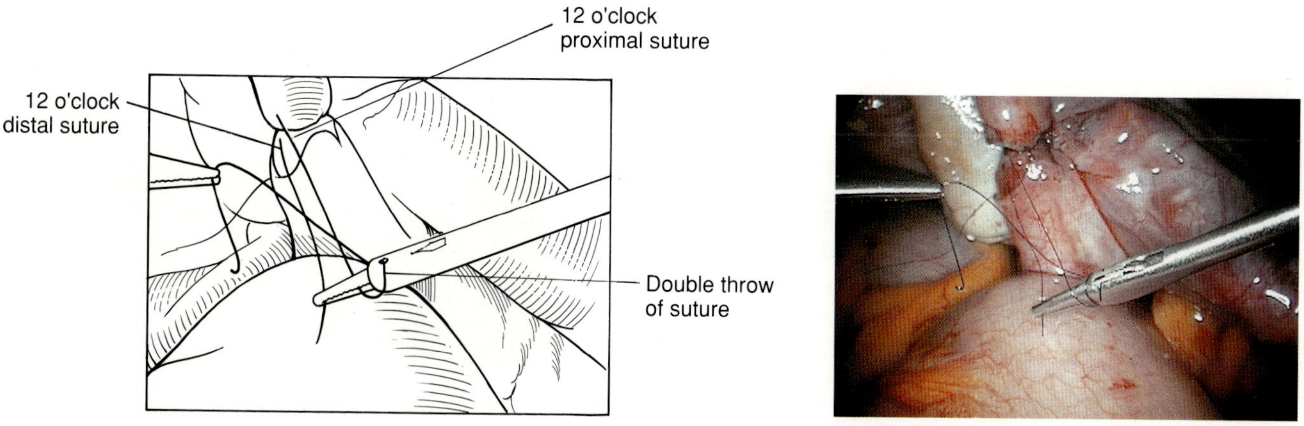

FIG. 32. The 9 o'clock suture is left untied. The 12 o'clock suture is now tied. The first double throw is shown.

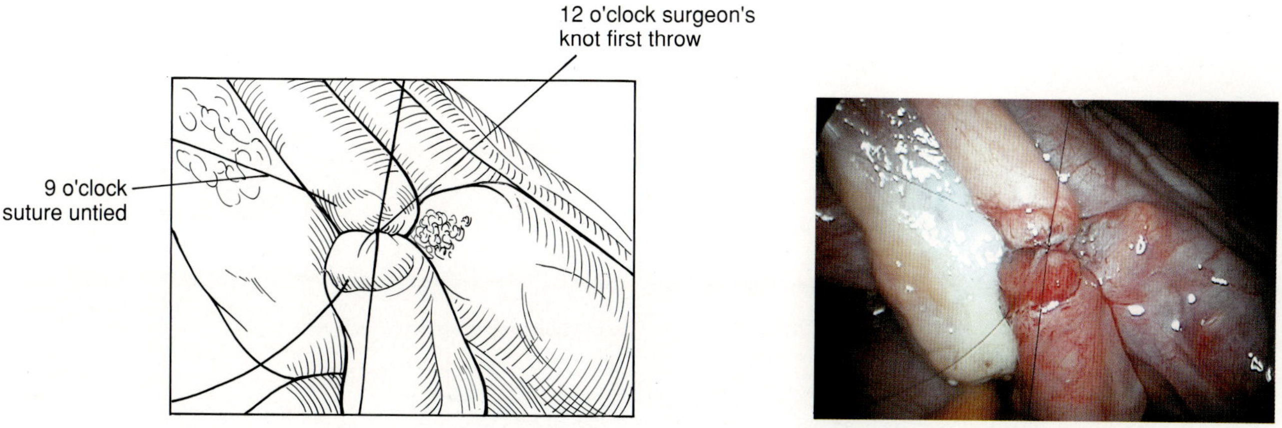

FIG. 33. The surgeon's knot is cinched tight. On the left, the 9 o'clock suture is seen not yet tied.

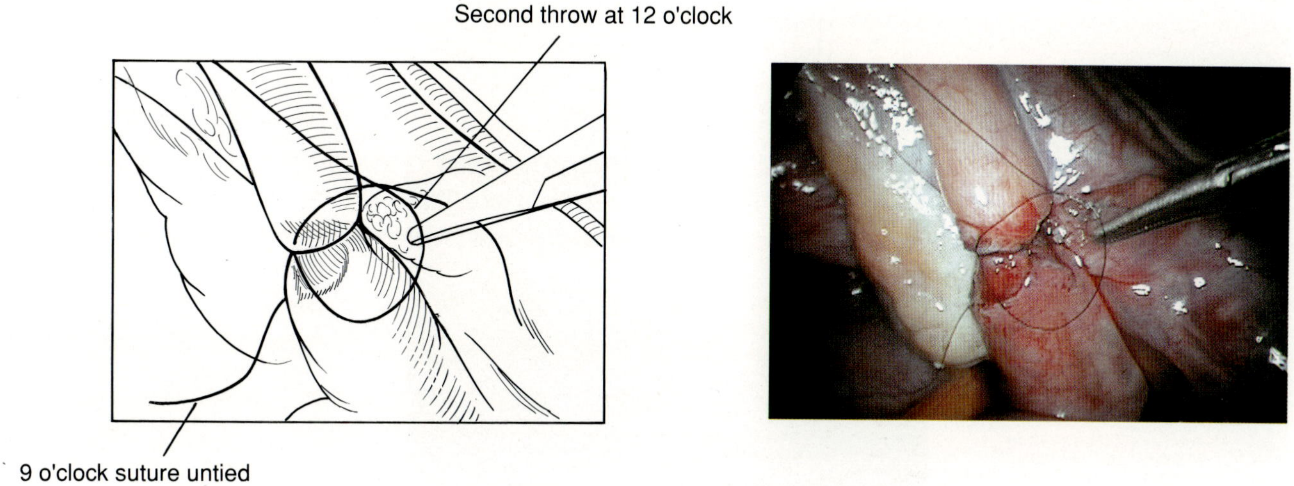

FIG. 34. A single, counterclockwise throw has been made for the second knot at 12 o'clock.

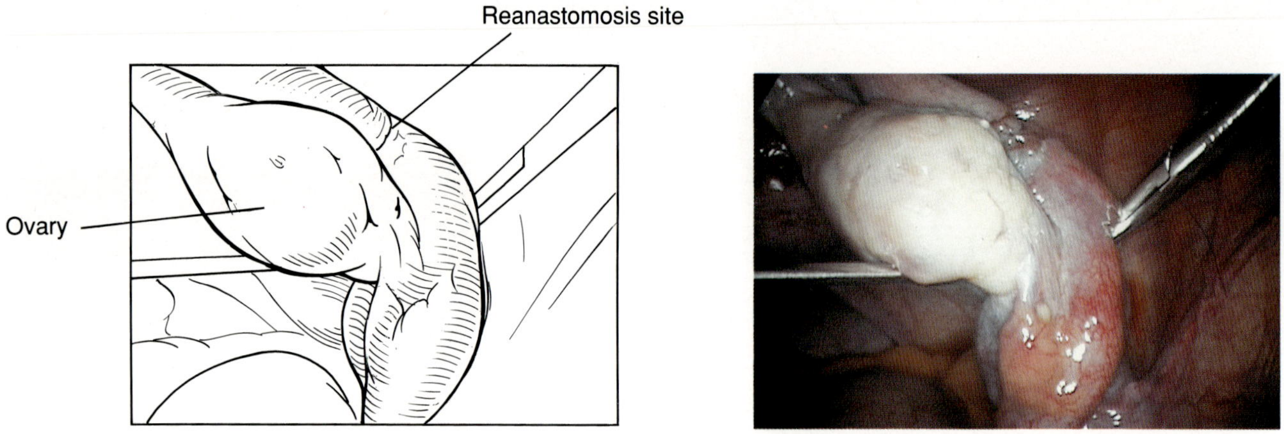

FIG. 35. All muscularis sutures have been tied and methylene blue is injected to confirm patency.

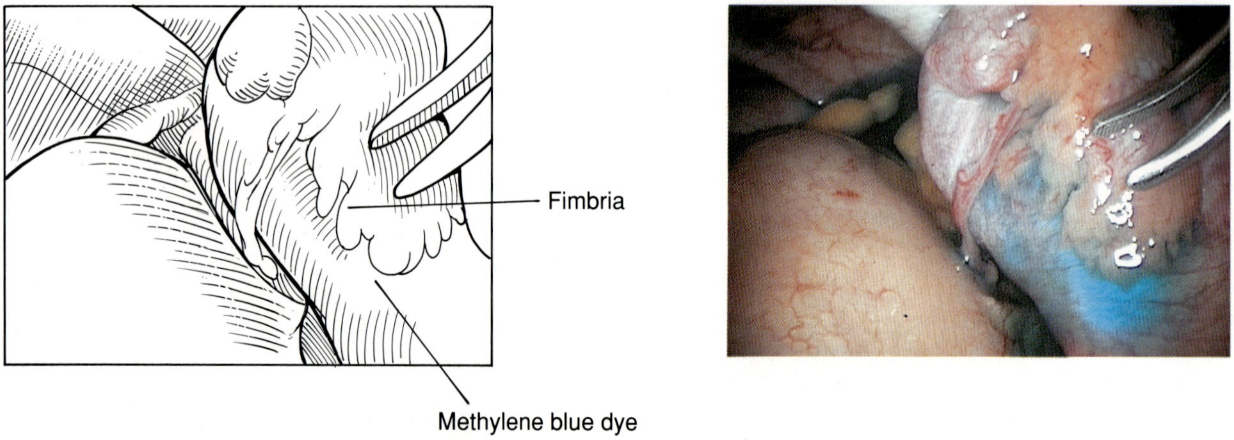

FIG. 36. Patency is established with low chromopertubation pressure.

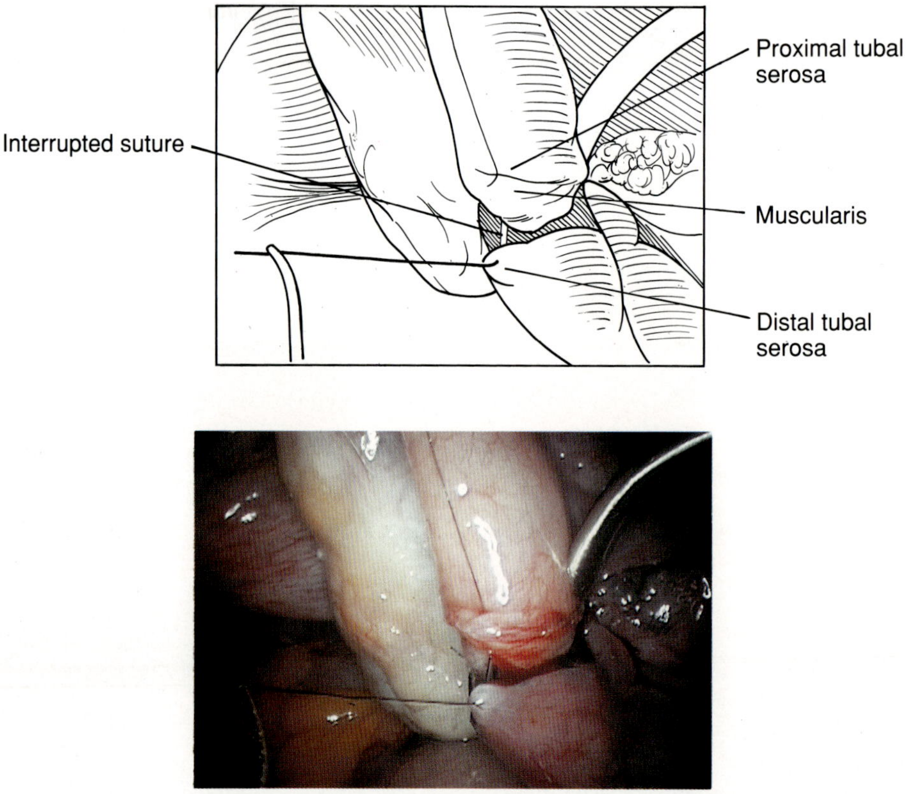

FIG. 37. 7-0 nylon is used for closure of the serosa with interrupted sutures.

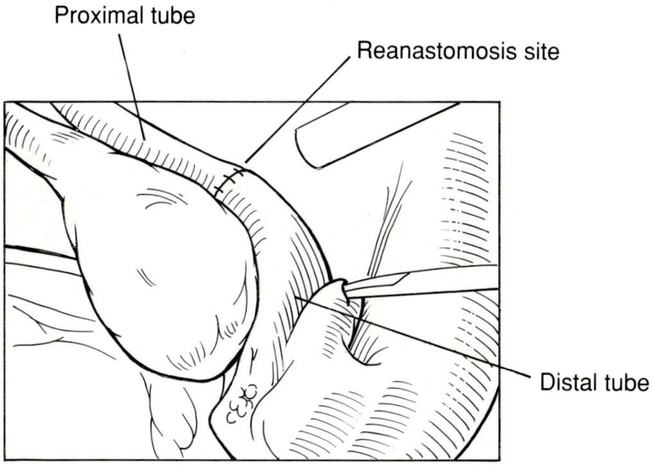

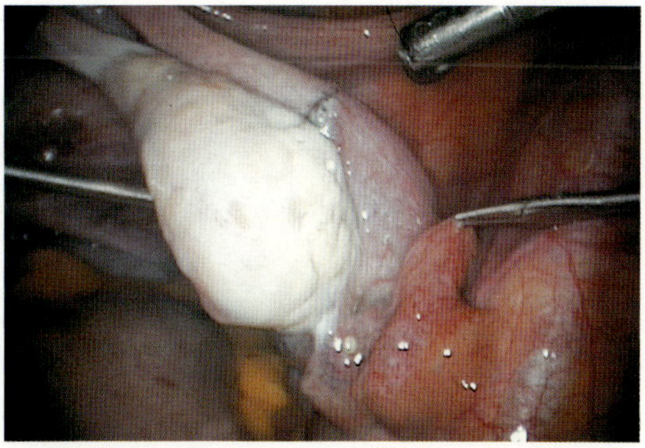

FIG. 38. Serosal closure is complete.

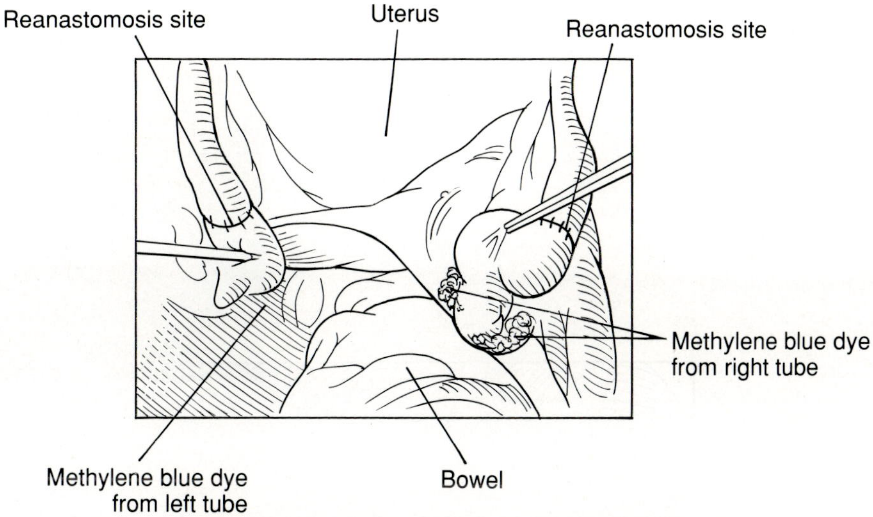

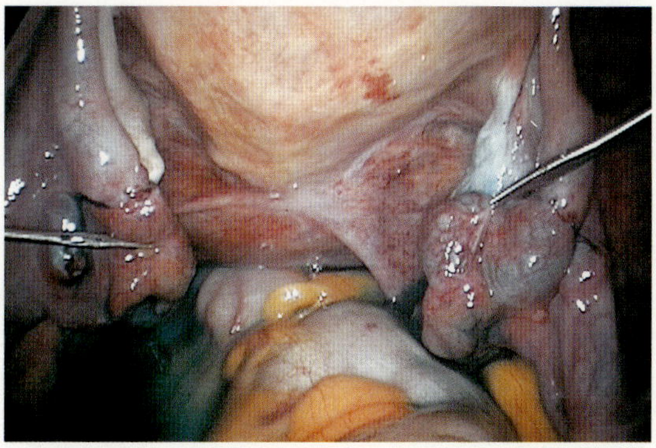

FIG. 39. Bilateral tubal anastomosis is completed with bilateral patency and no leakage at anastomotic site.

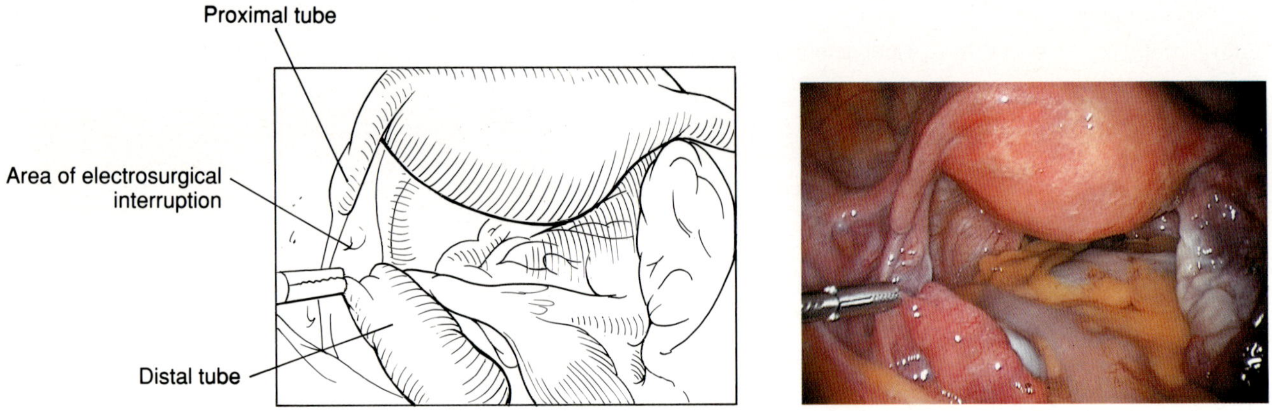

FIG. 40. Left tube showing midtubal electrosurgical interruption.

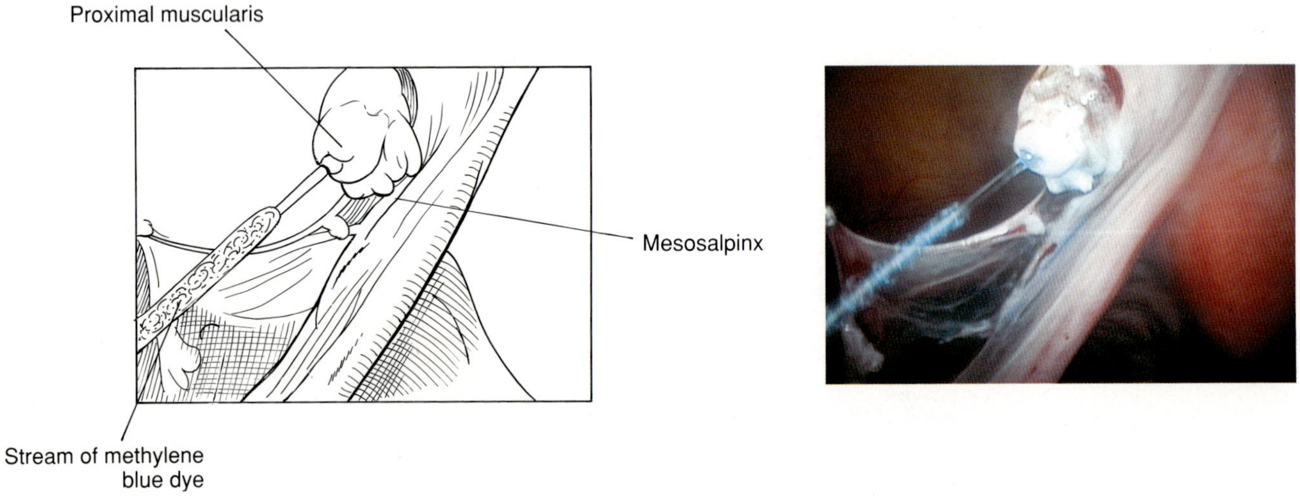

FIG. 41. Proximal patency is established. Good retrograde flow is achieved after isthmic excision.

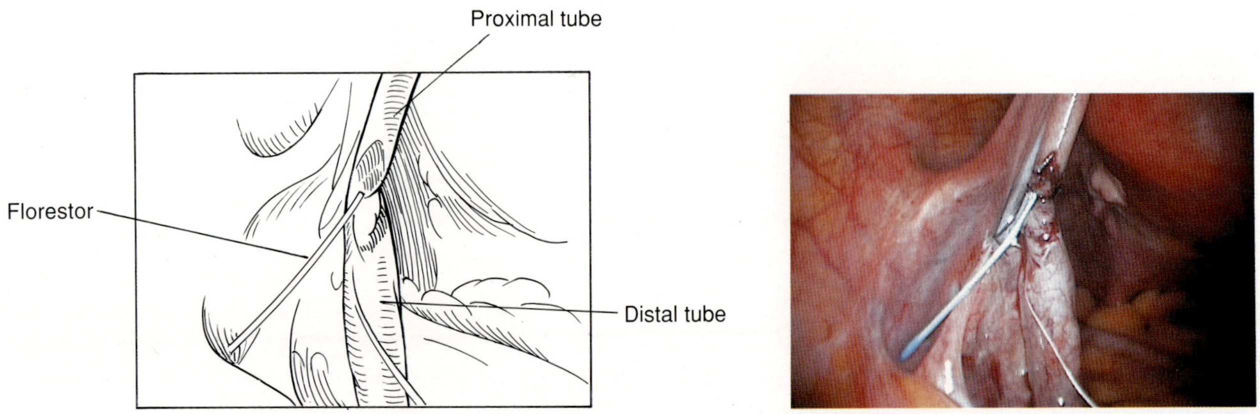

FIG. 42. Florestor 1.25 mm inserted into proximal and later distal tube.

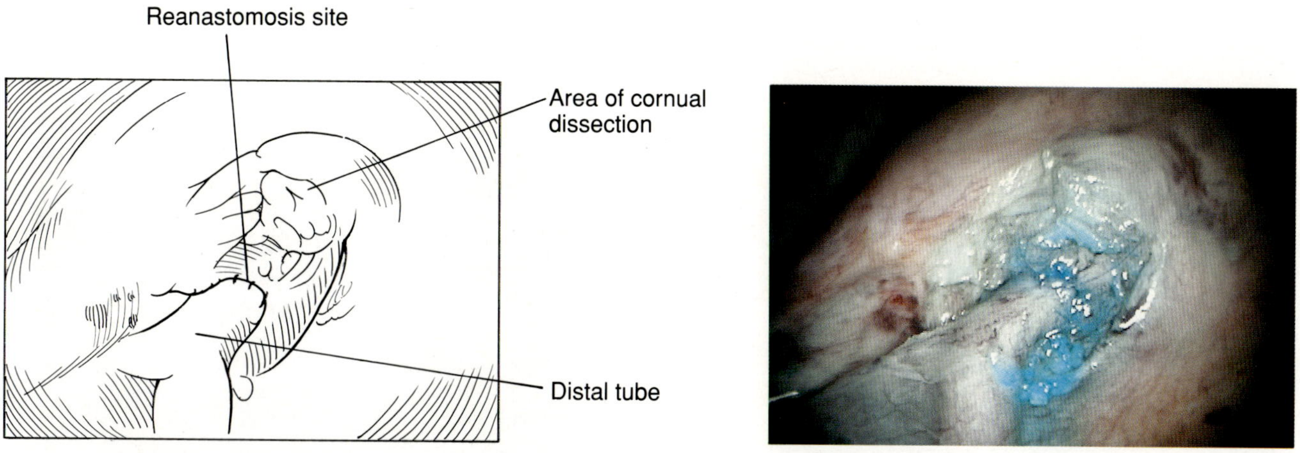

FIG. 54. The tubal anastomosis is complete and the stent has been removed. Four 8-0 sutures have been placed in the muscularis at 3, 6, 9, and 12 o'clock.

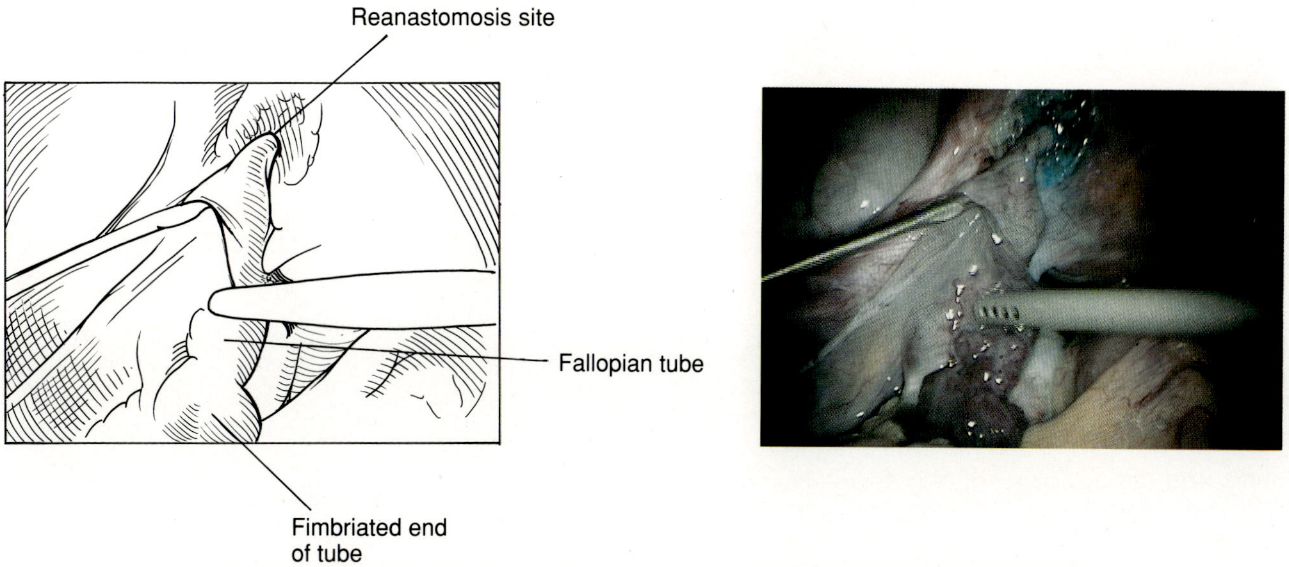

FIG. 55. Panoramic view of the completed anastomosis prior to uterine muscle closure.

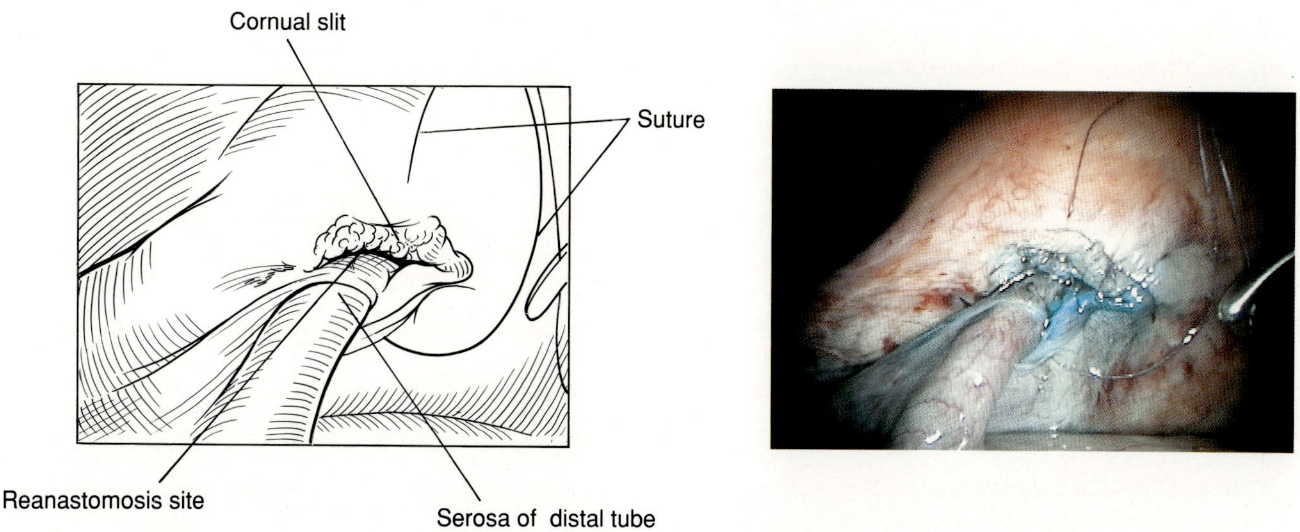

FIG. 56. 6-0 Vicryl is used to close the cornual slit, and the most lateral stitch will incorporate the serosa of the distal tube.

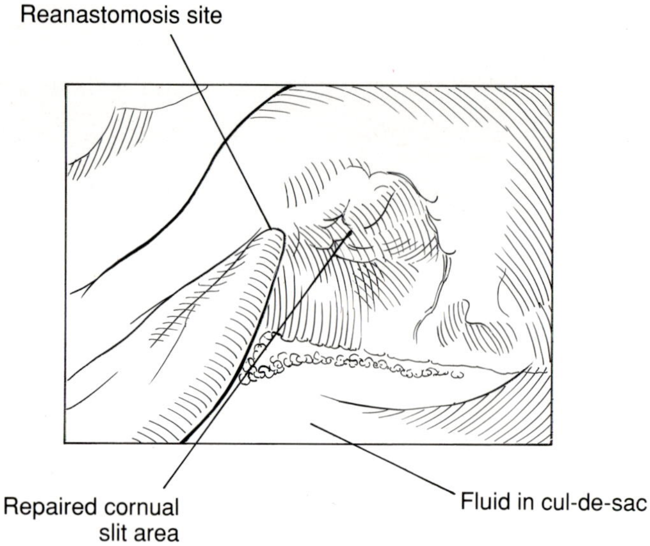

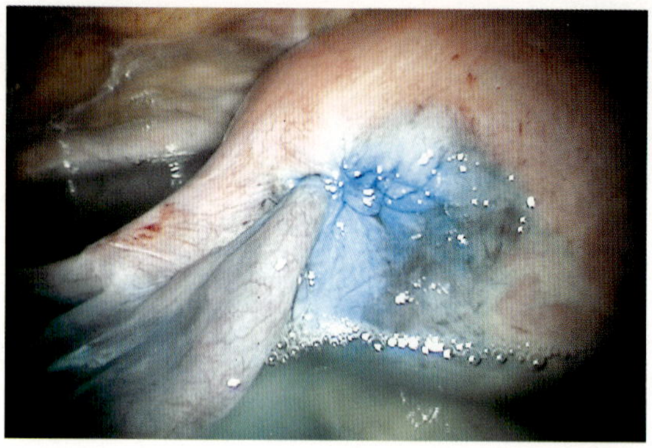

FIG. 57. Completed juxtauterine tubal anastomosis.

of photos, 40–45, depict the technique of isthmic–ampullary tubal anastomosis with the use of Florestor. Finally, Figs. 46–57 depict a juxtauterine–isthmic anastomosis.

COMMENTS

Reversal of sterilization is still the preferred treatment over in vitro fertilization for this indication because of the former's superior pregnancy outcome. Further, in women over 40 years of age, the dismal results of IVF contrast with the experience of reversal in obtaining a 45% intrauterine pregnancy rate (12).

The adhesioreductive advantages of operative laparoscopy compared to laparotomy have been well documented (13–16). Therefore, the performance of tubal anastomosis laparoscopically adds this potential benefit, in addition to the well-known economic and low-morbidity advantages of minimally invasive surgery.

The use of a minilaparotomy for microsurgical anastomosis has conferred outpatient benefits while maintaining excellent pregnancy rates; however, the patient population is highly selective (17). With laparoscopic tubal anastomosis all patients are eligible, with the greatest advantage to be gained by women who have had previous surgeries, e.g., for cesareans, pelvic inflammatory disease (PID), ruptured appendices etc., where the mobilization can be performed laparoscopically. Furthermore, excess weight is not a contraindication, as it is in minilaparotomy (17).

ALTERNATIVE TREATMENT

Previous reported attempts at exclusive laparoscopic tubal anastomosis have attempted to circumvent microsuturing by employing fibrin glue (18) or macrosutures (19,20). The former reported no pregnancies whereas the latter had 2 pregnancies out of 20 initially (19), with a later total of six (35%) (20). Many other innovations have been tried, but pregnancy outcomes have not been reported (21).

OUTCOME

We started using 8-0 sutures for rabbit anastomosis beginning in 1990 to determine the feasibility of exactly reproducing classic microsurgery, and in 1992 started human studies with IRB approval. The operating time decreased from $5\frac{1}{2}$ hr to $2\frac{1}{2}$ hr after the early cases, and all patients were discharged within 24 hr with the later patients discharged in 3–6 hr. Preliminary results have been encouraging with an intrauterine pregnancy rate of 60% after 6–12 months follow-up. There were no ectopic pregnancies. Results in 1993 are given in Table 3.

TABLE 3. *Laparoscopic tubal anastomosis results, 1993*

Total number of cases	10[a]
Age (28–42)	33.8 ± 4.7 years
Sterilization interval	7.4 ± 1.8 years
Follow-up	11.4 ± 3.5 months
Intrauterine pregnancy	6[b]
Procedure length	
1–5	5.9 ± 0.5 hr
6–10	3.1 ± 1.28 hr

[a] >40 years 1, male factor 1.
[b] 7 in 6 patients.
Presented at First Asia Pacific Congress on Endoscopic Surgery, Singapore, 1993.

ADDENDUM

Twenty-eight cases of sterilization reversal were performed between 1992 and 1994. The mean age was approximately 33.7 years old. Intrauterine pregnancy was achieved in 20 patients (71.4%) with one ectopic pregnancy (3.6%). The surgery/pregnancy interval was 4.35 (±$\frac{2}{3}$ months). The procedure length was 3.1 (±1.28 hours) and postoperative stay ranged from 2 to 26 hours.

HIGHLIGHTS

For laparoscopic microsurgery to be consistently reproducible, further development in instrumentation is necessary. The video capability is already here in terms of resolution and magnification and future zoom features would aid magnification without having to bring the laparoscope too close to the working field. The current genre of three-dimensional cameras is unsuitable for microsurgery.

Laparoscopic microsurgery is an attainable objective and preliminary results for tubal anastomosis is encouraging. This will be the last bastion of open microsurgery to be replaced by laparoscopy. In the process, however, we should not abandon the sound principles established by the pioneers of microsurgery, which has guided the success of reproductive surgery.

It is our hope that classical microsurgery will fulfill its greatest aspirations for reproductive surgery by its reinvention though laparoscopy.

ACKNOWLEDGMENTS

Columbia Hospital, Milwaukee, Wisconsin for its help in instituting the initial IRB approved trial, and the Hospital's Laparoscopy Team for their cooperation during the early cases. Thank you to Karl Storz for providing the illustrations.

REFERENCES

1. Swolin K. *Fifty fertilatiasoperationen. Vols 1, 2.* Microsurgical Concepts for Infertility Surgery, 1967.
2. Gomel V. *Tubal reconstruction by microsurgery* (abstracts). 8th World Congress on Fertility and Sterility, Buenos Aires, Argentina, 1974, Abstract No. 39.
3. Gomel V. Tubal reconstruction by microsurgery. *Fertil Steril* 1977;28:59.
4. Winston RML. Microsurgical tubocornual anastomosis for reversal of sterilization. *Lancet* 1977;1:284.
5. Winston RML. In: Chamberlin G, ed. *Tubal infertility.* London: Blackwell Scientific; 1983.
6. Gomel V. *Microsurgery in female infertility.* Boston: Little, Brown, 1983:239.
7. Xue P, Fa YY. Microsurgical reversal of female sterilization: long-term follow-up of 117 cases. *J Reprod Med* 1989;34(7):451–455.
8. Hogdall CK, Nielsen J, Ovlisen B. Reversal of female sterilization using macro technique. *Acta Obstet Gynecol Scand* 1989;68(8): 737–741.
9. Bai BC, Park CM, Kwak HM, Whang YW. Government-funding program on reversal of total sterilization. *Asia-Oceania J Obstet Gynaecol* 1992;18(1):73–80.
10. Langer M, Hick P, Nemeskeri N, Schneider B, Ringerl M. Psychological sequelae of surgical reversal or of IVF after tubal ligation. *Int J Fertil Menop Stud* 1993;38(1):44–49.
11. Gillett WR, Martin WL, Romans SE. Reversal of female sterilization: outcome of 210 referrals. *N Z Med J* 1993;106(955):173–175.
12. Trimbos-Kemper TCM. Reversal of sterilization in women over 40 years of age: a multicenter survey in the Netherlands. *Fertil Steril* 1990;53(3):575–577.
13. Luciano AA, Maier DB, Koch EI, Nulsen JC, Whitman GF. A comparative study of postoperative adhesions following laser surgery by laparoscopy versus laparotomy in the rabbit model. *Obstet Gynecol* 1989;74:220.
14. Nezhat CR, Nezhat FR, Metzger DA, Luciano AA. Adhesion reformation after reproductive surgery by videolaseroscopy. *Fertil Steril* 1990;53(6):1008–1011.
15. Lundorff P, Hahlin M, Kallfelt B, Thorburn J, Lindblom B. Adhesion formation after laparoscopic surgery in tubal pregnancy: a randomized trial versus laparotomy. *Fertil Steril* 1991;55(5).
16. Maier DB, Nulsen JC, Klock A, Luciano AA. Laser laparoscopy versus laparotomy in lysis of pelvic adhesions. *J Reprod Med* 1992;37(12):965–968.
17. Silva PD, Schaper AM, Meisch JK, Schauberger CW. Outpatient microsurgical reversal of tubal sterilization by a combined approach of laparoscopy and minilaparotomy. *Fertil Steril* 1991;55(4):696–699.
18. Sedbon E, Delajolinieres JB, Boudouris O, Madelenat P. Tubal desterilization through exclusive laparoscopy. *Human Reprod* 1989;4:158.
19. Reich H. Laparoscopic reversal of sterilization (abstract). Presented at the Second World Congress of Gynecologic Endoscopy, Clairemont-Ferrand, France, June 5–8, 1989.
20. Reich H, McGlynn F, Parente C, Sekel L, Levie M. Laparoscopic tubal anastomosis. *J Am Assoc Gynecol Laparosc* 1993;1(1):16–19.
21. Tsin DA, Mahmood D. Laparoscopic and hysteroscopic approach for tubal anastomosis. *J Laparoendosc Surg* 1993;3(1):63–66.

Endoscopic Management of Gynecologic Disease,
edited by G.D. Adamson and D.C. Martin.
Lippincott-Raven Publishers, Philadelphia © 1996.

CHAPTER 14

Laparoscopic Treatment of Endometriosis

G. David Adamson

It has become increasingly possible in the past decade to treat endometriosis at the time of diagnostic laparoscopy. Treatment can be accomplished through therapeutic laparoscopic techniques utilizing scissors, electrosurgical instruments, lasers, suture, and staplers (1). Some techniques are simple and can be performed by most gynecologists. However, laparoscopic treatment of advanced endometriosis can be technically demanding, requiring significant levels of knowledge, training, skill, and experience. Sophisticated equipment and well-trained, highly motivated assistants are also necessary. With the appropriate facilities, the experienced surgeon can perform complex endometriosis operations including extensive peritoneal dissection, cul-de-sac and rectovaginal dissection, resection of invasive bowel endometriosis, appendectomy, treatment of invasive ovarian endometriosis and endometriomas, oophorectomy, removal of tubal endometriosis, resection of bladder endometriosis, resection of ureteral endometriosis, removal of uterine endometriosis, uterosacral nerve ablation, presacral neurectomy, laparoscopy-assisted vaginal hysterectomy, and adhesiolysis. Requirements for surgery, surgical principles, operative techniques, and results need to be considered to provide optimal surgical treatment.

DEFINITION

Endometriosis is a pathologic condition in which the endometrium, consisting of endometrial glands and stroma, is found in ectopic or abnormal positions outside the endometrial cavity and uterine musculature. The usual location of this endometriosis is in the pelvis, but endometriosis has also been found in many extrapelvic sites including omentum, small intestine, appendix, anterior abdominal wall, surgical scars, diaphragm, lung, urinary tract, musculoskeletal, and neural systems (2–7). This chapter addresses the laparoscopic treatment of pelvic and bowel endometriosis. Treatment of extrapelvic or extraabdominal endometriosis should almost always be performed in conjunction with a medical or surgical specialist who is knowledgeable about the extrapelvic organ system. Endoscopic treatment may be useful in such areas as the diaphragm, lung, and musculoskeletal system.

PREVALENCE AND INCIDENCE

The prevalence and incidence of endometriosis depends on the population of women being studied. The range is 1–50% depending on surgical series (8). It has been reported to occur in 10–15% of women undergoing diagnostic laparoscopy, 2–5% of women undergoing tubal sterilization, 30–40% of infertile women having laparoscopy, and 14–53% of women with pelvic pain (9–18).

PATHOPHYSIOLOGY

Endometriosis is an enigmatic disease. There are several theories that attempt to describe the pathogenesis of endometriosis, the most popular being the retrograde menstruation theory, metaplasia theory, and hematogenous and lymphatic spread theory (19,20,21). Each of these and other possible etiologies may contribute variably to endometriosis in different patients (4). Altered immunity may also play a role (4,22). There are numerous factors that appear to affect whether a woman will have

G. D. Adamson: Department of Gynecology and Obstetrics, Stanford University School of Medicine, Stanford, California 94305; Department of Obstetrics, Gynecology, and Reproductive Sciences, University of California San Francisco, San Francisco, California 94143; and Fertility Physicians of Northern California, Palo Alto, California 94301.

this disease, the severity of the disease, symptoms, and response to treatment. These factors include genetics (familial predisposition), hormonal status (estrogen level, duration and amount of menstrual flow), lifestyle (weight and smoking), contraceptive use (oral contraceptives), obstetric history (number of pregnancies and lactation), anatomic factors (cervical stenosis), treatment history (prior medical or surgical treatment), race, and possible exposure to environmental toxins (19,20,23).

CLINICAL PRESENTATION

Endometriosis presents primarily as pelvic pain in about 80% of patients, infertility in about 20%, or ovarian endometrioma in less than 5% of cases (14). There is also a large incidence of asymptomatic disease, about 10–40% (16,24). Endometriosis may occur anytime after puberty, including adolescence (13,25,26).

It is generally held that pain symptoms of endometriosis do not correlate with severity of disease (21). Pain may occur as a result of secretion of irritating factors (e.g., histamine), adhesions that cause scarring or retraction, leaking endometriomas, compression of other visceral structures (e.g., bowel), compression of uterosacral nodules, and/or invasion of the urinary or gastrointestinal tract (21,27). Endometriosis is probably associated with infertility even in patients with minimal and mild disease, and a cause–effect relationship almost certainly exists for moderate and severe disease (18,21,28,29). Infertility could be caused by anatomic distortion and tubal obstruction, impaired ovarian function, luteinized unruptured follicle syndrome, peritoneal macrophages and a peritoneal inflammatory response, immunosuppression factors, peritoneal fluid prostaglandins, or other unknown factors (30,31). Endometriosis may also be associated with intraluminal pathology (32). Studies over-

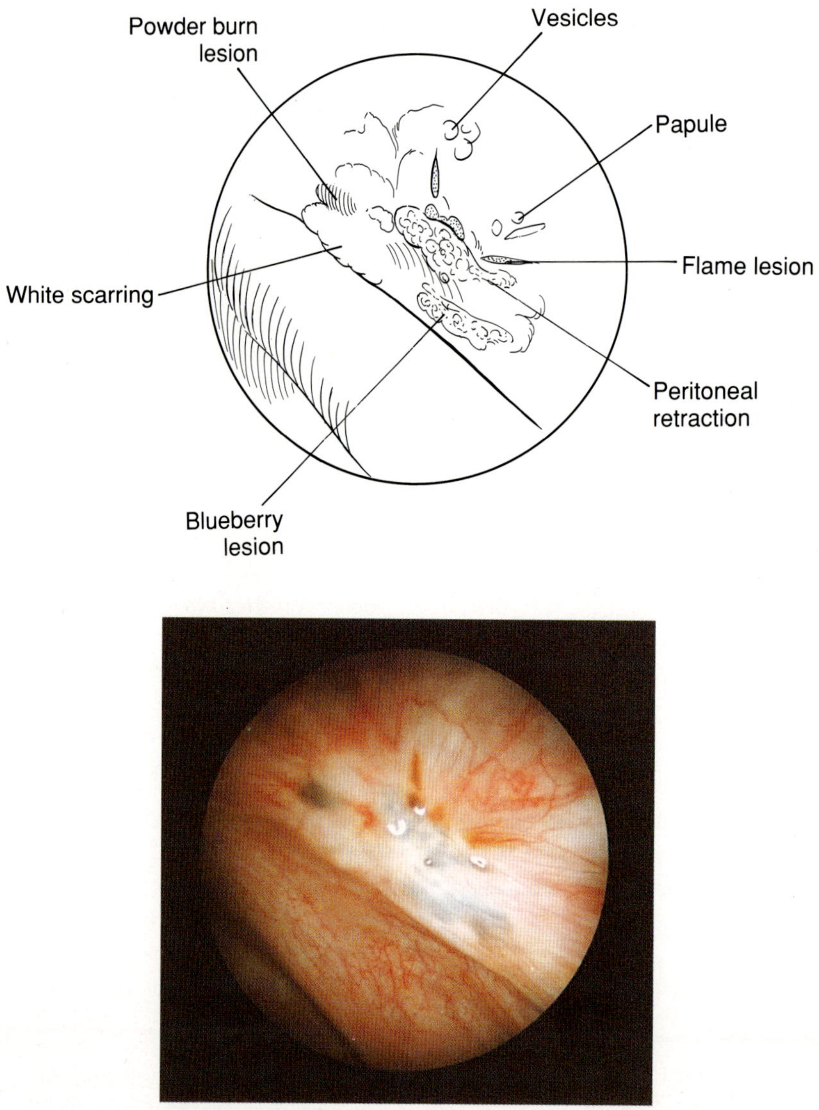

FIG. 1. Endometriosis lesion with multiple morphologic presentations.

all do not support an association between endometriosis and increased spontaneous abortion rates (21).

Endometriosis lesions occur throughout the pelvis. They tend to be more frequently in the posterior cul-de-sac and the ovary, and less frequently on the fallopian tubes (4,33–35). Endometriosis is almost certainly a progressive disease, but the rate of progression and nature of lesions may be very variable from patient to patient (36,37). Lesions can have many different appearances, including early superficial vesicular, papular, flame-like lesions, or brownish staining. Later lesions may include the classical bluish or powder burn lesions and whitish scarred lesions (Fig. 1). Eventually, endometriomas and invasive lesions, some being quite deep and nodular, develop. Combinations of these lesions are seen frequently (14,27,33,36–38). In addition, adhesions develop as a result of the inflammatory process caused by longstanding endometriosis with more extensive and dense adhesions developing over time. Complete cul-de-sac obliteration can result from longstanding invasive and adhesive disease.

Current staging systems often do not reflect the nature or extent of disease. Deep invasive peritoneal nodules and extensive superficial endometriosis may constitute advanced disease and yet have an American Fertility Society stage of only mild disease (39). Numerous studies have shown that current staging systems have limited correlation with the degree of infertility or pain (27, 40–45).

DIAGNOSIS

The diagnosis of endometriosis is suggested by several symptoms, including dysmenorrhea, dyspareunia (especially with aching following coitus), dyschezia, dysuria, mittelschmerz, or focal or generalized pelvic pain. Hematuria and hematochezia may also be symptoms of endometriosis. About 30% of patients with endometriosis do not have any pain. Signs of endometriosis include tenderness or nodularity in the posterior cul-de-sac, especially on the uterosacral ligaments, anterior cul-de-sac nodularity, adnexal masses from endometriomas, and reduced mobility or fixation of the pelvis due to pelvic adhesions (14,27,46).

Tests that may assist in the diagnosis of endometriosis include ultrasonography to evaluate the adnexa for endometriomas and the uterus for myomas or adenomyosis (47). Color and pulsed Doppler sonography may have increased utility in the future (48). Magnetic resonance imaging (MRI) or computerized tomography (CT) scan are currently rarely helpful, but further evaluation of their utility is ongoing (35,49,50). Hysterosalpingography cannot diagnose endometriosis but may help identify other pelvic pathology. CA-125 may occasionally be helpful in following the course of endometriosis after diagnosis and treatment, but the high false-positive and false-negative rate give it little utility in the initial diagnostic workup (51,52). Preoperative consultations with gastroenterologists, urologists, or other specialists as indicated should be scheduled to help ensure that laparoscopy produces the maximum benefits for the patient (14).

Currently the only definite test for endometriosis is diagnostic laparoscopy. Biopsy of lesions may sometimes be necessary to confirm the diagnosis of endometriosis and should always be performed if the surgeon is uncertain of the diagnosis.

The differential diagnosis includes pelvic inflamma-

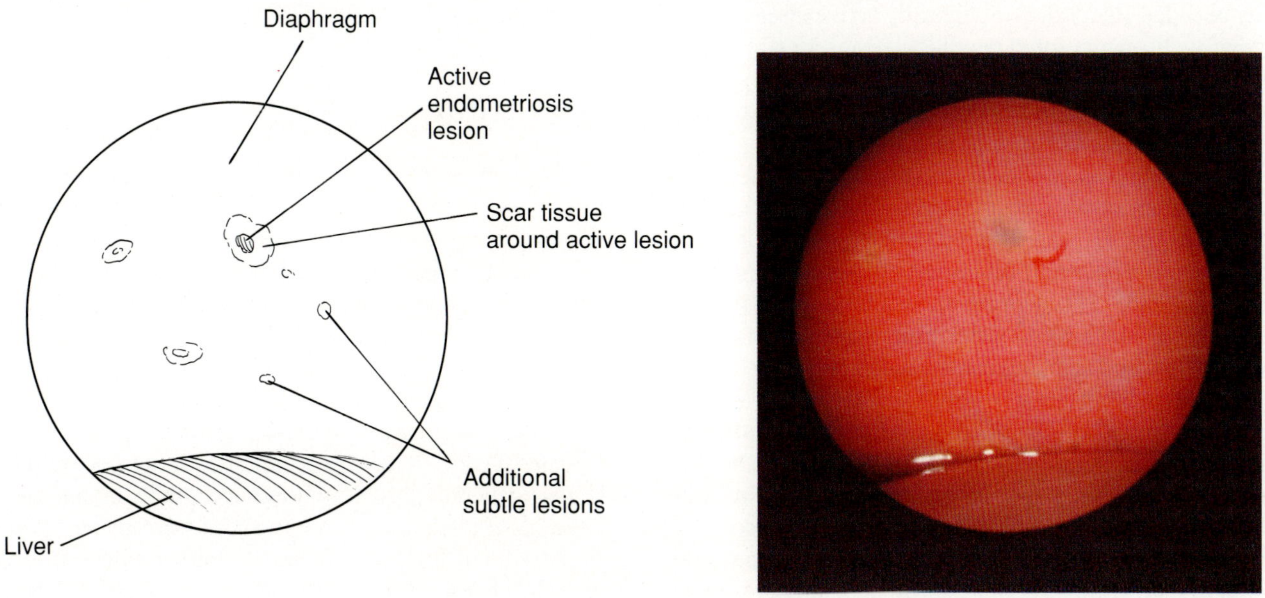

FIG. 2. Endometriosis of the diaphragm.

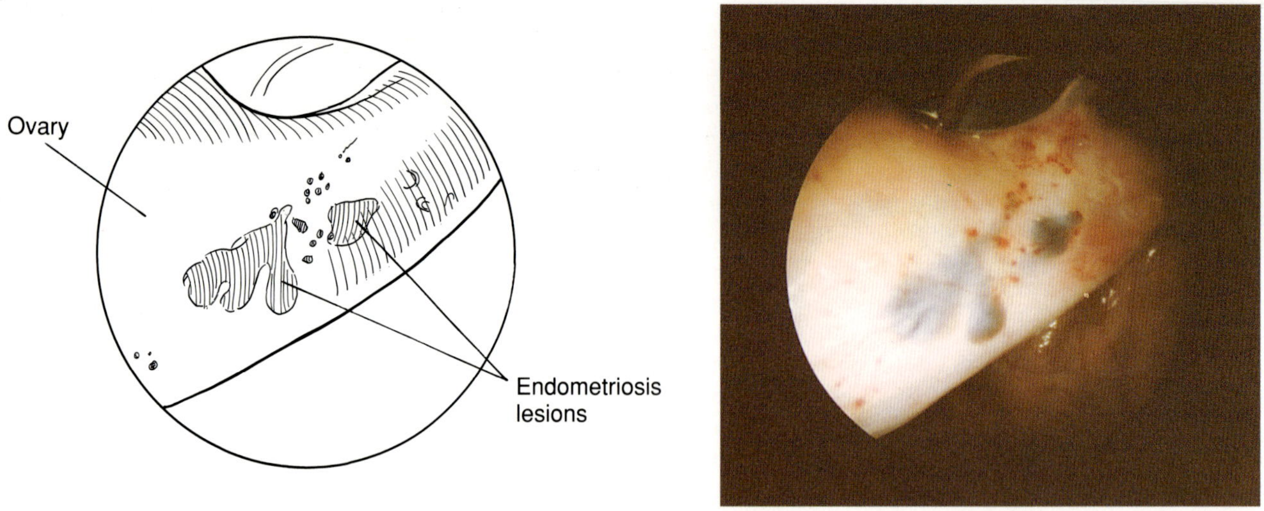

FIG. 3. Endometriosis in a postmenopausal woman receiving hormone replacement therapy.

tory disease, adenomyosis, myomas, benign ovarian tumors, malignant ovarian tumors (rare), pelvic pain of undetermined etiology, and normal pelvis. It should be emphasized to patients that diagnosis requires laparoscopy but that endometriosis is not always found at laparoscopy even when it has been suggested by the history, physical examination, and preoperative testing.

It has been estimated that the diagnosis of endometriosis has been missed in more than 7% of patients, and the extent of disease has been underestimated in as many as 50% of patients (17). Subtle lesions can be missed even by experienced laparoscopists (27,53). Other lesions such as old suture, ovarian cancer, carbon deposits from prior laser surgery, and hemangiomas may look like endometriosis (38,54). The surgeon must recognize the classical powder burn or blueberry lesion, white scar tissue that may be older, less endocrinologically active disease, clear or slightly brown-colored papillary lesions, or strawberry or flame-like lesions of recently developed, highly active endometriosis. Peritoneal pockets may also be associated with endometriosis (55).

A thorough and systematic examination of the pelvis and abdomen under direct vision without the camera at the beginning of surgery is essential in all patients to identify and document all endometriotic lesions (Figs. 2 and 3) (36,38,53). A probe should be used to palpate carefully all surfaces to determine depth of invasion. Contraction and scarring can be identified by tethering of the surrounding tissue to nonpliable tissue. All areas to be treated should be identified for subsequent treatment. Biopsy of peritoneum with frozen section may be helpful in confirming the diagnosis and determining optimal treatment. Findings should be carefully recorded even though current staging systems do not always accurately predict postoperative pain relief or pregnancy rate (40, 56–58).

INDICATIONS

Indications for laparoscopy to diagnose endometriosis include infertility of more than 1 year duration without other symptoms, or possibly after 6 months if the patient has symptoms or is older than 35. Patients with pelvic pain which has not responded after 3 months of nonsteroidal antiinflammatory drugs (NSAIDs) and/or 3 months of oral contraceptives are candidates for laparoscopy. Patients who present with adnexal masses suspected as being an endometrioma should have laparoscopy if the lesion does not resolve itself by 3 months, or sooner if there are concomitant symptoms such as pain or other factors that make surgery appropriate (59,60). The objectives of surgery are to remove or destroy implants, relieve symptoms, maintain or restore fertility, and avoid or delay recurrence of symptoms.

CONTRAINDICATIONS

Contraindications to surgery include multiple repeat operations at short intervals to treat lesions. If appropriate surgery is performed, it is uncommon for endometriotic lesions to recur within a few months (43,61). Repeat surgery for adhesiolysis is indicated in selected patients, usually those with infertility. Repeat surgery may be indicated after an appropriate interval if symptoms recur and are not treatable with medical therapy. Laparoscopy may be repeated to perform gamete intrafallopian transfer (GIFT) in selected patients. Surgery should not be performed in patients with unacceptably high medical or surgical risks. Laparoscopy should not be performed in patients at high risk for bowel injury unless an open technique or a technique designed to avoid bowel injury is utilized. Laparotomy is an appropriate approach for

TABLE 1. *Comparison of laparoscopic treatment of endometriosis for infertility with other treatment modalities*

	Entire patient population $n = 579$		Endometriosis-only subset[a] $n = 258$	
Treatment comparison	Increased pregnancy rate when treated laparoscopically (%)	*p* value	Increased pregnancy rate when treated laparoscopically (%)	*p* value
Laparoscopy vs. no treatment[b]	7	0.83	−14	0.64
Laparoscopy vs. medical treatment[b]	42	0.088	101	0.007
Laparoscopy vs. laparotomy	29	0.13	87	0.031

[a] Endometriosis-only subset = at least one fallopian tube and fimbria normal, and normal male factor.
[b] All patients receiving no treatment or medical treatments had minimal or mild disease.

many surgeons when laparoscopy may be too hazardous or the surgeon may not have the requisite skills or facilities to perform operative laparoscopy.

ALTERNATIVE TREATMENTS

Alternatives to laparoscopic treatment of endometriosis include no treatment for young patients with minimal symptoms or for women who have just completed a course of medical treatment. Minimal or mild pain symptoms may be successfully treated with NSAIDs and/or oral contraceptives. Other endocrinologic treatment includes progestins, danazol, or gonadotropin-releasing hormone (GnRH) agonists. It should be noted that pelvic pain associated with endometriosis is effectively treated by medical treatment and that all of the different medical treatments have similar efficacy (62–67). Laparoscopic treatment is also effective in treatment of pelvic pain (68,69). Danazol and GnRH agonists should not be used in the treatment of endometriosis unless the diagnosis has been confirmed at laparoscopy.

For infertility patients, no treatment is as effective as surgical treatment for minimal and mild disease (Table 1, Fig. 4) (70,71). Surgical treatment is required for more advanced disease with invasive nodular disease, endometriomas, and adhesions (59). Medical treatment, either alone or following surgery, does not improve pregnancy rates and should not be used in patients whose only symptom is infertility (64,70,71).

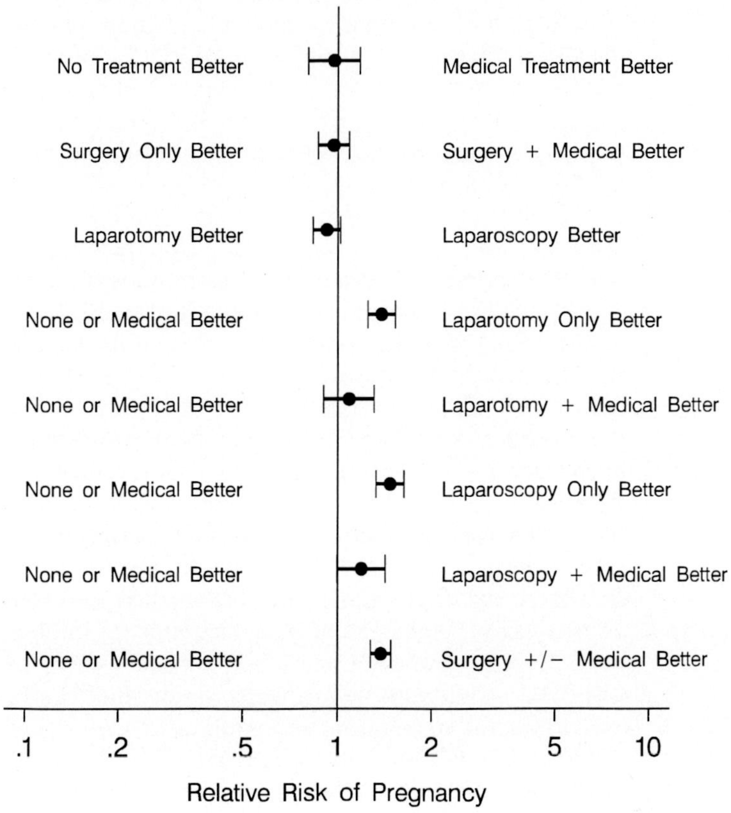

FIG. 4. Summary of meta-analysis estimates of relative risk of pregnancy (point estimate and 95% confidence interval) for different endometriosis treatment comparisons.

The approach to each patient must be individualized depending on her symptoms, signs, age, type and extent of disease, and the desire for fertility. Many patients prefer no treatment or medical treatment before surgery. However, surgery is often the most appropriate approach. Most patients prefer to retain as many of their reproductive organs as possible, but for some oophorectomy and/or hysterectomy will be a better option. Laparoscopy will generally be the preferred surgical approach, but laparotomy may be appropriate for some cases, especially those requiring extirpation of large endometriomas, extensive enterolysis, enterostomy, or bowel resection (72,73). Alternatives to treatment, or treatment in combination with surgery, such as the use of GnRH agonists preoperatively to treat severe endometriosis, should be considered and implemented as indicated (74).

EXPERIENCED SURGEON

Laparoscopic treatment of endometriosis requires a surgeon who is familiar with the pathophysiology of endometriosis and possible therapeutic options, including no treatment, medical therapy, laparotomy, or laparoscopic surgery, and who can integrate this knowledge with surgical judgement and technique (Table 2).

Initially, didactic and hands-on experience through residency and fellowship training, courses, preceptorships, and assisting in the operating room are needed. Each surgeon must then acquire laparoscopic experience treating minimal, mild, and moderate endometriosis before advancing to more complex procedures. Surgeons need to have a comprehensive understanding of normal and diseased pelvic anatomy, different surgical techniques, and the principles and application of mechanical, electrosurgical, and laser energy. Surgeons need to develop hand–eye coordination working from a video monitor with different instruments. Most important, each surgeon needs to develop an appreciation of the limitations of operative laparoscopy in his or her hands, since surgical procedures are usually more complex and difficult to perform at laparoscopy than at laparotomy (75).

TABLE 2. *Surgical principles in the treatment of endometriosis*

Knowledge of disease and treatment modalities
Experienced surgeon
Adequate facilities, personnel, and equipment
Appropriate patient selection
Informed consent
Proper patient position
Careful pelvic evaluation
Maximum exposure
Use of magnification
Minimum tissue trauma
Excellent hemostasis
Removal of all diseased tissue
Avoidance of foreign body material
Confirmation of tissue pathology

ADEQUATE FACILITIES, PERSONNEL, AND EQUIPMENT

Several principles regarding the setting for laparoscopic treatment of endometriosis can be stated. Laparoscopic technology has increased dramatically in the past few years. The facility needs an adequate sized operating room for the equipment and adequate time for performance of the operation. Backup support, such as the ability to perform a laparotomy, provide a blood transfusion, or transfer the patient to an acute care hospital from an ambulatory care facility, is mandatory.

Trained and motivated personnel, preferably who have worked together with the surgeon, are important for more complex cases. A well-trained anesthesiologist who is familiar with laparoscopic anesthesia is required. More complex cases can almost always be performed faster, better, and more safely with an assistant surgeon, preferably one who is also an experienced laparoscopist and who has worked with the surgeon. Facilities for frozen section tissue diagnosis also should be available.

Necessary equipment includes an operative laparoscope with good optics, a high-resolution video camera with appropriate light source, and at least one, preferably two, high-resolution video monitors. Other equipment includes a hand-operated irrigation and aspiration system; high-flow automatic regulating carbon dioxide (CO_2) insufflator; and 5-mm instruments for probing, grasping, cutting, unipolar and bipolar coagulating, irrigating, hydrodissecting, needle aspirating, ligating, suturing, and stapling. It is generally preferable to have most of the instruments 5 mm in size so that they can be moved from one puncture site to another during the operation (Fig. 5). However, several techniques require the use of, or are easier with, 10- to 12-mm instruments. These include CO_2 gas recirculators (Sun Medical, Arlington, TX), scissors, sutures, graspers, morcellators, staplers, and plastic bags for tissue removal. Adapters to reduce a 10- to 12-mm sheath opening to 5 mm increase the versatility of the larger ports. Instruments to perform open laparoscopy, minilaparotomy, and colpotomy should also be available. Rectal probes, ring forceps for the vagina, Valtchev retractor, and Foley catheters for rectal injection of dilute betadine solution or for occlusion of the vagina are sometimes needed when bowel endometriosis is being treated. Indigo carmine for intravenous injection when ureteral or bladder injury is suspected should also be available. Sterile milk can be used to test the small bowel for perforations.

The choice of energy source used to perform surgery is primarily dependent on the surgeon. The CO_2 laser has

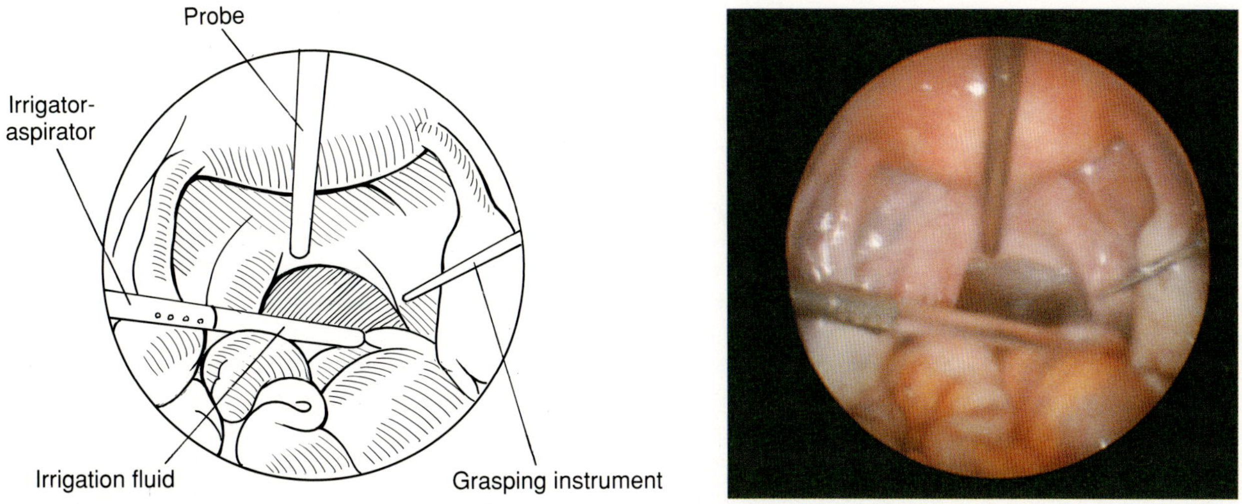

FIG. 5. Laparoscopic portals (3) for irrigator-aspirator, probe, and grasping instruments to evaluate pelvis.

the advantage of being very precise and not causing thermal injury away from the site of impact. The new Ultrapulse laser also provides very high power, which allows for faster dissection and for the ability to vary the amount of power and the amount of coagulating effect. This laser is therefore very desirable for precise work around the bowel, ureter, and other critical structures. Some surgeons prefer the neodymium:yttrium-aluminum-garnet (Nd:YAG), argon, or potassium deuterium phosphate (KTP-532) lasers because of the ability to use fibers and their coagulating effect (76). This coagulating effect would seem to be much less desirable when performing more precise dissection. Many surgeons prefer electrosurgery because of their familiarity with it and its easy availability. A major difficulty with unipolar electrosurgery is the risk of injury to other organs from unrecognized electrical burns. Some surgeons prefer scissors dissection, which is widely available. Scissors dissection can be fairly hemorrhagic, and a common difficulty with scissors is that they do not cut well. This problem has largely been overcome with the use of disposable instruments; however, these can be very expensive (1). Several innovative instruments for stapling, suturing, and bowel anastomosis currently are only available as disposable instruments. Their cost is sometimes justified by benefits provided to the patient through their use (see the chapter by Sanfilippo and Adamson "Operating Room Setup").

LAPAROSCOPIC ABDOMINAL APPROACHES

The patient undergoing endometriosis surgery who is at risk for moderate, severe, or bowel disease requires an empty bowel and bladder, as well as an empty stomach, at the time of surgery. The patient's history should be evaluated for indications for open laparoscopy. These could include previous laparotomy with complications, abdominal adhesions, previous bowel disease and/or peritonitis, colostomy, obesity, pelvic kidney, or metastatic disease. A few gynecologists prefer routine use of open laparoscopy because of theoretically increased safety of the procedure. However, open laparoscopy does increase the time required to enter the abdominal cavity and can hinder mobility of the laparoscopic sheath. Alternatives include new transparent trocars, with cutting blades, which function under direct vision. Pneumoperitoneum can be created in the upper abdominal midaxillary lines, suprapubically, or through the posterior vaginal fornix in selected patients. Direct trocar insertion may also be an appropriate technique in some circumstances.

PATIENT POSITION

At laparoscopy the patient is placed in a modified lithotomy position with her arm at her side on the side where the surgeon stands. The other arm may be extended if carefully supported in the appropriate position. Trendelenburg position will help to move the bowel out of the pelvis after the Veress needle and pneumoperitoneum has been established. The legs need to be well supported and padded and, if supported under the knees, mobilized approximately every 2 hr to help prevent compression injury to the nerves.

VISUALIZATION

Contemporary laparoscopes, light sources, and video equipment afford an excellent view of the pelvis for both the surgeon, operative assistants, and other operating room personnel (42). The six-to-eight times magnification provided by the laparoscope when in close proximity to lesions may be particularly important for diagnosis of the multiple morphologic presentations of endometriosis, for operating on the bowel, ureter, or vessels; or for salpingolysis, ovariolysis, fimbrioplasty, and salpingostomy (17,36,77). Although magnification is not as great as that provided by the operating microscope, this is probably only a limiting factor in performing tubal reanastomosis and possibly fimbrioplasty. The laparoscope's angle of view of the pelvis affords superior visualization in the cul-de-sac, under the ovaries, and in the upper abdomen relative to laparotomy. A very high level of operative precision can be attained because of this improved visualization. This precision can be enhanced by palpation with instruments to ascertain tissue consistency.

Careful systematic initial evaluation of the pelvis and abdominal cavity is mandatory prior to performing operative laparoscopy. Important anatomic landmarks and structures need to be identified. These include the ureters, uterine vessels, uterosacral ligaments, infundibulopelvic ligaments, external iliac vessels, bowel, bladder, fallopian tubes, ovaries, and uterus. The surgeon should appreciate the normal and abnormal anatomy and areas of greatest surgical risk. The type and degree of endometriosis should be determined and optimal surgical approach decided on. Potential increased equipment needs for the operation can be given to the circulating staff who will be able to anticipate the surgeon's requirements. Additional puncture sites should be placed as soon as the surgeon feels they may be necessary. Having adequate puncture sites is critical to the success of operative laparoscopy. For treatment of advanced endometriosis, three lower quadrant incisions are often appropriate.

Visualization of the pelvis under direct vision without the camera at the beginning and end of surgery will facilitate diagnosis of subtle disease, such as various types of endometriotic lesions, and confirm their removal. The

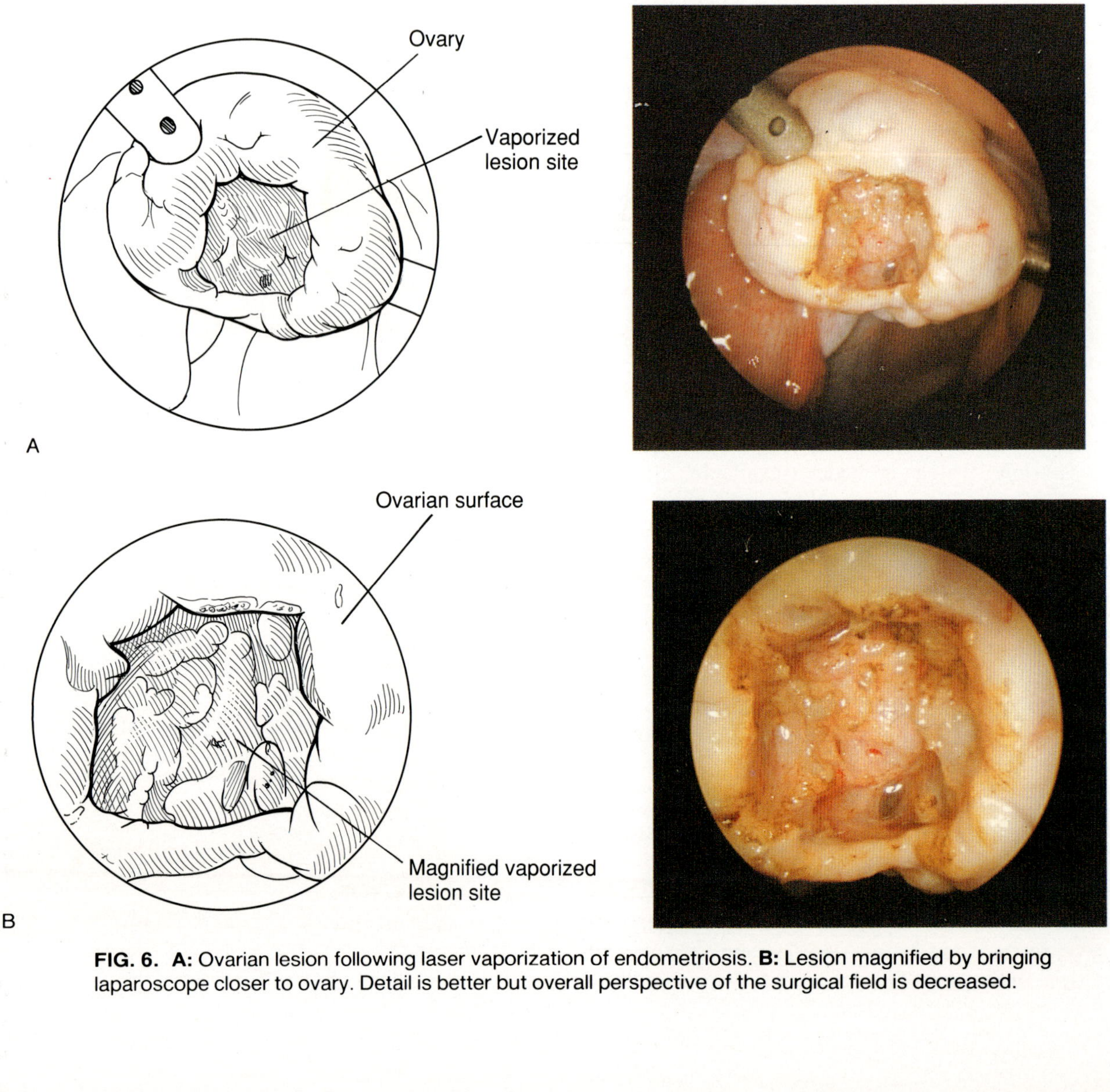

FIG. 6. A: Ovarian lesion following laser vaporization of endometriosis. **B:** Lesion magnified by bringing laparoscope closer to ovary. Detail is better but overall perspective of the surgical field is decreased.

laparoscope magnifies tissue so that when the laparoscope is about 1 cm from the tissue the magnification is approximately six times, at 2 cm four times, at 3 cm two times, and at 4 cm no magnification. At greater than 4 cm demagnification or the appearance of a smaller structure appears through the laparoscope. As magnification increases, visualization is improved in the observed area, but the overall perspective of the surgical field is decreased (Fig. 6A,B).

It is also important to recognize that operative laparoscopy has associated with it some unique disadvantages and complications not associated with laparotomy. The laparoscopic view is two-dimensional rather than three-dimensional as at laparotomy. Also, the resolution of the video monitor is not as good as direct vision at laparotomy. The surgeon must control the surgical field almost entirely through the two-dimensional video monitor, a more difficult process than operating at laparotomy. Coordination of intraoperative movements with the assistant surgeon is also more difficult. Fatigue can occur more easily because of the need to view the monitor in one place at all times (75).

PRINCIPLES OF SURGICAL TECHNIQUES

Surgical techniques utilized at operative laparoscopy attempt to maximize exposure, minimize trauma, and produce the desired result in the minimum amount of time. Hemostasis must be carefully maintained at all times and the appropriate instruments freely used in the different sites as necessary. Irrigation and aspiration can significantly assist in good visualization and in the maintenance of a clean surgical field. Irrigation fluid should be physiologic, such as Ringer's lactate. Irrigation with nonelectrolytic solutions, such as glycine, through the

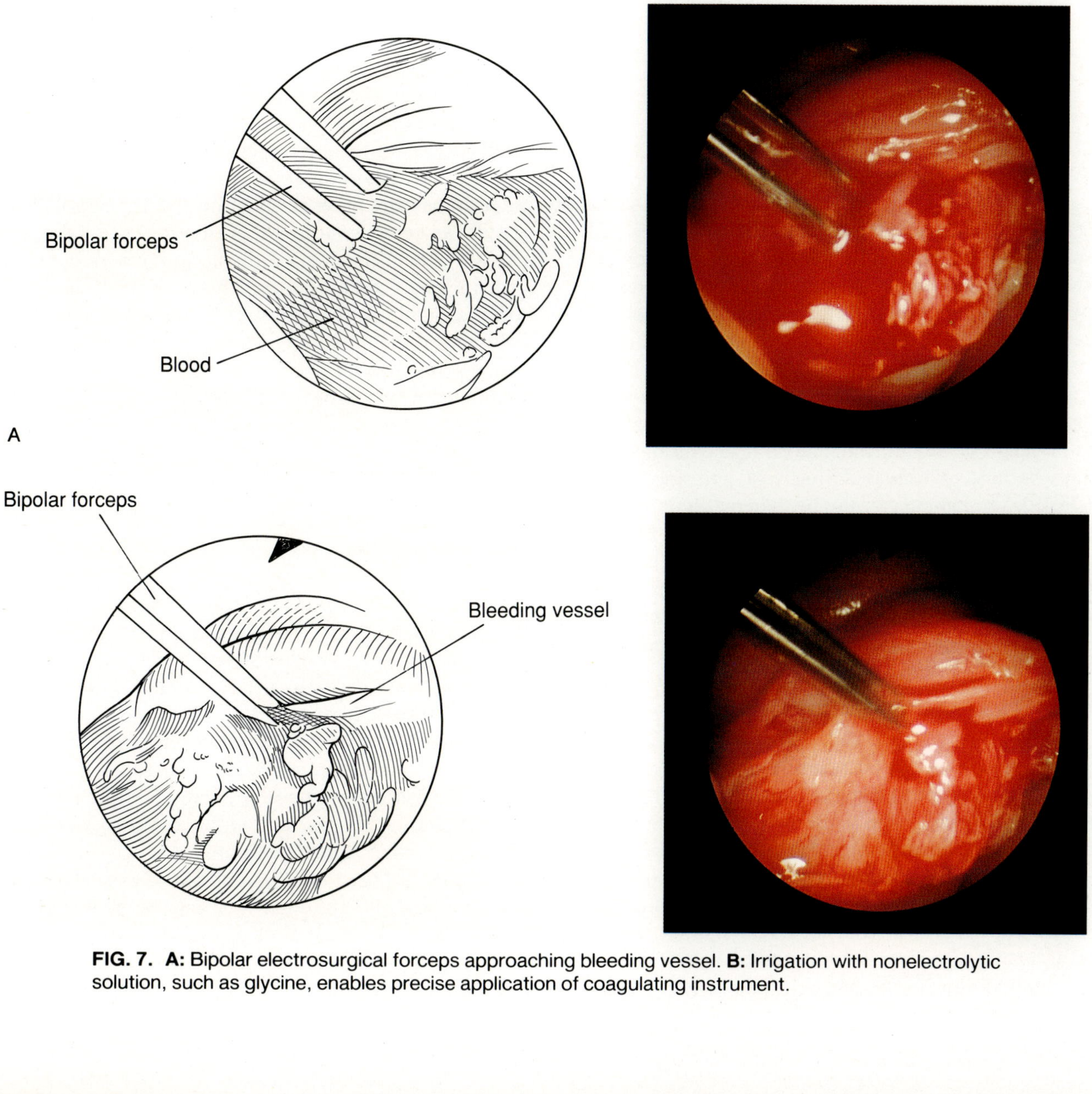

FIG. 7. A: Bipolar electrosurgical forceps approaching bleeding vessel. **B:** Irrigation with nonelectrolytic solution, such as glycine, enables precise application of coagulating instrument.

coagulating instruments greatly facilitates identification and coagulation of vessels because the blood can be irrigated away while coagulating (Fig. 7A,B).

The most important principle in operative laparoscopy is control of the surgical field. This requires good visualization of all pelvic structures and awareness of all anatomic structures and normal tissue, as well as knowledge of the location and extent of diseased tissue. For increased risk procedures it is necessary to evaluate whether the benefit of the procedure outweighs the risk. For some surgeons this may occur relatively frequently. Alternative methods of treatment should be carried out in such situations. It is important to recognize that at operative laparoscopy the surgeon is working without binocular vision and also with a camera placed at a distance from the surgical field. In addition, instruments are being used rather than hands to grasp. Laser energy effects have to be appreciated in advance on a theoretical basis and are not directly related to usual surgical senses. Therefore, the apparent control of the surgical field is less than one has at laparotomy, although the actual degree of control can be maximized significantly with surgical experience.

SIMULTANEOUS DIAGNOSIS AND TREATMENT

Diagnostic laparoscopy provides a relatively safe and simple method of diagnosing most anatomic gynecologic disease states. The choice of therapy can also be determined at the time of diagnostic laparoscopy. When appropriate, operative laparoscopy enables treatment to be initiated and possibly completed at the same time. Medical and surgical treatment modalities sometimes have the same results, but surgical treatment completed at the time of diagnosis has a distinct advantage over medical therapy because of decreased time, cost, and side effects (70,78,79). The patient can also be spared a second operation (laparotomy) if operative laparoscopy can be performed at the time of diagnosis (80). However, it is more important to give the patient the best operation possible in the particular surgeon's hands rather than to compromise by performing a poor operation at laparoscopy.

TISSUE TRAUMA

Operative laparoscopy offers several advantages to laparotomy with respect to surgical tissue trauma. The abdominal cavity is not open to the drying air of the operating room, preserving tissue integrity. This is especially true when copious irrigation is performed throughout the procedure. The tissue is also not cooled by room air at laparoscopy, further reducing tissue trauma. However, at laparoscopy tissue can be cooled by CO_2 gas at room temperature if constant irrigation is not carried out. Tissue is not exposed to foreign bodies such as talc from gloves. Most importantly, under ideal circumstances, tissue is not grasped, squeezed, or abraded by handling and packing off of the bowel as occurs at laparotomy. This maintains serosal integrity and probably reduces the risk of de novo adhesion formation. These advantages are especially pronounced when treating disease that is difficult to visualize at laparotomy, such as under the ovaries and deep in the cul-de-sac. However, despite the fact that palpation of structures can be performed with instruments, tactile sense is less than that which can be obtained digitally at laparotomy.

ADHESION FORMATION

It is possible that operative laparoscopy produces superior results to laparotomy with respect to the reformation of adhesions removed at the initial surgery, but this has not yet been demonstrated conclusively (81). However, studies strongly suggest that de novo adhesion formation is less frequent following operative laparoscopy compared with laparotomy (81–83). The apparent reduced de novo adhesion formation may be due to reduced tissue trauma or to a reduction in oozing from small vessels immediately after surgical injury due to the increased intraabdominal pressure created by the pneumoperitoneum. Earlier ambulation and absence of packing off the bowel could theoretically result in less ileus and subsequent mechanical disruption of early-forming adhesions by bowel peristalsis. Perhaps the single most important preventive measure is meticulous surgical technique at the initial procedure (84). Second-look laparoscopy remains the primary method of diagnosing and treating reformed or de novo adhesions (85,86).

LAPAROSCOPIC TREATMENT OF ENDOMETRIOSIS LESIONS

Treatment of Peritoneal Disease

The first step in treating peritoneal lesions is to obtain adequate visualization. Mobilization of the uterus may be assisted by using weights on a cervical tenaculum attached to an intracervical device, as well as with transabdominal probes. Anterior cul-de-sac treatment must be accompanied by continuous bladder drainage, and posterior cul-de-sac treatment requires adequate mobilization of the ovaries and bowel by transabdominal instruments including probes, fans, and graspers, as well as by use of the Trendelenburg position.

Treatment of peritoneal lesions can be by sharp resection with scissors, although this may be hemorrhagic. Destruction by unipolar electrosurgery carries the risk of damage to deeper structures unless fine-needle tips are used. Microbipolar electrosurgery can effectively destroy

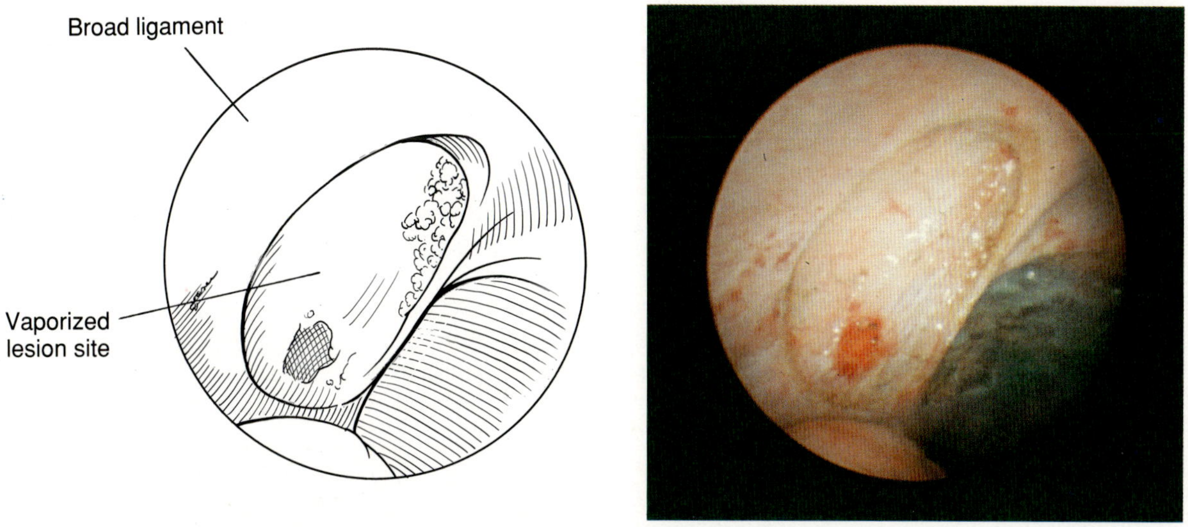

FIG. 8. Base of left broad ligament showing clean lesion with minimal injury to remaining tissue following complete CO_2 laser vaporization of endometriosis.

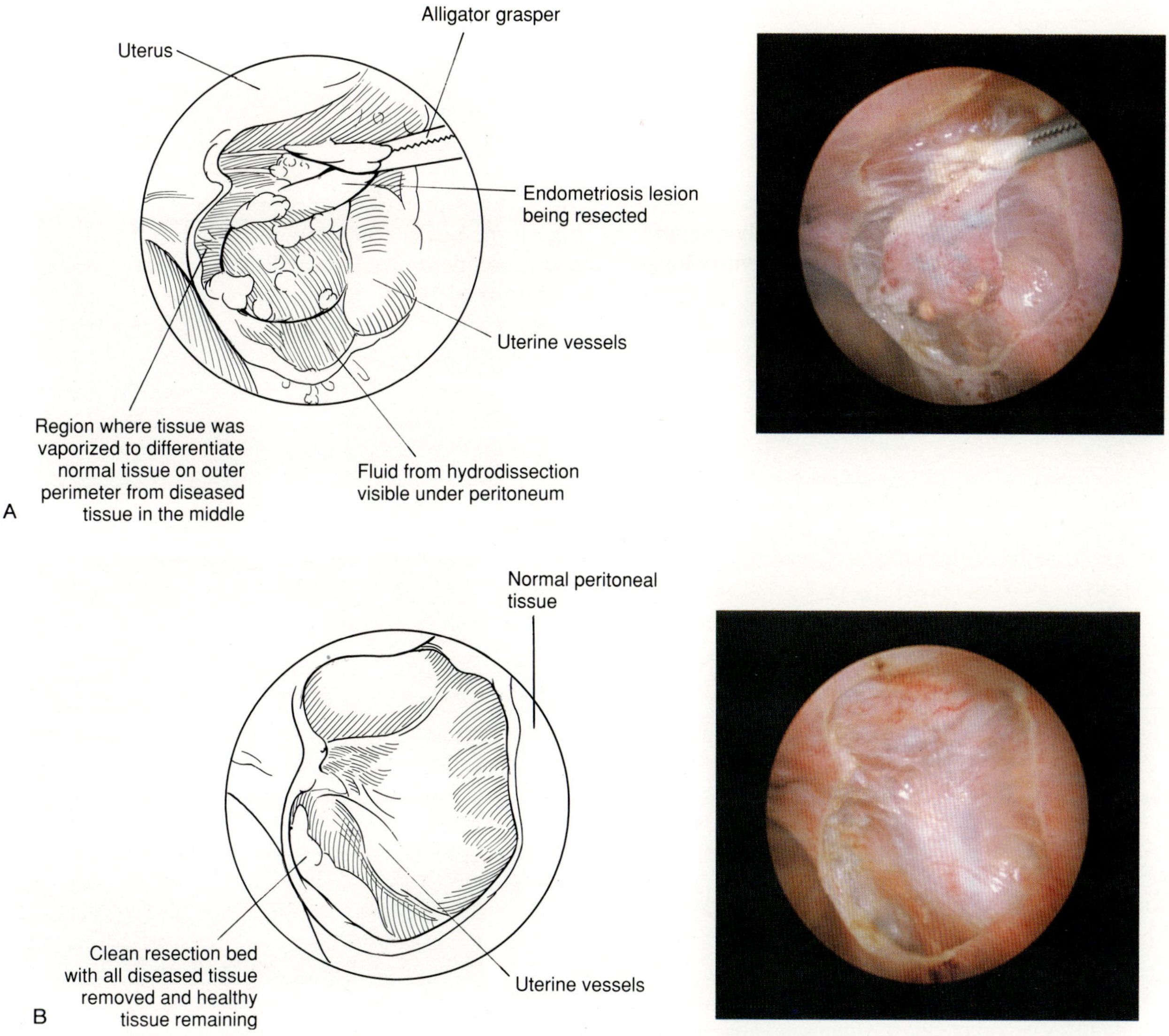

FIG. 9. A: Peritoneal endometriosis lesion on right broad ligament being resected after hydrodissection under peritoneum and circumscription of entire lesion to be removed. **B:** Resected area showing minimal injury to residual tissue.

small lesions, as can fiber laser energy. Endocoagulation and fulguration can destroy superficial lesions. However, the extent of destruction cannot be determined precisely with these thermal but nonvaporizing modalities, resulting in possible inadequate treatment, overtreatment, or risk of injury to contiguous structures.

With the CO_2 laser the endometriotic lesion can be vaporized or resected with precision. A continuous wave, superpulse, or ultrapulse waveform can be used. The laser settings depend on the type of laser, type of waveform, spot size, surgeon's skill, and risk of injury to contiguous structures. Hydrodissection, which involves the injection of irrigating fluid under the peritoneum or other structures, can help to protect deeper structures from injury by the CO_2 laser beam and allow higher power settings and faster dissection to be performed safely. Hydrodissection does not protect against injury when fiber lasers such as argon, KTP-532, or Nd:YAG are used because the energy from these lasers will pass through fluid.

Hydrodissection may also allow easier identification of tissue planes. A small hole is initially made in the peritoneum, through which irrigating fluid is injected under high pressure. The next step after hydrodissection is to circumscribe the lesion with the laser beam, scissors, or electrosurgical instrument. With the CO_2 laser, the depth of penetration can be controlled by pulsing the beam with the foot pedal to vary the amount of energy delivered to the tissue. This circumscription ensures that all of the diseased tissue will be removed and that only healthy tissue will be at the edges of the treated region. Smaller lesions can then be completely vaporized inside the circumscribed area (Fig. 8). Larger lesions can be removed faster and more cleanly by sharp resection of the entire peritoneum (Fig. 9A,B). At least one and sometimes two graspers can be utilized to elevate the edge of the peritoneum from the subperitoneal tissues, thereby identifying a plane for dissection. Both standard and micrograspers or alligator graspers can be used.

When endometriosis is deeply invasive over the ureter

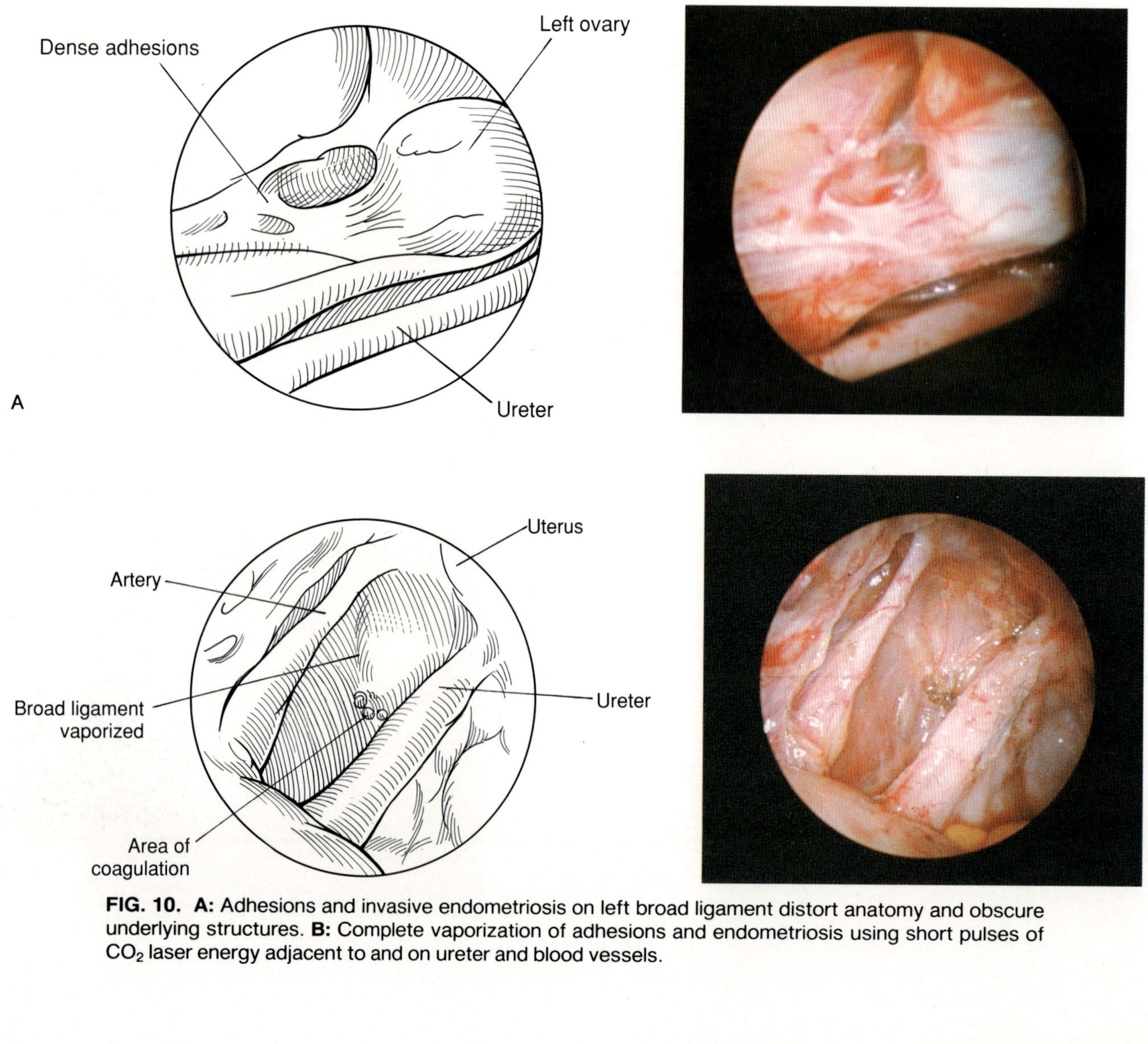

FIG. 10. A: Adhesions and invasive endometriosis on left broad ligament distort anatomy and obscure underlying structures. **B:** Complete vaporization of adhesions and endometriosis using short pulses of CO_2 laser energy adjacent to and on ureter and blood vessels.

or broad ligament vessels, planes may be difficult or impossible to identify and the surgeon must dissect with extreme care. Hydrodissection, while frequently very helpful, often does not create a clear plane when endometriosis invasion is severe. In addition, traction on the peritoneum can cause underlying structures, such as ureter or blood vessels, to be elevated toward the area of dissection. Lower power density for continuous wave or energy density per pulsed wave as well as greater caution need to be exercised when performing such dissection. Short pulses of laser or electrical energy can be delivered by the foot pedal, or small bites can be taken with scissors (Fig. 10A,B). When normal anatomy is very difficult to identify, a helpful approach is to begin dissection away from the lesion at a point where normal anatomy can be ascertained. Sometimes it is useful to identify the ureter and vessels at the pelvic brim and dissect inferiorly with the ureter under direct vision (Fig. 11A,B). Areas of greatest risk while performing peritoneal vaporization and resection include the ureters throughout their course, the internal iliac vein near its bifurcation, the external iliac vessels, the superior aspect of the broad ligaments just beneath the ovary, and the cardinal ligament where the ureter and vessels have changing anatomic relationships. The goal is always to remove all diseased tissue. Both visual inspection and palpation with instruments help confirm that only healthy, pliable, nonindurated tissue is left in the bed of the resection.

Adhesiolysis should be performed using a titanium rod as backstop if possible, hydrodissection of deeper tis-

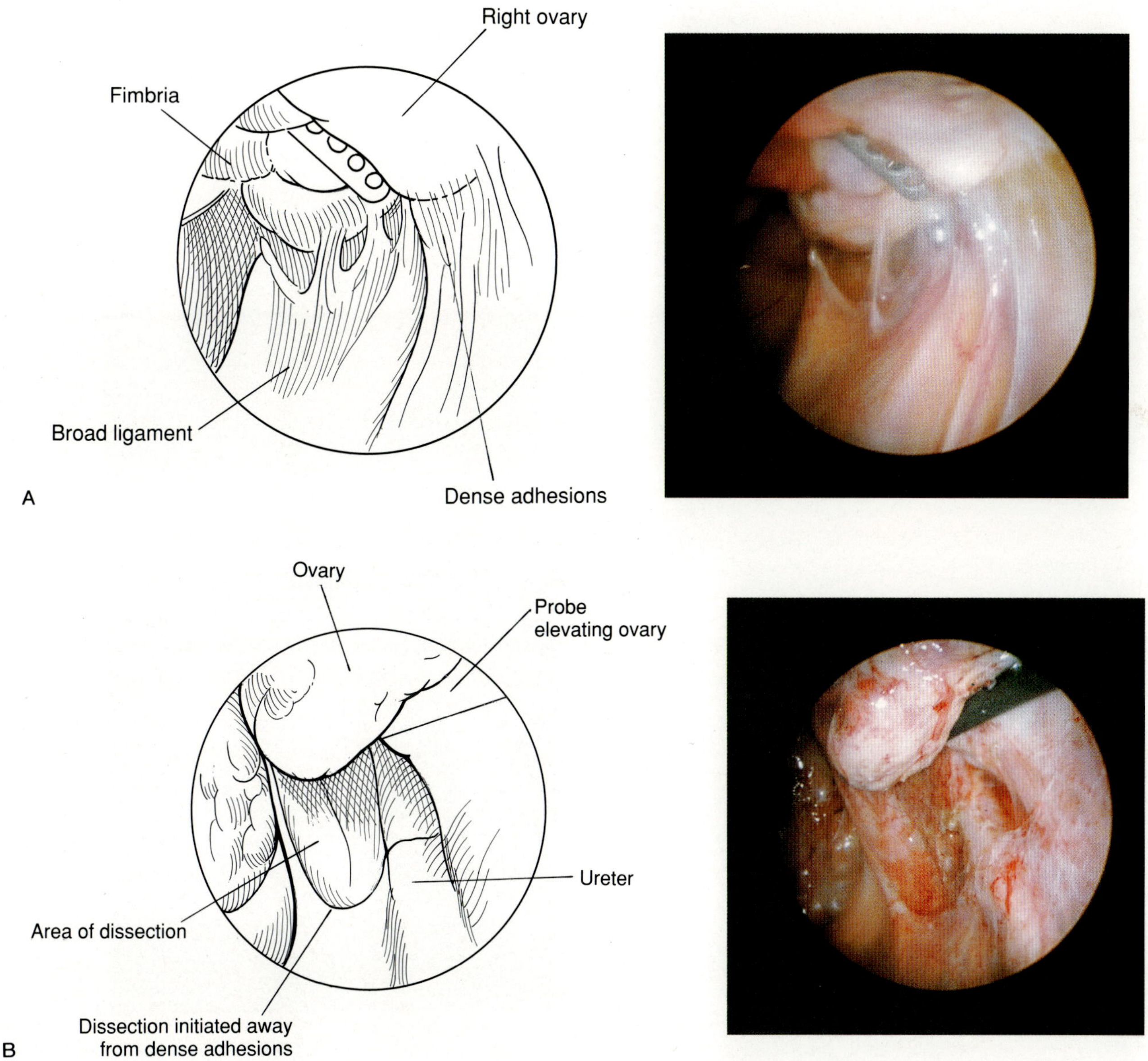

FIG. 11. **A:** Dense adhesions attaching right ovary to right broad ligament near ureter. **B:** Adhesiolysis over ureter completed after initiation of dissection at pelvic brim to identify ureter.

sues when not possible, or very carefully using short pulses of energy when neither technique is feasible because of very dense adhesions (Fig. 12A,B). Traction should be obtained through use of probes to improve visualization. Graspers should be used only on tissue that is to be removed, whenever possible, so as to minimize tissue injury to structures that are not being removed. When graspers are used on tissue that is not going to be resected, the tissue least vulnerable to forming adhesions or having its function reduced because of subsequent adhesion formation should be grasped.

After all of the endometriosis has been resected and hemostasis obtained, the patient should be placed in reverse Trendelenburg position to allow any fluid in the upper abdomen to flow into the pelvis where it can be evacuated. Then the pneumoperitoneum should be evacuated for the intraabdominal gas pressure to reach zero. This allows "bleeders" which may have been tamponaded by the pneumoperitoneum to bleed. After 3 min, the pneumoperitoneum should be reestablished and bleeding vessels identified and coagulated before the operation is terminated. The identification of bleeding vessels is facilitated by placing fluid in the cul-de-sac and looking for "trailers" of blood in the fluid from bleeding vessels (Fig. 13).

It is difficult to evaluate results of treatment of peritoneal disease, since published studies do not directly address this aspect of surgical treatment and the studies suffer from methodologic weaknesses (83). A recent review of laparoscopic treatment of endometriosis re-

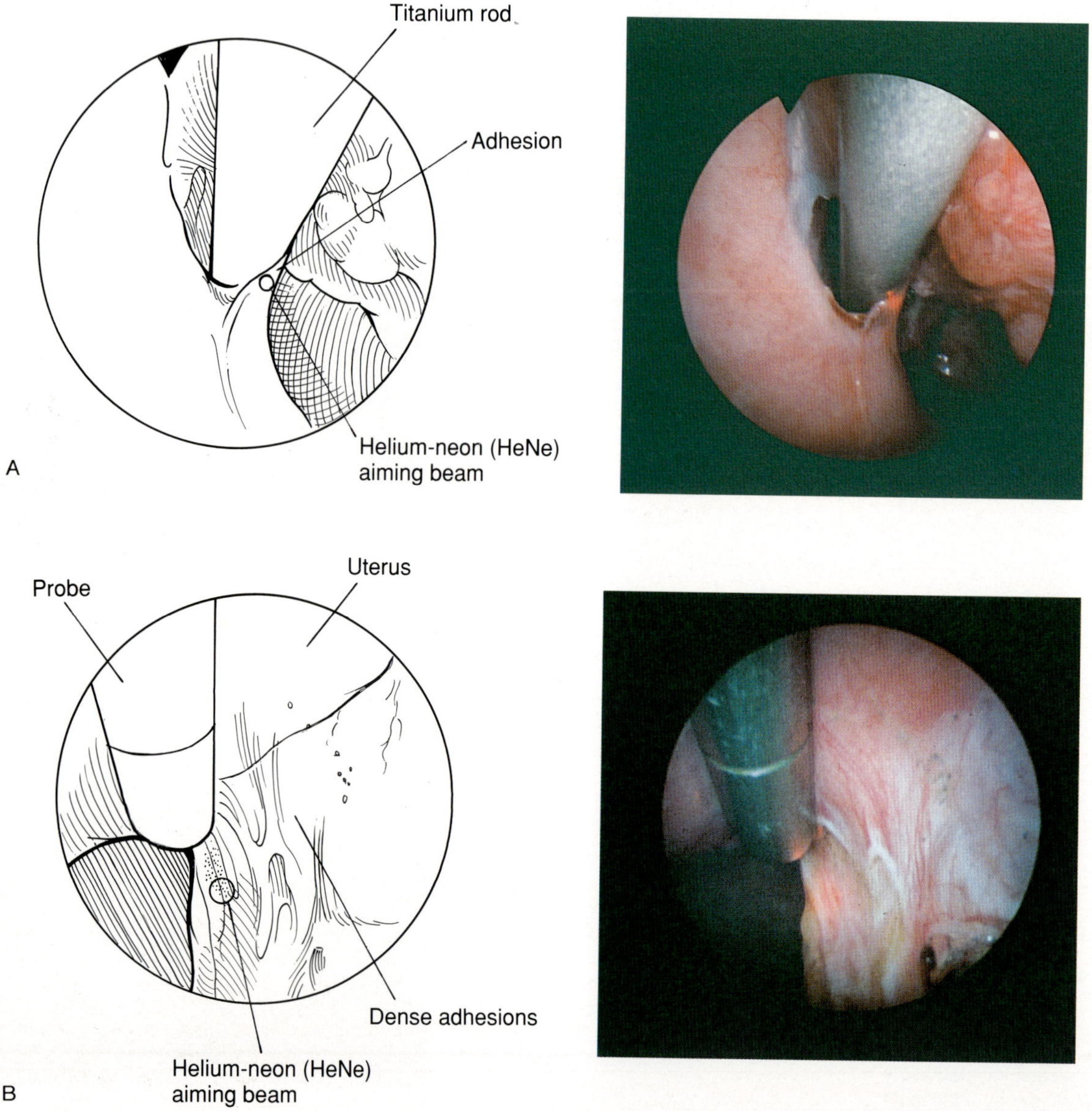

FIG. 12. A: Adhesiolysis using titanium rod backstop. **B:** Dense adhesiolysis using short pulses of CO_2 laser energy.

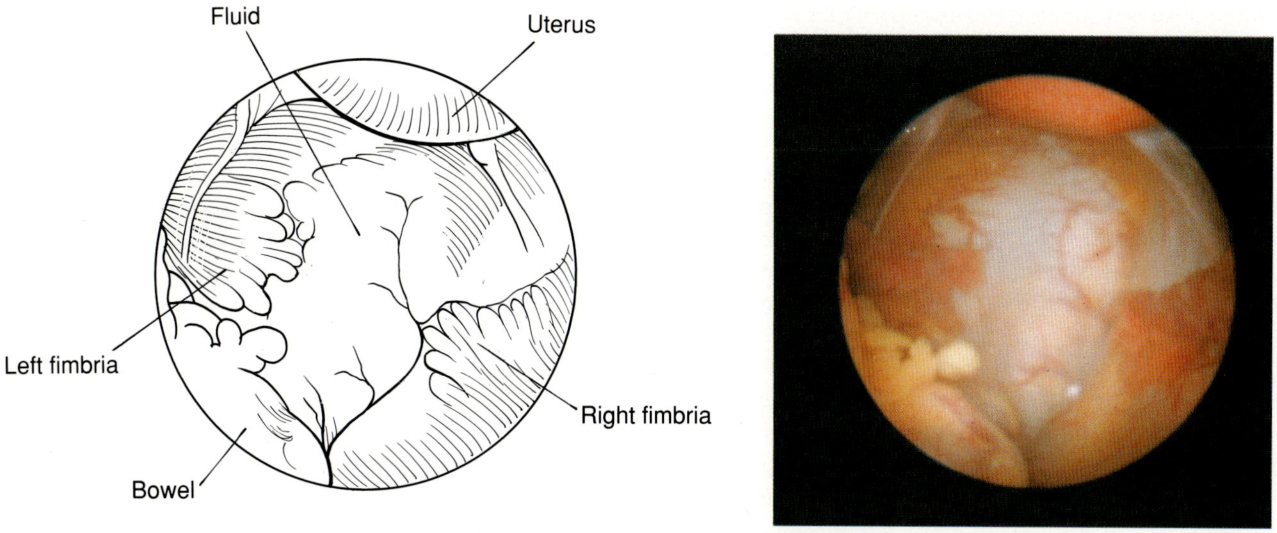

FIG. 13. Physiologic fluid placed in the cul-de-sac to facilitate identification of bleeding vessels.

ported pregnancy rates for minimal and mild disease after laparoscopic electrocoagulation of 64% and 52%, respectively (87). Treatment with CO_2 laser vaporization was reported to result in a 59% pregnancy rate for minimal and 58% for mild disease (87). The author's experience is reflected in Table 3 (70). It is not known as to whether patients with extensive and/or invasive peritoneal disease alone will have pregnancy rates higher or lower than those reported in these studies.

The amount of pelvic pain reduction postperitoneal disease resection is even more difficult to evaluate because of the additional problem of quantifying pain and isolating its causes. One study reported a 41% total relief of pain, 35% partial, and 24% failure rate overall. However, the nature and location of lesions and the grading scale were not reported (88). Another study reported that 67% of patients were pain-free (43). Pain symptomatology appears to be related to the dimension of invasive endometriotic lesions (45). Sutton et al. reported a prospective randomized trial of laser laparoscopy in the treatment of pelvic pain associated with endometriosis that showed 62.5% improved at 6 months in the treated group compared with 22.6% in the control group (89).

It is not yet clear as to what the effect will be of the increasing trend to resect completely all disease rather than treat it simply by coagulation, fulguration, or laser without resection (23). In a recent study, 61% of patients had clinically recognized lesions penetrating deeper than 2 mm, 43% had lesions penetrating deeper than 3 mm, and 25% had lesions penetrating deeper than 5 mm. The deepest lesion was 15 mm. Coagulation or laser vaporization to 5 mm would have missed endometriotic lesions in one quarter of patients (90). Another study confirmed the frequent presence of deep lesions, which were active 68% of the time. Deep lesions infiltrated through loose connective tissue septa into the fibromuscular tis-

TABLE 3. *Estimated cumulative life table pregnancy rates by stage of endometriosis*

	Entire patient population					Endometriosis-only subset[a]				
		Pregnant in 3	% Pregnant				Pregnant in 3	% Pregnant		
	No.	years	1 Year	2 Years	3 Years	No.	years	1 Year	2 Years	3 Years
All	579	274	36.9 ± 2.2	53.6 ± 2.4	61.7 ± 2.6	258	130	39.7 ± 3.3	57.4 ± 3.6	65.8 ± 3.8
Minimal	161	91	49.8 ± 4.3	64.9 ± 4.5	73.7 ± 4.6	91	49	44.8 ± 5.7	61.2 ± 6.0	70.5 ± 6.1
Mild	185	89	38.0 ± 3.8	55.6 ± 4.3	62.3 ± 4.6	101	49	40.9 ± 5.2	54.9 ± 5.7	63.1 ± 6.4
Moderate	142	63	31.1 ± 4.2	50.5 ± 4.9	57.4 ± 5.1	49	26	35.6 ± 7.5	60.3 ± 8.3	71.1 ± 8.1
Severe	91	31	22.0 ± 4.6	35.8 ± 5.9	46.7 ± 6.6	17	6	18.6 ± 9.7	42.6 ± 13.6	42.6 ± 13.6
All minimal/ mild	346	180	43.4 ± 2.3	59.8 ± 3.1	67.7 ± 3.3	192	98	42.7 ± 3.9	58.0 ± 4.2	66.8 ± 4.4
All moderate/ severe	233	94	27.5 ± 3.1	44.7 ± 3.8	53.2 ± 4.0	66	32	30.9 ± 6.1	55.4 ± 7.2	63.2 ± 7.2

[a] Endometriosis-only subset = at least one fallopian tube and fimbria normal, and normal male factor.

sue and always stopped at the underlying fat tissue. Very deep implants (>10 mm) were found exclusively in patients with pain whereas superficial implants were found most frequently in patients with infertility (83%) (91). The results of these studies suggest that the most precise energy source available, namely, the CO_2 laser, should have some advantages in performing complete resection and vaporization of peritoneal lesions. However, good surgical technique should enable the surgeon to effect adequate and safe resection with other energy sources.

Treatment of Noncystic Ovarian Endometriosis

The ovary frequently has superficial lesions similar to those on the peritoneum and/or invasive endometriosis lesions less than 1 cm in diameter and not classically defined as endometriomas (Fig. 14A). These superficial lesions should be vaporized or coagulated with the minimal amount of thermal injury created in the surrounding ovary, since adhesions form very easily following ovarian injury. Intermittent pulsing of the laser beam by means of the foot pedal can facilitate this technique. Care should be taken not to create serious thermal injury near the fimbria or fimbria ovarica, as this might compromise distal tubal mobility and/or function. Power density of laser or electrosurgery should be reduced if necessary to minimize thermal injury (Fig. 14B). Deeper lesions should be completely resected and/or vaporized using appropriate meticulous technique to minimize ovarian injury (Fig. 15A,B). All suspicious lesions should be evaluated to ensure that all endometriosis is ablated. Deeper, noncystic lesions especially need to be completely extirpated (Fig. 15C). Injury to the vascular supply of the ovary should be avoided. It is always necessary to elevate

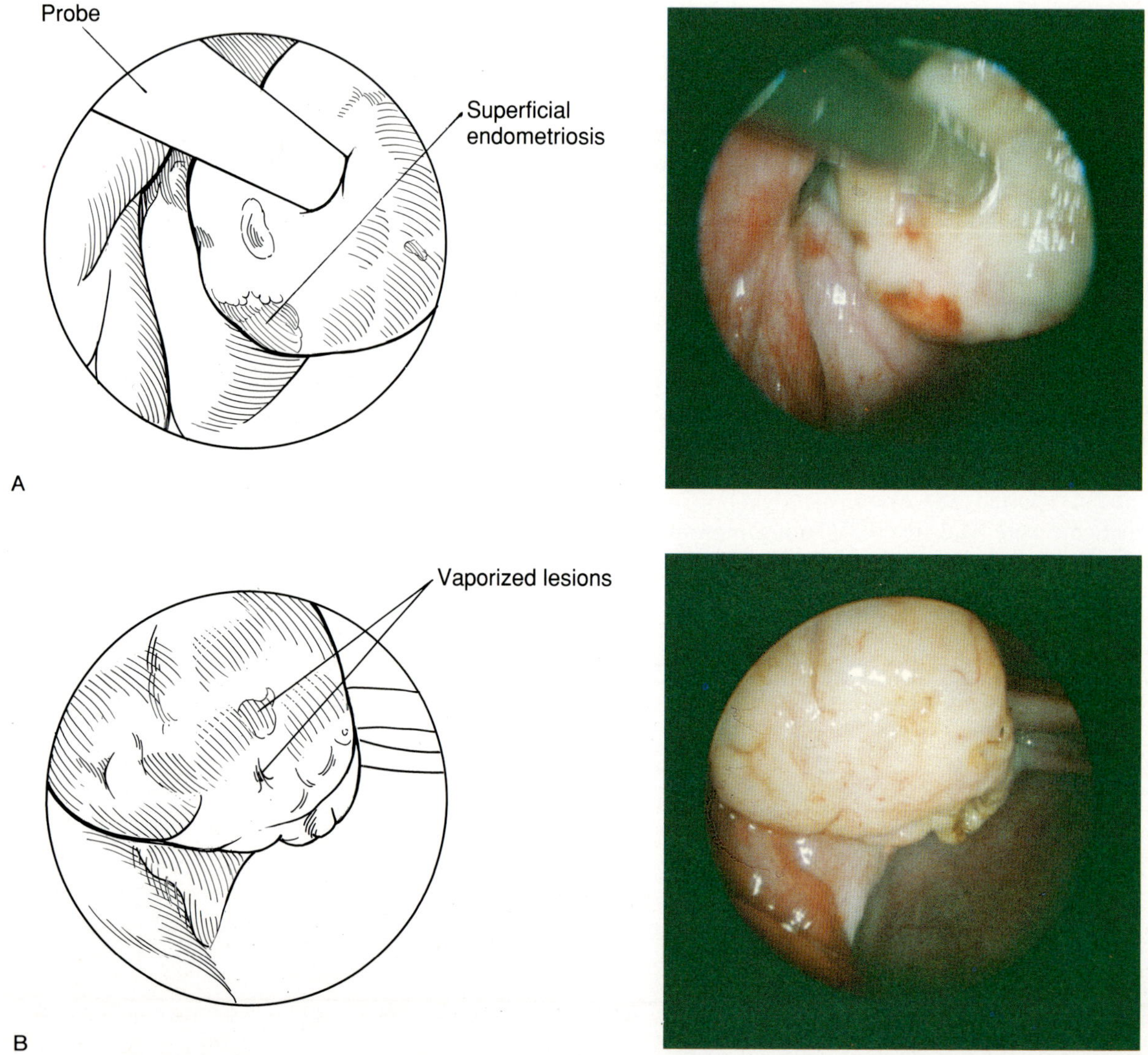

FIG. 14. A: Superficial endometriosis lesions on left ovary. **B:** Vaporized lesions showing minimal thermal injury to ovary.

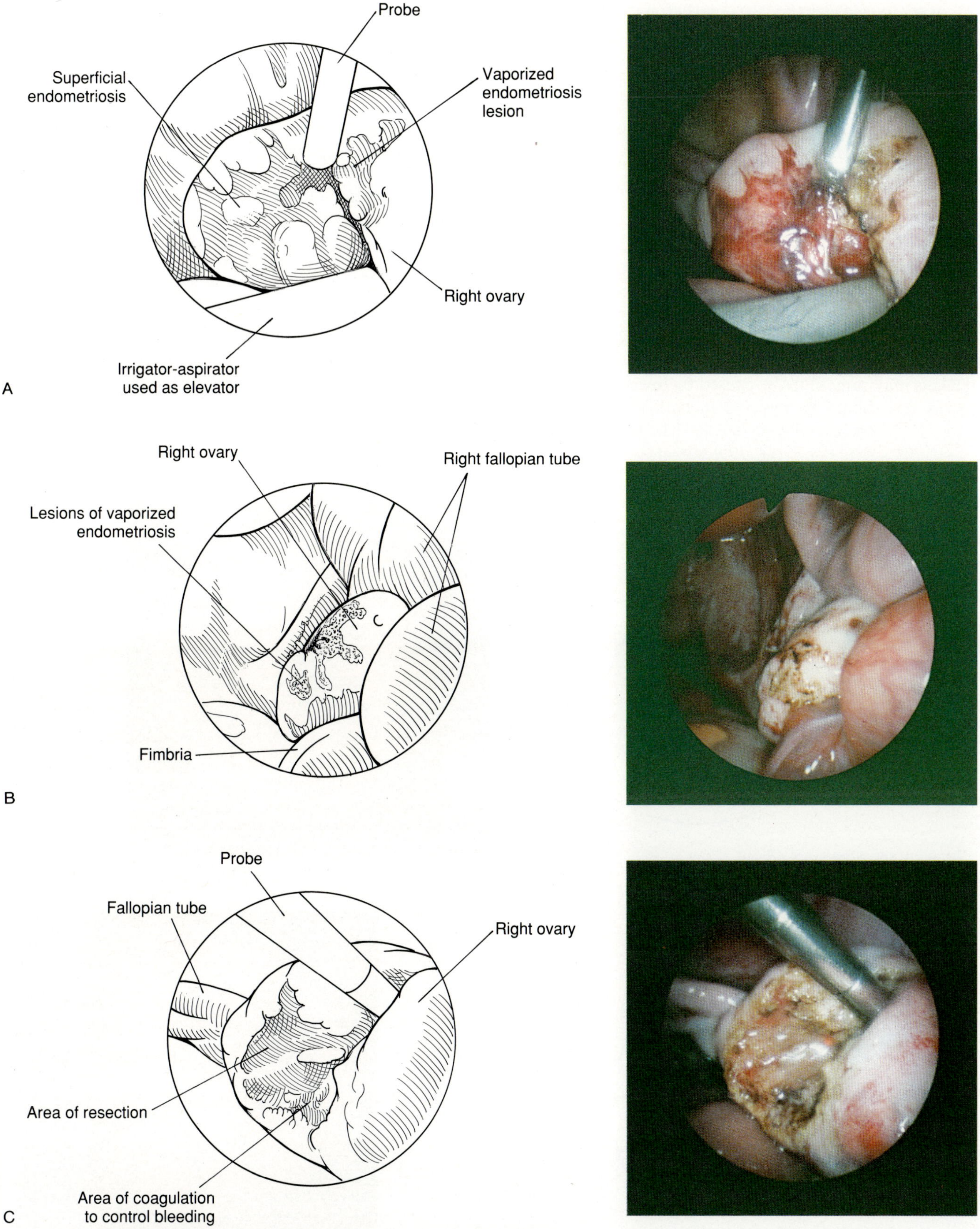

FIG. 15. A: Superficial and invasive lesion on medial aspect of right ovary. **B:** Vaporized lesions from Fig. 15A showing minimal injury to ovary. **C:** Undersurface of ovary from Fig. 15A showing complete vaporization of invasive endometriosis.

the ovary to visualize the lateral surface lying against the upper surface of the broad ligament. Inability to elevate the ovary almost always implies that adhesions and/or endometriosis lesions are under the ovary. Such disease should be treated by vaporization, resection, and/or coagulation until all the disease is removed and complete mobilization of the ovary is possible.

Cul-de-Sac and Rectovaginal Dissection

An area where some of the deepest invasion and most difficult dissection may occur is the posterior cul-de-sac and rectovaginal septum. Here active endometriosis can be found deep in the fibromuscular tissue (27,91). Such disease can cause pain and possibly infertility. Peritoneal pockets may sometimes be caused by invasive endometriosis and should be resected in patients with pelvic pain. These pockets may be deeper than initially appreciated, and dissection needs to be performed carefully with copious hydrodissection to avoid injury to deeper structures (Fig. 16A,B). Martin pioneered the use of excisional techniques for endometriosis resection and first reported on the laparoscopic approach to infiltrating cul-de-sac endometriosis (Fig. 17) (92). As experience was gained, more of the procedure was performed laparoscopically rather than vaginally. Two of seven patients had deep sigmoid colon lesions requiring laparotomy for focal colon excision and repair. Redwine also reported new techniques for laparoscopic en bloc resection of obliterated cul-de-sac endometriosis (93). Reich et al. reported on 100 patients with partial or complete cul-de-sac obliteration secondary to deep fibrotic endometriosis and described their technique in detail (see below) (94). These techniques and the author's are similar (Fig. 18A–C). This involves circumscribing the entire lesion, then freeing the anterior rectum from the uterus and loose areolar tissue of the rectovaginal septum. The visible and

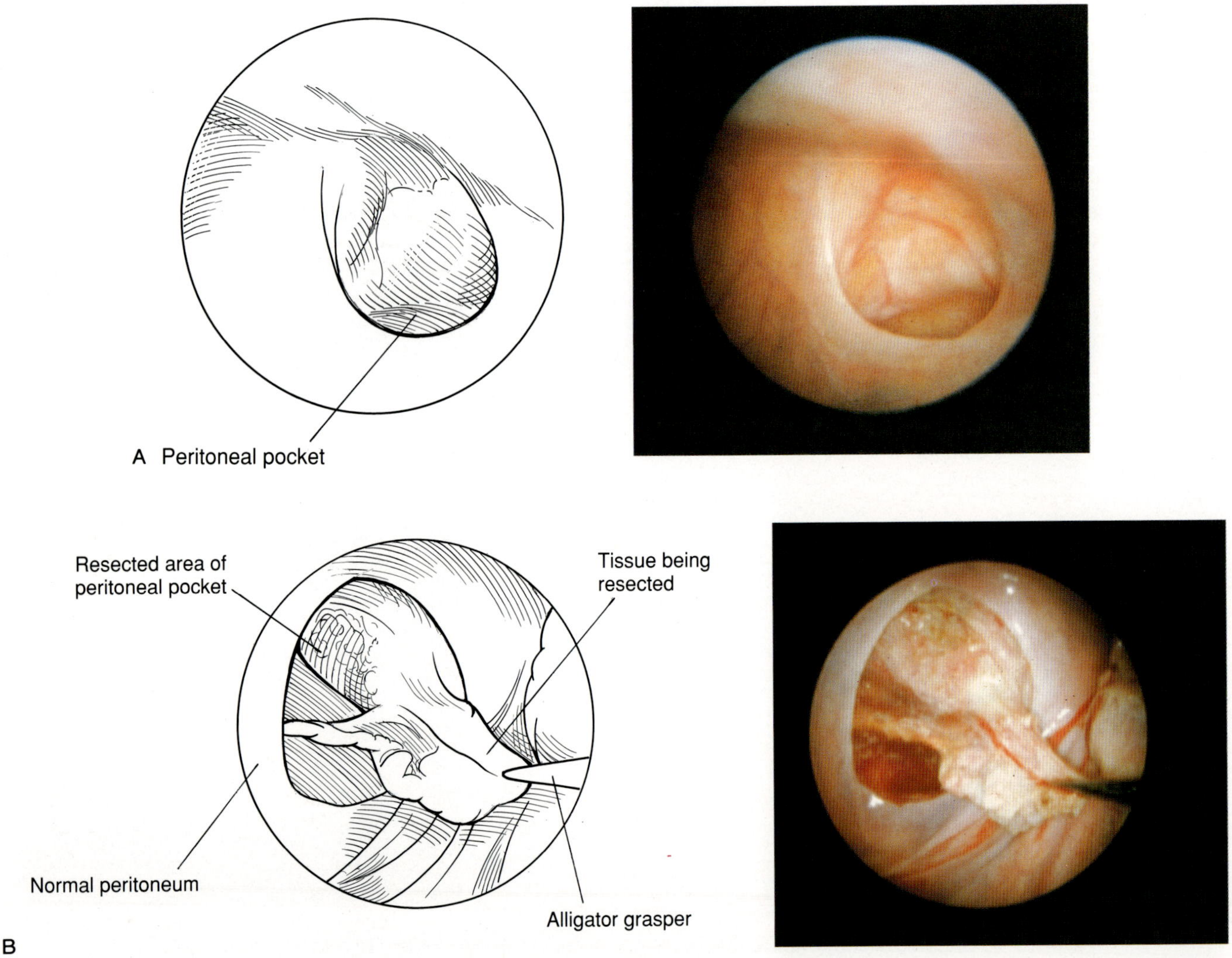

FIG. 16. **A:** Peritoneal pocket medial to right uterosacral ligament. **B:** Resection of peritoneal pocket.

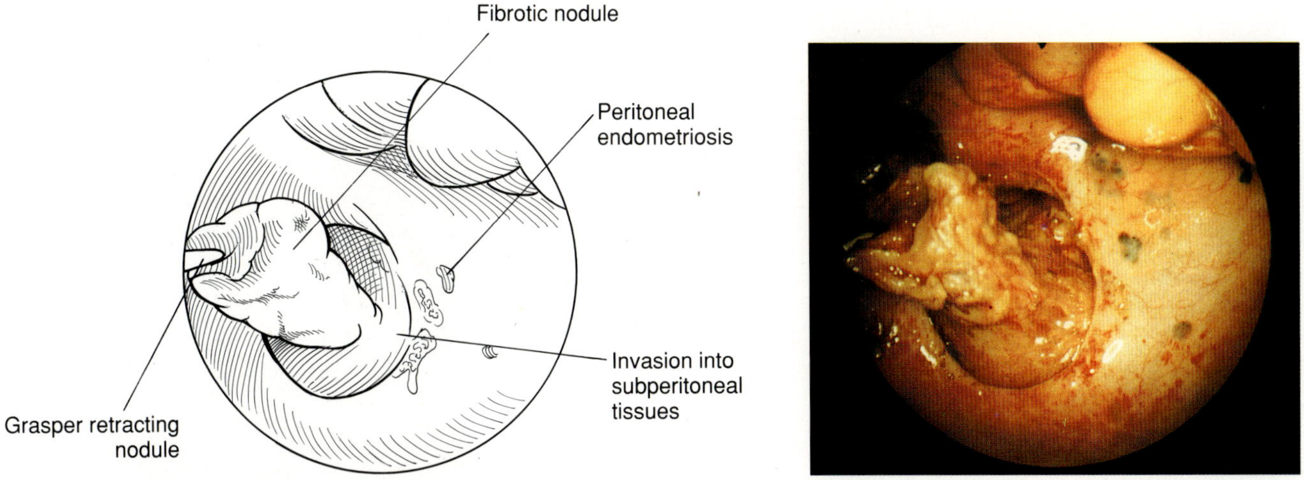

FIG. 17. Resection of deeply infiltrating fibrotic nodule in posterior cul-de-sac. From Dan Martin, M.D.

palpable deep fibrotic endometriosis on the bowel is then vaporized and/or excised working from the perimeter with healthy tissue toward the endometriotic lesion. Use of a sponge on a ring forceps inserted into the posterior vaginal fornix, placement of a rectal probe, use of a Valtchev retractor for anteversion of the uterus, and frequent intraoperative rectovaginal examinations help to determine pelvic anatomy. Dissection is carried out bluntly with scissors, electrosurgery, and/or laser, with copious use of aquadissection (hydrodissection) to help identify tissue planes and perform dissection. Lesions extending through the posterior vaginal wall can be dissected en bloc with a 30-cc Foley bag in the vagina to maintain the pneumoperitoneum. The vagina can be closed vaginally or laparoscopically. Deep rectal muscularis defects can be closed with 2-0 suture. Reich sometimes plicates the uterosacral ligaments and lateral rectal peritoneum across the midline to reperitonealize the anterior rectum. If there is any question regarding bowel integrity, a 30-cm^3 Foley catheter can be passed per rectum, the rectosigmoid compressed with a laparoscopic bowel clamp above the site of dissection, and a dilute solution of betadine injected while the pelvis is filled with irrigating solution. Reich reported an average operating time of 3 hr, with one case lasting 8 hr.

Pregnancy was achieved in 34 of 46 infertile couples (74%) (94). Of the women who conceived, 13 of 34 (38%) had more than one laparoscopy. Five of six women who underwent three laparoscopies conceived. Of women with pelvic pain, 41 of 46 (89%) had significant relief 6 months after laparoscopy. Complications included anemia in two patients, corneal abrasion in one, and transient unilateral brachial plexus injury in one. A complete 3-day bowel preparation with soft diet, fluid diet, clear liquid diet, Golytely or Colyte, is mandatory for mechanical cleaning of the bowel before this type of dissection is attempted. Reich emphasized the need to remove all evident endometriosis, or at least as much as possible, and the desirability of avoiding bowel resection, a potentially morbid procedure. The author has compared laparoscopy vs. laparotomy for treatment of complete endometriotic posterior cul-de-sac obliteration (95). In a series of 27 patients with extensive disease and infertility, life table pregnancy rates were 29.6% at 1 and 2 years in 11 patients treated laparoscopically, compared with 0% at one year, and 23.7% at 2 years in 16 patients treated at laparotomy (Table 4). No serious complications occurred in the author's reported series or subsequent cases to date involving cul-de-sac and rectovaginal dissection, including those in which the bowel has been sutured following enterostomy. No patients have required transfusion, management in intensive care, or reoperation. One patient was readmitted for 24 hr for intravenous antibiotics because of suspected infection. Thorough informed consent including discussion of other options, adequate bowel preparation, and surgical skill and experience are mandatory before such operations should be attempted, as they can be technically demanding (96). The literature results support the conclusion that laparoscopic treatment of advanced endometriosis requiring cul-de-sac and rectovaginal dissection can provide satisfactory results equivalent to those obtained at laparotomy when

TABLE 4. *Complete endometriotic posterior cul-de-sac obliteration: estimated life table pregnancy rates*

% Pregnant (years)	Laparoscopy	Laparotomy
1	29.6 ± 14.4	0 ± 0.0
2	29.6 ± 14.4	23.7 ± 12.2

$p = 0.084$ (Breslow statistic).

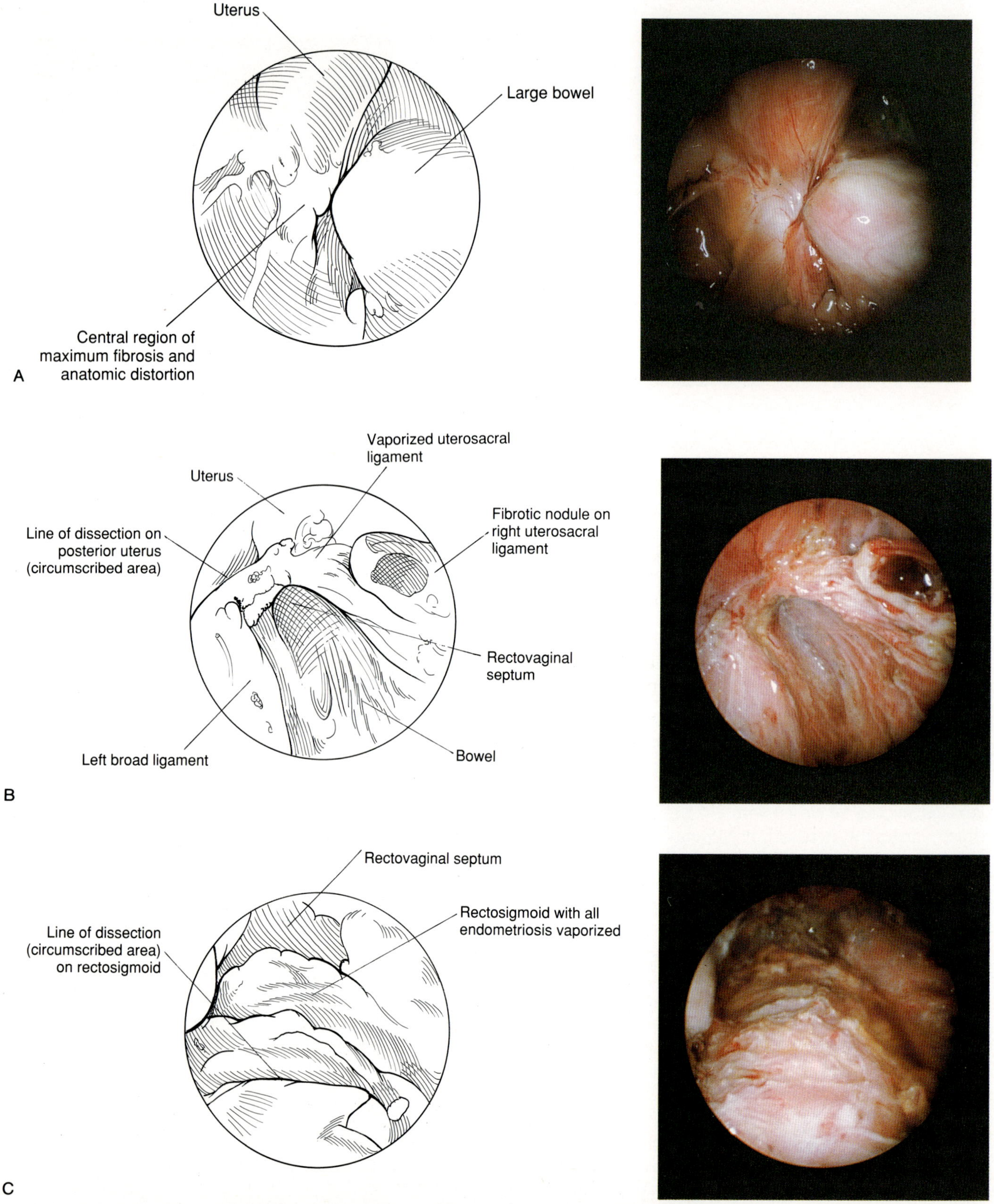

FIG. 18. A: Posterior cul-de-sac and rectovaginal invasive endometriosis causing marked anatomic distortion and obliteration. **B:** Dissection of posterior cul-de-sac by circumscription, vaporization, and identification of fibrotic lesion for resection. **C:** Restoration of normal posterior cul-de-sac anatomy following dissection, vaporization, and resection of adhesions, endometriosis, and fibrotic lesions.

performed by very experienced endoscopists (92–95, 97). All of the surgeons reporting on this technique emphasize the need for complete resection of the diseased tissue.

Resection of Invasive Bowel Endometriosis

Superficial and mildly invasive large bowel endometriosis lesions can be treated effectively and safely with the CO_2 laser because of its great precision (Fig. 19). Use of other energy sources for more than superficial lesions carries a high risk of unrecognized transmural thermal injury with subsequent bowel perforation. Only very superficial small bowel lesions should be treated unless the surgeon is prepared to perform laparoscopic resection and repair. The potential catastrophic consequences of unrecognized transmural bowel injury mandate that such a cautious approach be taken.

Aggressive surgical management of advanced colorectal endometriosis has been shown to be effective and safe when performed at laparotomy (98). Martin reported in 1988 on two patients who required focal colon excision and repair at laparotomy as a result of significant endometriotic bowel lesions found at the time of laparoscopic treatment of invasive cul-de-sac disease (92). However, it is increasingly possible to resect endometriotic nodules infiltrating the anterior rectus muscularis (Fig. 20A–C) (94). An assistant's finger in the rectum can help with dissection. Repair can be performed laparoscopically with suture when the rectal lumen is not entered. When it is entered, the bowel should be repaired in two layers in the usual fashion. If the hole in the rectum is low and the vagina has also been entered, transvaginal closure may also be performed. This assumes, of course, that a complete mechanical bowel preparation has been performed prior to surgery. In some cases, a single suture layer of 2-0 Vicryl or similar suture with large bites may be appropriate.

Recently, cases have been reported of complete bowel resection of severe endometriosis and reanastomosis performed endoscopically using suture or staplers (99,100). These procedures have been performed by or with the assistance of general surgeons. Problems with misfiring of the stapling instrument, requirement for laparotomy, anastomosis failure with resultant morbidity, and long-term sequelae requiring permanent colostomy mandate that this procedure still be considered investigational unless traditional abdominal general surgical techniques are duplicated at laparoscopy. Technological advances and increased clinical experience will undoubtedly ensure that laparoscopic bowel resection and reanastomosis will become a commonly performed procedure for rectosigmoid endometriotic disease. Resection and repair of small or large bowel endometriotic lesions higher in the gastrointestinal tract will also become more amenable to laparoscopic treatment as more gynecologists and general surgeons become familiar with performing these procedures in a routine fashion endoscopically rather than at laparotomy (Fig. 21). When considering surgical treatment of bowel lesions, gynecologists should consider their own expertise and consult general surgeons and gastroenterologists preoperatively and intraoperatively as dictated by the patient's best interests (see the chapter by Redwine, "Treatment of Bowel Lesions").

Appendectomy

Many gynecologists perform appendectomy for benign conditions, including appendiceal endometriosis.

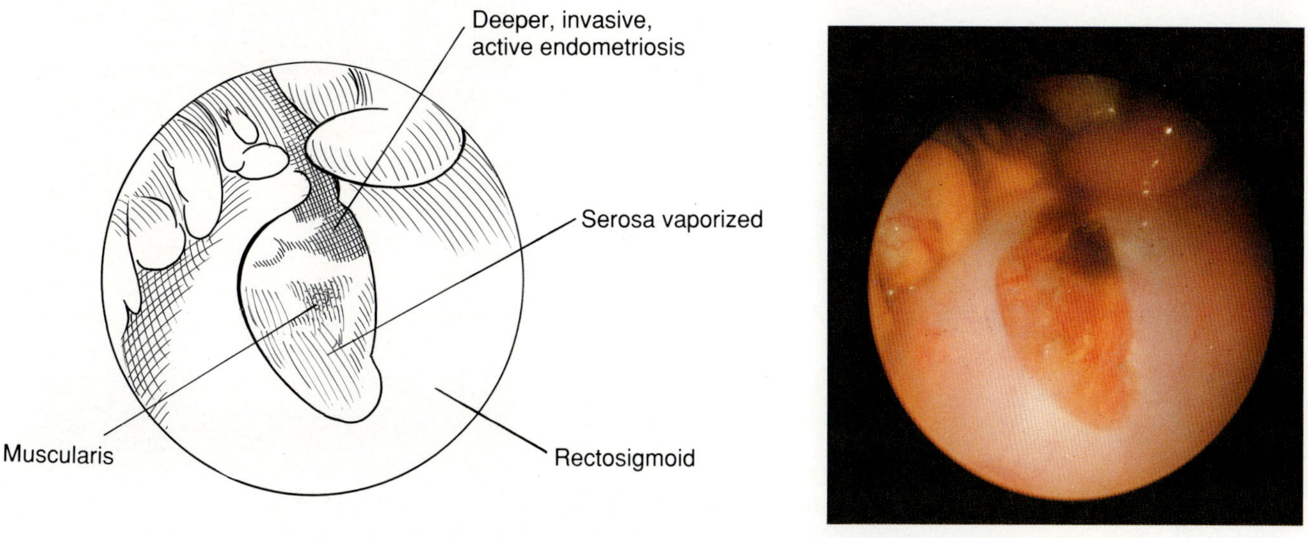

FIG. 19. Mildly invasive endometriosis on rectosigmoid treated with CO_2 laser.

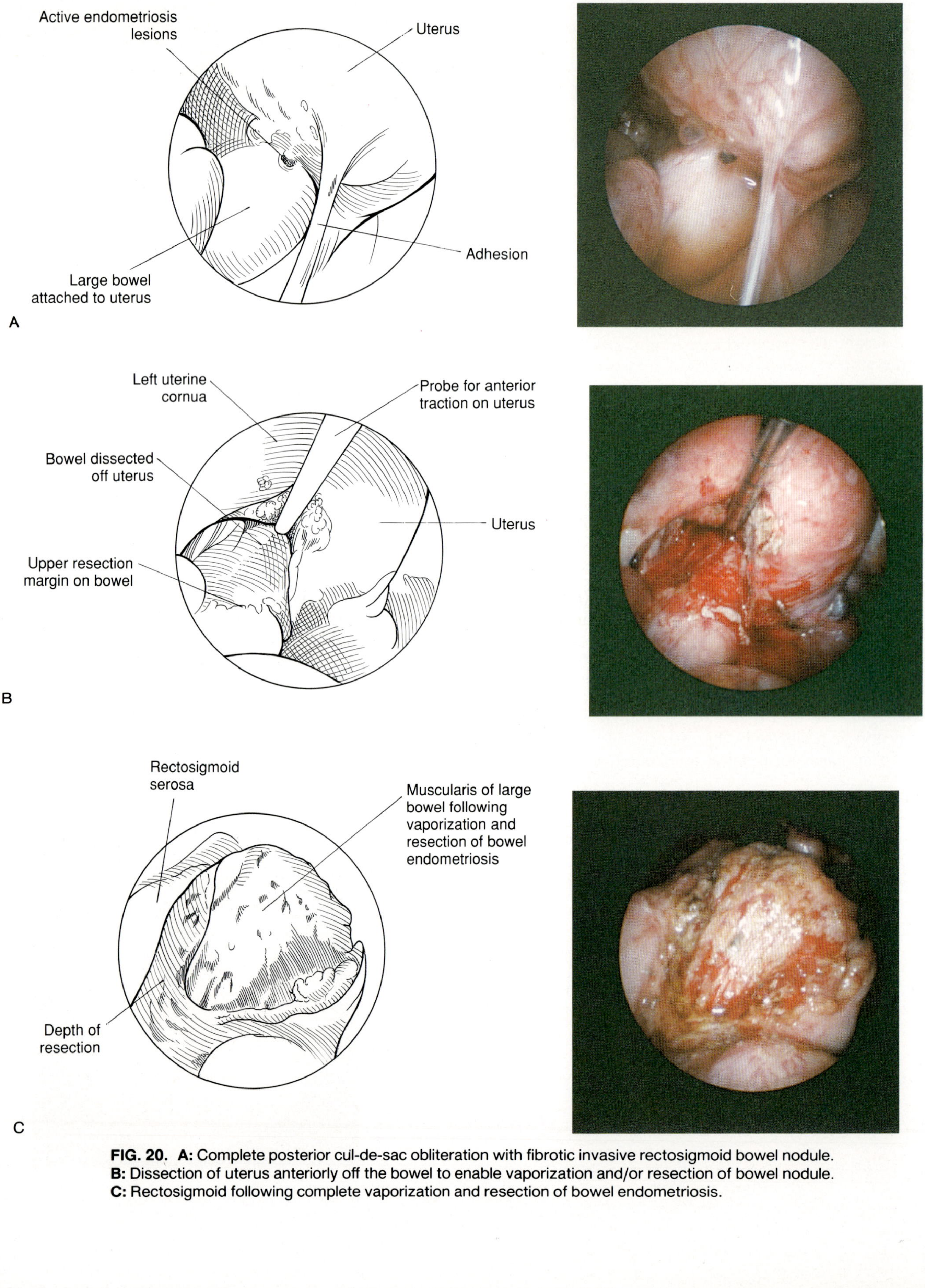

FIG. 20. **A:** Complete posterior cul-de-sac obliteration with fibrotic invasive rectosigmoid bowel nodule. **B:** Dissection of uterus anteriorly off the bowel to enable vaporization and/or resection of bowel nodule. **C:** Rectosigmoid following complete vaporization and resection of bowel endometriosis.

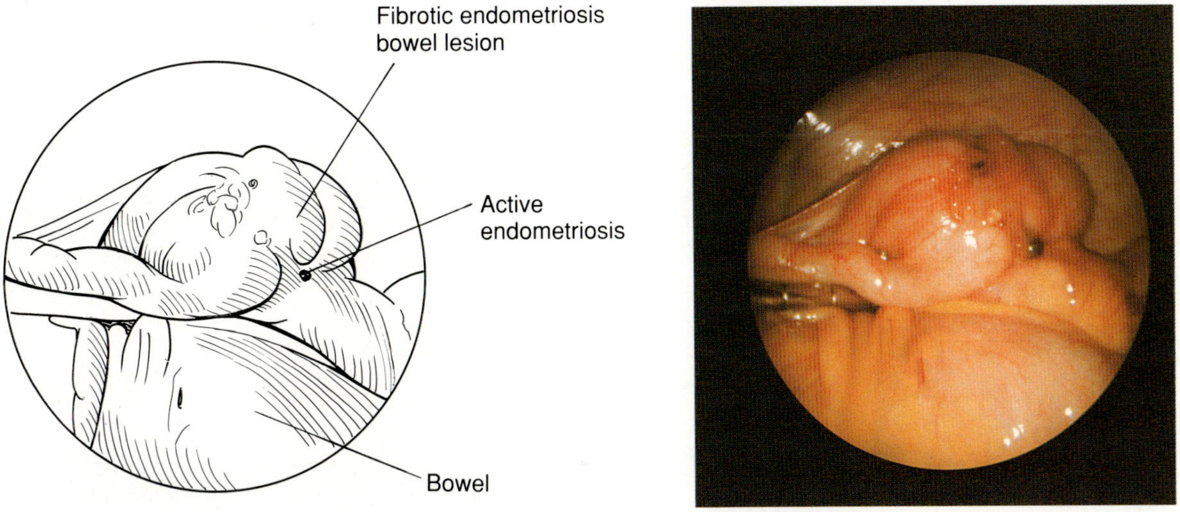

FIG. 21. Ascending colon endometriotic lesion causing obstruction. Bowel resection subsequently performed with stapling device laparoscopically.

The role of incidental appendectomy in the routine gynecology patient without appendiceal disease is more controversial, and few reproductive surgeons recommend incidental appendectomy in the infertility patient. Appendectomy can be performed safely and quickly at laparoscopy using automatic stapling devices (101). A more traditional approach can also be used (Fig. 22A,B). The appendix is grasped at its tip and bipolar electrosurgery, clips, or suture used to obtain hemostasis before cutting the appendiceal vessels at the base of the appendix. Care must be exercised not to injure the cecum. Two endoloops are then placed at the base of the appendix on top of each other and a third 5 mm distally. A grasper or endoloop can then be placed at the appendiceal tip and the appendix transected between the ligatures and removed. Microbipolar electrosurgery carefully applied to the residual stump will sterilize the raw surface. The stump does not need to be buried. Routine postappendectomy care should be provided. Results have been reported to be equivalent to those at laparotomy (102) (see the chapter by Kurtz and Daniell, "Appendectomy").

Ovarian Endometriomectomy

Laparoscopic treatment of ovarian endometriomas has been controversial because of concern that diagnosis of an ovarian cancer could be missed, that contamination of the pelvis with an ovarian cancer could result in reduced survival, and that unnecessary laparoscopic surgery might be performed in a cancer patient who needs laparotomy (103,104). This issue was highlighted by a questionnaire review that collected 42 cases of ovarian masses treated laparoscopically that were eventually determined to be malignant (105). Capsule rupture and delay of treatment raised concern about the appropriateness of the laparoscopic approach to adnexal masses. While delay of treatment can be avoided, capsule rupture will inevitably occur in at least some patients who have an ovarian malignancy treated laparoscopically. Whether or not such rupture affects prognosis has been actively debated (106,107). A set of guidelines for laparoscopic surgery in the management of ovarian cysts was recently presented by a group of gynecologic oncologists, reproductive endocrinologists, and ultrasonographers (108). Ultrasonography may be the most helpful technique (47,109). These have been summarized in Table 5. It should be noted that CA-125 is not very sensitive or specific and is most useful as a marker of disease progression. Additional studies that some consider might be helpful include MRI or CT scan, carcinoembryonic antigen, needle aspiration for cytology, and ovarian cystoscopy and biopsy. Such diagnostic procedures are not infallible (110). The patient should be informed that the risk of an ovarian neoplasm being malignant increases with age from 8% at less than 20 years, to 35% at ages 40–49, with the risk of low malignant potential neoplasms being 0% and 6%, respectively (111). Other problems with laparoscopic ovarian cystectomy include possible sequelae such as adhesions or seeding from dermoid cysts or mucinous cystadenomas.

However, most adnexal masses are not malignant. Therefore, many experienced laparoscopists believe that by following careful guidelines the risk of unwittingly treating an adnexal malignancy at laparoscopy can be reduced to one in several hundred patients. Since the actual extent of injury to the patient should a malignancy be opened is controversial, many laparoscopists feel that adnexal masses, and in particular endometriomas, can reasonably be approached laparoscopically (59,86,112–

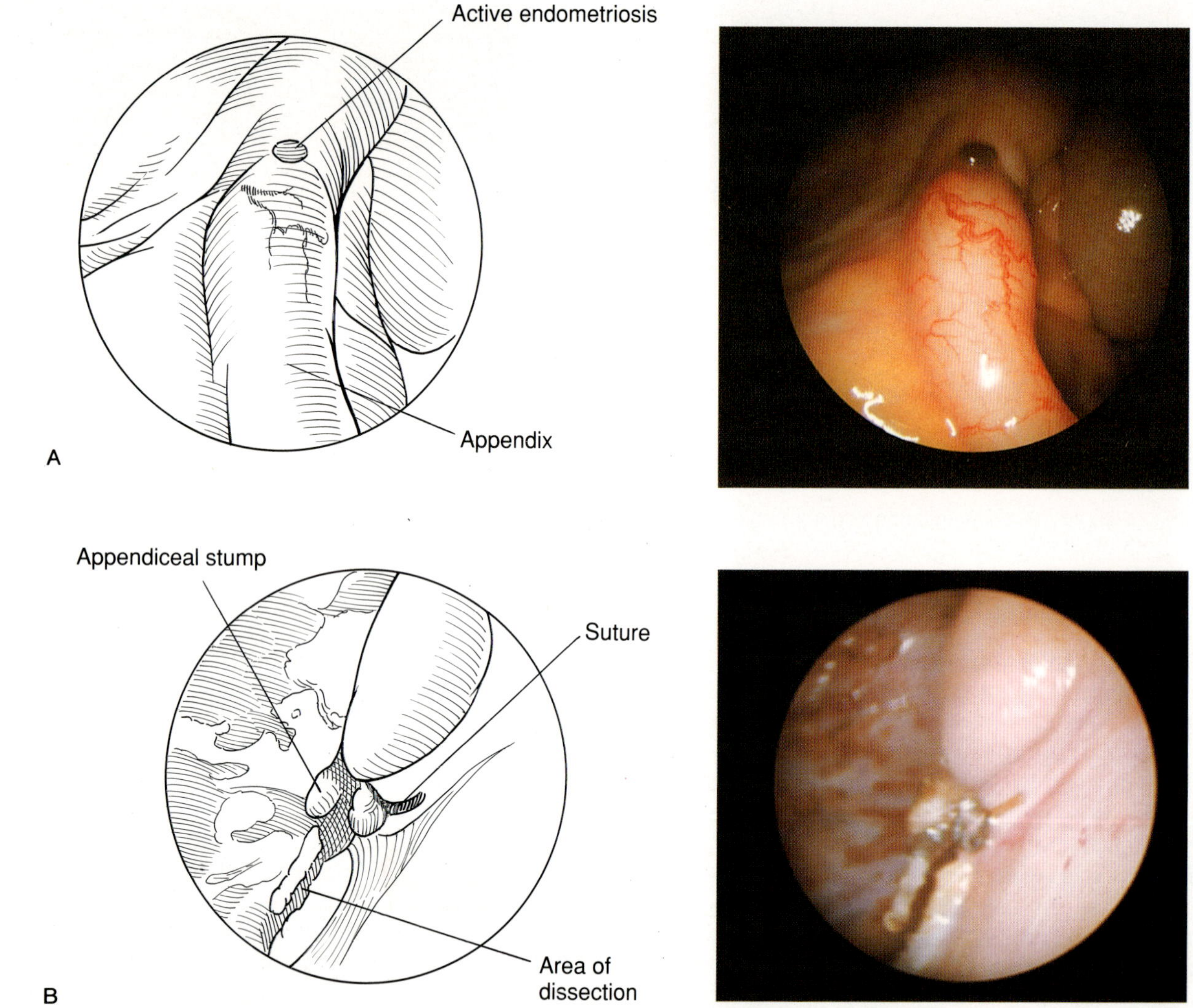

FIG. 22. **A:** Appendiceal endometriosis. **B:** Appendiceal stump following appendectomy with electrosurgery and endoloops.

TABLE 5. *Guidelines for laparoscopic surgery in the management of ovarian cysts*

History
Differential diagnosis
Cancer (personal and family)
Physical examination
Size, consistency, fixation
Ultrasonography
Size, unilocular, unilateral, completely cystic, smooth border, peritoneal fluid
Tumor markers
CA-125, α-fetoprotein, hCG
Informed consent
Intraoperative procedures
Peritoneal washings
Exploration of all peritoneal surfaces and biopsy as indicated
Exploration of ovarian mass for external excrescences or other suspicious findings
Frozen section
Laparotomy
Immediate for suspicious or confirmed malignant masses
Avoidance of cyst rupture

114). Some surgeons have recommended simple puncture and drainage of endometriomas, but this approach fails approximately half of the time (115–117). A more successful approach involves drainage of the cyst followed by electrosurgical or laser ablation of the cyst wall using argon or Nd:YAG lasers (118,119). Brosens and Puttemans suggested that only the base of the endometrioma needs to be coagulated or vaporized resulting in loss of blood supply to the endometriotic cyst wall and its resolution (59,120). Others have recommended complete resection of the cyst wall because this can result in less thermal injury to the ovary and greater assurance of complete removal of the endometriotic tissue as well as a pathology specimen (86,112,121). Resection of an endometrioma is performed after it has been drained revealing the classical "chocolate" material (Figs. 23A, 24A). Copious irrigation and aspiration should be performed to remove all of the endometrioma fluid from the abdominopelvic cavity. Grasping instruments are placed on the ovarian cortex and on the cyst wall to establish a

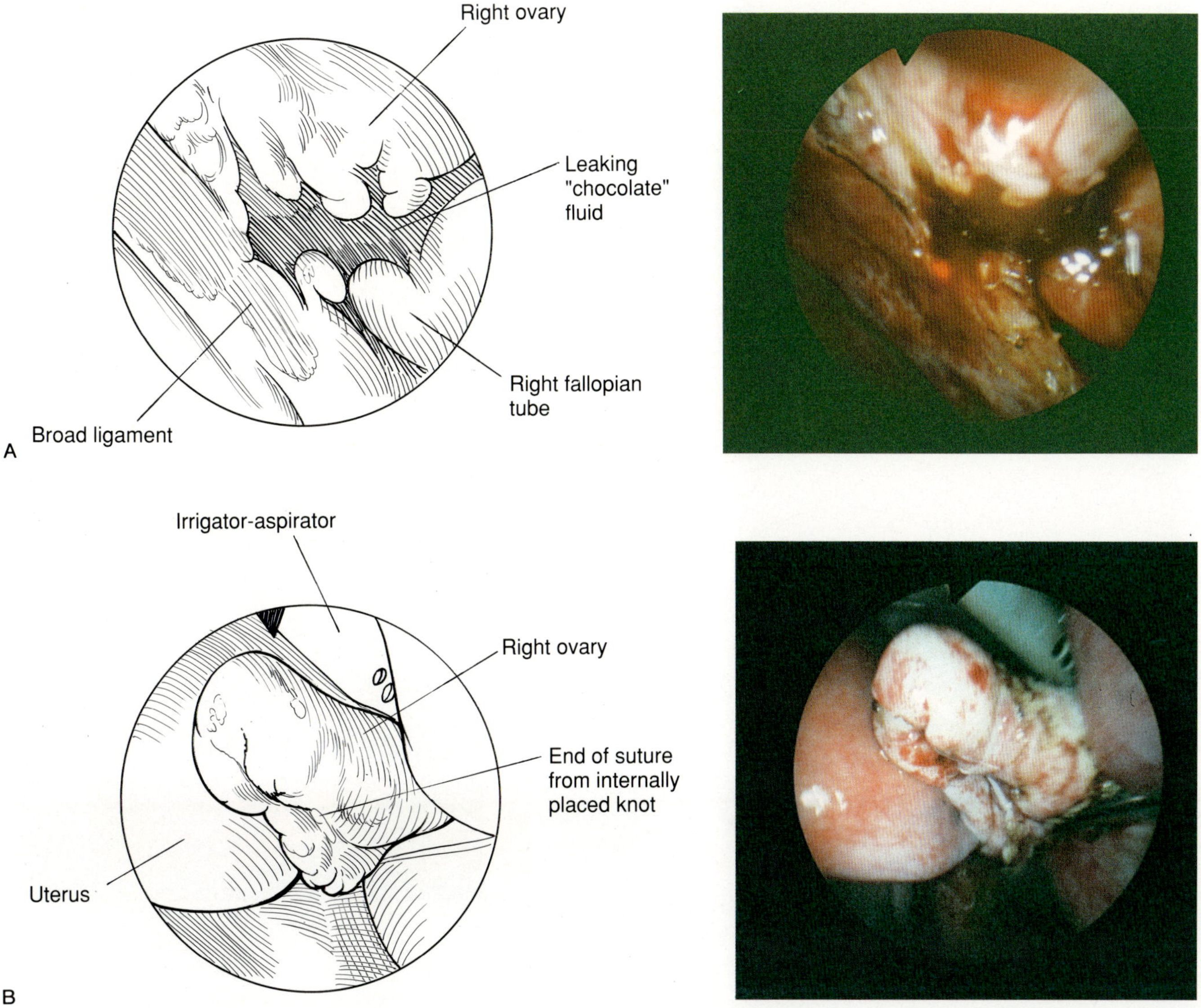

FIG. 23. A: Leaking right ovarian endometrioma. **B:** Suture placed in right ovary following endometrioma resection.

tissue plane (Fig. 24B). Hydrodissection can be helpful in developing tissue planes, especially in larger endometriomas. Blunt dissection can be performed, if possible without creating bleeding, or sharp dissection can be performed.

Traction placed on the cyst wall and ovarian cortex should be gentle to prevent tearing. Copious irrigation and microbipolar coagulation of small bleeding vessels enhances the ease of dissection by improving visualization of the tissue plane. The incision in the cyst wall should be made at the weakest point of the cyst, usually the inferior aspect of the ovary. Dissection should attempt to leave healthy uninjured ovary in apposition to tubal fimbria (Figs. 23B, 24C). The dissection is optimally performed with the cyst in a pouch to ensure that the contents of the cyst cannot leak into the pelvic cavity. After resection, the base of the ovary can be vaporized or coagulated if any small fragments of cyst wall remain. Although some surgeons have recommended suture closure of the ovary, most feel that this is unnecessary (114). Use of sutures is generally associated with greater adhesion formation. Should an ovary be widely opened, one or two deep resorbable sutures may help bring the ovarian edges into closer apposition (Fig. 23B).

For large endometriomas, one possible approach is drainage at laparoscopy followed by 3 months of ovarian suppression with danazol or a GnRH agonist and a second laparoscopy for cyst wall resection when the endometrioma is smaller. This has the obvious disadvantage of requiring medical treatment and a second operation, with the attendant costs, risks, and side effects, as well as several months longer to complete treatment. This ap-

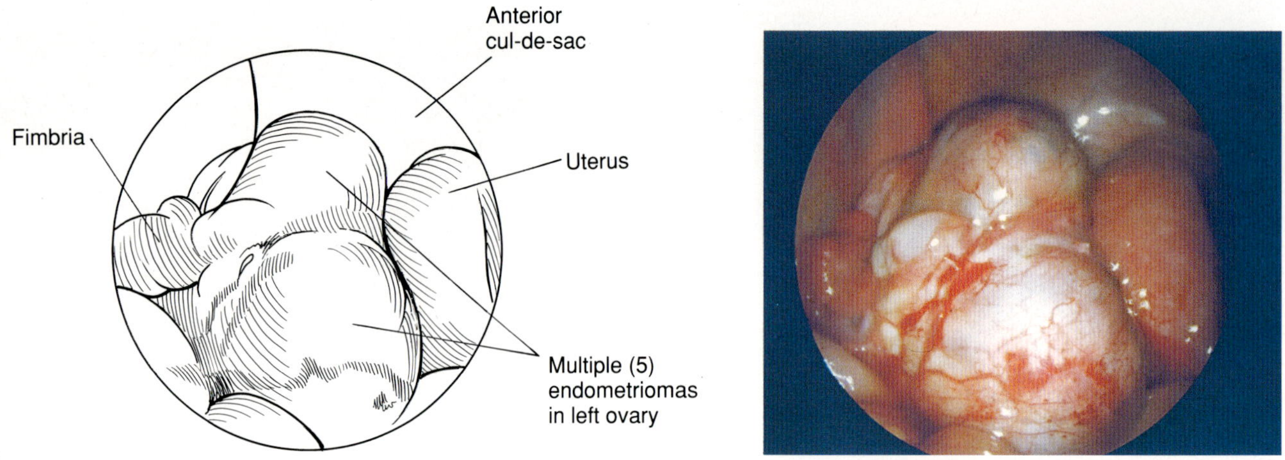

A

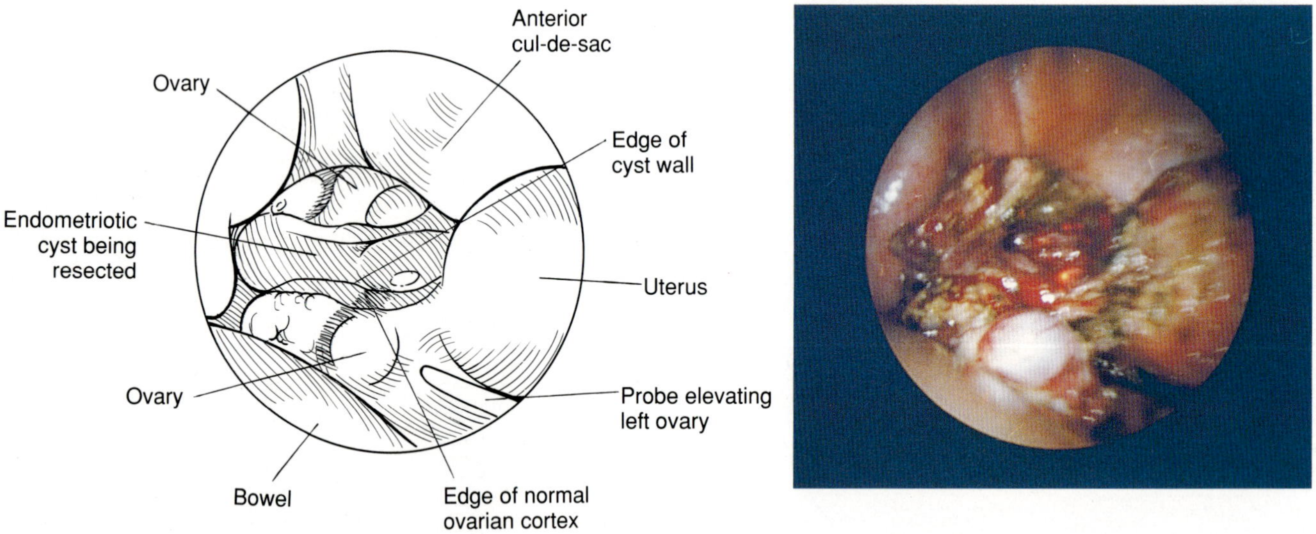

B

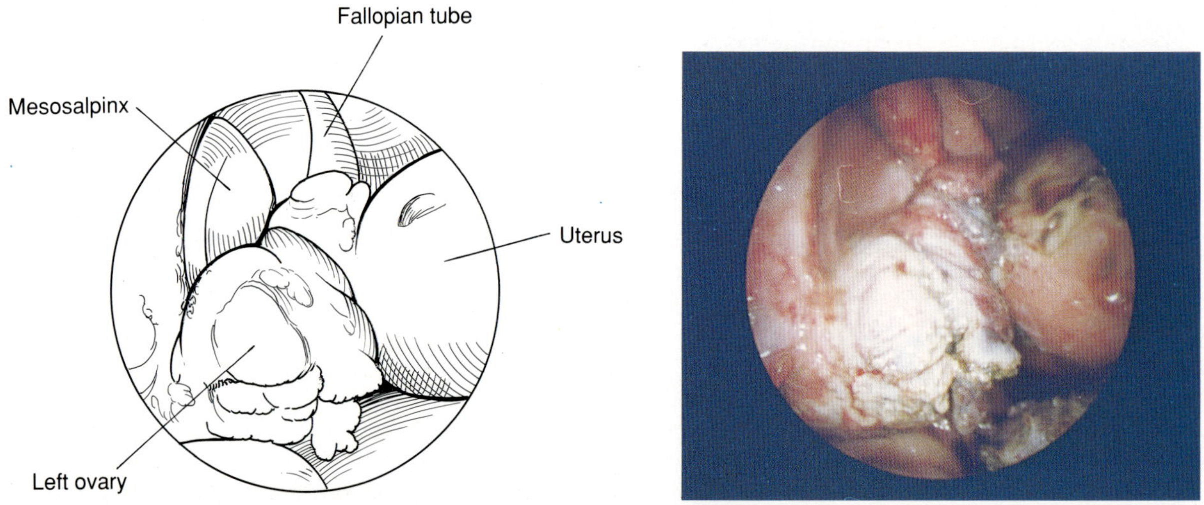

C

FIG. 24. A: Left ovary with five endometriomas. **B:** Left ovarian multiple endometriomectomy in progress. **C:** Completion of multiple endometriomectomy with single suture to appose ovarian edges.

proach may also be unsuccessful (122). Another suggested approach is a combination laparoscopy and minilaparotomy (123).

Results of laparoscopic endometrioma treatment for infertility patients have shown 12 of 23 (52%) pregnant and 26 of 52 (50%) pregnant (114,121). The author's prospective cohort study comparing laparoscopy to laparotomy treatment of endometriomata showed an estimated cumulative percent pregnant at 3 years of 52% for the laparoscopy group and 46% for the laparotomy group (Fig. 25) (112). Pregnancy rates were not affected by the size or number of endometriomata. With respect to pain relief, Reich and McGlynn reported 19 of 31 (61%) patients having pain relief, 9 requiring further extirpative operations, and 3 lost to follow-up (121). Five additional women with hypermenorrhea had relief of symptoms. Ovarian function after conservational surgery appears to be normal (124). Recurrence occurs in less than 10% of resected endometriomas, with de novo adhesion formation in approximately 20% and partial recurrence of dense adhesions in approximately 80% (86,114).

Oophorectomy

Oophorectomy is rarely indicated for treatment of ovarian endometriosis. However, in cases where multiple operations for endometriomas have already been performed, when pain has not responded to prior therapies, when extensive adhesions have persisted despite prior surgeries, or when the ovary is functionally destroyed, either unilateral or bilateral oophorectomy may be indicated. Complete mobilization of the ovary prior to removal is necessary. Several methods can be utilized including coagulation and incision, endoloop sutures, clips, or a laparoscopic stapling device (Fig. 26A,B). Careful identification of the ureter is essential to avoid injury. The ovary can then be morcellated using a morcellator, scissors, or laser, or brought out through a colpotomy or minilaparotomy incision. Small plastic bags to enclose the ovary can prevent spill of cystic fluid and facilitate removal. Ovarian remnants can also be removed. This surgery can be technically demanding because of extensive adhesions and frequent attachment to the ureter. The fallopian tube can easily be included in the extirpated specimen should this be technically easier and clinically appropriate. Other endometriotic disease should be resected at the time of oophorectomy. Postoperative serum follicle-stimulating hormone and/or estradiol levels can establish that bilateral oophorectomy has removed all of the ovarian tissue. This type of surgery must be performed very carefully in order to avoid ovarian remnant syndrome. Fewer than 10% of patients should have ongoing pelvic pain following oophorectomy if patients are appropriately selected (125).

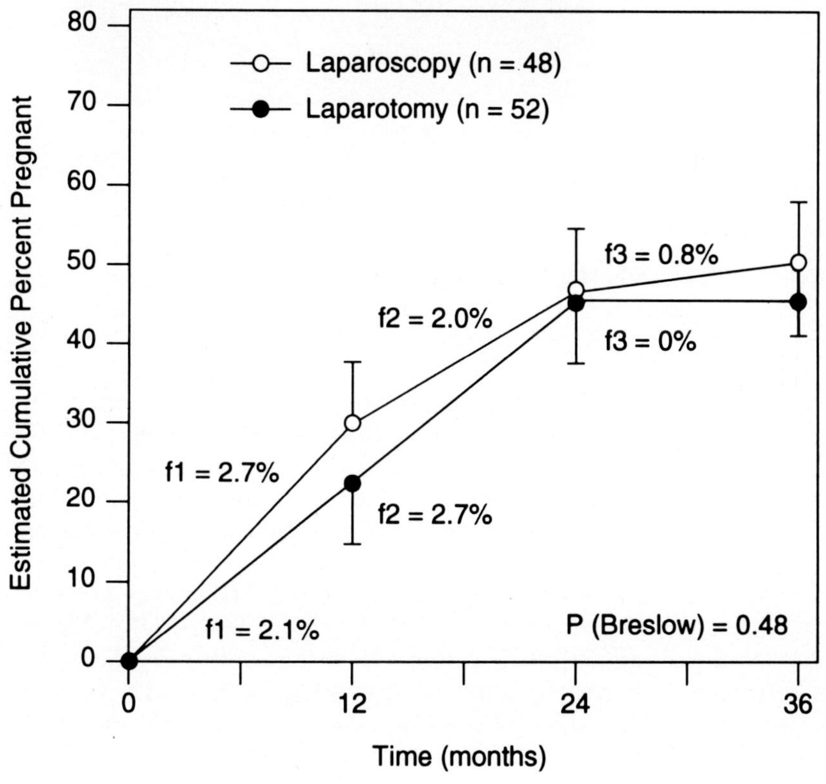

FIG. 25. Life table estimates of cumulative pregnancy rates for CO_2 laser laparoscopy and laparotomy in 12-month intervals after endometrioma resection. Bars indicate standard error, *f* is monthly fecundity for each separate year.

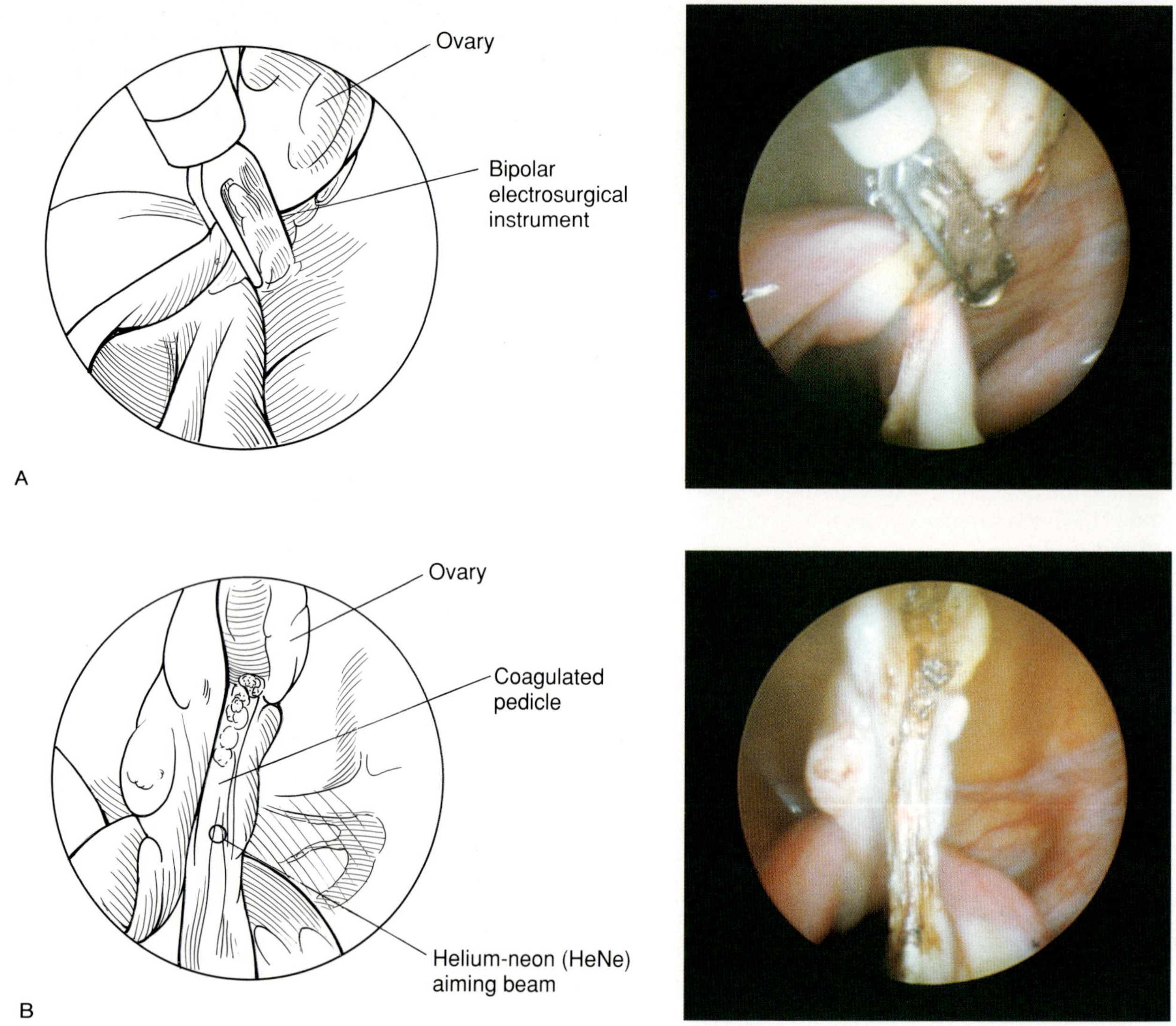

FIG. 26. A: Bipolar coagulation of right ovarian pedicle prior to incision. **B:** Retraction and incision of mesovarium.

Tubal Endometriosis Treatment

Tubal endometriosis is frequently superficial but it can also become deeply invasive. In the proximal tube, this may require resection and reanastomosis at laparotomy. More distally, the tube can become grossly distorted and adherent to the ovary, and occasionally obstructed in the ampulla, or distorted in the fimbrial region to create a distal obstruction. Vaporization using power and pulse settings to minimize thermal injury and to control depth of CO_2 laser beam penetration can provide excellent results (Fig. 27A–C). Other lasers and mechanical or electrosurgical dissection are not as precise or thorough as that which can be achieved with the CO_2 laser. Suturing of the tube is rarely required. Results have not been reported but in the author's experience appear favorable.

Bladder Endometriosis Resection

The uterovesical fold can have deeply invasive endometriosis because of the presence of fibromuscular tissue and its dependent position (91). The bladder itself can also have deep lesions. Resection can be performed following circumscription of the lesion with scissors, laser, or electrosurgery, copious use of hydrodissection, and sharp resection and/or vaporization. The bladder can be filled with indigo carmine through the Foley catheter to check for any defects (Fig. 28A). Partial thickness defects can be closed in a single layer (Fig. 28B). Full-thickness defects can be closed with a standard two-layer closure. Cystoscopy can be performed if necessary. The bladder should be drained with a catheter postoperatively for 7–10 days if full-thickness resection has been performed.

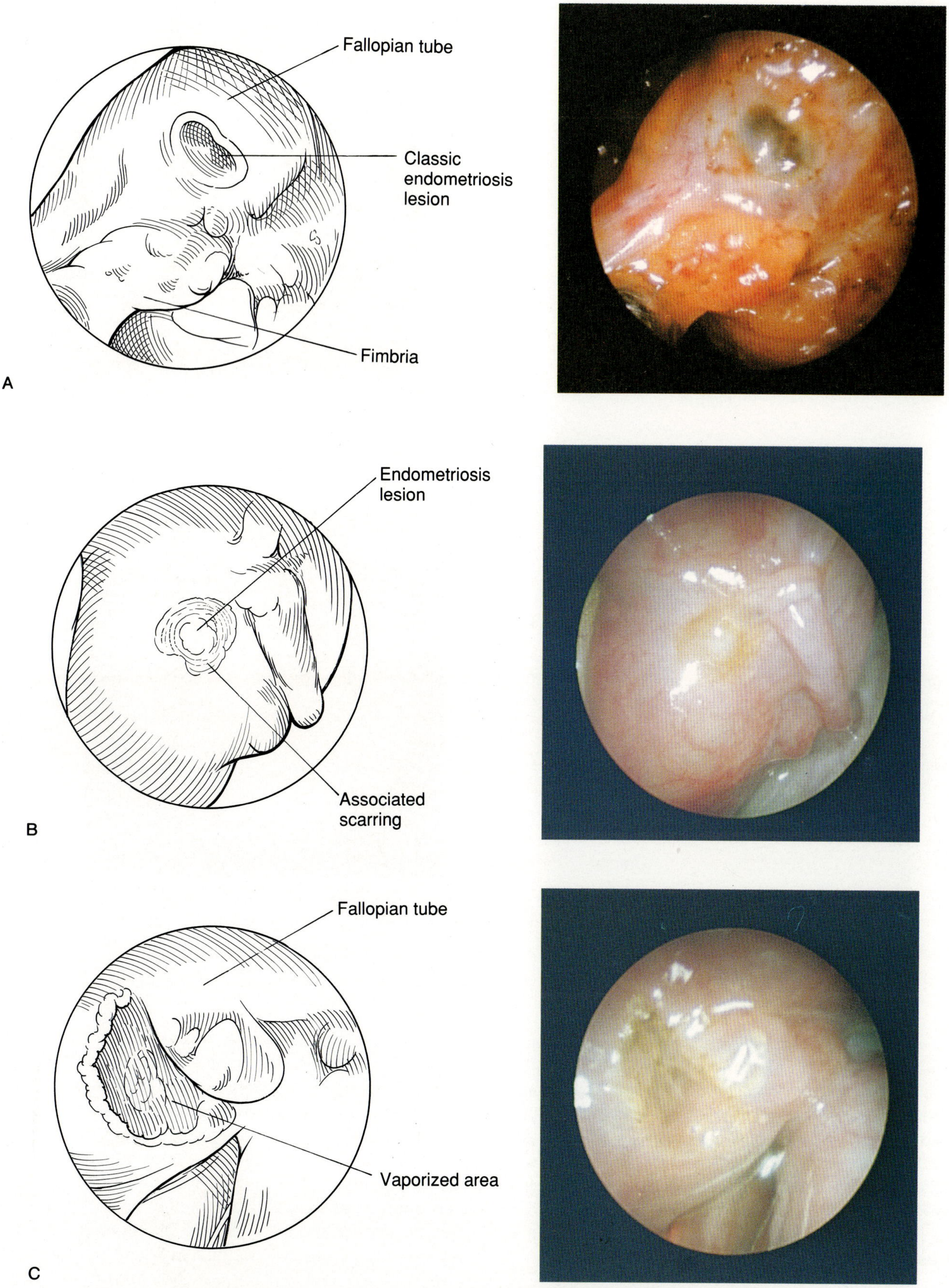

FIG. 27. A: Mildly invasive endometriosis of the distal fallopian tube. **B:** Right distal fallopian tube papule and brownish lesion with associated invasive scarring. **C:** Lesion in Fig. 27B following vaporization.

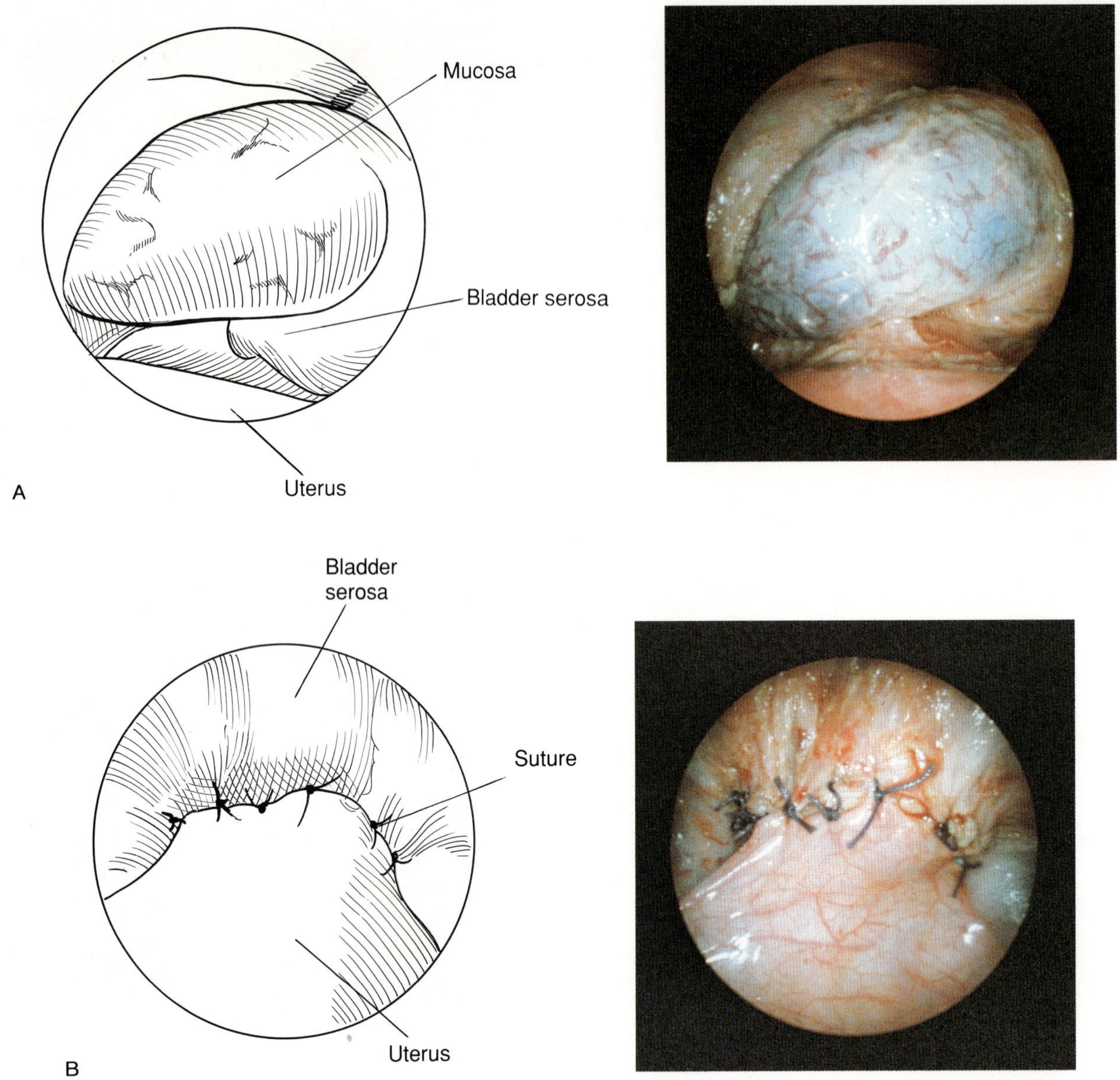

FIG. 28. A: Indigo carmine showing through mucosa of bladder following resection of anterior cul-de-sac endometriosis invading completely through the bladder muscularis layer. **B:** Repair of bladder muscularis with single layer of interrupted sutures.

Care must be taken when dissecting deep lesions laterally not to injure vessels or the ureter. The bladder can be checked postoperatively with an intravenous pyelogram and/or cystoscopy to ensure that appropriate healing has occurred. Successful partial cystectomy has been reported with subsequent pregnancy (126). Endometriotic bladder lesions must be differentiated from endocervicosis of the bladder (127).

Ureteral Endometriosis Resection

Endometriosis is frequently found near the ureter and often causes distortion of its course through the pelvis. However, even when endometriosis invasion is extensive and severe, rarely does it actually cause loss of function through kinking or obstruction (128,129). In these cases a surgical approach is warranted. Diagnosis is facilitated by preoperative intravenous pyelogram and/or cystoureteroscopy. Intraoperative intraureteral catheters are preferred by only a few surgeons. Careful dissection using appropriate power setting and energy sources will often free up a ureter and allow normal functioning. Ureterolysis should be initiated in an area where normal anatomy is clearly visible. This is usually around the pelvic brim or just superior to the uterosacral ligament. The CO_2 laser's precision is particularly useful for this type of

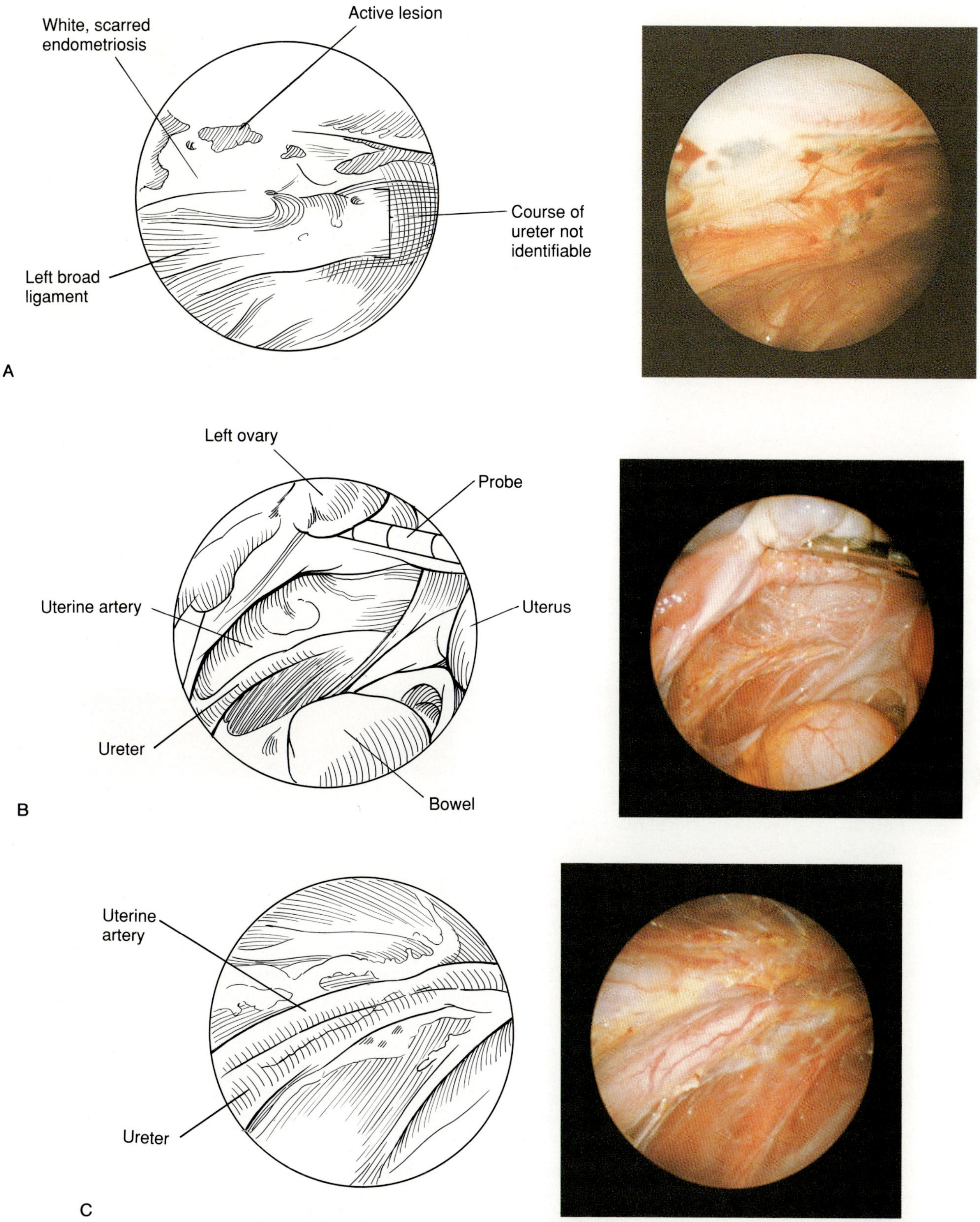

FIG. 29. **A:** Left broad ligament endometriosis overlying ureter. **B:** Complete vaporization and resection of broad ligament endometriosis reveals course of ureter and uterine artery. **C:** Close-up view with magnification of ureter and uterine artery demonstrating precision and clean dissection following CO_2 laser vaporization of invasive endometriosis.

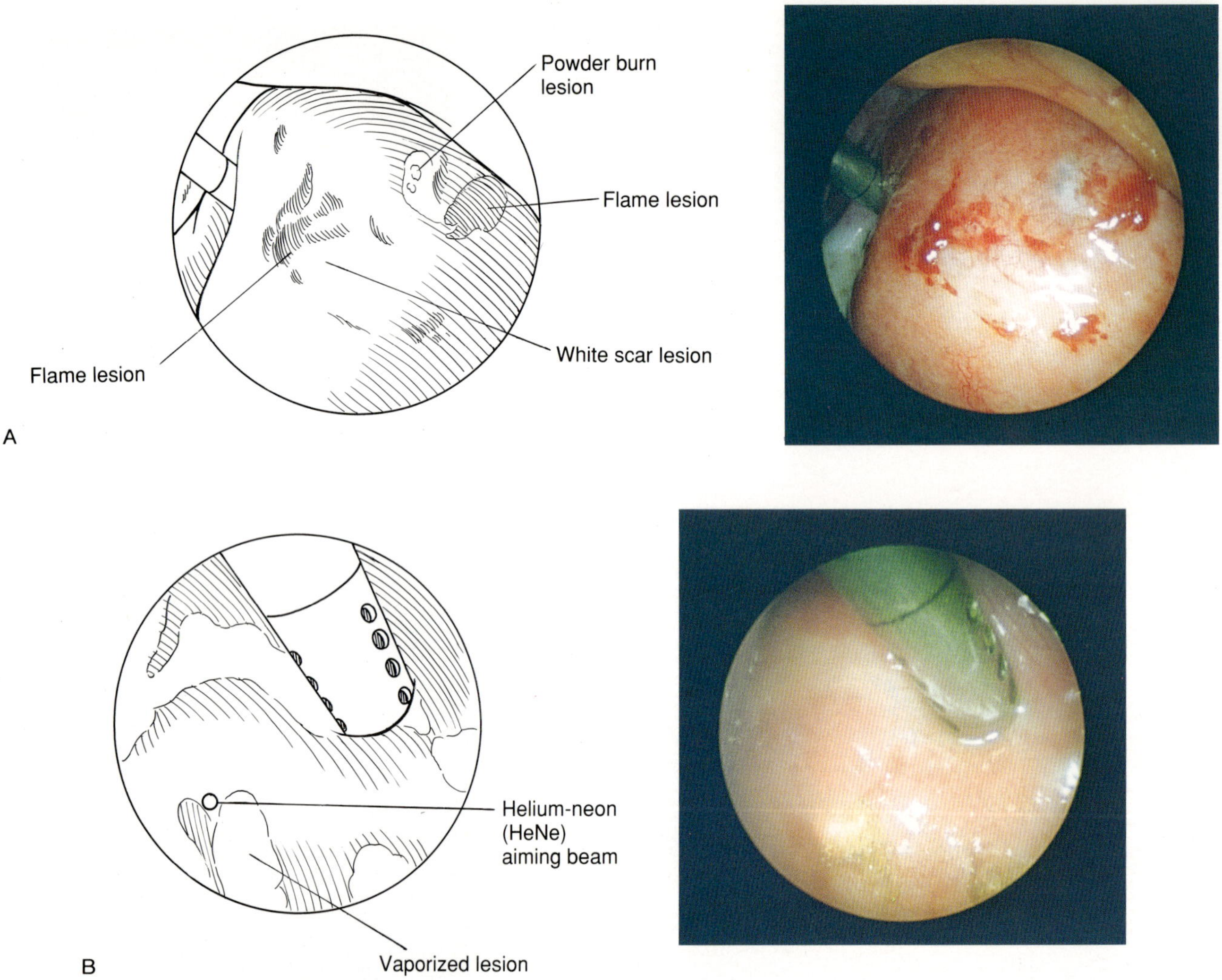

FIG. 30. **A:** Uterine fundus with multiple morphologically variable lesions. **B:** Uterine fundus following vaporization of endometriosis lesions.

dissection and vaporization using short pulses of laser energy (Fig. 29A–C). Complications of ureteral endometriosis resection include pelvic leakage of urine and fistula formation (130). Indigo carmine (10 cm^3) should be injected intravenously and the urinary catheter bag observed for blue dye after approximately 5–10 min. The ureter should then be carefully evaluated for evidence of perforation by examination under clear irrigating fluid in the cul-de-sac. If complete obstruction exists or a large injury has occurred to the ureter, resection of the diseased tissue and ureteral reanastomosis has been reported at laparoscopy (131). However, urologic consultation in such cases would seem to be mandatory for most gynecologists.

Uterine Endometriosis Treatment

The uterus infrequently has endometriosis attached to it except at the uterovesical fold and between the uterosacral ligaments at the posterior aspect of the cervix when posterior cul-de-sac obliteration occurs (Fig. 30A,B). Identification of the fibrotic endometriosis lesion from the normal cervical tissue both anteriorly and posteriorly can be difficult. Normal tissue is more pliable, less white in color, and more vascular. Bipolar electrosurgery can be used to coagulate the small vessels, which bleed when normal tissue is resected or vaporized. Hemostasis is more difficult when uterine endometriosis is treated. The usual principles of complete circumscription of the lesion preceding resection or vaporization should be followed.

Laser Uterosacral Nerve Ablation (LUNA)

LUNA is an operation that developed from Doyle's procedure to destroy the sensory fibers to the cervix and lower uterine segment (132). The indication for this procedure is midline pelvic pain, and it is frequently considered for patients with endometriosis and pain (133) (see the chapter by Feste, "Laser Uterosacral Nerve Ablation"). Care needs to be taken to identify and avoid the ureter, which is usually 1–2 cm lateral although possibly closer if cul-de-sac distortion is present. Blood vessels are just lateral to the uterosacral ligament and bowel medially. The uterosacral ligament may be resected in the course of resecting endometriosis involving the ligament. Traction placed on the uterus helps to define the ligaments. The lesion should then be circumscribed before resection because the anatomy changes as the ligament is resected.

Presacral Neurectomy

Presacral neurectomy has been a controversial procedure for many years but is frequently considered for women with endometriosis (133). Reported results have varied (46,133,134). This may be due to inappropriate and/or variable patient selection and/or incomplete resection of the nerve plexus. Presacral neurectomy is only indicated for severe midline dysmenorrhea (134) (see the chapter by Feste and Wilson, "Presacral Neurectomy").

Uterine Suspension

Uterine suspension is a controversial procedure used as treatment for deep dyspareunia, chronic pelvic pain, and to elevate the uterus away from extensively resected areas postsurgically. Suspension can be performed by plicating the uterosacral ligaments, or the round ligaments, or by elevating the round ligaments or uterus to the anterior abdominal wall. No well-controlled studies support the efficacy of this procedure and reported results vary widely (135). Postoperative discomfort may result, and care needs to be taken not to create pockets into which small bowel could pass and result in bowel obstruction. In addition, the effect of suspension is almost invariably temporary. The role of this procedure in laparoscopic treatment of endometriosis is unclear at this time.

Laparoscopy-Assisted Vaginal Hysterectomy

Laparoscopy-assisted vaginal hysterectomy (LAVH) was recently reported as a superior method of performing vaginal hysterectomy when significant pelvic pathology, such as endometriosis, requires diagnosis and treatment, or when oophorectomy is desired but adnexal masses or adhesions hinder or prevent that procedure at vaginal hysterectomy (136–138). LAVH has become controversial because it appears to have been used inappropriately by some surgeons. In addition, this procedure can be technically demanding and complications occur easily with inexperienced laparoscopists. The usual surgical approaches for laparoscopy and hysterectomy surgery need to be followed during performance of LAVH. The major benefit of LAVH is its capability of converting an abdominal hysterectomy into a vaginal hysterectomy. Although the vast majority of patients with endometriosis and pelvic pain obtain pain relief following hysterectomy, some patients will not (139,140). All patients need careful preoperative counseling regarding the efficacy of hysterectomy and/or oophorectomy and issues involved with hormonal replacement therapy (see the chapter by Reich, "Hysterectomy").

Adhesiolysis

Endometriosis is frequently associated with significant pelvic adhesions. Such adhesions can distort fimbrial–ovarian relationships, thereby reducing fertility (70, 141). Adhesions can also distort normal anatomic relationships causing organ dysfunction and sometimes pain. Principles of adhesiolysis include operating in the midproliferative phase, good exposure, gentle tissue handling, removal of only adhesions causing dysfunction, copious irrigation, removal of ischemic tissue, nonuse of sutures, fluid flotation, and early postoperative ambulation. During lysis, hydrodissection and gentle traction can help to identify tissue planes and facilitate dissection. Tissue should be touched only when necessary and then moved with a probe rather than grasped. If grasped, tissue that is being removed should be held rather than tissue being left, and the least traumatic instruments possible should be used. Power settings on energy sources should be set at appropriate levels so as to minimize contiguous thermal damage. Laser beams should be backstopped as necessary with titanium rods or irrigation fluid.

Hemorrhage can facilitate adhesion formation when the fibrin clot provides a matrix for invasion by fibroblasts. Use of magnification and bipolar electrosurgery can reduce oozing, as can avoidance of aspirin and NSAIDs for several weeks before surgery. It is also important to control bleeding quickly at laparoscopy because bleeding that would ordinarily be insignificant at laparotomy can quickly obscure the surgeon's view, resulting potentially in the need for laparotomy or transfusion. Hemostasis can also be improved by coagulating or isolating a vessel before cutting it. Hemostasis may be facilitated by use of the CO_2 laser as well as fiber lasers. The microbipolar and large bipolar forceps should also be available at all times. The maintenance of hemostasis

TABLE 6. *Potential benefits of preoperative GnRH agonists on adhesion formation following operative endoscopy*

Causes of adhesion formation	Potential benefits of GnRH agonists
Tissue trauma	Smaller incisions
	Fewer incisions
	Decreased tissue dissection
	Decreased bleeding in tissue
	Hysterectomy less likely with myomectomy
	Laparoscopic/hysteroscopic approach more likely
	Avoidance of uterine cavity at laparotomy for myomectomy
	Shorter operating time with smaller myomas
Infection	Endoscopic or vaginal approach more likely
	Decreased tissue dissection
	Shorter operating time with smaller myomas
Ischemia	Decreased sutures with smaller myomas
	Decreased need for coagulation
	Decreased tissue dissection
	Decreased operative blood loss
	Availability of autologous donation
Denuded surface apposition	Decreased tissue dissection
	Better visualization, decreased tissue manipulation
	Fewer incisions
	Smaller incisions
	Hysteroscopic approach
Foreign body	Decreased need for sutures
	Laparoscopic/hysteroscopic approach
	Decreased operative blood loss
Hemorrhage	Decreased dissection
	Decreased bleeding
	Reduced operating time
	Better visualization
	Laparoscopic/hysteroscopic approach

increases the surgeon's ability to perform the surgery without using clips, staples, sutures, or Roeder loops, which are foreign bodies that can increase adhesion formation. It is possible that the multiple end-organ effects caused by the hypoestrogenism associated with GnRH agonist use may result in an improved pelvic milieu and fewer postoperative adhesions (Table 6).

Many adjunctive therapies to prevent adhesion reformation have been used. These include dextran, fibrinolytic and anticoagulant regimens, and antiinflammatory agents, progesterone, NSAIDs, antihistamines, and barrier methods. The principle of barriers is that they prevent direct apposition of tissue surfaces, which therefore cannot become fused together by fibrin. Currently two barriers are being extensively studied: oxidized regenerated cellulose (Interceed Tc-7, Ethicon, Somerville, NJ) and expanded polytetrafluoroethylene (PTFE, Gore-Tex, W. L. Gore and Associates, Flagstaff, AZ). Both have shown promise in some studies but the optimal clinical role of these barriers is still to be determined (142).

Operative laparoscopy reduces adhesions but reformation has been shown to occur at 66% of sites at which adhesions were originally lysed (81). However, laparoscopic treatment of tubal adhesions has been shown to be associated with increased pregnancy rates in endometriosis patients (70). Second-look laparoscopy enables evaluation of results and lysis of any reformed adhesions, with the expectation that on average only half will recur (85). It is not known as to whether patients undergoing laparoscopic adhesiolysis for endometriosis have similar results. Clinical studies and basic science data show no consistent superiority of laser surgery over conventional adhesiolysis either with respect to relief of pain, pregnancy rates, or subsequent adhesion reformation. However, some reconstructive surgeons feel that lasers, and especially the newer ultrapulse lasers, provide increased capabilities to the surgeon to perform extensive pelvic adhesiolysis with minimal damage to normal tissues (see the chapter by Shamma and Diamond, "Postoperative Adhesion Development After Operative Laparoscopy: Evaluation After Early Second-Look Procedure").

RECURRENCE OF ENDOMETRIOSIS

Recurrence rates of endometriosis are likely related to initial stage of the disease, adequacy of initial documen-

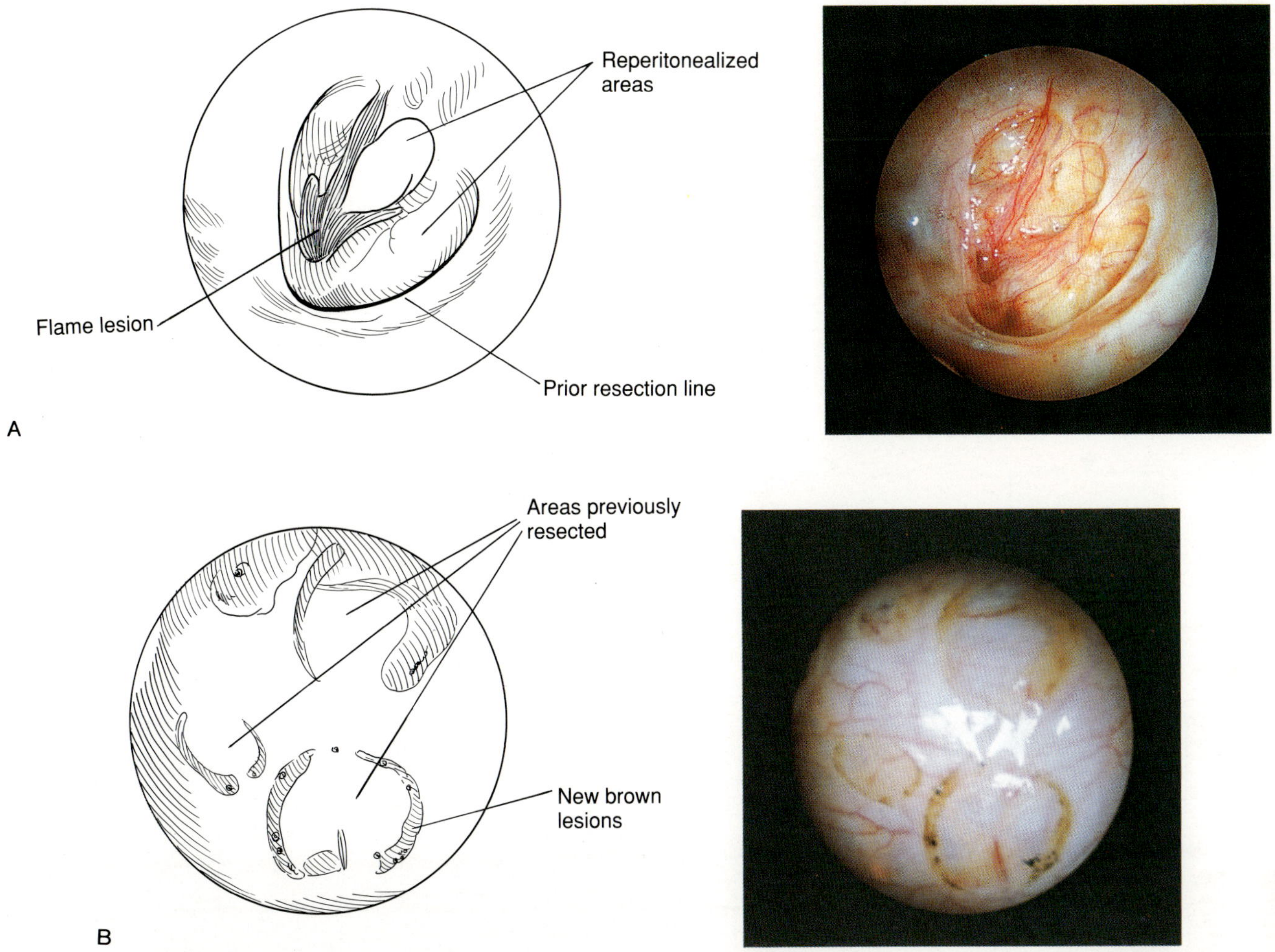

FIG. 31. A: Recurrence of flame lesions endometriosis on reperitonealized area previously completely resected. **B:** Recurrence of superficial brownish staining on reperitonealized area previously completely resected.

tation of disease, adequacy of treatment, occurrence of pregnancy postoperatively, use of concomitant hormonal treatments, risk factors for endometriosis, and adequacy of follow-up. Approximate recurrence rate following medical treatment is 30% (143,144). Most studies do not have sufficiently detailed findings and data to differentiate between the amount of initial and subsequent disease, persistence of lesions or appearance of new ones, and the sequelae of endometriosis, such as pain and infertility, compared with initial symptoms of the disease. The absence of correlation between symptoms and findings further complicates the issue (145,146). More recent data suggest that approximately 20% of patients have recurrence over 5 years following complete extirpation of the disease (61,147). Superficial disease may occur earlier even in areas where complete extirpation of endometriosis was performed (Fig. 31A,B).

CONCOMITANT TREATMENT MODALITIES

Laparoscopic treatment of endometriosis appears to be at least equivalent to or superior to no treatment, medical treatment, or laparotomy (Table 1, Fig. 4) (70, 148–150).

Laparoscopic treatment of endometriosis may sometimes be combined with medical therapy involving danazol or GnRH agonists. The purpose of combined treatment is to improve treatment success or facilitate surgical procedures (Table 6). Preoperative medical treatment suppresses ovulation so that functional cysts will not be present or confused with endometriosis. Potential advantages include a reduced volume of endometriotic tissue, the destruction of which may be effected in a shortened operating time. The reduced volume of tissue may also result in less risk of injury to ureters, blood vessels, and bowel. Metastatic or extensive superficial

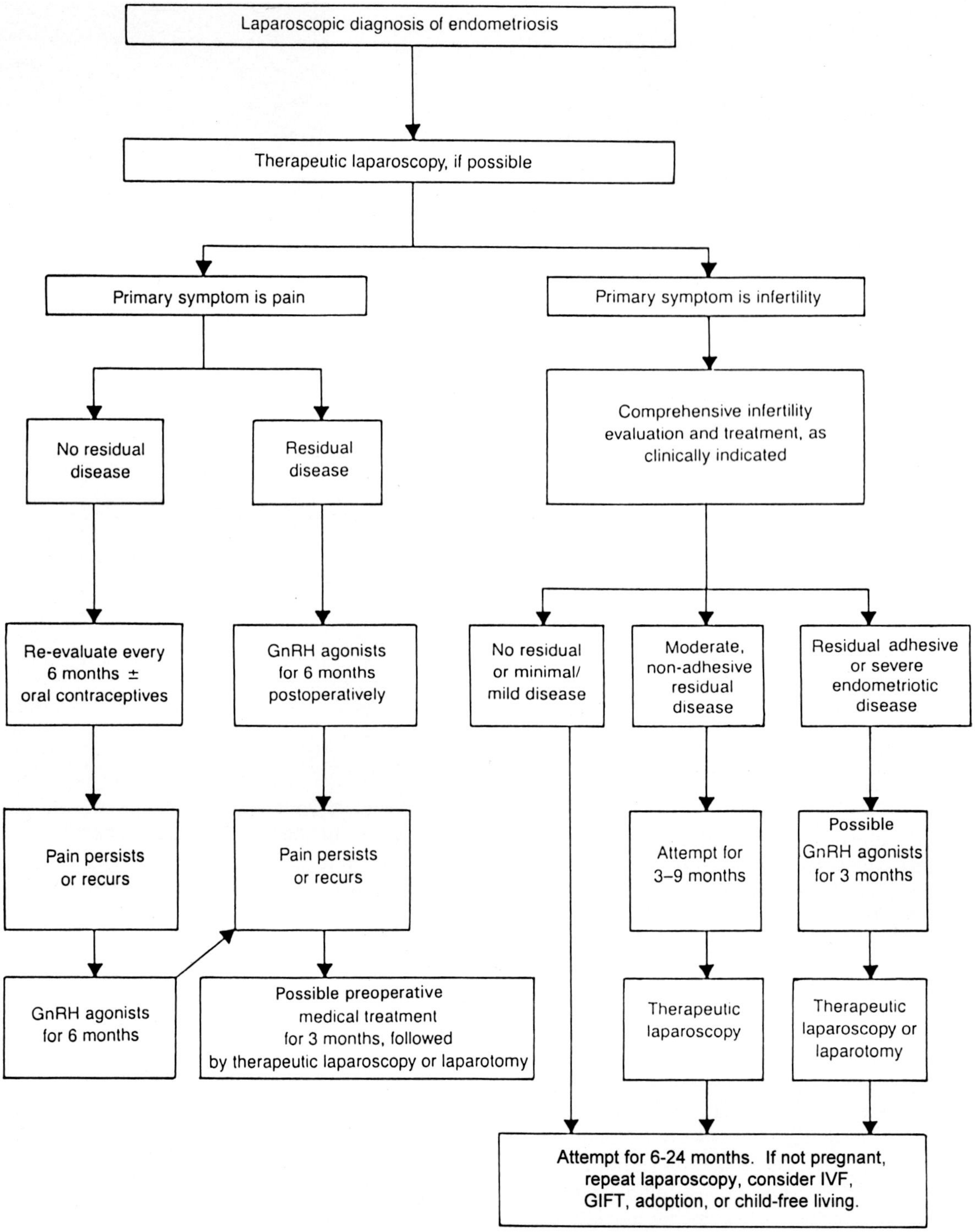

FIG. 32. Postlaparoscopy management of endometriosis.

disease will be treated. The reduced vascularity in the pelvis may result in reduced inflammation and postoperative adhesions, although this has not been proven. There may be a slight reduction in endometrioma size. Adenomyosis will be reduced and filmy adhesions may become lysed. Other uses of GnRH agonists prior to surgery include reduction of symptoms, increased time for adequate preoperative evaluation, easier scheduling of surgery, and even delay or avoidance of surgery for a woman nearing menopause. Potential disadvantages of preoperative medical treatment include the changed appearance of endometriosis, which might make it more difficult to diagnose; drug cost and side effects; delay of diagnosis; and delay in attempting pregnancy (151). Postoperative medical treatment may be indicated if complete resection of disease has not been accomplished for treatment of microscopic or metastatic disease, or for treatment of pain.

Pregnancy rates with laparoscopy alone appear to be equal to or higher than those of medical therapy alone (Fig. 4) (64,70,87,141). Therefore, because of the additional financial and time cost, preoperative medical therapy should probably be reserved for patients with severe symptomatology, to facilitate surgery scheduling when necessary, or for patients with known severe disease where medical treatment may allow for a better pelvic milieu for reconstructive surgery. It is unknown as to what, if any, effect preoperative medical treatment has on subsequent pregnancy rates. Postoperative medical treatment may be indicated for patients with severe refractory pelvic pain or in whom disease has not been completely extirpated but should be avoided whenever possible in infertility patients because of the inability to conceive while taking the medication. Postoperative medical treatment does not improve pregnancy rates (Fig. 4) (70,71). Overall, the available data do not support the routine perioperative use of GnRH agonists or other hormonal therapies, but these may be of value in selected patients (152).

POSTLAPAROSCOPY PATIENT MANAGEMENT

Management plans should be based on surgical results, prognosis, and the patient's desires (Fig. 32) (60, 153–155). Other infertility factors such as ovulation, male, and cervical factor should be treated as clinically indicated. Hysterosalpingogram may be performed 3–12 months postoperatively for diagnostic and possibly therapeutic purposes in selected patients. Controlled ovarian hyperstimulation may be used to increase pregnancy rates (156). A repeat laparoscopy should be performed 9–24 months postoperatively if the patient has not conceived and if the overall clinical situation and prognosis justifies a repeat operation. If the patient had a limited prognosis following the initial surgery or has additional important fertility problems, then IVF, GIFT, adoption, or child-free living should be seriously considered as alternative approaches (60,96,157).

Patients with chronic pelvic pain frequently need adjunctive therapy. This may be symptomatic, such as analgesics or NSAIDs; hormonal, such as GnRH agonists, progestins, or oral contraceptives; changes in activities of daily living, such as diet and exercise; and/or referral to a pain clinic for comprehensive diagnosis and treatment including nerve blocks, analgesic cocktails, biofeedback, and psychological support (158). This comprehensive approach to the patient's pain should be explained to her prior to surgery and reinforced postoperatively.

Endometriosis patients with infertility and/or pain may find helpful educational materials and support from the Endometriosis Association in Milwaukee, Wisconsin and/or Resolve in Boston, Massachusetts.

CRITIQUE

Even those who are critical of the role of laparoscopy in the treatment of endometriosis and feel that "there is insufficient evidence to recommend laparoscopy over laparotomy for correction of infertility resulting from tubal injury or endometriosis" have stated that "there was suggestive, but not yet proven, evidence that laparoscopic surgery with laser techniques may be superior to laparotomy in the management of infertility resulting from moderate and severe endometriosis" (83). The author of this chapter also did not consider economic or postsurgical recovery factors in reaching his conclusions and felt that there were no good studies available to determine the relative merits of laparoscopy or laparotomy for the treatment of pain. Data subsequent to those available for Gant's 1992 paper strongly support the major role of laparoscopic surgery in the treatment of endometriosis.

HIGHLIGHTS

Laparoscopic treatment of endometriosis has become a surgical possibility because of pioneering gynecologic surgeons and technological developments. Laparoscopic management can produce pregnancy rates equivalent or superior to laparotomy and other treatment modalities (Table 1, Fig. 4) (42,70,95,112,141,159,160).

Numerous studies suggest some improvement in pelvic pain following certain surgical procedures for advanced endometriosis and some good studies support the potential role of laparoscopy in performing such surgeries. Complication rates with laparoscopy appear to be equivalent to or lower than at laparotomy, although strict comparative data are not available (83,161).

Overall it is clear that operative laparoscopy for treatment of endometriosis is appropriate in many clinical situations. However, these procedures can be complex, and it is mandatory that patient selection be based on sound clinical indications and performed by experienced laparoscopists who have their patient's best interest as their only criteria for operating. Further technological improvements, more experience, better designed studies, and responsible discussion of results will enable laparoscopic surgeons to provide even better care for their patients with endometriosis.

REFERENCES

1. Johns DA. Reusable instruments for operative laparoscopy. *Infertil Clin North Am* 1993;4(2):233–238.
2. Cowart CL, London SN. Extrapelvic endometriosis. *Infertil Reprod Med Clin North Am* 1992;3(3):731–746.
3. Mitchell GW. Extrapelvic endometriosis. In: Schenken RS, ed. *Endometriosis: contemporary concepts in clinical management.* Philadelphia: JB Lippincott; 1989:307–328.
4. Schenken RS. Pathogenesis. In: Schenken RS, ed. *Endometriosis: contemporary concepts in clinical management.* Philadelphia: JB Lippincott; 1989:1–48.
5. Koger KE, Shatney CH, Hodge K, McClenathan JH. Surgical scar endometrioma. *Surg Gynecol Obstet* 1993;177(3):243–246.
6. Carta F, Guiducci G, Fulcheri E, Bernucci C, Rivano C. Radicular compression by extradural spinal endometriosis. Case report. *Acta Neurochirurgica* 1992;114(1–2):68–71.
7. Markham SM. Extrapelvic endometriosis. In: Thomas E, Rock J, eds. *Modern approaches to endometriosis.* Boston: Kluwer Academic; 1991:151–182.
8. Wheeler JM. Epidemiology and prevalence of endometriosis. *Infertil Reprod Med Clin North Am* 1992;3(3):545–549.
9. Hasson HM. Incidence of endometriosis in diagnostic laparoscopy. *J Reprod Med* 1976;16:135.
10. Strathy JH, Molgaard CA, Coulam CB. Endometriosis and infertility: a laparoscopic study of endometriosis among fertile and infertile women. *Fertil Steril* 1982;38:667.
11. Norwood GE. Sterility and fertility in women with pelvic endometriosis. *Clin Obstet Gynecol* 1960;3:456.
12. Dmowski WP. Current concepts in the management of endometriosis. *Obstet Gynecol Annu* 1981;10:279.
13. Hurd SJ, Adamson GD. Pelvic pain: endometriosis as a differential diagnosis in adolescents. *Adol Pediatr Gynecol* 1992;5:3–7.
14. Pittaway DE. Diagnosis of endometriosis. *Infertil Reprod Med Clin North Am* 1992;3(3):619–631.
15. Vercellini P, Fedele L, Bianchi S, Candiani GB. Pelvic denervation for chronic pelvic pain associated with endometriosis: fact or fancy? *Am J Obstet Gynecol* 1991;165(3):745–749.
16. Acosta A, Buttram VC, Besch PK, Malinak LR, Franklin RR, Vanderheyen JP. A proposed classification of pelvic endometriosis. *Obstet Gynecol* 1973;12:49.
17. Martin DC, Hubert GD, Vander Zwaag R, el-Zeky FA. Laparoscopic appearance of peritoneal endometriosis. *Fertil Steril* 1989;51(1):63–67.
18. Vercellini P, Crosignani PG. Minimal and mild endometriosis. Is there anything new under the sun? *J Reprod Med* 1993;38(1):49–52.
19. Haney AF. The pathogenesis and aetiology of endometriosis. In: Thomas E, Rock J, eds. *Modern approaches to endometriosis.* Boston: Kluwer Academic; 1991:3–19.
20. Schenken RS. Pathogenesis of endometriosis. *Infertil Reprod Med Clin North Am* 1992;3(3):531–544.
21. Burns WN, Schenken RS. Pathophysiology. In: Schenken RS, ed. *Endometriosis: contemporary concepts in clinical management.* Philadelphia: JB Lippincott; 1989:83–126.
22. Corson SL. *Endometriosis, the enigmatic disease.* Durant, OK, Essential Medical Information Systems, Inc., 1992;103.
23. Koninckx PR, Martin D. Treatment of deeply infiltrating endometriosis. *Curr Opin Obstet Gynecol* 1994;6(3):231–241.
24. Dmowski WP, Cohen MR. Antigonadotropin (danazol) in the treatment of endometriosis. Evaluation of post-treatment fertility and three year follow-up data. *Am J Obstet Gynecol* 1978;41:130.
25. Davis GD, Thillet E, Lindemann J. Clinical characteristics of adolescent endometriosis. *J Adol Health* 1993;14(5):362–368.
26. Howard FM. The role of laparoscopy in chronic pelvic pain: promise and pitfalls. *Obstet Gynecol Surv* 1993;48(6):357–387.
27. Koninckx PR, Martin DC. Deep endometriosis: a consequence of infiltration or retraction or possibly adenomyosis externa? *Fertil Steril* 1992;58(5):924–928.
28. Inoue M, Kobayashi Y, Honda I, Awaji H, Fujii A. The impact of endometriosis on the reproductive outcome of infertile patients. *Am J Obstet Gynecol* 1992;167(1):278–282.
29. Toma SK, Stovall DW, Hammond MG. The effect of laparoscopic ablation or danocrine on pregnancy rates in patients with stage I or II endometriosis undergoing donor insemination. *Obstet Gynecol* 1992;80(2):253–256.
30. Hirata J, Kikuchi Y, Imaizumi E, Tode T, Nagata I. Endometriotic tissues produce immunosuppressive factors. *Gynecol Obstet Invest* 1994;37(1):43–47.
31. Bowman MC, Cooke ID, Lenton EA. Investigation of impaired ovarian function as a contributing factor to infertility in women with pelvic adhesions. *Human Reprod* 1993;8(10):1654–1656.
32. Bowman MC, Cooke ID. Comparison of fallopian tube intraluminal pathology as assessed by salpingoscopy with pelvic adhesions. *Fertil Steril* 1994;61(3):464–469.
33. Brosens IA. The endometriotic implant. In: Thomas E, Rock J, eds. *Modern approaches to endometriosis.* Boston: Kluwer Academic; 1991:21–31.
34. Ramzy I. Pathology. In: Schenken RS, ed. *Endometriosis: contemporary concepts in clinical management.* Philadelphia: JB Lippincott; 1989:49–82.
35. Pauerstein CJ. Clinical presentation and diagnosis. In: Schenken RS, ed. *Endometriosis contemporary concepts in clinical management.* Philadelphia: JB Lippincott; 1989:127–44.
36. Redwine DB. Age-related evolution in colour appearance of endometriosis. *Fertil Steril* 1987;48(6):1062–1063.
37. Redwine DB. The distribution of endometriosis in the pelvis by age groups and fertility. *Fertil Steril* 1987;47(1):173–175.
38. Jansen RP, Russell P. Non-pigmented endometriosis: clinical, laparoscopic, and pathologic definition. *Am J Obstet Gynecol* 1986;155(6):1154–1159.
39. American Fertility Society. Classification of endometriosis. *Fertil Steril* 1985;43:351.
40. Adamson GD, Frison L, Lamb EJ. Endometriosis: studies of a method for design of a surgical staging system. *Fertil Steril* 1982;38(6):659–666.
41. Fedele L, Parazzini F, Bianchi S, Arcaini L, Candiani GB. Stage and localization of pelvic endometriosis and pain. *Fertil Steril* 1990;53(1):155–158.
42. Nezhat C, Crowgey S, Nezhat F. Videolaseroscopy for the treatment of endometriosis associated with infertility. *Fertil Steril* 1989;51(2):237–240.
43. Sutton CJG. Laser laparoscopy of the treatment of endometriosis. In: Thomas E, Rock J, eds. *Modern approaches to endometriosis.* Boston: Kluwer Academic; 1991:199–219.
44. Groff TR. Classifications. In: Schenken RS, ed. *Endometriosis: contemporary concepts in clinical management.* Philadelphia: JB Lippincott; 1989:145–168.
45. Ripps BA, Martin DC. Correlation of focal pelvic tenderness with implant dimension and stage of endometriosis. *J Reprod Med* 1992;37(7):620–624.
46. Ripps BA, Martin DC. Focal pelvic tenderness, pelvic pain, and dysmenorrhea in endometriosis. *J Reprod Med* 1991;36(7):470–472.
47. Mais V, Guerriero S, Ajossa S, Angiolucci M, Paoletti AM, Melis GB. The efficiency of transvaginal ultrasonography in the diagnosis of endometrioma. *Fertil Steril* 1993;60(5):776–780.

48. Kurjak A, Kupesic S. Scoring system for prediction of ovarian endometriosis based on transvaginal color and pulsed Doppler sonography. *Fertil Steril* 1994;62(1):81–88.
49. Siegelman ES, Outwater E, Wang T, Mitchell DG. Solid pelvic masses caused by endometriosis: MR imaging features. *AJR* 1994;163(2):357–361.
50. Sugimura K, Takemori M, Sugiura M, Okizuka H, Kono M, Ishida T. The value of magnetic resonance relaxation time in staging ovarian endometrial cysts. *Br J Radiol* 1992;65(774):502–506.
51. Garzetti GG, Ciavattini A, Tranquilli AL, Arduini D, Romanini C. Serum CA-125 concentration in endometriosis patients: role of pelvic and peritoneal irritation. *Gyn Endocrinol* 1994;8(1):27–31.
52. Koninckx PR, Muyldermans M, Moerman P, Meuleman C, Deprest J, Cornillie F. CA 125 concentrations in ovarian "chocolate" cyst fluid can differentiate an endometriotic cyst from a cystic corpus luteum. *Human Reprod* 1992;7(9):1314–1317.
53. Stripling MC, Martin DC, Chatman DL, Zwaag RV, Poston WM. Subtle appearance of pelvic endometriosis. *Fertil Steril* 1988;49(3):427–431.
54. Martin DC, Vander Zwaag R. Excisional techniques for endometriosis with the CO_2 laser laparoscope. *J Reprod Med* 1987;32: 753.
55. Chatman DL, Zbella EA. Pelvic peritoneal defects and endometriosis: further observations. *Fertil Steril* 1986;46(4):711–714.
56. Olive DL. Classification of endometriosis. *Infertil Reprod Med Clin North Am* 1992;3(3):633–643.
57. American Fertility Society. Management of endometriosis in the presence of pelvic pain. *Fertil Steril* 1993;60:952–955.
58. Damario MA, Rock JA. Evaluating the American Fertility Society's Classification for endometriosis. *Contemp Ob/Gyn* 1994;15: 57–67.
59. Brosens IA. New principles in the management of endometriosis. *Acta Obstetrica Gynecologica Scand* (Suppl) 1994;159:18–21.
60. Adamson GD. Management of endometriosis. II. Surgical approaches. *Female Patient* 1991;16:59–66.
61. Redwine DB. Conservative laparoscopic excision of endometriosis by sharp dissection: life table analysis of reoperation and persistent or recurrent disease. *Fertil Steril* 1991;56(4):628–634.
62. Adamson GD, Kwei L, Edgren RA. Pain of endometriosis: effects of nafarelin and danazol therapy. *Int J Fertil* 1994;39(4):215–217.
63. Henzl MR, Corson SL, Moghissi K, Buttram VC, Berqvist C, Jacobson J. Administration of nasal nafarelin as compared with oral danazol for endometriosis. A multicenter double-blind comparative trial. *N Engl J Med* 1988;318(8):485–489.
64. Hughes EG, Fedorkow DM, Collins JA. A quantitative overview of controlled trials in endometriosis-associated infertility. *Fertil Steril* 1993;59(5):963–970.
65. Hurst BS, Schlaff WD. Treatment options for endometriosis: medical therapies. *Infertil Reprod Med Clin North Am* 1992;3(3): 645–655.
66. Bayer SR, Seibel MM. Medical treatment: danazol. In: Schenken RS, ed. *Endometriosis: contemporary concepts in clinical management.* Philadelphia: JB Lippincott; 1989:169–188.
67. Olive DL. Medical treatment: alternatives to danazol. In: Schenken RS, ed. *Endometriosis: contemporary concepts in clinical management.* Philadelphia: JB Lippincott; 1989:189–212.
68. Sutton CJG, Hill D. Laser laparoscopy in the treatment of endometriosis. A 5 year study. *Br J Obstet Gynaecol* 1990;97(2):181–185.
69. Davis GD, Thillet E, Wilks R. Laparoscopic treatment of advanced endometriosis. Pain. *Infertil Reprod Med Clin North Am* 1993;4(2):337–344.
70. Adamson GD, Hurd SJ, Pasta DJ, Rodriguez BD. Laparoscopic endometriosis treatment: is it better? *Fertil Steril* 1993;59(1):35–44.
71. Adamson GD, Pasta DJ. Surgical treatment of endometriosis-associated infertility: meta-analysis compared with survival analysis. *Am J Obstet Gynecol* 1994;171:1488–1505.
72. Luciano AA, Manzi D. Treatment options for endometriosis: surgical therapies. *Infertil Reprod Med Clin North Am* 1992;3(3): 657–682.
73. Redwine DB. Treatment of endometriosis-associated pain. *Infertil Reprod Med Clin North Am* 1992;3(3):697–720.
74. Silverberg KM. Combination therapy for endometriosis. *Infertil Reprod Med Clin North Am* 1992;3(3):683–695.
75. Adamson GD. Advantages of laparoscopic and laser surgery. *Infertil Reproductive Med Clin North Am* 1993;4(2):239–254.
76. Dlugi AM, Saleh WA, Jacobsen G. KTP/532 laser laparoscopy in the treatment of endometriosis-associated infertility. *Fertil Steril* 1992;57(6):1186–1193.
77. Adamson GD. Diagnosis and clinical presentation of endometriosis. *Am J Obstet Gynecol* 1990;162(2):568–569.
78. Younger JB. Endometriosis. *Curr Opin Obstet Gynecol* 1993; 5(3):333–339.
79. Luciano AA, Lowney J, Jacobs SL. Endoscopic treatment of endometriosis-associated infertility. Therapeutic, economic and social benefits. *J Reprod Med* 1992;37(7):573–576.
80. Bruhat MA, Mage G, Chapron C, Pouly JL, Canis M, Wattiez A. Present-day endoscopic surgery in gynecology. *Eur J Obstet Gynecol Reprod Biol* 1991;41(1):4–13.
81. Operative Laparoscopy Study Group. Postoperative adhesion development after operative laparoscopy: evaluation at early second-look procedures. *Fertil Steril* 1991;55(4):700–704.
82. Diamond MP, Daniell JF, Feste J, et al. Adhesion reformation and de novo adhesion formation after reproductive pelvic surgery. *Fertil Steril* 1987;47(5):864–866.
83. Gant NF. Infertility and endometriosis: comparison of pregnancy outcomes with laparotomy versus laparoscopic techniques. *Am J Obstet Gynecol* 1992 Apr;166(4):1072–1081.
84. Guerre EF, Diamond MP. Adhesion prevention: does anything work? *Infertil Reprod Med Clin North Am* 1993;4(2):275–287.
85. Jansen RP. Early laparoscopy after pelvic operations to prevent adhesions: safety and efficacy. *Fertil Steril* 1988 Jan;49(1):26–31.
86. Canis M, Mage G, Wattiez A, Chapron C, Pouly JL, Bassil S. Second-look laparoscopy after laparoscopic cystectomy of large ovarian endometriomas. *Fertil Steril* 1992;58(3):617–619.
87. Cook AS, Rock JA. The role of laparoscopy in the treatment of endometriosis. *Fertil Steril* 1991;55(4):663–680.
88. Canis M, Mage G, Manhes H, Pouly JL, Wattiez A, Bruhat MA. Laparoscopic treatment of endometriosis. *Acta Obstet Gynecol Scand* (Suppl) 1989;150:15–20.
89. Sutton CJG, Ewen SP, Whitelaw N, Haines P. Prospective, randomized double-blind controlled trial of laser laparoscopy in the treatment of pelvic pain associated with minimal, mild, and moderate endometriosis. *Fertil Steril* 1994;62:696–700.
90. Martin DC, Hubert GD, Levy BS. Depth of infiltration of endometriosis. *J Gynecol Surg* 1989;5:55.
91. Cornillie FJ, Oosterlynck DJ, Lauweryns JM, Koninckx PR. Deeply infiltrating pelvic endometriosis: histology and clinical significance. *Fertil Steril* 1990;53(6):978–983.
92. Martin DC. Laparoscopic and vaginal colpotomy for the excision of infiltrating cul-de-sac endometriosis. *J Reprod Med* 1988; 33(10):806–808.
93. Redwine DB. Laparoscopic en bloc resection for treatment of the obliterated cul-de-sac in endometriosis. *J Reprod Med* 1992; 37(8):695–698.
94. Reich H, McGlynn F, Salvat J. Laparoscopic treatment of cul-de-sac obliteration secondary to retrocervical deep fibrotic endometriosis. *J Reprod Med* 1991;36(7):516–522.
95. Adamson GD, Hurd SJ, Rodriguez BD, et al. Laparoscopy versus laparotomy for treatment of posterior cul-de-sac obliteration. Abstract, American Association of Gynecologic Laparoscopists, Chicago, IL, September 24–27, 1992.
96. Adamson GD. Management of endometriosis. I. Pharmacologic therapies. *Female Patient* 1991;16:35–40.
97. Nezhat C, Nezhat F, Pennington E. Laparoscopic treatment of infiltrative rectosigmoid colon and rectovaginal septum endometriosis by the technique of videolaparoscopy and the CO_2 laser. *Br J Obstet Gynaecol* 1992;99(8):664–667.
98. Bailey HR, Ott MT, Hartendorp P. Aggressive surgical management for advanced colorectal endometriosis. *Dis Col Rect* 1994;37(8):747–753.
99. Phillips EH, Franklin M, Carroll BJ, Fallas MJ, Ramos R, Rosenthal D. Laparoscopic colectomy. *Ann Surg* 1992;216(6):703–707.

100. Redwine DB, Sharpe DR. Laparoscopic segmental resection for the sigmoid colon for endometriosis. *J Laparoendosc Surg* 1991;1(4):217–220.
101. Daniell JF, Gurley LD, Kurtz BR, Chambers JF. The use of an automatic stapling device for laparoscopic appendectomy. *Obstet Gynecol* 1991;78(4):721–723.
102. Nowzaradan Y, Barnes JP Jr, Westmoreland J, Hojabri M. Laparoscopic appendectomy: treatment of choice for suspected appendicitis. *Surg Laparosc Endosc* 1993;3(5):411–416.
103. Vancaillie TG. The role of laparoscopy in the surgical treatment of ovarian cysts. *Infertil Reprod Med Clin North Am* 1993;4(2): 305–319.
104. Anderson R. Endoscopic treatment of ovarian cysts. The oncologists' view. *Infertil Reprod Med Clin North Am* 1993;4(2):321–336.
105. Maiman M, Seltzer V, Boyce J. Laparoscopic excision of ovarian neoplasm subsequently found to be malignant. *Obstet Gynecol* 1991;77(4):563–565.
106. Dembo AJ, Davy M, Stenwig AE, Berle EJ, Bush RS, Kjorstad K. Prognostic factors in patients with stage I epithelial ovarian cancer. *Obstet Gynecol* 1990;75(2):263–273.
107. Webb MJ, Decker DG, Massey E, et al. Factors influencing survival in stage I ovarian cancer. *Am J Obstet Gynecol* 1973;116: 222.
108. Seltzer VL, Maiman M, Boyce A, et al. Laparoscopic surgery in the management of ovarian cysts. *Female Patient* 1992;17:16.
109. Obwegeser R, Deutinger J, Bernascheck G. The risk of malignancy with an apparently simple adnexal cyst on ultrasound. *Arch Gynecol Obstet* 1993;253(3):117–120.
110. Markuly SN, Fanning J, Hindman TL, Galle PC, Ertmoed E, Hilgers RD. False-positive malignant peritoneal cytology associated with pelvic endometriosis. *J Am Osteop Assoc* 1994;94(2): 157–161.
111. Koonings PP, Campbell K, Mishell DR Jr, Grimes DA. Relative frequency of primary ovarian neoplasms: a 10-year review. *Obstet Gynecol* 1989;74(6):921–926.
112. Adamson GD, Subak LL, Pasta DJ, Hurd SJ, von Franque O, Rodriguez BD. Comparison of CO_2 laser laparoscopy with laparotomy for treatment of endometriomata. *Fertil Steril* 1992;57(5):965–973.
113. Bateman BG, Kolp LA, Mills S. Endoscopic versus laparotomy management of endometriosis. *Fertil Steril* 1994;62:690–695.
114. Wood C, Maher P, Hill D. Diagnosis and surgical management of endometriomas. *Aust N Z J Obstet Gynaecol* 1992;32(2):161–163.
115. Fragenheim H. The range and limits of operative laparoscopy in the diagnosis of sterility. In: Philips J, Downey CA, eds. *Endoscopy in gynecology*. St. Louis: American Association of Gynecologic Laparoscopists; 1978:276.
116. Aboulghar MA, Mansour RT, Serour GI, Sattar M, Ramzy AM, Amin YM. Treatment of recurrent chocolate cysts by transvaginal aspiration and tetracycline sclerotherapy. *J Assist Reprod Genet* 1993;10(8):531–533.
117. Giorlandino C, Taramanni C, Muzii L, Santillo E, Nanni C, Vizzone A. Ultrasound-guided aspiration of ovarian endometriotic cysts. *Int J Gynaecol Obstet* 1993;43(1):41–44.
118. Keye WR Jr., Hansen LW, Astin M, et al. Argon laser therapy of endometriosis: a review of 92 consecutive patients. *Fertil Steril* 1987;47:208.
119. Kojima E, Morita M, Otaka K, Yano Y. Nd:YAG laser laparoscopy for ovarian endometriomas. *J Reprod Med* 1990;35(6):592–596.
120. Brosens IA, Puttemans PJ. Double-optic laparoscopy: salpingoscopy, ovarian cystoscopy and endo-ovarian surgery with the argon laser. *Bailliere's Clin Obstet Gynaecol* 1989;3(3):595.
121. Reich H, McGlynn F. Treatment of ovarian endometriomas using laparoscopic surgical techniques. *J Reprod Med* 1986;31(7): 577–584.
122. Vercellini P, Vendola N, Bocciolone L, Colombo A, Rognoni MT, Bolis G. Laparoscopic aspiration of ovarian endometriomas. Effect with postoperative gonadotropin releasing hormone agonist treatment. *J Reprod Med* 1992;37(7):577–580.
123. Goldenberg M, Oelsner G, Bider D, Admon D, Rabinowich O, Mashiach S. A new approach to ovarian cystectomy: a combined laparoscopic and extra-abdominal microsurgical technique. *Gynecol Obstet Invest* 1994;37(3):196–198.
124. Sayegh R, Garcia CR. Ovarian function after conservational ovarian surgery: a long-term follow-up study. *Int J Gynaecol Obstet* 1992;39(4):303–309.
125. Redwine DB. Endometriosis persisting after castration: clinical characteristics and results of surgical management. *Obstet Gynecol* 1994;83(3):405–401.
126. Dubuisson JB, Chapron C, Aubriot FX, Osman M, Zerbib M. Pregnancy after laparoscopic partial cystectomy for bladder endometriosis. *Human Reprod* 1994;9(4):730–732.
127. Clement PB, Young RH. Endocervicosis of the urinary bladder. A report of six cases of a benign müllerian lesion that may mimic adenocarcinoma. *Am J Surg Pathol* 1992;16(6):533–542.
128. Patel A, Thorpe P, Ramsay JW, Shepherd JH, Kirby RS, Hendry WF. Endometriosis of the ureter. *Br J Urol* 1992;69(5):495–498.
129. Lam AM, French M, Charnock FM. Bilateral ureteric obstruction due to recurrent endometriosis associated with hormone replacement therapy. *Aust N Z J Obstet Gynaecol* 1992;32(1):83–84.
130. Steckel J, Badillo F, Waldbaum RS. Uretero-fallopian tube fistula secondary to laparoscopic fulguration of pelvic endometriosis. *J Urol* 1993;149(5):1128–1129.
131. Nezhat C, Nezhat F, Green B, et al. Laparoscopic treatment of obstructed ureter due to endometriosis by resection and ureteroureterostomy: a case report. *J Urol* 1992;148(3):865–868.
132. Doyle JB. Paracervical uterine denervation by transection of the cervical plexus for relief of dysmenorrhea. *Am J Obstet Gynecol* 1955;70:11.
133. Gutmann JN, Olive DL. LUNA, laparoscopic presacral neurectomy. *Infertil Reprod Med Clin North Am* 1993;4(2):371–387.
134. Tjaden B, Schlaff WD, Kimball A, Rock JA. The efficacy of presacral neurectomy for the relief of midline dysmenorrhea. *Obstet Gynecol* 1990;76(1):89–91.
135. Grimes DA. Frontiers of operative laparoscopy: a review and critique of the evidence. *Am J Obstet Gynecol* 1992;166(4):1062–1071.
136. Reich H, DeCaprio J, McGlynn F. Laparoscopic hysterectomy. *J Gynecol Surg* 1989;5:23.
137. Johns DA. Laparoscopy assisted vaginal hysterectomy. *Infertil Reprod Med Clin North Am* 1993;4(2):389–402.
138. Reich H. Laparoscopic hysterectomy. *Surg Laparosc Endosc* 1992;2(1):85–88.
139. Walters MD. Definitive surgery. In: Schenken RS, ed. *Endometriosis: contemporary concepts in clinical management*. Philadelphia: JB Lippincott; 1989:267–278.
140. Davis GD, Wolgamott G, Moon J. Laparoscopically assisted vaginal hysterectomy as definitive therapy for stage III and IV endometriosis. *J Reprod Med* 1993;38(8):577–581.
141. Adamson GD, Lu J, Subak LL. Laparoscopic CO_2 laser vaporization of endometriosis compared with traditional treatments. *Fertil Steril* 1988;50(5):704–710.
142. Adamson GD. Laser surgery for adhesions in advanced endoscopic and laser surgery. American Association of Gynecologic Laparoscopists, Santa Barbara, CA, April 25–27, 1991;24.
143. Barbieri RL, Evans S, Kistner RW. Danazol in the treatment of endometriosis: analysis of 100 cases with a 4-year followup. *Fertil Steril* 1982;37(6):737–746.
144. Dmowski WP. Danazol in the treatment of endometriosis and infertility. *Prog Clin Bio Res* 1982;112(Part B):167–186.
145. Schenken RS, Malinak LR. Reoperation after initial treatment of endometriosis with conservative surgery. *Am J Obstet Gynecol* 1978;131:406.
146. Williams TJ, Pratt JH. Endometriosis in 1000 consecutive coeliotomies, incidence and management. *Am J Obstet Gynecol* 1977;120:245.
147. Wheeler JM, Malinak LR. Recurrent endometriosis: incidence, management, and prognosis. *Am J Obstet Gynecol* 1983;146(3): 247–253.
148. Barbieri RL. Gonadotropin-releasing hormone agonists: treatment of endometriosis. *Clin Obstet Gynecol* 1993;36(3):636–641.
149. Kauppila A. Changing concepts of medical treatment of endometriosis. *Acta Obstet Gynecol Scand* 1993;72(5):324–336.
150. Barbieri RL. Hormone treatment of endometriosis: the estrogen

threshold hypothesis. *Am J Obstet Gynecol* 1992;166(2):740–745.

151. Adamson GD. Use of GnRH agonists to improve results of operative laparoscopy and hysteroscopy. In: Polan ML, Henzl MR, eds. *Infertil Reprod Med Clin North Am* 1993;4(1):65–81.
152. Kaplan CR, Schenken RS. Combination medical and surgical treatment. In: Schenken RS, ed. *Endometriosis: contemporary concepts in clinical management.* Philadelphia: JB Lippincott; 1989:279–292.
153. Witt BR, Barad DH. Management of endometriosis in women older than 40 years of age. *Obst Gynecol Clin North Am* 1993;20(2):349–363.
154. Olive DL. Conservative Surgery. In: Schenken RS, ed. *Endometriosis: contemporary concepts in clinical management.* Philadelphia: JB Lippincott; 1989:213–248.
155. Vancaillie T, Schenken RS. Endoscopic surgery. In: Schenken RS, ed. *Endometriosis: contemporary concepts in clinical management.* Philadelphia: JB Lippincott; 1989:249–265.
156. Kemmann E, Ghazi D, Corsan G, Bohrer MK. Does ovulation stimulation improve fertility in women with minimal/mild endometriosis after laser laparoscopy? *Int J Fertil Menop Stud* 1993;38(1):16–21.
157. Schenken RS, Riehl RM. In vitro fertilization/embryo transfer and gamete intrafallopian transfer. In: Schenken RS, ed. *Endometriosis: contemporary concepts in clinical management.* Philadelphia: JB Lippincott; 1989:293–306.
158. Walker E, Katon W, Harrop-Griffiths J, Holm L, Russo J, Hickock LR. Relationship of chronic pelvic pain to psychiatric diagnoses and childhood sexual abuse. *Am J Psychiatry* 1988;145(1):75–80.
159. Adamson GD. The choice of therapy for the operative treatment of endometriosis is endoscopic laser surgery. *J Gynecol Surg* 1991;7(2):129–131.
160. Olive DL, Martin DC. Treatment of endometriosis-associated infertility with CO_2 laser laparoscopy: the use of one- and two-parameter exponential models. *Fertil Steril* 1987;48:18.
161. Peterson HB, Hulka JF, Phillips JM. American Association of Gynecologic Laparoscopists 1988 membership survey on operative laparoscopy. *J Reprod Med* 1990;35(6):587–589.

Endoscopic Management of Gynecologic Disease,
edited by G.D. Adamson and D.C. Martin.
Lippincott-Raven Publishers, Philadelphia © 1996.

CHAPTER 15

Ovarian Cystectomy

Daniel C. Martin

The decision to perform an ovarian cystectomy, the removal of an ovarian cyst, is based on preoperative and intraoperative findings and predicated on informed consent. Although these decisions are more readily made for a patient with a known cyst who has been evaluated preoperatively, ovarian cystectomy is sometimes decided on intraoperatively. This possibility is considered in all patients prepared for laparoscopy.

PREOPERATIVE DECISIONS

The major decision to be made preoperatively is whether the patient should have a cystectomy or an oophorectomy. This decision is based on various combinations of physical exam, age, history, ultrasonography, and tumor markers. Concern regarding spill of a malignancy (1–6), a dermoid cyst (7), or a mucinous cyst (8) may be important. However, spilling may not be clinically significant (9), whereas missing the diagnosis of a cancer, delaying definitive therapy, and incomplete staging are more dangerous (7,10–12). Furthermore, castrating a young patient for a benign disease has significant health and medical/legal implications. In a reproductive age range patient, hysterectomy and oophorectomy should *not* be performed for a frozen section diagnosis of borderline or low-grade malignancy.

Preoperative assessment by ultrasonography (13), magnetic resonance imaging (14), or tumor markers, such as CA 125, α-fetoprotein, and chorionic gonadotropin (15), are particularly useful in postmenopausal patients (16). These tests may be helpful in select patients of reproductive age.

Informed consent generally covers the possibility of immediate laparotomy and hysterectomy. In young patients desiring to preserve fertility, the decision is generally reached to get permanent sections rather than basing a laparotomy and hysterectomy on a frozen section.

Informed consent can be very difficult due to the wide range of risks associated with this type of care. Retrospective reviews have shown a risk of iatrogenic rupture of a malignant neoplasm at laparoscopy from 0.06% (17) to 100% (10) (see Table 1). However, using laparotomy instead of laparoscopy does not guarantee that incomplete staging and delay in therapy will not occur (5,12).

Unilocular, simple cysts and dermoid cysts in young patients are generally treated by cystectomy. This is particularly true with a simple cyst revealed on sonogram and a negative CA 125 when the patient desires preservation of fertility. In Herrmann's series, 100% of simple cysts < 10 cm were benign whereas 90% of simple cysts > 10 cm were benign. Furthermore, benign cysts in reproductive age range patients often have sonograms with cystic and solid components. Herrmann found cystic and solid components in 58% of the benign cysts as opposed to 93% of malignant cysts (18). In my practice, benign, cystic, ovarian endometriomas have had sonogram reports of a 10.1-cm cystic and solid mass and a 9-cm solid mass. On the other hand, a cystic and solid mass accompanied by an elevated CA 125 level in a menopausal patient (16) is highly predictive of cancer and should generally be handled by oophorectomy with preparation for immediate staging accompanied by hysterectomy, contralateral adnexectomy, omental biopsy or excision, pelvic cytology and upper abdominal cytology.

Oophorectomy is frequently indicated when there is a problem with lateral pelvic pain following previous conservative surgery for this pain. Furthermore, oophorectomy may be the best approach for dermoid cysts and mucinous cystadenomas. Rupture of a mucinous cystadenoma may result in pseudomyxoma peritonei (8). Inadvertent spilling of a dermoid may result in peritonitis

D. C. Martin: Department of Obstetrics and Gynecology, University of Tennessee, Baptist Memorial Hospital, Memphis, Tennessee 38103.

TABLE 1. *Risk of rupture of malignant cysts*[a]

Study	Number of patients	Number of cyst ruptures	Percentage
Maiman (10)	42	42	100
Peterson (17)	5075	3	0.06

[a] Varies according to type of analysis. Maiman examined the records of patients with known cancer, whereas Peterson studied laparoscopy in any patient with an ovarian cyst.

(7). Many dermoid cysts can be diagnosed preoperatively, and we may develop sonographic, color Doppler or other studies capable of distinguishing mucinous cystadenomas in the future.

As an adjunctive concern, there is the worry that aggressive use of laparoscopy may result in treatment of functional cysts that would otherwise resolve spontaneously.

A patient who is at high risk for bowel adhesions or bowel involvement of endometriosis has a bowel preparation. Self-bloodbanking is encouraged. When a patient may have an appendix involved with endometriosis or tumor, appendectomy with the increased potential for hospitalization is discussed.

Laparoscopic ovarian cystectomy is associated with decreased hospitalization and recovery time compared to the procedure being done by laparotomy. There also appears to be a decreased incidence of new adhesion formation (19,20) and improved patient acceptance and sense of well-being. The overall costs have been reported as less by Levine (21) but may be greater if the surgeon uses lasers and disposable equipment (22,23).

Once the decision is made to perform a cystectomy, then the decisions regarding laparoscopy or laparotomy will depend on the nature of the cyst but will be more influenced by the surgeon's experience. No-spill techniques for oophorectomy are available involving a sacking technique with exteriorization prior to drainage or morcellation. These techniques have been used by urologists to resect kidneys with no spill into the abdominal cavity (24) and are discussed later in this chapter.

INTRAOPERATIVE DECISIONS

When ovarian cysts are densely adherent to the bowel or broad ligament, these commonly recur when lysed (19,20). In infertility patients, these dense adhesions are frequently avoided. In patients with pelvic pain who desire to preserve the ovary, the cyst is resected and either an Interceed Tc-7 (Johnson and Johnson) or Gore-Tex (W.L. Gore and Associates) barrier is placed. Gore-Tex is used in infertility surgery when patients understand and accept the need for a second laparoscopy for removal of the barrier. Laparotomy can also be considered, as these dense adhesions may be too dense for control at laparoscopy.

Ovarian cancer may present with dense adhesions and external surface excrescences. A frozen section is taken in this situation, and plans are made accordingly. In infertility patients, the most common plan is to obtain peritoneal washings, examine the omentum and diaphragm, perform additional biopsies of upper lesions, stop the surgery, wait for permanent sections, and then discuss the findings with the patient and an oncologist. Areas of the diaphragm below the level of the air pocket can frequently be visualized by running irrigation solution through the operating channel of the operating laparoscope. This opens the space immediately in front of the optics and allows visualization of deeper structures than can be seen in the air pocket. In select patients, particularly postmenopausal patients, in whom informed consent has included the immediate performance of exploratory laparotomy with total abdominal hysterectomy and bilateral salpingoophorectomy, surgery can proceed based on frozen section results.

INSTRUMENTATION

Mechanical, electrosurgical, thermal, and laser techniques are used by different surgeons. The basic mechanical instruments are atraumatic blunt probes, irrigators, aspirators, scissors, and graspers. The probes used for

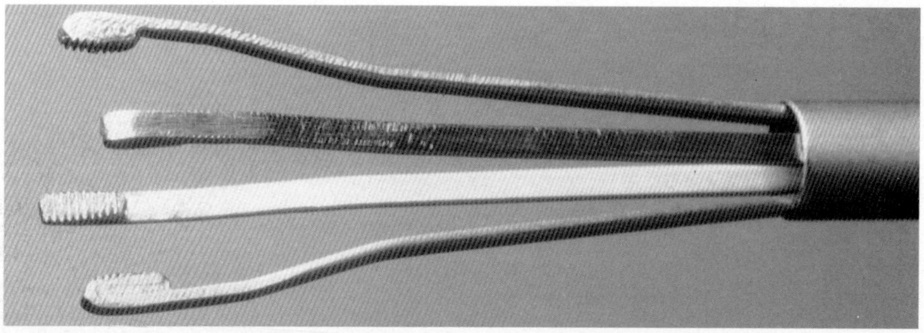

FIG. 1. Hasson's multiprong atraumatic grasping forcep is one of several specialized instruments useful in mobilizing and controlling the ovary during dissection and laparoscopic surgery.

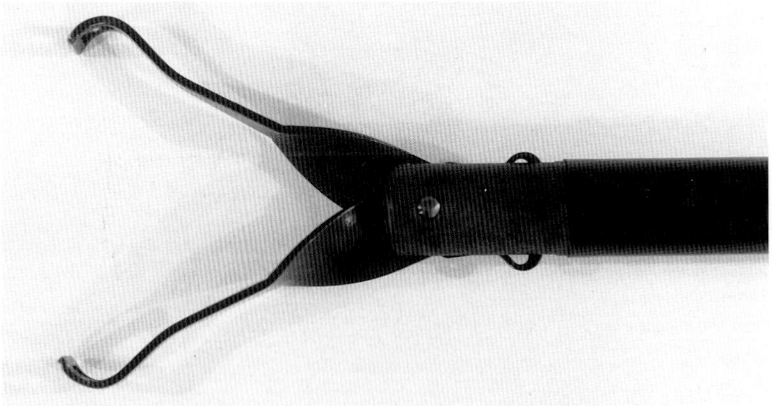

FIG. 2. Disposable Babcock clamps (U.S. Surgical, Norwalk, CT) are available for fixation of the uterovarian ligament at laparoscopy.

manipulation are smooth so as to avoid pulling tissue into the hinges. These have centimeter markings for measuring structures in the pelvis. An angled hinge increases the surgeon's ability to manipulate structures and to measure tissue.

The grasping forceps used for ovarian cystectomy can be atraumatic, toothed, or multipronged. Atraumatic forceps frequently do not grasp sufficiently to stabilize the ovary and may result in more inadvertent trauma due to the multiple manipulations necessary to hold the ovary in place. On the other hand, toothed forceps cause a defined injury but may result in less bruising. Multipronged atraumatic forceps have been reported to provide the advantages of atraumatic holding while giving more stabilization than simpler atraumatic forceps (Fig. 1). Disposable equipment, such as laparoscopic Babcock clamps, can be used to stabilize the ovary (Fig. 2). Although disposable equipment is expensive (23), it is available, sterile, and reliable.

Irrigation and aspiration systems are used for lavage and dissection (25,26). In addition to specifically designed systems, standard blood pressure cuffs can be used with a spiked Corson probe (Cabot Medical, Langhorne, PA) for irrigation. Straight suction to the wall can be used. When the aspiration system is also used to eliminate laser plume, protective filters are placed in the line to prevent the hydrocarbons in the plume from depositing in the system pipes. If this material accumulates in the pipes, the latter can occlude and require major repair.

Although cysts generally are not closed, suturing techniques (27,28) can be useful when closure of a cyst wall is indicated. Intraovarian suturing is discussed later in this chapter.

Monopolar electrosurgery can be used for incision or vaporization. On the other hand, bipolar electrosurgery is used for hemostasis by desiccating tissue (29,30). Monopolar delivery at high power density can vaporize tissue in a fashion very similar to that of lasers (31–34).

Endocoagulation is used to avoid electrosurgery and the risk of electrosurgical burn (35). Although it is possible to produce a thermal burn inadvertently, this should be a rare clinical occurrence due to endocoagulation's slow mechanism of action as compared to electrosurgical or laser techniques. However, thermal coagulation is a slow technique and can increase the operating time.

The four lasers most commonly used in gynecology are the carbon dioxide (CO_2), argon, potassium-trideuterium-phosphate (KTP), and neodymium:yttrium-aluminum-garnet (Nd:YAG) (36,37). The CO_2 laser produces the most predictable what-you-see-is-what-you-get effect using no-touch techniques. However, mirror alignment and smoke plume can be difficult to control. The CO_2 laser appears to be the most commonly used laser for both external and internal gynecologic use.

Argon, KTP, and Nd:YAG lasers can be directed through quartz fibers. All three of these lasers have a greater intrinsic depth of penetration than the CO_2 laser; the Nd:YAG laser has the greatest penetration. However, this depth of penetration is most apparent at the low power densities used for coagulation. On the other hand, high power densities are created with small fibers and artificial tips. The high power densities are associated with decreased thermal coagulation. Very small tips and high power density can create a thermal coagulation zone similar to that of the CO_2 laser (38–40).

Like any equipment or technique that has been closely monitored, lasers have been associated with complications. These include hypothermia, emphysema, hemorrhage, transfusion, laparotomy, colostomy, urinary leak, and death (41).

NO-SPILL TECHNIQUES

Spill is avoided when it appears to be important for patient care, such as when there is a possibility of ovarian cancer or teratoma. Although oophorectomy offers the best protection against this possibility, slow dissection of a cyst out of the ovary also decreases the chance of spill. Slow dissection involves countertraction, spreading with

TABLE 2. *Fenestration recurrence rate*[a]

	Number	Recurrent
Removal	13	1 (8%)
Fenestration alone	9	8 (89%)

[a] Hasson (43) demonstrated a decreased recurrence following stripping as compared to fenestration of ovarian endometriomas.

atraumatic forceps, and use of water under pressure. When the cyst is successfully shelled out, it is placed in a sack, the neck of the sack and the trocar sleeve is pulled out of the abdominal wall, and the sack is then decompressed or the cyst morcellated within the sack. General surgeons have used large cannulas (4 cm) to remove spleens intact and this may be reasonable for certain cysts in gynecology. Minilaparotomy and colpotomy in conjunction with a sack have also been discussed as approaches to remove cysts (42).

FENESTRATION AND CYSTECTOMY

Fenestration of cysts may be reasonable when a cyst has clear fluid and flat lining compatible with a functional cyst. However, fenestration alone has a higher recurrence rate than does removal (43) (Table 2). When the inside lining is compatible with endometriosis, stripping or sharp dissection appear to be more reasonable (44,45). Coagulating the inner lining may decrease recurrence (46).

CHOCOLATE CYSTS OF THE OVARY

Chocolate cysts of the ovary can be endometrioma, residual of a hemorrhagic corpus luteum, or nonspecific on histology. When these are opened and examined, the general appearance of an endometrioma is a mottled lining with red or brown areas on a white fibrotic base (47). On the other hand, corpus lutea tend to have a smoother, more uniformly brown or yellow–brown lining. Biopsies for confirmation of endometriosis are best taken from the red streaks of tissue coming off the base. Biopsies of the brown areas frequently show hemosiderin and can be associated with aging corpus lutea, corpus albicans, and endometriomas. The chance that observation of the wall will result in missing a cancer is small (2), but the consequences are significant (4,10); biopsy is used to decrease this possibility. Preoperative sonography and serologic markers may aid in clinical decisions regarding specific patients (13,15).

Stripping techniques can be used to remove the entire capsule for complete histologic analysis. Although stripping techniques produce a more complete specimen for histologic analysis, they are more difficult and may not be more effective for endometriosis than biopsy followed by coagulation (46). In addition, stripping removes not only the pseudocapsule but also a thin rim of healthy ovary immediately adjacent to the capsule (Fig. 3). With large endometriomas, this small rim may have adequate volume to compromise the overall function of the ovary.

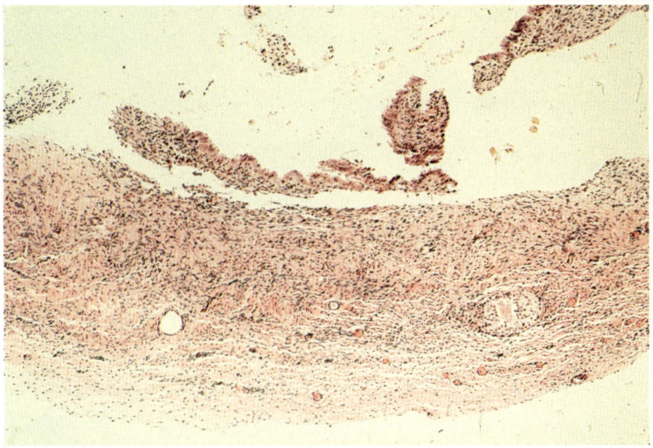

FIG. 3. This endometrioma, which has been stripped, has glands and stroma on the inner lining, a scarred pseudocapsule, and then healthy ovarian stroma with eggs and developing follicles on the outside rim.

Chocolate cysts of less than 5 mm have little or no fibrotic reaction (Fig. 4) and tend to be irregular in their infiltration (47). These are generally biopsied and then coagulated or vaporized (Fig. 5). For those cysts measuring 5–20 mm, various techniques determined by the appearance are used as the procedure progresses. When the cysts are >2 cm, the fibrotic reaction is prominent and stripping of the pseudocapsule is accomplished slowly (Fig. 6). This stripping also removes a rim of healthy ovary. Two grasping forceps are usually all that is needed. However, for cysts exceeding 4 cm, a third grasping forcep or a transabdominal suture to hold the tissue

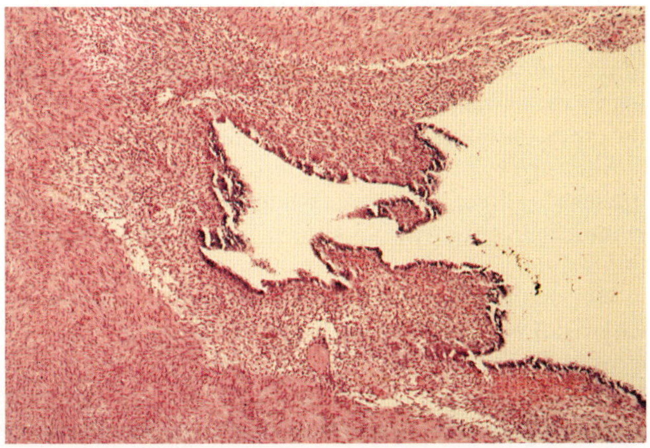

FIG. 4. Small endometriomas have irregular infiltration, and the stroma of the endometriosis is immediately adjacent to the stroma of the ovary with no intervening pseudocapsule.

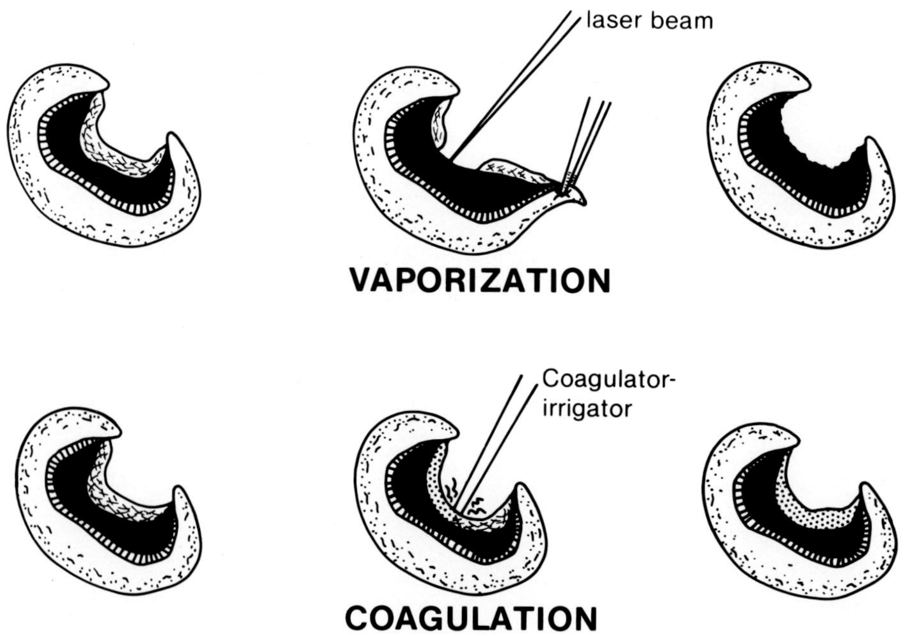

FIG. 5. Small endometriomas first are biopsied and then the base vaporized or coagulated. (From Martin DC, ed. *Intra-abdominal laser surgery*. 2nd ed. Memphis: Resurge Press; in preparation.)

to the anterior abdominal wall may increase visualization and control.

As the stripping approaches the hilum, special attention and care is used to avoid the hilar vessels. When stripping is difficult in this area, the capsule is generally amputated above the hilar vessels and the remnant base is coagulated. When these cysts have been greater than 5 cm, laparoscopies have taken up to 5 hr (41,48). The glands and stroma of large cysts are usually on the surface of the inner lining (as evident in Fig. 7). The depth of penetration of the stroma into the inner lining capsule has been measured to be as deep as 1.5 mm (Fig. 8). Treating these large chocolate cysts by biopsy and coagulation followed by exams and sonograms may help preserve healthy ovarian tissue (46). However, this treatment increases the risk of missing an ovarian cancer (2).

In the management of these chocolate cysts, an incision is made at the most dependent portion so that the walls tend to collapse back together at the end of the procedure. Sutures are generally avoided as suturing has been shown to increase adhesions both in peritoneum (49–52) and in ovaries (48,53–57). Furthermore, the highest pregnancy rate reported with ovarian cystectomy at laparoscopy was 92% by Reich and McGlynn (58) when no other factors were present and no sutures used. This is similar to Martin's report of an 80% pregnancy rate following treatment of severe endometriosis using laser and no sutures (59). When ovarian suturing is needed, laparotomy with true intracapsular, subcortical closure is preferred (60–62). The use of fibrin glue has been suggested to avoid the ischemic sequelae of suturing (46,63). This glue is not available in the United States.

Sutures may be needed to preserve the fimbrial–gonadal relationship when the fimbria ovarica allows the tubal ostium to be >4 cm away from the ovary (61). These may be used when thermal or laser coagulation of the serosa would not constrict this area successfully. Although 7.0 suture is preferred, 6.0 is easier to handle at laparoscopy.

OTHER CYSTS

Rupture of a mucinous cystadenoma may result in pseudomyxoma peritonei (8), whereas spill of a dermoid cyst may result in diffuse peritonitis (7). If a dermoid cyst or a mucinous cystadenoma is spilled during a cystectomy, the patient and table must be reversed to put the head in an up position to keep the fluid in the pelvis. The pelvic volume is approximately 20–80 cm^3 and spill into the upper abdomen can occur rapidly with irrigation (44) (Fig. 9). Furthermore, dermoid cysts can have malignant components (Fig. 10).

Major concerns at the opposite extremes are that oophorectomy may be more reasonable than ovarian cystectomy (64) and aggressive use of laparoscopy may result in treatment of functional cysts that would otherwise resolve spontaneously.

ADHESIONS

Laparoscopic techniques result in fewer new adhesions than do laparotomy techniques (20,65,66). There have been many studies suggesting and denying that

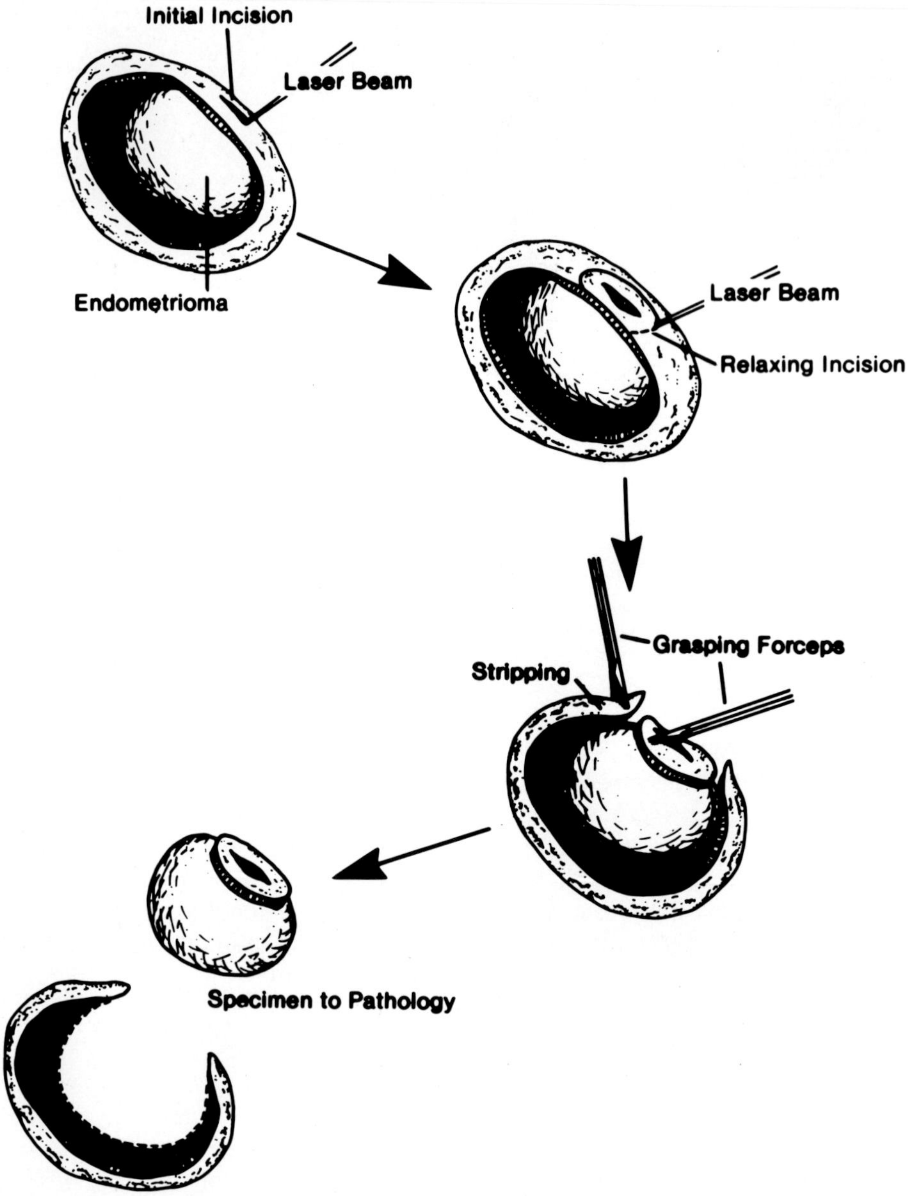

FIG. 6. Larger endometriomas can be removed by stripping. An initial incision is made in a dependent portion to facilitate spontaneous closure. Once the initial incision is made and the endometrioma drained, a relaxing incision is made to facilitate grasping of the specimen. The surgeon slowly strips the specimen out trying to preserve as much of the healthy ovary as possible. This specimen is then sent in its entirety to pathology.

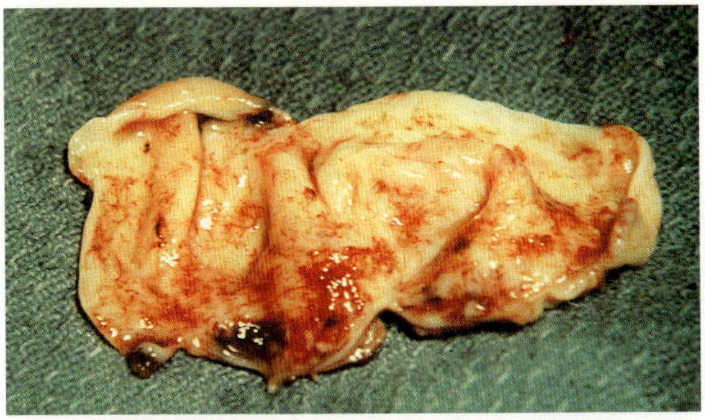

FIG. 7. The most common appearance of an endometrioma that has been opened and washed is an irregular mottled red and brown appearance. The red areas contain the highest yield for glands and stroma on histologic sectioning. The brown areas are generally hemosiderin-laden and nondiagnostic. The white lining is a scarred pseudocapsule.

multiple agents help in adhesion prevention. Of the agents suggested, there are two that are FDA-approved. The first is Interceed (Tc-7) (67) and the other is Gore-Tex (68). The advantage of Interceed is that it can be cut into small pieces and laid into the pelvis through a laparoscope. At this time, Gore-Tex still requires suturing, is not absorbable, and, when used in infertility patients, requires a second operation for removal in order to allow egg transit. Comparative studies between Interceed and Gore-Tex are needed.

In treating patients with known pelvic and/or abdominal adhesions, the insertion techniques are more important than usual (69–72). Increased preparation of the patient for the possibility of bowel damage includes informed consent and bowel preparation.

Filmy adhesions can be lysed by several techniques (41,73–76). Although blunt dissection and lysis has been advocated, there is the worry that the abraded surfaces,

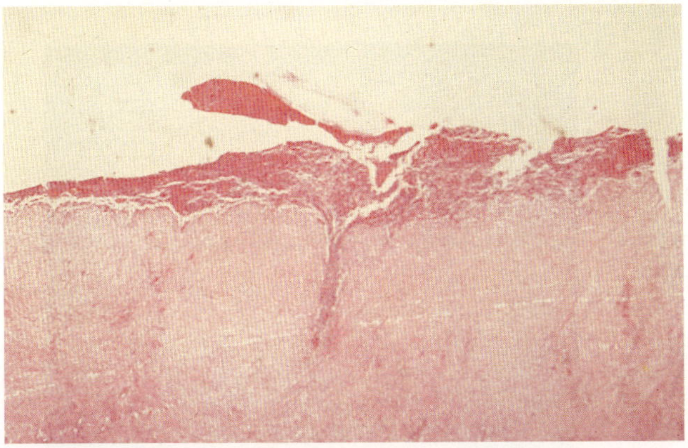

FIG. 8. In close examinations of the pseudocapsule, infiltration of the stromal component has been measured as deep as 1.5 mm into the pseudocapsule. At this depth, coagulation is still effective.

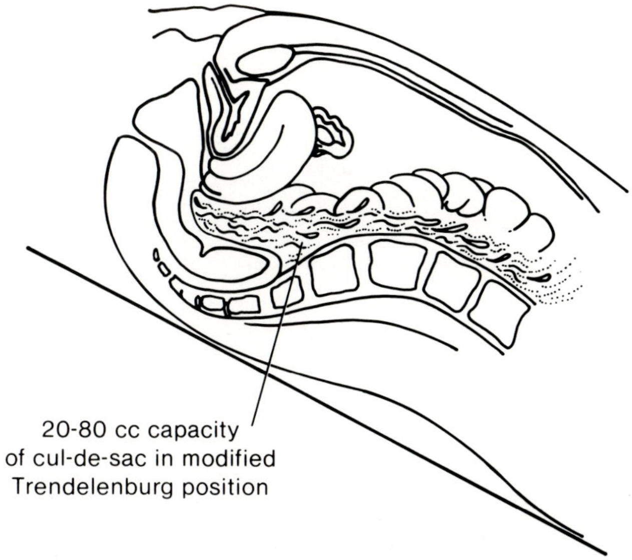

FIG. 9. The capacity of the cul-de-sac in modified Trendelenburg position is generally from 20 to 80 cm^3. If a teratoma or other worrisome cyst is spilled, the patient should be moved into a head-up position to keep the fluid in the pelvis.

with their oozing and biochemical activity, may adhere more readily than surfaces that are cleanly cut and hemostatic. Past data suggest that adhesions are more common with ischemic tissue than with dead tissue (41, 49–52).

Scissors and coagulation are very useful for upper abdominal incisions from the omentum and epiploic fat to the anterior abdominal wall. These are progressively cut and coagulation is used when bleeding occurs. Many of these adhesions are avascular. A significant area of concern is that the adhesions that are seen through the laparoscope can sometimes hide bowel on the other side. Care is taken to identify both sides of the adhesions when possible. This sometimes includes placing the laparoscope through a lower port in order to get a view from the other side. Furthermore, while trying to avoid the bowel, surgeons have made their dissections so far anterior that the bladder has been entered. This complication requires minilaparotomy, repair of the bladder, and indwelling catheterization.

Dense adhesions are more difficult to control with scissors and coagulation and there is an increased chance that bowel is hidden in these. Slow dissection with electrosurgical knife or with lasers is generally performed (73,76,77).

STEIN–LEVENTHAL SYNDROME

The treatment of Stein–Leventhal syndrome at laparoscopy has been performed by microcyst puncture, biopsy of the multiple microcystic areas, furrowing of the ovary, and true wedge resection (41,53,55,74,75,78–80).

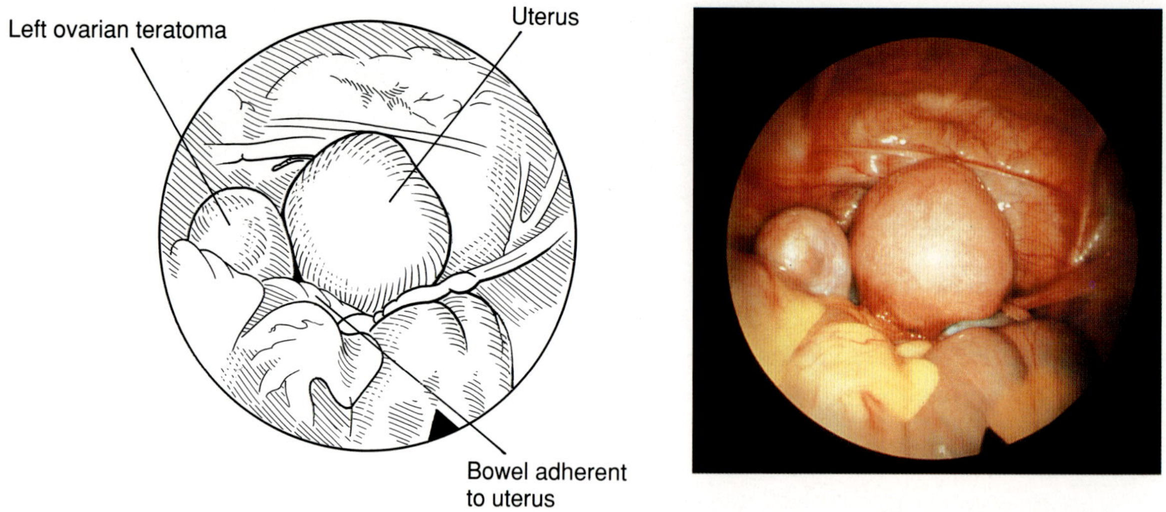

FIG. 10. This patient has extensive endometriosis completely obliterating the cul-de-sac with the bowel adherent to the uterine fundus. In addition, there is a 4-cm teratoma of the left ovary. This was removed at laparotomy because of the extensive endometriosis. There was a 1 cm grade I immature teratoma within an otherwise mature teratoma. With this removed intact, the patient's prognosis is excellent.

Following treatment there is a decrease in testosterone and luteinizing hormone (53,80). Postoperative pregnancy rates have been from 52% to 57% (53,55,80).

APPENDECTOMY

When cysts are on the right side, particularly in patients who have chronic right pain, appendectomy is considered as an elective procedure. Furthermore, the chance of an unexpected finding, such as endometriosis or other tumor, is considered (Fig. 11).

MARCAINE-MORPHINE BLOCKS

As outpatient procedures become increasingly complex, involving multiple incisions at laparoscopy and minilaparotomy, deadening of incisional pain with marcaine-morphine blocks increases the patients' comfort at home and their sense of well-being postoperatively. A solution of 2 mg of morphine per 10 ml of 0.25% marcaine is injected into the incision. The amount varies from 10 ml for two to three small incisions to 30 ml for a large laparotomy incision. This is very similar to the marcaine blocks used by anesthesiologists in long-term pain therapy (48).

COMPLICATIONS

Complications are those of surgery in general. These occur both at laparotomy and at laparoscopy. When there are dense adhesions to the bowel, lysing these may result in bowel laceration, which requires suturing (81).

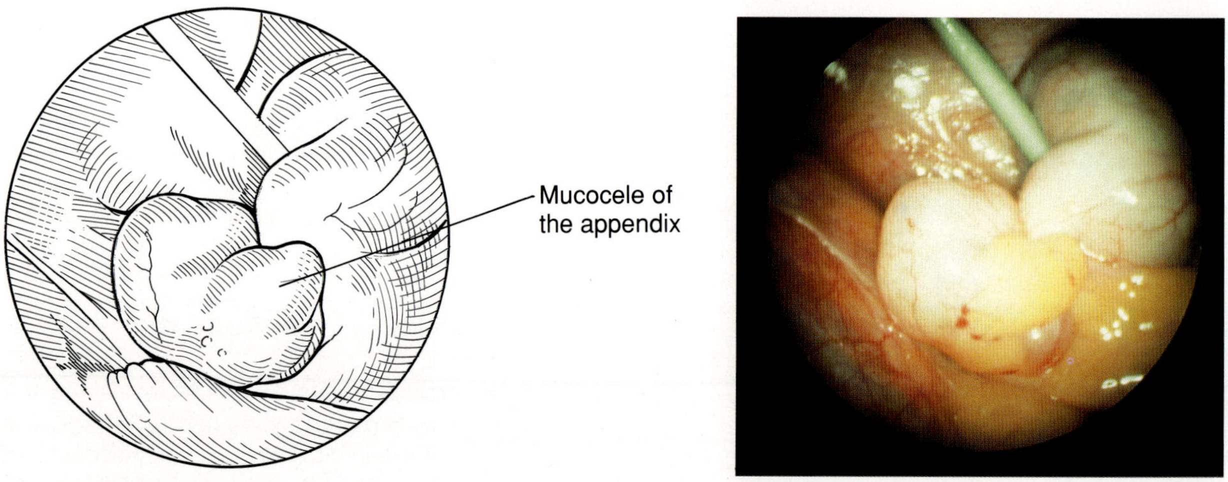

FIG. 11. This mucocele of the appendix can present as a small pelvic cyst on sonography associated with chronic right lower quadrant pain.

The chance of bowel laceration can be decreased by applying traction on the tissues, thereby pushing the ovary away from the colon, and dissecting against the ovary itself.

With large cysts, damage to the hilar vessels results in increased chance of hemorrhage and loss of the ovary. When these cysts are endometriomas, it appears reasonable to dissect the cyst back to the area near the hilar vessels and then resect the cyst at this level. The remnant wall is then coagulated intact over the hilar vessels.

Although many authors stress the risk of adhesion formation, there appears to be a decreased appearance of new adhesions when cystectomy is performed laparoscopically. Donnez states that using glue to close the defect results in future decreased adhesions (46).

Bleeding points generally are coagulated, although sutures and loops can be used. At the end of the procedure, the air pocket is withdrawn so that the intraabdominal pressure is below the venous pressure. The area is then reinsufflated to check for any bleeding occurring at normal intraabdominal pressure. When the surgeon is worried about the possibility of a delayed bleed, a drain can be placed and left in the abdomen for 2 hr. The drain is removed in the recovery room as long as the patient has no evidence of excess bleeding (81,82).

Delayed treatment of ovarian cancer is discussed earlier in this chapter. However, this possibility cannot be overemphasized at laparoscopy or laparotomy. Maiman et al. (10) discussed this possibility at laparoscopy, and Trimbos et al. (5) documented that surgical staging was complete in only 53% of cases after one or two laparotomies.

HIGHLIGHTS

Bipolar coagulators, unipolar electrosurgery, thermal cautery, and lasers can be used to coagulate, vaporize, or excise tissue. Combining these techniques is better than concentrating on any one of them. Changes in the use of this equipment have been rapid, and attending update courses is essential in developing and maintaining optimal techniques.

REFERENCES

1. Nezhat C, Nezhat F. Comparison of different treatment methods of endometriomas by laparoscopy (letter to the editor). *Obstet Gynecol* 1992;79:315.
2. Parker WH, Berek JS. Management of selected cystic adnexal masses in postmenopausal women by operative laparoscopy: a pilot study. *Am J Obstet Gynecol* 1990;163:1574–1577.
3. Piver MS, Lele SB, Bakshi S, Parthasarathy KL, Emrich LJ. Five and ten year estimated survival and disease-free rates after intraperitoneal chromic phosphate; stage I ovarian adenocarcinoma. *Am J Clin Oncol* (CCT) 1988;11(5):515–519.
4. Schwartz PE. An oncologic view of when to do endoscopic surgery. *Clin Obstet Gynecol* 1991;34:467–472.
5. Trimbos JB, Schueler JA, van Lent M, Hermans J, Fleuren GJ. Reasons for incomplete surgical staging in early ovarian carcinoma. *Gynecol Oncol* 1990;37:374–377.
6. Webb MJ, Decker DG, Mussey E, Williams TJ. Factors influencing survival in stage I ovarian cancer. *Am J Obstet Gynecol* 1973;116:222–228.
7. Parker WH. Management of ovarian cysts by operative laparoscopy. *Contemp Ob/Gyn,* November 1991:47–48.
8. Rutledge FN. Neoplastic ovarian tumors. In: Te Linde RW, Mattingly RF, Thompson JD, eds. *Operative gynecology.* 6th ed. Philadelphia: JB Lippincott; 1985:877–907.
9. Dembo AJ, Davy M, Stenwig AE, Berle EJ, Bush RS, Kjorstad K. Prognostic factors in patients with stage I epithelial ovarian cancer. *Obstet Gynecol* 1990;75:263–273.
10. Maiman M, Seltzer V, Boyce J. Laparoscopic excision of ovarian neoplasms subsequently found to be malignant. *Obstet Gynecol* 1991;77:563–565.
11. Morales AJ, Murphy AA. Operative laparoscopy in gynecology. *Curr Probl Obstet Gynecol* 1992;March/April:73–102.
12. Young RC. Initial therapy for early ovarian carcinoma. *Cancer* 1987;60:2042–2049.
13. Fleischer AC. Transabdominal and transvaginal sonography of ovarian masses. *Clin Obstet Gynecol* 1991;34:433–442.
14. Scoutt LM, McCarthy SM. Imaging of ovarian masses: magnetic resonance imaging. *Clin Obstet Gynecol* 1991;34:443–451.
15. Schwartz PE. Ovarian masses: serologic markers. *Clin Obstet Gynecol* 1991;34:423–432.
16. Berchuck A, Boente MP, Bast RC. The use of tumor markers in the management of patients with gynecologic carcinomas. *Clin Obstet Gynecol* 1992;35:45–54.
17. Peterson HB, Hulka JF, Phillips JM. American Association of Gynecologic Laparoscopists' 1988 membership survey on operative laparoscopy. *J Reprod Med* 1990;35:587–589.
18. Herrmann UJ, Locher GW, Goldhirsch A. Sonographic patterns of ovarian tumors: prediction of malignancy. *Obstet Gynecol* 1987;69:777–781.
19. Diamond MP, Daniell JF, Feste J, et al. Adhesion reformation and de novo adhesion formation after reproductive pelvic surgery. *Fertil Steril* 1987;47:864–866.
20. Diamond MP, Daniell JF, Johns DA, et al. Postoperative adhesion development after operative laparoscopy: evaluation at early second-look procedures. *Fertil Steril* 1991;55:700–704.
21. Levine RL. Economic impact of pelviscopic surgery. *J Reprod Med* 1985;30:655–659.
22. Jordan AM. Hospital charges for laparoscopic and open cholecystectomy (letter to the editor). *JAMA* 1991;266:3425.
23. Voyles CR, Petro AB, Meena AL, Haick AJ, Koury AM. A practical approach to laparoscopic cholecystectomy. *Am J Surg* 1991;161:365–370.
24. Clayman RV, Kavoussi LR, Soper NJ, et al. Laparoscopic nephrectomy: initial case report. *J Urol* 1991;146:278–282.
25. Nezhat C, Nezhat FR. Safe laser endoscopic excision or vaporization of peritoneal endometriosis. *Fertil Steril* 1989;52:149–151.
26. Reich H. Laparoscopic treatment of extensive pelvic adhesions, including hydrosalpinx. *J Reprod Med* 1987;32:736–742.
27. Clarke HC. Laparoscopy—new instruments for suturing and ligation. *Fertil Steril* 1972;23:274–277.
28. Marrero MA, Corfman RS. Laparoscopic use of sutures. *Clin Obstet Gynecol* 1991;34:387–394.
29. Levy BS, Soderstrom RM. Electrical techniques in sterilization. In: Martin DC, ed. *Manual of endoscopy.* Santa Fe Springs: American Association of Gynecologic Laparoscopists, 1990:57–61.
30. Reich H, Vancaillie TG, Soderstrom RM. Electrical techniques. In: Martin DC, ed. *Manual of endoscopy.* Santa Fe Springs: American Association of Gynecologic Laparoscopists, 1990:105–112.
31. Luciano AA. Effects of electrosurgery and lasers on tissue. In: Martin DC, ed. *Manual of endoscopy.* Santa Fe Springs: American Association of Gynecologic Laparoscopists, 1990:23–30.
32. Luciano AA, Whitman G, Maier DB, Randolph J, Maenza R. A comparison of thermal injury, healing patterns, and postoperative adhesion formation following CO_2 laser and electromicrosurgery. *Fertil Steril* 1987;48:1025–1029.
33. Martin DC. Tissue effects of lasers. *Semin Reprod Endocrinol* 1991;9(2):127–137.
34. Martin DC. Tissue effects of lasers and electrosurgery. In: Sanfilippo JS, Vitale G, Perissat J, eds. *Atlas of laparoscopic general surgery.* Philadelphia: JB Lippincott; in press.
35. Semm K, Friedrich ER, eds. *Operative manual for endoscopic abdominal surgery.* Chicago: Year Book; 1987.

36. Harris DM, Werkhaven JA. Biophysics and applications of medical lasers. *Arch Otolaryngol Head Neck Surg* 1989;3:91–123.
37. Martin DC, Diamond MP, Yussman MA. Laser laparoscopy for infertility surgery. In: Sanfilippo JS, Levine RL, eds. *Operative gynecologic endoscopy.* New York: Springer-Verlag; 1989:211–235.
38. Joffe SN, Brackett KA, Sankar MY, Daikuzono N. Resection of the liver with the Nd:YAG laser. *Surg Gynecol Obstet* 1986;163:437–442.
39. Joffe SN, Foster J, Schroder T, Brackett K. Splenic resection with the contact Nd:YAG laser system. *J Ped Surg* 1988;23:829–834.
40. Shirk GJ. Use of the Nd:YAG laser for the treatment of endometriosis. *Am J Obstet Gynecol* 1989;160:1344–1351.
41. Martin DC, Diamond MP. Operative laparoscopy: comparison of lasers with other techniques. *Curr Probl Obstet Gynecol Fertil* 1986;9:563–601.
42. Hulka JF, Reich H. *Textbook of laparoscopy.* Philadelphia: WB Saunders; 1994:181–185.
43. Hasson HM. Laparoscopic management of ovarian cysts. *J Reprod Med* 1990;35:863–867.
44. Martin DC. Laparoscopic treatment of ovarian endometriosis. *Clin Obstet Gynecol* 1991;34:452–459.
45. Nezhat C, Winer WK, Nezhat F, Nezhat C. Laparoscopic treatment of endometriosis with laser and videocamera augmentation (videolaseroscopy). *J Gynecol Surg* 1989;5:163–169.
46. Donnez J, Nisolle M, Karaman Y, et al. CO_2 laser laparoscopy in peritoneal endometriosis and in ovarian endometrial cyst. *J Gynecol Surg* 1989;5:361–366.
47. Martin DC, Berry JD. Histology of chocolate cysts. *J Gynecol Surg* 1990;6:43–46.
48. Martin DC. Therapeutic laparoscopy. In: Martin DC, ed. *Laparoscopic appearance of endometriosis.* 2nd ed. vol 1. Memphis: Resurge Press; 1990:21–29.
49. Elkins TE, Stovall TG, Warren J, Ling FW, Meyer NL. A histologic evaluation of peritoneal injury and repair: implications for adhesion formation. *Obstet Gynecol* 1987;70:225–228.
50. Ellis H. The cause and prevention of postoperative intraperitoneal adhesions. *Surg Gynecol Obstet* 1971;133:497–511.
51. Ellis H. Internal overhealing: the problem of intraperitoneal adhesions. *World J Surg* 1980;4:303–306.
52. Nezhat CR, Nezhat FR, Metzger DA, Luciano AA. Adhesion reformation after reproductive surgery by videolaseroscopy. *Fertil Steril* 1990;53:1008–1011.
53. Armar NA, McGarrigle HHG, Honour J, Holownia P, Jacobs HS, Lachelin GCL. Laparoscopic ovarian diathermy in the management of anovulatory infertility in women with polycystic ovaries: endocrine changes and clinical outcome. *Fertil Steril* 1990;53:45–49.
54. Brumsted JR, Deaton J, Lavigne E, Riddick DH. Postoperative adhesion formation after ovarian wedge resection with and without ovarian reconstruction in the rabbit. *Fertil Steril* 1990;53:723–726.
55. Daniell JF, Miller W. Polycystic ovaries treated by laparoscopic laser vaporization. *Fertil Steril* 1989;51:232–236.
56. De Leon FD, Edwards M, Heine MW. A comparison of microsurgery and laser surgery for ovarian wedge resections. *Int J Fertil* 1990;35:177–179.
57. Portuondo JA, Melchor JC, Neyro JL, Alegre A. Periovarian adhesions following ovarian wedge resection or laparoscopic biopsy. *Endoscopy* 1984;16:143–145.
58. Reich H, McGlynn F. Treatment of ovarian endometriomas using laparoscopic surgical techniques. *J Reprod Med* 1986;31:577–584.
59. Martin DC. CO_2 laser laparoscopy for endometriosis associated with infertility. *J Reprod Med* 1986;31:1089–1094.
60. Batt RE, Udagawa SM, Wheeler JM. Endometriosis: microconservative surgery. In: Hunt RB, ed. *Atlas of female infertility surgery.* St. Louis: Mosby–Year Book, 1992:454–481.
61. Cohen BM. Surgery of the ovary, including anatomic derangements of the fimbrial-gonadal ovum-capture mechanism. In: Hunt RF, ed. *Atlas of female infertility surgery.* St. Louis: Mosby–Year Book, 1992:389–402.
62. Cook AS, Rock JA. The role of laparoscopy in the treatment of endometriosis. *Fertil Steril* 1991;55:663–680.
63. Adamyan LV, Myinbayev OA, Kulakov VI. Use of fibrin glue in obstetrics and gynecology: a review of the literature. *Int J Fertil* 1991;36:76–88.
64. Johns A. Laparoscopic oophorectomy/oophorocystectomy. *Clin Obstet Gynecol* 1991;34:460–466.
65. Luciano AA, Maier DB, Koch EI, Nulsen JC, Whitman GF. A comparative study of postoperative adhesions following laser surgery by laparoscopy versus laparotomy in the rabbit model. *Obstet Gynecol* 1989;74:220–224.
66. Lundorff P, Thorburn J, Hahlin M, Källfelt B, Lindblom B. Adhesion formation after laparoscopic surgery in tubal pregnancy: a randomized trial versus laparotomy. *Fertil Steril* 1991;55:911–915.
67. Diamond MP, Linsky CB, Cunningham T, et al. Adhesion reformation: reduction by the use of Interceed (TC7) plus heparin. *J Gynecol Surg* 1991;7:1–6.
68. Boyers S, Diamond M, DeCherney A. Reduction of postoperative pelvic adhesions in the rabbit with GORE-TEX® surgical membrane. *Fertil Steril* 1988;49:1066–1070.
69. Hasson HM. Open techniques for equipment insertion. In: Martin DC, ed. *Manual of endoscopy.* Santa Fe Springs: American Association of Gynecologic Laparoscopists, 1990:23–29.
70. Jarrett JC. Laparoscopy: direct trocar insertion without pneumoperitoneum. *Obstet Gynecol* 1990;75:725–727.
71. Kaali SG, Bartfai G. Direct insertion of the laparoscopic trocar after an earlier laparotomy. *J Reprod Med* 1988;33:739–740.
72. Kleppinger RK. Closed techniques for equipment insertion. In: Martin DC, ed. *Manual of endoscopy.* Santa Fe Springs: American Association of Gynecologic Laparoscopists, 1990:15–22.
73. Daniell JF. Laparoscopic enterolysis for chronic abdominal pain. *J Gynecol Surg* 1989;5:61–66.
74. Gomel V. Operative laparoscopy: time for acceptance. *Fertil Steril* 1989;52:1–11.
75. Murphy AA. Operative laparoscopy. *Fertil Steril* 1987;47:1–18.
76. Sutton C, MacDonald R. Laser laparoscopic adhesiolysis. *J Gynecol Surg* 1990;6:155–159.
77. Nager CW, Murphy AA. Ectopic pregnancy. *Clin Obstet Gynecol* 1991;34:403–411.
78. Gadir AA, Mowafi RS, Alnaser HMI, Alrashid AH, Alonezi OM, Shaw RW. Ovarian electrocautery versus human menopausal gonadotrophins and pure follicle-stimulating hormone therapy in the treatment of patients with polycystic ovarian disease. *Clin Endocrinol* 1990;33:585.
79. Kojima E, Yanagibori A, Otaka K, Hirakawa S. Ovarian wedge resection with contact Nd:YAG laser irradiation used laparoscopically. *J Reprod Med* 1989;34:444–446.
80. Sumioki H, Utsunomyiya T, Matsuoka K, Korenaga M, Kadota T. The effect of laparoscopic multiple punch resection of the ovary on hypothalamo-pituitary axis in polycystic ovary syndrome. *Obstet Gynecol Survey* 1989;44:208–210.
81. Sutton C. The limitations of laparoscopic ovarian biopsy. *J Obstet Gynaecol Br Commonw* 1974;81:317–321.
82. Esposito JM, Rubino G. Bleeding after ovarian biopsy under laparoscopic vision. *Am J Obstet Gynecol* 1974;119:857–858.

Endoscopic Management of Gynecologic Disease,
edited by G.D. Adamson and D.C. Martin.
Lippincott-Raven Publishers, Philadelphia © 1996.

CHAPTER 16

Laparoscopic Myomectomy

Harrith M. Hasson

Laparoscopic myomectomy is the disengagement and removal of myomas and the management of the operative uterine defect by laparoscopic means. Myomectomy is becoming increasingly popular as a reproductive procedure. Patients who are not interested in fertility but wish to preserve their uteri are also requesting myomectomy rather than hysterectomy when surgery is indicated. The main disadvantages of traditional myomectomy using the laparotomy approach have been the association with considerable blood loss intraoperatively, prolonged morbidity postoperatively, and adhesion formation. With regard to these, laparoscopy may offer several distinct advantages over laparotomy.

Laparoscopy entails remote manipulation of tissues with instruments directed through a limited number of access points, which are made by small incisions into a distended closed abdomen. Surgery is conducted by observing and interacting with images displayed on a video monitor; these are processed by a camera connected to the laparoscope. With this approach, the abdominal wall is not impaired by a large incision and retraction thereof, the bowel is not traumatized by application of surgical sponges and retractors, and organs are not dried out by room air or touched by human hands. Furthermore, the magnification realized by videolaparoscopy facilitates careful microsurgical dissection of tissues and occlusion of blood vessels before they are transected. This results in less operative trauma and blood loss during surgery.

In our experience, laparoscopic myomectomy has been associated with reduced intra- and postoperative morbidity, shorter hospital stay and recovery time, earlier return to normal activities, fewer postoperative adhesions, better cosmetic scars, and improved documentation as compared to traditional abdominal myomectomy.

H. M. Hasson: Department of Obstetrics and Gynecology, Grant Hospital of Chicago; and Rush Medical College, Chicago, Illinois 60614-0898.

INDICATIONS AND CONTRAINDICATIONS

Uterine leiomyoma is the most common gynecologic tumor. It occurs in 20–25% of all women. It is the most common indication for hysterectomy in the United States, accounting for over 175,000 cases annually (1). Although myomectomy with uterine preservation is less common, 33,000 procedures were performed in the United States in 1988 (2).

Myomectomy by laparoscopy is indicated only if the lesion is associated with one or more of the following:

1. Infertility, including recurrent abortion, with or without associated factors.
2. Bleeding, pain, and pressure symptoms of significant nature and duration in patients wishing to conceive or to maintain childbearing potential or simply to preserve their uteri.
3. Pelvic mass with uterine size greater than 12 gestational weeks, a dominant myoma greater than 7 cm, or a rapidly growing tumor.

Laparoscopic myomectomy is generally contraindicated under the following circumstances:

1. A patient's medical condition, including degree of obesity, makes it inadvisable to maintain her in Trendelenberg position with her abdomen distended with gas for an extended period of time.
2. Uterine size greater than 18 gestational weeks or dominant myoma greater than 15 cm.
3. Patient has advanced disease with diffuse leiomyomatosis or more than six significant myomas ≥3 cm.
4. Patient has a submucous myoma protruding more than 50% into the endometrial cavity.

In cases of unsuspected adenomyosis, it is best to refrain from dissecting the mass beyond making the diagnosis, since there are no cleavage planes.

PREOPERATIVE ASSESSMENT AND PREPARATION

The diagnosis of leiomyoma is usually made by pelvic examination and confirmed by ultrasound. Although ultrasound remains the primary imaging modality for the evaluation of myomas, it has certain technical limitations. It is not accurate in patients with excessive obesity (3), congenital uterine anomalies (4) or in those with marked uterine enlargement or submucous lesions (5). Many of these difficulties are overcome with magnetic resonance imaging (MRI). MRI appears to be capable of localizing the position of lesions within the uterus (3–5), predicting their number (4,5), and discovering degenerative changes occuring within the lesions (4,5). Furthermore, MRI has been successfully utilized to differentiate between leiomyomas and adenomyosis. In one report, the imaging modality correctly distinguished adenomyosis from leiomyomas in 92 of 93 patients (6). In that study, 71 of the patients had leiomyomas only, 16 had adenomyosis, and 6 had both lesions. The endometrial cavity should be evaluated with hysteroscopy or hysterosalpingography (HSG), and endometrial sampling should be performed as indicated.

Medical treatments are employed to reduce myoma size prior to surgery. DeCherney et al. (7) noted significant reductions in the size of myomas when the patients were treated with 800 mg of danazol daily for 6 months. Measurements were made by ultrasound and repeated at 3 and 6 months. Currently, use of this pharmacologic agent has been largely supplanted by gonadotropin-releasing hormone agonists (GnRHa).

GnRHa and their more potent analogs represent promising though temporary therapeutic modalities for the treatment of leiomyomas, mainly through induction of a reversible state of hypogonadotropic hypogonadism. Initial administration causes a burst of released gonadotropins from the pituitary gland, which in turn causes a flare of estrogen production from the ovary. Continued administration of GnRHa induces a state of desensitization to further stimulation and down-regulation of gonadotropic receptors in the pituitary. This results in sustained suppression of gonadotropins and marked abatement of ovarian steroidogenesis. Follicular maturation and growth is arrested and a state of hypoestrogenism ensues. GnRHa may have an additional inhibitory role on the growth of leiomyomas through direct action on specific GnRH binding sites in the tumors (8).

Inducing a hypoestrogenic state with GnRH-a has several advantages, some disadvantages, and temporal limitations. Ovulation is inhibited (9–12); the ensuing amenorrhea or hypomenorrhea improves the patients hematologic profile (10–12). Reductions in the volume and vascularity of myomas and the host uterus relieves associated symptoms, reduces intraoperative blood loss, and facilitates removal of the tumor masses during laparoscopic surgery. Shrinkage of the uterine volume was reported to have a mean of 36% at 12 weeks and 45% at 24 weeks (12) and a range of 35–57% (13). Less intraoperative blood loss was noted in patients treated with GnRH-a as compared with controls in groups of patients managed with conventional abdominal hysterectomy (14) (235 vs. 350 ml) and conventional abdominal myomectomy (10) (213 vs. 302 ml). The same benefits are expected with laparoscopic myomectomy.

The induced hypoestrogenic state has several unpleasant side effects, including vasomotor flushes, insomnia, mood changes, headache, and vaginal dryness (9–13). A larger concern relates to the potential of trabecular bone loss with long-term administration. However, studies indicate that women treated with GnRHa for 6 months or less suffer no irreversible decreases in bone density (12). Preoperative GnRHa therapy should not be given for longer than 6 months, especially since it has been shown that near maximal benefits are achieved by 12 weeks (9,12).

Apprehensions about effects on lipid metabolism linger. Freidman et al. (12) reported small increases in total cholesterol and low density lipoprotein (LDL) cholesterol in patients treated with leuprolide acetate. Mean concentrations of high-density lipoprotein (HDL) cholesterol did not change. The degree of risk of an adverse cardiovascular occurence due to the small cholesterol changes during the 3- to 6-month treatment period is not known (12). Other concerns include delay in the diagnosis of uterine sarcoma (11,15–17), concealment of small myomas (18), and degeneration of large myomas necessitating piecemeal enucleation (11). Following termination of GnRHa therapy, menses usually return within 3 months and leiomyomas return to pretreatment size within 6 months (10,12).

Current GnRHa formulations available in the United States include leuprolide acetate depot 3.75 mg to be administered intramuscularly every 4 weeks and nafarelin acetate nasal spray 400 μg to be administered twice daily. As compared to the intranasal route, the depot formulation appears to have a more reproducible suppression effect and an improved compliance rate (13).

MYOMECTOMY AND MALIGNANCY

Uterine leiomyosarcomas are rare mesenchymal tumors that arise within a myoma or de novo from the myometrium (19). The incidence of sarcomatous degeneration in surgically removed leiomyomas is between 0.1% and 0.5% (20,21). The incidence increases steadily from the fourth to the sixth decade of life (21). The fundamental criterion for assessing malignancy of the tumor is the number of mitotic figures per unit of tissue. Authorities differ in their justification of the diagnosis of leiomyosarcoma: the number of mitotic figures varies from 5 per 10 high-power fields (H-PF) (21,22) to 10 per 10 H-PF (21,22) to 2 per any H-PF (19). The degree of

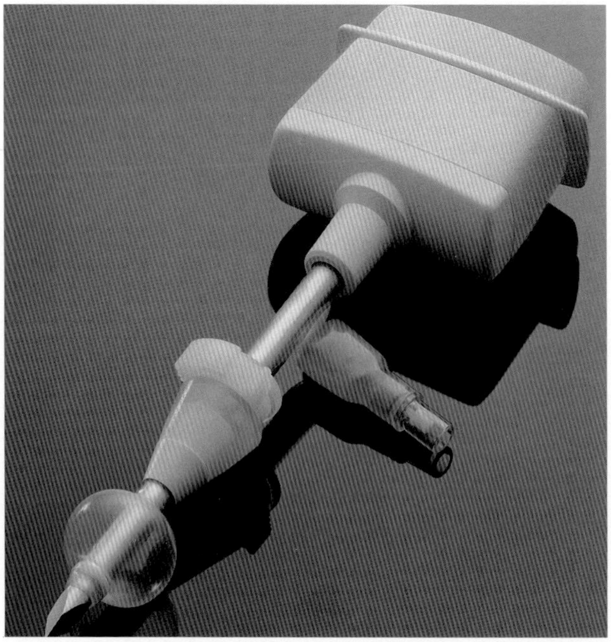

FIG. 1. Stable access cannula (SAC). Marlow Surgical Technologies, Willoughby, OH.

malignancy is directly related to the number of mitotic figures per H-PF. It has been reported that patients with lesions arising in leiomyomas have significantly better prognoses than those with primary myosarcoma (19). It was also shown that patients younger than 50 years of age have significantly better prognoses than older patients (23). In another study, the 5-year survival of premenopausal patients was 93%, that of postmenopausal patients 50% (19). The finding of unsuspected leiomyosarcoma in a laparoscopic myomectomy specimen poses a difficult therapeutic dilemma in younger patients wishing to conceive. Although hysterectomy is a safer approach, preserving the uterus may be a viable alternative if the patient understands and accepts the risk. Only one of six patients who had myomectomy alone for leiomyosarcoma arising in a myoma developed recurrence (19).

With the increased popularity of GnRHa therapy for preoperative preparation of patients with symptomatic leiomyomas, some of the patients presumed to have myomas may actually have sarcomas. The effect of GnRHa on sarcomatous lesions is variable. After 3 months of therapy, the uterine mass did not change in size in a 46-

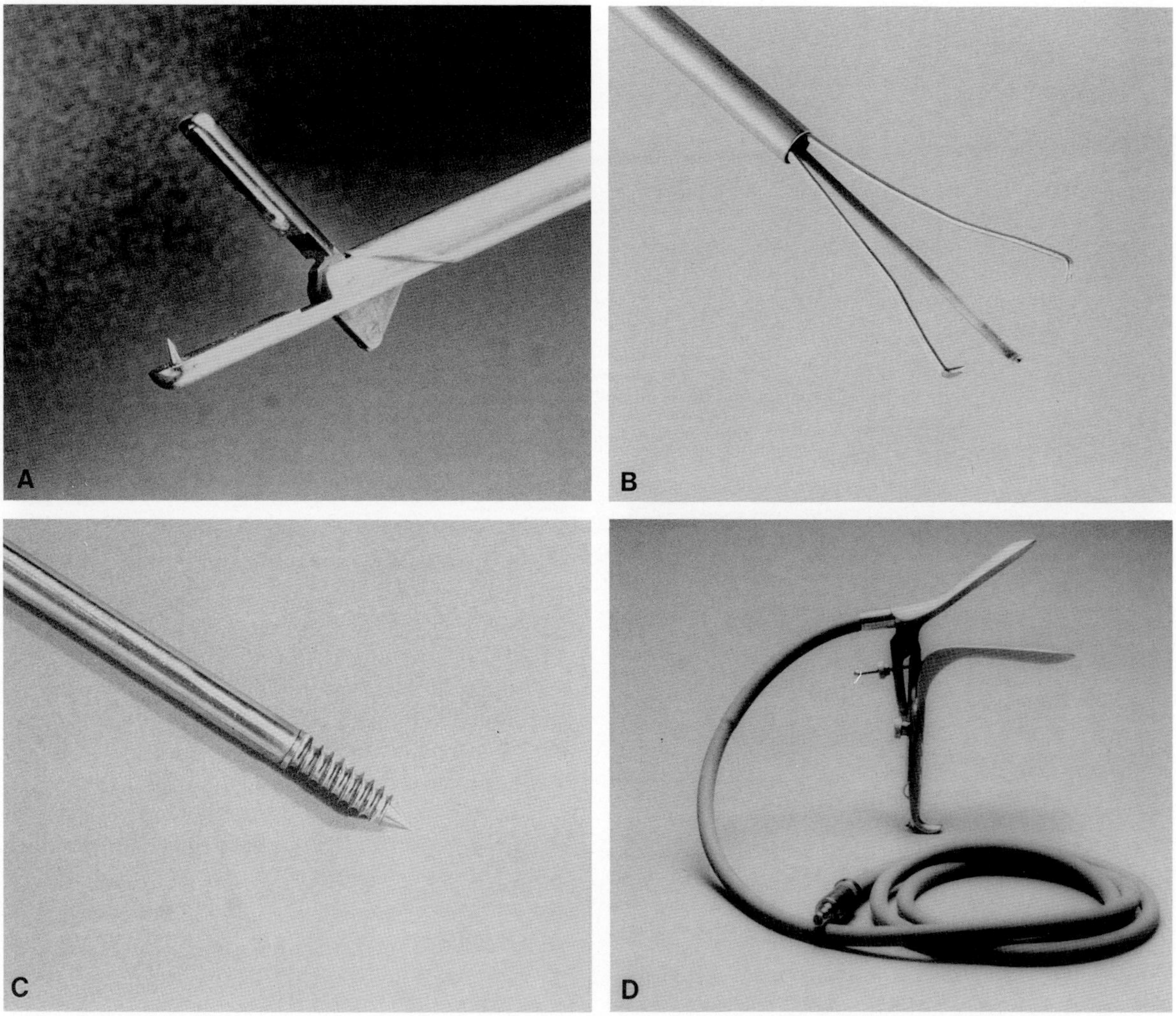

FIG. 2. Special instruments for laparoscopic myomectomy. **A**: Toothed forceps. **B**: Bulldog grasper. **C**: Myoma drill, 5 mm. **D**: Vaginal speculum with fiberoptic light. (From ref. 29, with permission.)

year-old woman (15) and grew larger in a 39-year-old patient who also experienced irregular uterine bleeding during the treatment (16). In a third report of patients with leiomyosarcoma who received GnRHa therapy, a 41-year-old woman with a 10-cm mass consistent with leiomyoma started bleeding profusely after 2 months of therapy (17). These reports imply that the occurrence of irregular or profuse uterine bleeding, the lack of a shrinkage response, or the presence of a paradoxical growth response during GnRHa treatment of leiomyomas suggests the possibility of malignancy and calls for further evaluation or prompt surgical management.

The direct inhibitory effect of GnRHa on myomatous tissue as well as the reduced blood supply to the tumor secondary to the hypoestrogenic state may cause intense degenerative changes in larger myomas. Such alterations, previously noted with progestin therapy (24), were associated with cellular transmutations including augmented mitotic activity (25). Laborious piecemeal enucleation of affected tumors during laparoscopic myomectomy is one anticipated difficulty with GnRHa–dependent degeneration; Meyer et al. (15) point out another: the potential for a more complicated diagnosis of malignancy.

INSTRUMENTATION

Laparoscopic myomectomy requires the availability of an appropriate video camera system and laparoscope, an electronic high-flow insufflator, and a properly functioning electrocautery unit. According to Semm, other energy sources, such as the CO_2 laser, fiberoptic lasers, and endocoagulation, are useful alternatives.

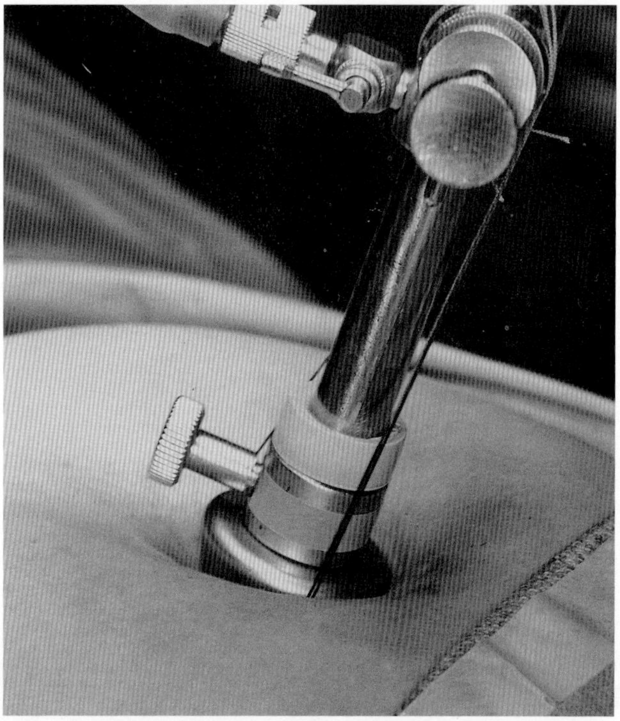

FIG. 3. Creation of an airtight seal following pulling of the fascial sutures snugly into the holders of the open laparoscopy cannula. (From ref. 41, with permission.)

Instruments needed for this operation include cannulas to secure stable access to the operative field (see Fig. 1); appliances to effect uterine elevation; and tools for incision, cutting, grasping, manipulating and suturing. Other preferred implements include a plastic pouch to collect and retrieve multiple tumor specimens and a vaginal speculum with attached fiberoptic light to furnish brilliant illumination of the vaginal apex during vaginal extraction. Other instruments that I prefer include a holding forceps with a spike, a Bulldog grasper, and a myoma drill to hold, fix, and manipulate the tumor mass (see Fig. 2). Open laparoscopy is used routinely to gain primary access to the abdomen (Fig. 3).

PROCEDURE

Many of the steps of this procedure call for coordinated movements between two individuals. In patients with deep intramural, cervical, or broad ligament lesions, the availability of a capable associate surgeon or assistant is indispensable. Laparoscopic myomectomy requires three ancillary access ports in the midline, right and left lower quadrants of the abdomen. The position of the points of access depends on the size of the uterus: the larger the uterus, the higher the points of entry. The steps of the procedure may be divided into disengaging the myoma from its uterine bed, managing the uterine defect, and removing the myoma(s) from the abdomen.

1. Disengaging the myomas. Hemostasis is accomplished during laparoscopic myomectomy by injecting vasopressin, 10 μm diluted in 40 ml of normal saline, subserosally into the myometrium at the base of the myoma and the pseudocapsule, thereby covering the incisional site, and by coagulating blood vessels before they are severed during dissection. Precise coagulation is assisted by the magnification afforded by video laparoscopy. Although not always possible, a vertical uterine incision in the midline places it in the relatively avascular area of the uterus (see Fig. 4). More than one myoma can be removed from one extended vertical midline incision. Additional vertical incisions are placed as needed. (I do not use transverse incisions except for pedunculated myomas, which are excised at the base of the pedicle.)

The incision is carried through the pseudocapsule into the myoma until the characteristic pearly white, whorly appearance of the leiomyoma is clearly appreciated. At this point it is helpful to fix and manipulate the tumor by turning the myoma drill into the substance. Against such force of traction, countertraction applied at the cut edges of the pseudocapsule helps to identify connective tissue bridges connecting the myoma to the host uterus. Many

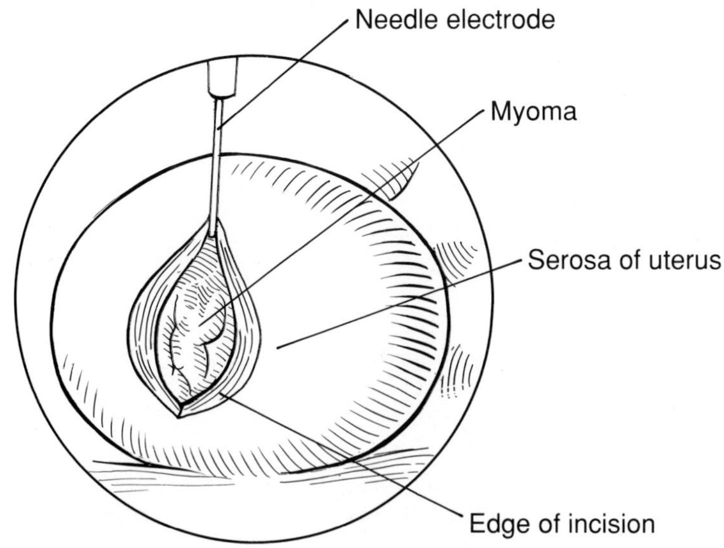

FIG. 4. Vertical uterine incision made with a unipolar cautery needle electrode.

of these bridges are avascular. Some contain feeding and drainage vessels. Although much of the blood supply to the myoma is localized within a major vascular pedicle, radiographic studies have shown that blood supply to the tumor comes from more than one internal nutrient artery and in the form of peripheral vessels (20). Placing a probe in the proper cleavage plane between the uterus and myoma and firmly—but gently—prying the tumor out of its bed is a useful procedure to facilitate disengagement, (see Fig. 5). This maneuver simply breaks up small avascular connecting bridges and allows the tumor to emerge from its bed. Vascular bridges and pedicles are coagulated preferably with bipolar cautery before they are cut. Once the myoma is substantially out of its bed, the myoma drill is replaced by the grasper and strong secure traction is applied in various directions to clearly expose remaining bridges as well as the primary vascular pedicle (see Fig. 6). Following coagulation, these are cut and the myoma is freed from its uterine bed.

At times, following incision of the pseudocapsule, the familiar whorled appearance and rubbery consistency of a leiomyoma are replaced by a soft, spongy consistency and a homogeneous appearance of a degenerating mass of tissue. This may result from benign conditions that diminish blood supply to the tumor, such as use of GnRHa or malignant transformation. Benign degeneration cannot be differentiated from sarcomatous change by gross examination. In suspicious cases, the surgeon should obtain a frozen section.

2. *Managing the operative defect.* For pedunculated,

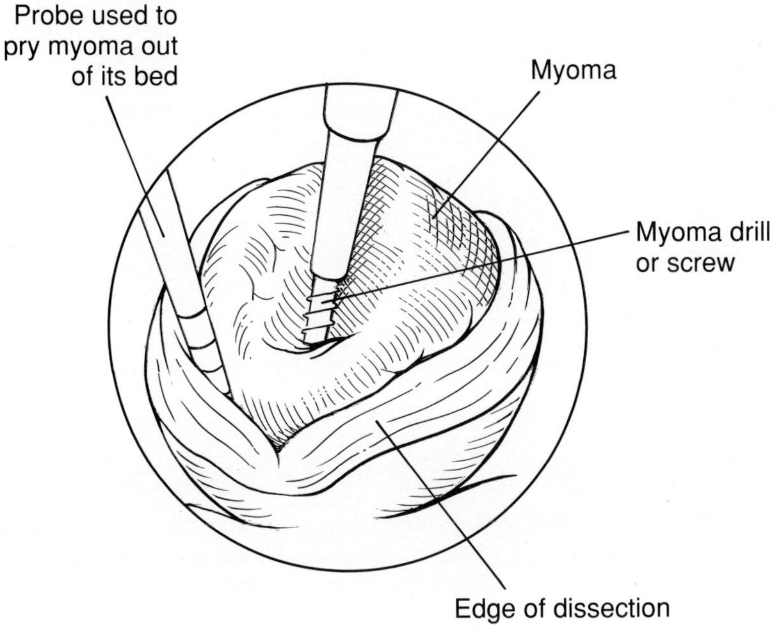

FIG. 5. The myoma is fixed and manipulated with a myoma drill and is pried out of its bed with a probe.

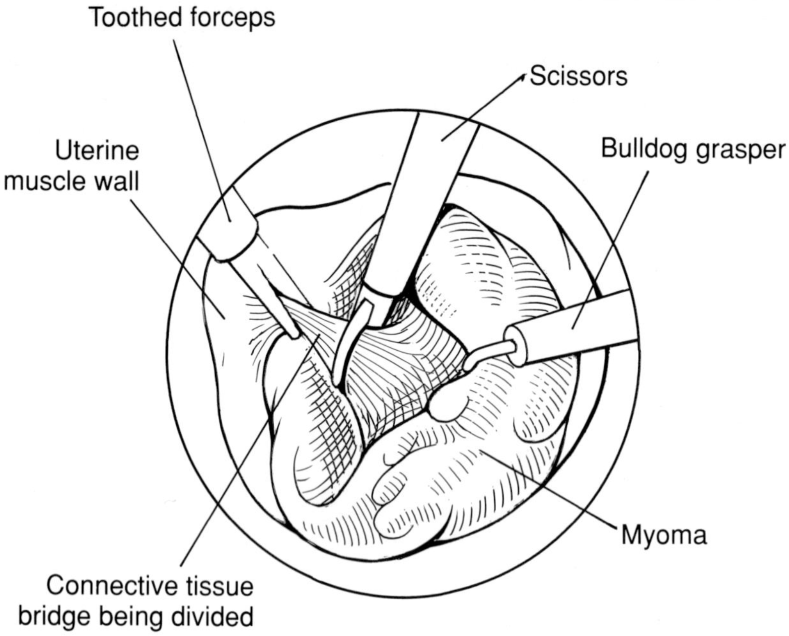

FIG. 6. Exposure of connective tissue bridges between tumor and uterus with traction and countertraction maintained with a Bulldog grasper and toothed forceps. (From ref. 29, with permission.)

subserosal, and intraligamentary leiomyomas, the edges of the operative site are coagulated to achieve hemostasis and the site is covered with Tc-7 (Interceed, Ethicon, Cincinnati, OH), as indicated. For superficial intramural tumors and following hemostasis (see Fig. 7), the uterine defect is approximated with one continuous suture using a baseball-type stitch that includes the serosa (see Fig. 8). The needle through the noose knot secures the beginning of the suture (see Fig. 9); and the half-hitch end knot secures the end (26) (see Fig. 10). Alternatively, a knot is formed on the suture line, a staple is applied inside the knot, the combination of a staple backed by a knot is used to secure the beginning of the suture line, and the end is secured with the application of one or more staples (27).

For deep intramural myomas (with or without a submucous component), we add one or more layers of interrupted sutures to close the myoma bed. A small curved needle, such as a CT-2 needle, with a 2-0 polyglactin suture is most suitable. The needle is rotated in the plane of the layer to be approximated and the suture is tied with extracorporeal Roeder loop knots or the throws are brought down individually with a knot pusher. While the surgeon sutures with a curved needle, it is best to lift the edge of the tissue to be sutured off the plane with a grasping forceps and to drive the needle in

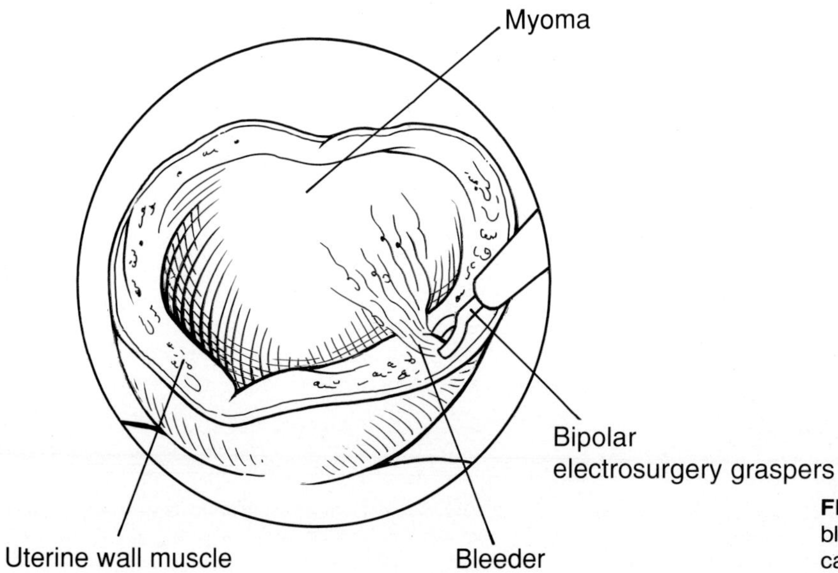

FIG. 7. Achieving hemostasis by coagulating bleeders at the wound edges with bipolar cautery.

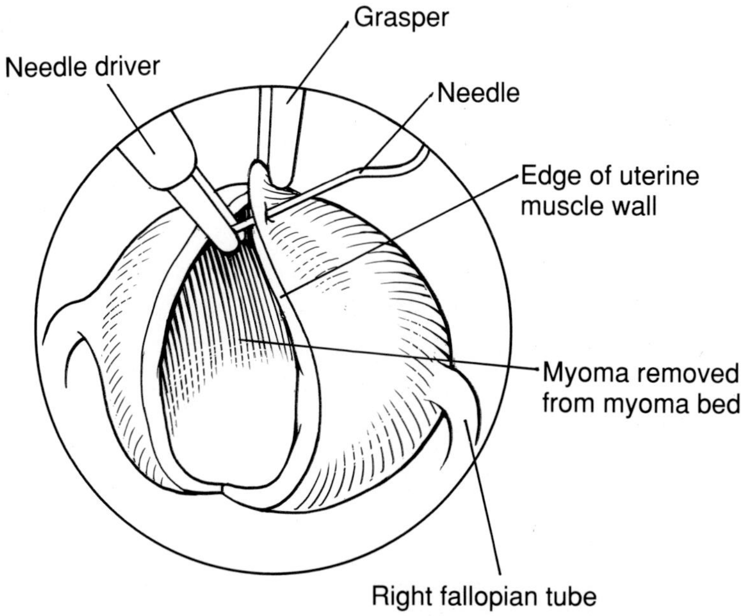

FIG. 8. Begining of a baseball stitch to close superficial uterine defect.

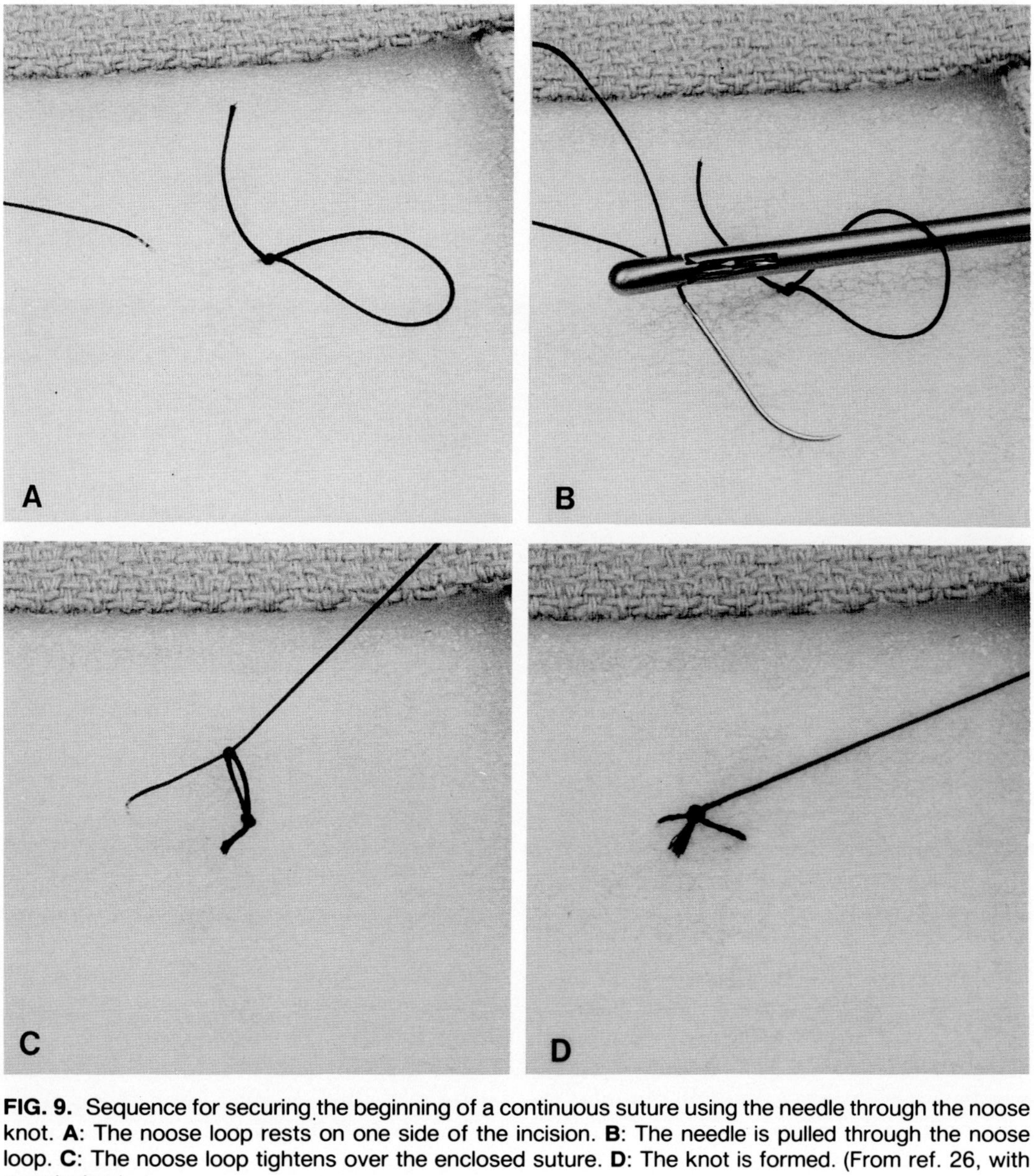

FIG. 9. Sequence for securing the beginning of a continuous suture using the needle through the noose knot. **A**: The noose loop rests on one side of the incision. **B**: The needle is pulled through the noose loop. **C**: The noose loop tightens over the enclosed suture. **D**: The knot is formed. (From ref. 26, with permission.)

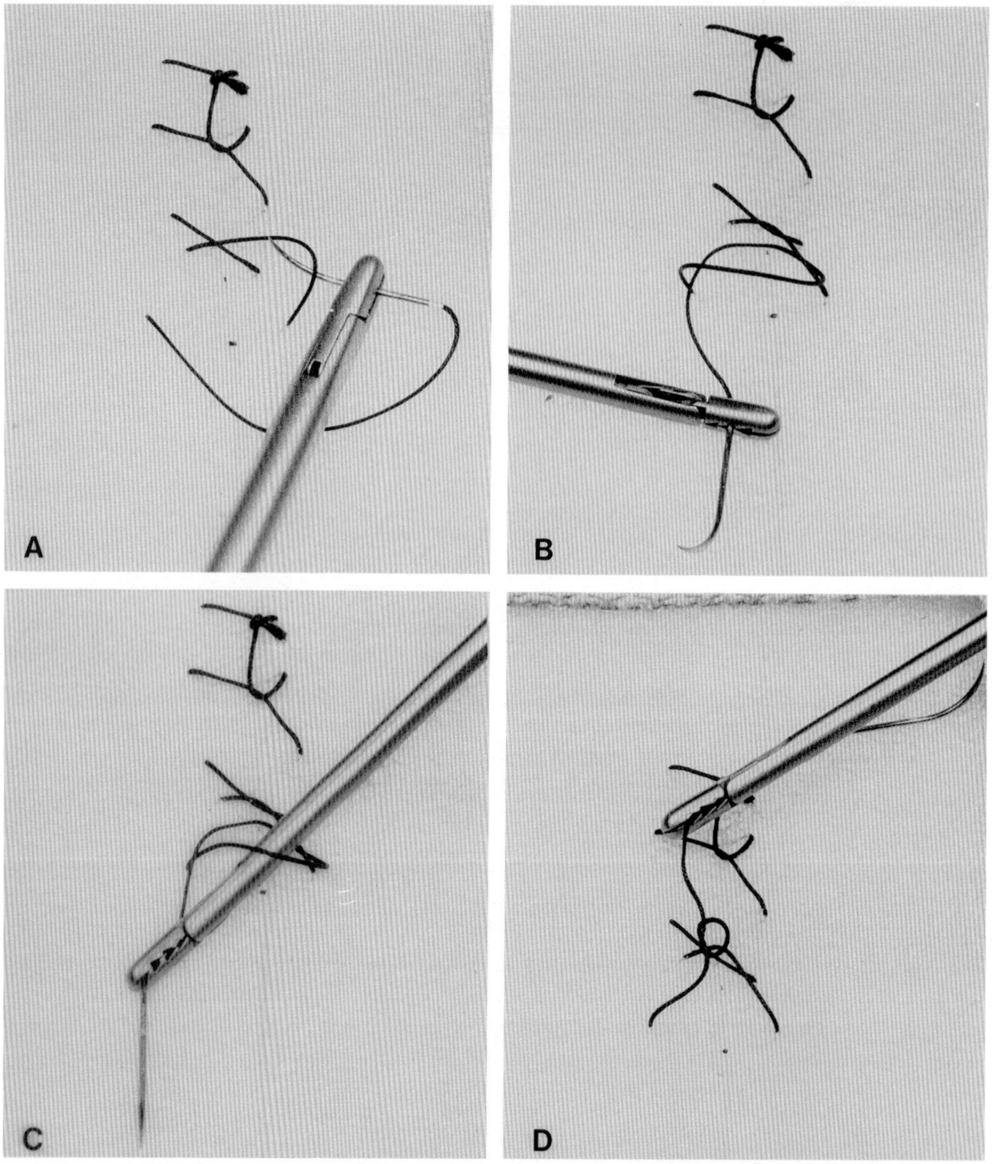

FIG. 10. Sequence for completing a continuous suture using the half-hitch end knot. **A**: The needle is passed under the loop of the last stitch. **B**: The second loop is formed within remaining suture. **C**: The knot-forming end of suture is pulled into the loop. **D**: The knot-forming end is pulled out of the loop to tighten the sliding knot over the enclosed suture. (From ref. 26, with permission.)

the plane using a twisting rotational movement. Whenever sutures are used, a layer of Interceed (Tc-7) should be applied to the dry, sutured site (see Fig. 11) to mitigate the development of adhesions.

We now follow the principle of using staples as markers for subsequent evaluation of the uterine scar by hysterosalpingogram (HSG), as described by Beyth and Ohel (28). One staple is applied to tissues beneath the serosa near each end of the incision, and additional staples are similarly placed along the length of the incision and spaced at regular intervals of 1.5 cm. Use of a curved needle requires the use of at least one 10-mm cannula to introduce the needle into and extract it out of the abdomen.

3. Removing the myoma(s). Following excision, individual myomas are stored in the cul-de-sac and then removed jointly by either an abdominal or a vaginal approach.

For one or two myomas ≤5 cm in size, we use the orange peel technique: the myoma is held securely on both ends with Bulldog or other toothed graspers, put on the stretch, and cut with a scissors so as to convert it to a long narrow strip of tissue (see Fig. 12). The myoma strips are removed though an 11-mm cannula.

For larger myomas in a patient with good vaginal elasticity and a wide vaginal fornix, we utilize the vaginal approach. We either tent the vagina cephalad with uterine dressing forceps and cut an incision, from above, be-

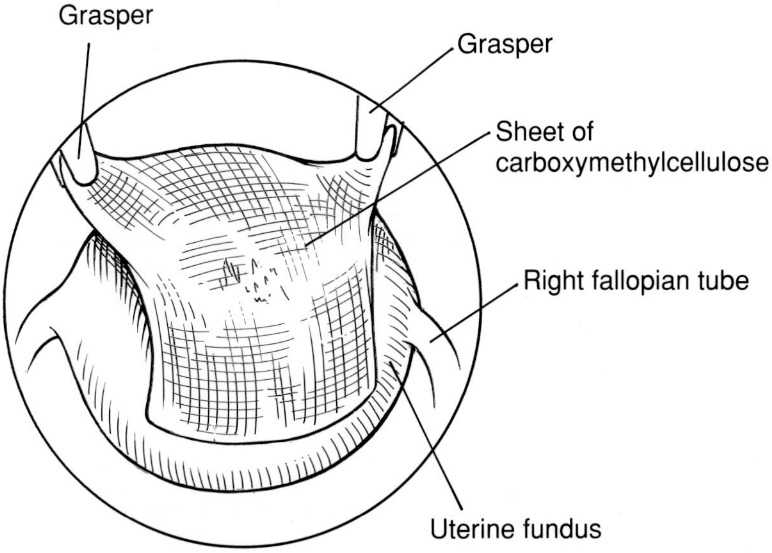

FIG. 11. Applying a sheet of Tc-7 over the operative site.

tween the slightly spread jaws of the forceps; or we push a myoma into the vaginal fornix from above and cut the incision, from below, using the vaginal bulge as a landmark (see Fig. 13). The incision may be enlarged and the specimen delivered into the vaginal defect from above, grasped with a tenaculum from below, and removed. The vaginal incision is closed from below with a continuous suture. Since the pressure in the abdomen is always higher than that of the vagina, the irrigation fluid and insufflation gas in the pelvis always move in one direction: from the pelvis to the vagina. Such circumstances recreate conditions of laminar flow and prevent abdominal contamination with vaginal flora.

For even larger myomas or large myomas in patients with inadequate vaginal elasticity or multiple myomas, we withdraw the tumors from the abdomen through a minilaparotomy incision using the externalization technique. An additional 10-mm cannula is introduced into the abdomen in the midline through a suprapubic incision placed at the pubic hair line. In the case of multiple myomas, a pouch is introduced into the abdomen through this extraction port and the stored myomas are

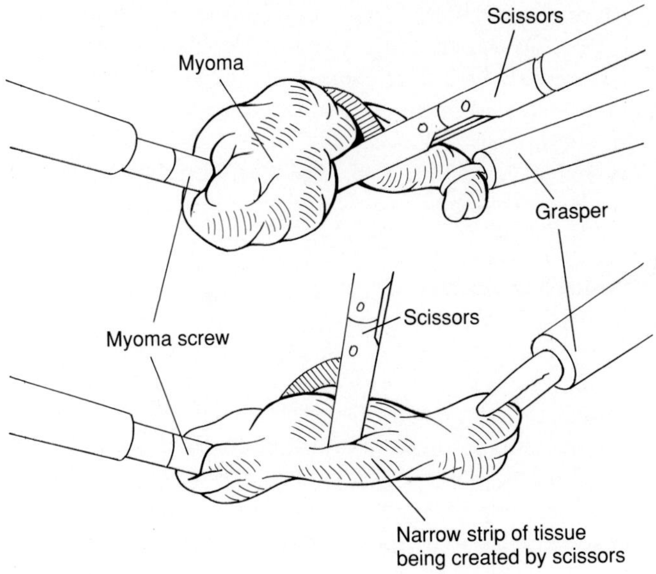

FIG. 12. Converting a myoma to a narrow strip of tissue with the "orange peel" technique. (From ref. 29, with permission.)

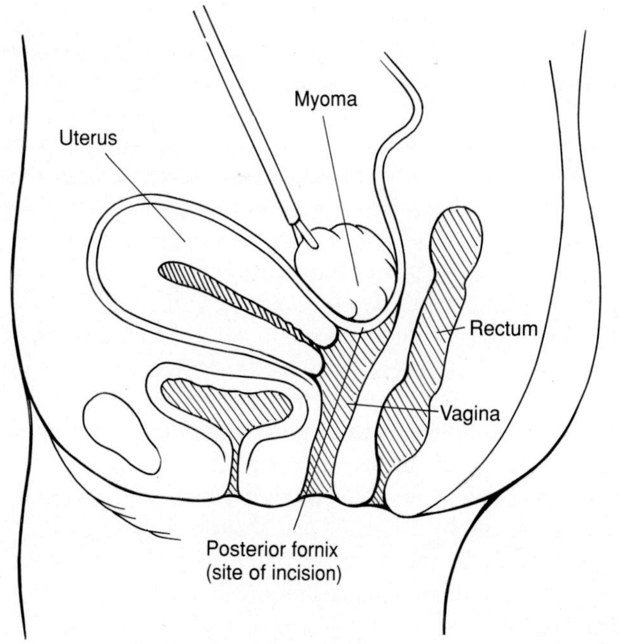

FIG. 13. Pushing the myoma from above to establish a bulge for safe vaginal incision, from below.

placed into the pouch, which is then closed and pulled up against the abdominal incision. In the case of one large tumor, a myoma drill is inserted into the abdomen through the extraction port and turned into the stabilized tumor to fix it securely. The mass is then pulled up against the incision. Two additional tumor masses can be captured and retained using Bulldog graspers introduced through each of the right and left ancillary ports.

In any case, the 10-mm skin incision is then enlarged to 3–5 cm according to the size of the mass, the fascial incision is similarly extended, the muscles are separated in the midline, the peritoneal defect is sought and enlarged with retractors, and the specimen is pulled from the abdomen with the use of one or more tenaculums. Masses captured by Bulldog graspers are brought under the enlarged extraction port and lifted out of the abdomen with one or more tenaculums. The prongs of the Bulldog grasper are retracted under vision and then the forceps are withdrawn from the abdomen. Larger specimens are morcellated *outside* of the abdomen after bringing the leading edge of the tumor out of the incisional gap. Following removal of the myomas, the fascia is approximated and the abdomen is reinflated for final inspection and lavage.

Another alternative is the use of the Semm 20-mm trocar and morcellation system. The trocar is introduced into the abdomen through a suprapubic incision. The tumor is grasped with a sharp grasper or is pinned with a corkscrew-type instrument; a cylinder with distal sharp teeth is brought down into the tumor mass to drill out a core or a cylinder of tissue; and the process is repeated until the myoma is completely removed.

CLINICAL EXPERIENCE

Preoperative Case Selection and Preparation

Our group previously reported our preliminary results in 56 patients (29). With increased experience based on more than 90 patients over a 4-year period, we have more clearly defined our case selection criteria. We use GnRHa in patients with leiomyomas larger than 6 cm in diameter and prefer to administer depot leuprolide acetate 3.75 mg in monthly injections until suppression of estradiol (E2) to levels less than 20 pg/ml is achieved for at least 2 months, provided that the duration of therapy does not exceed 6 months. The treatment is started in the midluteal or early follicular phase of the menstrual cycle but not at midcycle to avoid an excessive estrogen flare (9). Large uterine masses are shrunk down to 16–18 weeks gestation size with GnRHa therapy; larger masses cannot be removed laparoscopically because of space limitations.

The medical treatment is monitored with pelvic examination, monthly E2 assessment, and periodic ultrasound evaluations. We have not as yet used magnetic resonance imaging (MRI) for monitoring purposes. Although we have removed up to 14 myomas from one patient, we generally try to limit laparoscopic myomectomy to patients with four or fewer significant myomas (>3 cm). Freidman et al. (30) reported a significantly higher ultrasound recurrence rate for surgically treated patients with more than three leiomyomas when they were followed for 27–38 months. Interestingly, most of the recurrent myomas detected by ultrasound were not associated with clinical symptoms at the time of evaluation.

Operative Data

Generally, our estimated blood loss (EBL) is between 50 and 100 ml, depending on the number, size, and location of the leiomyomas. To date, no blood transfusions were given to any patient and there were no laparotomies. The mean EBL in our report was 75 ml (29). Other studies on laparoscopic myomectomy report comparable amounts of blood loss, with ranges of 5–200 (31) and 10–600 ml (32), and a mean of 78 ml (31). Reports on myomectomy by CO_2 laser laparotomy each give a higher mean EBL of 150 ml (33) and 200 ml (34). Studies on myomectomy by laparotomy without the use of lasers give even higher mean EBL values of 300 ml (35) and 311 ml (34).

Our operative time has continued to decrease with increasing experience and the development of better methods of tissue removal from the abdomen. Currently, the usual range is between 1 and 3 hr, depending on technical complexity. Tissue examinations of the leiomyomas have revealed various benign degenerative changes in about 30%, adenomyosis in 7%, and calcification in 5% of cases. To date, we have not encountered a leiomyosarcoma.

Postoperative Data

The hospital stay was a day or less in all but three patients. The reason for a second day of hospital stay was related to logistics in one patient (she needed to have bladder polyps surgery) and conservative follow-up in another (she was our first patient to undergo abdominal myomectomy through a minilaparotomy incision). The third patient had febrile morbidity associated with upper respiratory tract infection and significant subcutaneous emphysema. She stayed 4 days during which time her symptoms subsided. The most frequent complication—noted in four patients—was the development of subcutaneous emphysema from leakage of pneumoperitoneum gas around secondary sleeves into the subcutaneous space. The problem occurred during extended procedures where repeated instrument exchanges and manipulations over time caused the secondary incisions to stretch about the ancillary sleeves, thereby permitting CO_2 gas to permeate in the subcutaneous tissue plane. This was aggravated by the fact that the secondary sleeves were placed into loose incisions and, thus, were vulnerable to being pulled out of the abdomen with each unguarded instrument exchange. Replacing the sleeves into the abdomen with or without a trocar further compromised the integrity of the abdominal wall and accelerated the rate of gas leakage into the subcutaneous tissues. This problem ceased to occur after we began using the cannula shown in Fig. 1. Access to the subcutaneous space was occluded by the apposition of the device's cone against the balloon at the incisional site.

The occurrence of postoperative pelvic adhesions is a complex, multifactorial phenomenon. Although many of the factors are related to surgical technique, others are not. We strongly recommend routine second-look laparoscopy 3 weeks after surgery for all patients who have undergone laparoscopic myomectomy for reproductive reasons. At that time, the presence of adhesions and the condition of the repaired uterine defect are evaluated and a therapeutic adhesolysis is performed, as indicated. We also offer second-look laparoscopy to patients who had myomectomy for other indications, especially if they had multiple lesions and/or postuterine wall incisions. Our data indicate that laparoscopic myomectomy is associated with less adhesion formation than is myomectomy by laparotomy: of 28 patients undergoing second-look procedures, 30% had no adhesions and 70% had mild or moderate adhesions. In one study of 20 patients who had abdominal CO_2 laser myomectomy followed by second-look procedures, postoperative adhesions were noted in all patients: 75% were mild and 25% were moderate-to-severe (32). Technical considerations that appear to mitigate adhesion formation include securing excellent hemostasis at the operative site and covering the site with a sheet of Tc-7 if sutures are applied.

The condition of the uterine scar formation following laparoscopic removal of deep intramural leiomyomas is a cause of concern. Nezhat et al. noted uterine fistulas posteriorly in six patients who had deep intramural myomas (36). However, the uterine defect was not sutured in three patients and only the serosa was reapproximated in the other three patients (32). Harris (37) reported a case of uterine dehiscence at 34 weeks gestation in a patient who conceived 3 months after laparoscopic excision of a 3-cm myoma that was resected from the posterior uterine wall with electrocautery following retraction with a myoma screw. The serosa of the resulting uterine defect was reapproximated with 4-0 interrupted polyglycolic sutures. We advocate closing the uterine defect in layers, as previously described. In reproductive patients, we perform an hysterosalpingogram 4 months after surgery to evaluate the integrity of the uterine scar before allowing the patient to conceive. We have begun to apply staples in the operative site to provide objective means of measuring the thickness and length of the uterine wall at the incisional site, at the time of HSG (28). To date, we have not observed uterine fistulas in second-look procedures, including three cesarean sections for obstetric indications. Thirteen patients have had normal vaginal deliveries.

In our report, the conception rate for infertility patients was 71% (29). Two patients continuing pregnancy at the time of writing subsequently delivered—one by section and one normally, giving a live birth rate of 59%. These rates have remained substantially representative of our subsequent experience. This may be compared to a conception rate of 40% following abdominal myomectomy in 1,202 infertile patients as reported in an extensive review by Buttram and Reiter in 1981 (38). In more recent review of six studies of abdominal myomectomy in 132 infertile patients whose cases were reported after 1982, Verkauf (39) found a conception rate of 58%. The cases were divided into those with recurrent abortion with a conception rate of 69% (9 of 13), those in which leiomyomas were presumed to be the sole cause of infertility with a conception rate of 59% (47 of 79), and those cases in which the tumors were associated with other potential causes of infertility and having a conception rate of 50% (20 of 40). Such ranking of outcome is consistent with our experience. The rates of recurrence and reoperation following laparoscopic myomectomy are expected to be similar to those noted after abdominal myomectomy. An expected, higher recurrence rate for patients with multiple leiomyomas have already been alluded to. In their 1981 review of 3206 cases, Buttram and Reiter (38) recorded a recurrence rate of 15% and a retreatment rate of 10%, which included reoperation and radiation therapy. In a more recent review of seven studies totaling 185 patients, Verkauf (39) reported a recurrence rate of 8% and a reoperation rate of 7%. Candiani et al. (40) found the cumulative 10-year recurrence rate to be 27% by life table analysis. Clinically significant recurrences usually occurred 3 or more years after surgery (40). In a recent study of 62 patients having abdominal myomectomy, 1 had recurrence at 4 years and 3 at 5 years, leading to repeat myomectomy in 1 patient, hysterectomy in 2, and expectant therapy in the fourth (34). So far, only one of our patients has had a supracervical laparoscopic hysterectomy 3 years after laparoscopic myomectomy. Hysterectomy was performed for recurrent menometrohaggia; the pathology report showed adenomyosis and 2-min myomas, each 0.4 cm in diameter. Three patients have had recurrence in the form of small myomas without associated symptoms.

HIGHLIGHTS

Laparoscopic myomectomy is an attractive alternative to traditional myomectomy in selected cases. Patients with multiple leiomyomas (six or more lesions ≥3 cm) or large uterine size (>18 gestational weeks) may not be suitable candidates. Preoperative treatment with gonadotropin-releasing hormone agonists is recommended for lesions ≥7 cm.

The operative technique involves disengaging the myoma(s), securing hemostasis at the wound edges, approximating the myometrial defect, and withdrawing the specimen from the abdomen. Removing the tumor(s) can be time-consuming. Options include vaginal extraction using a colpotomy incision or abdominal removal using the orange peel or exteriorization technique or the Semm morcellator.

In my experience, outcomes related to operative blood loss, morbidity, hospital stay, and recovery time—as well as clinical effectiveness in terms of conception and recurrence rates—have been most satisfactory.

REFERENCES

1. Bachmann GA. Hysterectomy: a critical review. *J Reprod Med* 1990;35:839–862.
2. National Center for Health Statistics. Vital Health Statistics. National Hospital Discharge Survey. Series 13 No. 108; 1989.
3. Dudiak CM, Turner DA, Patel SK, et al. Uterine leiomyomas in the infertile patient: preoperative localization with MR imaging versus US and hysterosalpingography. *Radiology* 1988;167:627–630.
4. Hricak H, Tscholakoff D, Heinrichs L, et al. Uterine leiomyomas: correlation of MR, histopathologic findings and symptoms. *Radiology* 1986;158:385–391.
5. Zawin M, McCarthy S, Scoutt LM, et al. High-field MRI and US evaluation of the pelvis in women with leiomyomas. *Magn Reson Imag* 1990;4:371–376.
6. Togashi K, Ozasa H, Konishi I, et al. Enlarged uterus: differentiation between adenomyosis and leiomyoma with MR imaging. *Radiology* 1989;171:531–534.
7. DeCherney AH, Maheux R, Polan ML. A medical treatment for myomata uteri. *Fertil Steril* 1983;39:429–430 (abstract).
8. Wiznitzer A, Marback M, Hazum E, et al. Gonadotropin-releasing hormone specific binding sites in uterine leiomyomata. *Biochem Biophys Res Commun* 1988;152:1326–1331.
9. West CP, Lumsden MA, Lawson S, et al. Shrinkage of uterine fibroids during therapy with goserelin (Zoladex): a luteinizing hormone-releasing hormone agonist administered as a monthly subcutaneous depot. *Fertil Steril* 1987;48:45–51.
10. Friedman AJ, Rein MS, Harrison-Atlas D, et al. A randomized, placebo-controlled, double-blind study evaluating leuprolide acetate depot treatment before myomectomy. *Fertil Steril* 1989;52: 728–733.
11. Friedman AJ, Lobel SM, Rein MS, et al. Efficacy and safety considerations in women with uterine leiomyomas treated with gonadotropin releasing hormone agonists: the estrogen threshold hypothesis. *Am J Obstet Gynecol* 1990;163:1114–1119.
12. Friedman AJ, Hoffman DI, Comite F, et al. Treatment of leiomyomata uteri with leuprolide acetate depot: a double-blind, placebo-controlled multicenter study. *Obstet Gynecol* 1991;77: 720–725.
13. Rock JA. Gonadotropin-releasing hormone agonist analogs in the treatment of uterine leiomyomas. *J Gynecol Surg* 1991;7:147–153.
14. Lumsden MA, West CP, Baird DT. Goserelin therapy before surgery for uterine fibroids. *Lancet* 1987;1:36–37.
15. Meyer WR, Mayer AR, Diamond MP, et al. Unsuspected leiomyosarcoma: treatment with a gonadotropin-releasing hormone analogue. *Obstet Gynecol* 1990;75:529–531.
16. Loong EPL, Wong FWS. Uterine leiomyosarcoma diagnosed during treatment with agonist of luteinzing hormone releasing hormone for presumed uterine fibroid. *Fertil Steril* 1990;54:530–531.
17. Hitti IF, Glasberg SS, McKenzie C, et al. Uterine leiomyosarcoma with massive necrosis diagnosed during gonadotropin-releasing hormone analog therapy for presumed uterine fibroid. *Fertil Steril* 1991;56:778–780.
18. Fedele L, Vercellini P, Bianchi S, et al. Treatment with GnRH agonists before myomectomy and the risk of short-term myoma recurrence. *Br J Obstet Gynaecol* 1990;97:393–396.
19. Dinh TV, Woodruff JD. Leiomyosarcoma of the uterus. *Am J Obstet Gynecol* 1982;144:817–823.
20. Vollenhoven BJ, Lawrence AS, Healy DL. Uterine fibroids: a clinical review. *Br J Obstet Gynecol* 1990;97:285–298.
21. Leibsohn S, d'Ablaing G, Mishell RD, et al. Leiomyosarcoma in a series of hysterectomies performed for presumed uterine leiomyomas. *Am J Obstet Gynecol* 1990;162:968–976.
22. Berchuck A, Rubin S, Hoskins WJ et al. Treatment of uterine leiomyosarcoma. 1988;71:845–850.
23. Kahanpaa KV, Wahlstrom T, Grohn P, et al. Sarcomas of the uterus: a clinicopathological study of 119 patients. *Obstet Gynecol* 1986;67:417–424.
24. Goldzieher JW, Maqueo M, Ricaud L, et al. Induction of degenerative changes in uterine myomas by high dosage progestin therapy. *Am J Obstet Gynecol* 1966;96:1078–1087.
25. Segaloff A, Weed JC, Sternberg WH, et al. The progesterone therapy of human uterine leiomyomas. *J Clin Endocrinol* 1949;9: 1273–1291.
26. Hasson HM. Half-hitch knot for securing the end of continuous sutures. *Obstet Gynecol* 1992;80:724–726.
27. Rotman C. Personal communication, 1991.
28. Beyth Y, Ohel G. Postmyomectomy evaluation of uterine scar: a new hysterographic method. *Fertil Steril* 1983;39:564–565.
29. Hasson HM, Rotman C., Rana N, et al. Laparoscopic myomectomy. *Obstet Gynecol* 1992;80:884–888.
30. Friedman AJ, Daly M, Juneau-Norcross M, et al. Recurrence of myomas after myomectomy in women pretreated with leuprolide acetate depot or placebo. *Fertil Steril* 1992;58:205–208.
31. Daniell JF, Gurley LD. Laparoscopic treatment of clinically significant symptomatic uterine fibroids. *J Gynecol Surg* 1991;7:37–40.
32. Nezhat C, Nezhat F, Silfen SF, et al. Laparoscopic myomectomy. *Int J Fertil* 1991;36:275–280.
33. Starks GC. CO_2 laser myomectomy in an infertile population. *J Reprod Med* 1988;33:184–186.
34. McLaughlin DS. Metroplasty and myomectomy with CO_2 laser for maximizing the preservation of normal tissue and minimizing blood loss. *J Reprod Med* 1985;30:1–9.
35. Smith DC, Uhlir JK. Myomectomy as a reproductive procedure. *Am J Obstet Gynecol* 1990;162:1476–1479.
36. Nezhat C, Nezhat F, Silfen SF, et al. Laparoscopic myomectomy. Letter to the editor. *Int J Fertil* 1992;37:64.
37. Harris WJ. Uterine dehiscence following laparoscopic myomectomy. *Obstet Gynecol* 1992;80:545–546.
38. Buttram VC, Reiter RC. Uterine leiomyomata: etiology, symptomatology, and management. *Fertil Steril* 1981;36:433–445.
39. Verkauf BS. Myomectomy for fertility enhancement and preservation. *Fertil Steril* 1992;58:1–15.
40. Candiani GB, Fedele L, Parazzini F, et al. Risk of recurrence after myomectomy. *Br J Obstet Gynaecol* 1991;98:385–389.
41. Hasson HM. Open laparoscopy. In: Sciarra JJ, ed. *Gynecology and obstetrics,* vol. 6. Philadelphia: Harper and Row, 1992;1–10.

Endoscopic Management of Gynecologic Disease,
edited by G.D. Adamson and D.C. Martin.
Lippincott-Raven Publishers, Philadelphia © 1996.

CHAPTER 17

Polycystic Ovarian Syndrome

Mark W. Surrey and Eric S. Surrey

The association of amenorrhea, chronic anovulation, hirsutism, obesity, and infertility with enlarged sclerocystic ovaries was initially reported in 1939 by Stein and Cohen (1). Since its initial description, polycystic ovarian syndrome (PCOS) has become recognized as a multifaceted disorder. The hypothalamus, pituitary, adrenal glands, ovaries, and extraglandular tissues have all been implicated in the pathophysiology of PCOS (2). Although the etiology of this syndrome is controversial and clinical presentation is variable, a self-perpetuating cycle of endocrine imbalance is pathognomonic (3). Recent advances in the understanding of this imbalance have led to changing concepts about the clinical manifestation, evaluation, and medical and surgical management of PCOS (4).

PATHOPHYSIOLOGY

The pathophysiology of this phenomenon is controversial. Polycystic ovarian syndrome is commonly associated with inappropriately elevated luteinizing hormone (LH) secretion and relatively constant and low follicle-stimulating hormone (FSH) release. Increased responsiveness of LH release in response to gonadotropin-releasing hormone (GnRH) stimulation has been demonstrated (2,5). Luteinizing hormone elevation leads to a disproportionate stimulation of ovarian androgen secretion. Peripheral conversion of androgens to estrogens leads to an abnormal tonic elevation of the ratio of serum estrone to estradiol levels. This, in turn, results in further suppression of FSH release. Despite these abnormalities, PCOS patients seem to retain intact negative and positive feedback mechanisms in the hypothalamic-pituitary axis. Recently, investigators have demonstrated a significant role for insulin-like growth factors and insulin resistance in the pathophysiology of this syndrome (6). Whether the inherent abnormality in this disorder rests at the level of the ovary, hypothalamus, or pituitary has not been conclusively determined.

M. W. Surrey and E. S. Surrey: Center for Reproductive Medicine and Surgery, Beverly Hills, California 90210.

CLINICAL PRESENTATION

Clinical manifestations of PCOS include various menstrual disturbances ranging from amenorrhea to dysfunctional uterine bleeding, secondary to unopposed estrogenic stimulation of the endometrium. Mild hirsutism, acne, and obesity are associated with PCOS, but they are not necessary to the diagnosis of this syndrome. Obesity may be present in up to 40% of PCOS patients (7). Excess body fat contributes to the abnormal endocrine balance as a site for peripheral conversion of androgens to estrogens (8). Plasma-free testosterone levels are often increased despite normal total serum testosterone. Patients may also manifest elevations in serum prolactin and dehydroepiandrosterone sulfate (DHEA-S) levels.

Infertility in PCOS is due primarily to chronic anovulation. Ovulatory dysfunction may be responsible for 20% of infertility patients, and as many as 20% of these patients may have PCOS (6). Alterations in oocyte quality and corpus luteum function may be secondary to the chronically elevated androgen levels within the ovarian microenvironment, although this has not been clearly established.

DIFFERENTIAL DIAGNOSIS

The differential diagnosis of PCOS includes functional disorders of the thyroid, adrenal glands (Cushing's syndrome and congenital enzyme deficiencies), and ovary (hyperthecosis). Ovarian and adrenal neoplasms also should be suspected in the presence of overt signs of virilization.

MEDICAL THERAPY

Initial therapy of PCOS in the obese woman may begin with weight reduction. Weight loss decreases insulin resistance and may benefit gonadotropin secretion (9).

Patients with menstrual disturbances and who are not interested in conception may be administered progestins or combination oral contraceptives in an effort to oppose tonically elevated estrogen levels. This therapy also decreases the associated risk of endometrial hyperplasia secondary to unopposed estrogen exposure. Long-acting GnRH agonists have been shown to reduce ovarian androgen production and to ameliorate hirsutism (10).

Clomiphene citrate has been the most commonly used agent for inducing ovulation and should be the first line of therapy in the PCOS patient attempting pregnancy. By acting as a competitive inhibitor to circulating estrogens, GnRH and gonadotropin release is stimulated. Follicular maturation follows. The augmented estradiol levels cause a positive feedback on the hypothalamus and pituitary, resulting in an LH surge. The use of human chorionic gonadotropins (hCG) as an adjunct when the follicle diameter is 20 mm should improve ovulation rates to about 75% (11). It is interesting that despite these high ovulation rates, pregnancy occurs in only 40% of PCOS patients; this may reflect an inherent abnormality at the level of the oocyte (12). Abnormalities in cervical mucus production and endometrial thickness also have been described. The addition of dexamethasone 0.25–0.5 mg daily at bedtime has been advocated for clomiphene-resistant PCOS patients with elevated adrenal androgen levels (13).

Human menopausal gonadotropins (hMG) contain equivalent amounts of purified FSH and LH. Infertile patients with PCOS who fail to ovulate after clomiphene citrate therapy may respond to hMG with hCG. This therapy requires careful monitoring of follicular development by serial ultrasound examinations and measurement of serum estradiol. Polycystic ovarian syndrome patients are at relatively high risk of developing ovarian hyperstimulation syndrome following treatment due to inherently elevated baseline LH and estrogen levels with follicles at varying stages of maturation prior to initiation of gonadotropins (14). Conception rates in PCOS patients following hMG-hCG treatment are not as high as those reported among patients with hypothalamic amenorrhea (15). This may again reflect an inherent oocyte defect induced by chronic androgen elevation. Administration of purified FSH theoretically would provide a more physiologic approach to induce ovulation in the patients (4). The incidence of ovarian hyperstimulation syndrome is lower, but ovulation and conception rates have not been shown to be higher after its use.

Gonadotropin-releasing hormone agonists have been used in PCOS patients to down-regulate pituitary gonadotropes and, thus, reduce circulating androgen and estrogen levels. Subsequent to this suppression, hMG, FSH, or pulsatile GnRH can be administered with some improvement in results in otherwise unresponsive patients (16–20).

Bromocriptine lowers serum prolactin levels and has been used to induce ovulation in clomiphene-resistant PCOS patients with hyperprolactinemia. However, based on randomized trials, the efficacy of this therapy in PCOS patients with normal prolactin levels has not been consistently established (20,21).

SURGICAL MANAGEMENT

Whereas surgical therapy had originally been the only approach available to PCOS patients, its use is now largely reserved for patients who desire pregnancy and who are resistant to medical therapy (Fig. 1). In 1939, Stein and Cohen demonstrated that bilateral ovarian wedge resection performed at laparotomy frequently resulted in postoperative ovulation in patients with PCOS (22). In a classic study of hormonal changes after wedge resection, Judd and coworkers reported a profound but temporary reduction of aberrant ovarian sex steroid hormone secretion, a persistent postoperative reduction of circulatory testosterone levels, but no discernible effects on serum gonadotropin levels (23). Decreasing intraovarian androgen levels may allow for the initiation of folliculogenesis. Identifying such hormones as inhibin as well as various growth factors in follicular fluid suggests the hypothesis that an acute reduction in ovarian steroidogenesis may result from decreasing the overall volume of follicular fluid in the ovary. Other mechanisms that may result in ovulation after cystotomy in these patients may include the following:

1. Drainage of follicular fluid containing high androgen concentrations results in an acute reduction of intraovarian androgen levels.
2. Androgen production is significantly limited by coagulation and/or vaporization of the atretic follicles and surrounding stroma.
3. Local reduction of ovarian androgen production may decrease the inhibitory effect of androgens on normal folliculogenesis.
4. Lowered circulating ovarian androgen levels result in diminished peripheral conversion of androgen to estrogen and decreased positive feedback on LH production.
5. The secondary reduction of ovarian inhibin permits a rise of FSH secretion, which results in a normal LH/FSH ratio (24).

The most common complication of ovarian wedge resection is the development of postoperative adhesions. A significant number of patients undergoing second-look laparoscopy have developed periovarian adhesions to the site of wedge resections (25,26).

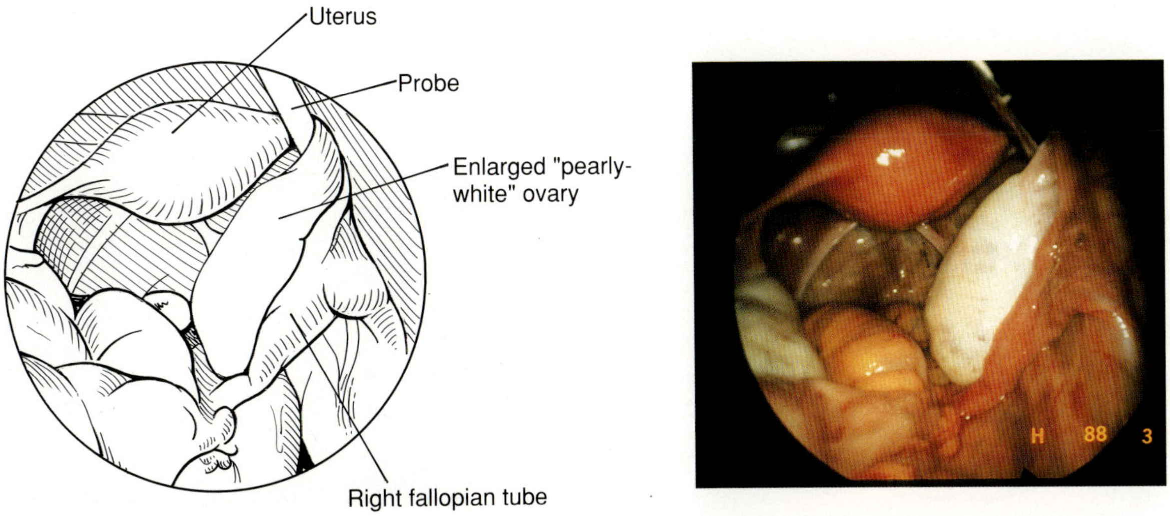

FIG. 1. Patient with Stein–Leventhal syndrome has enlarged ovaries. Figure shows the right ovary enlarged to the size of the uterus with the typical "pearly white" capsule.

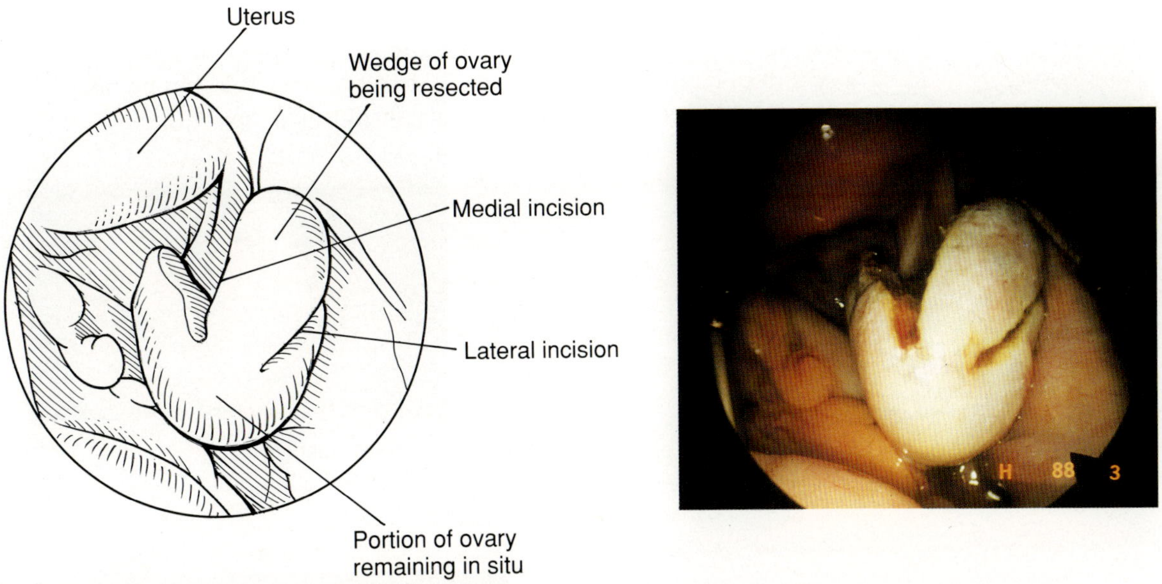

FIG. 2. A wedge-type incision is made and extended into the ovary at the end of the dissection.

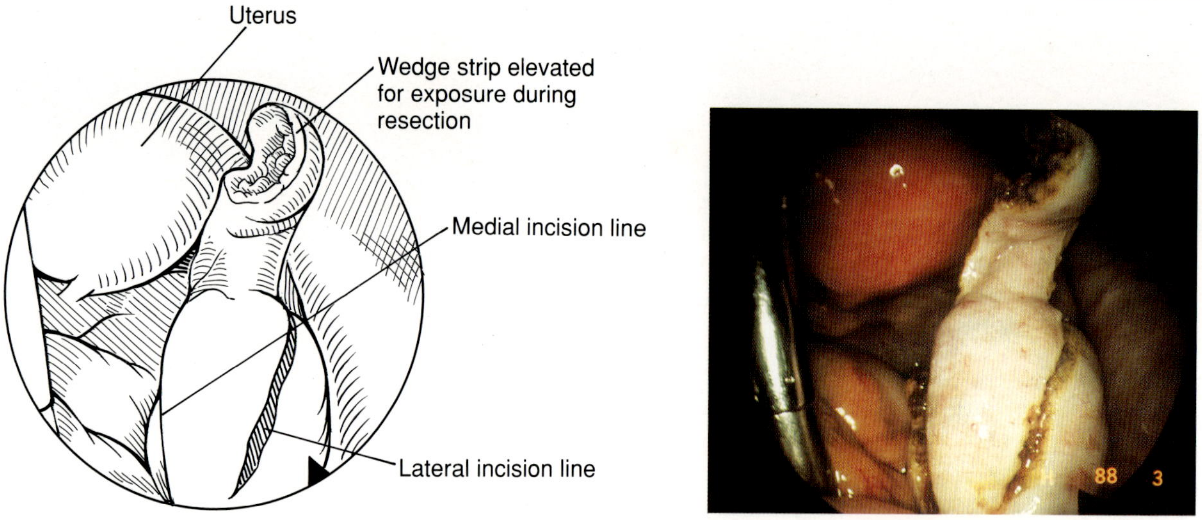

FIG. 3. The wedge strip is held up for retraction in the process of dissection.

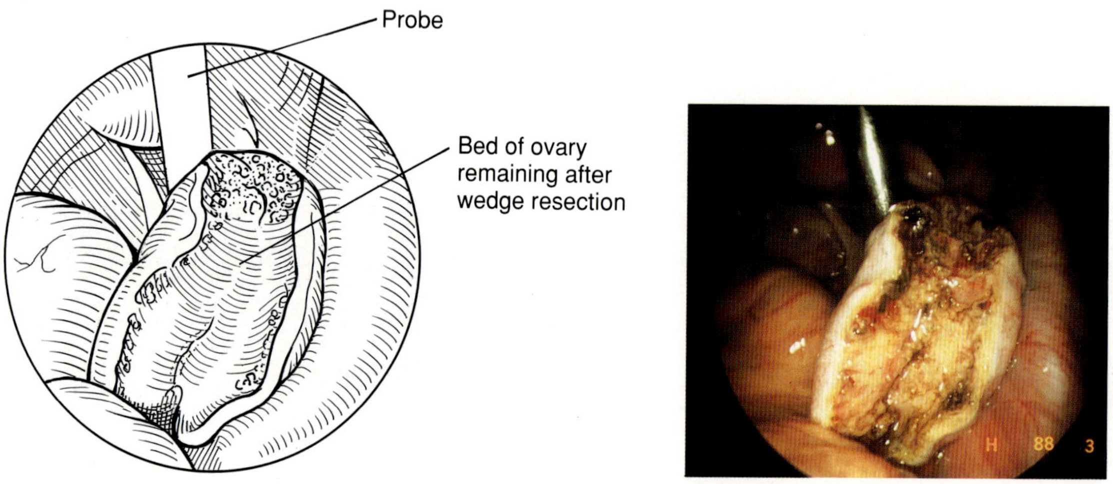

FIG. 4. Appearance of the ovary at the end of the dissection.

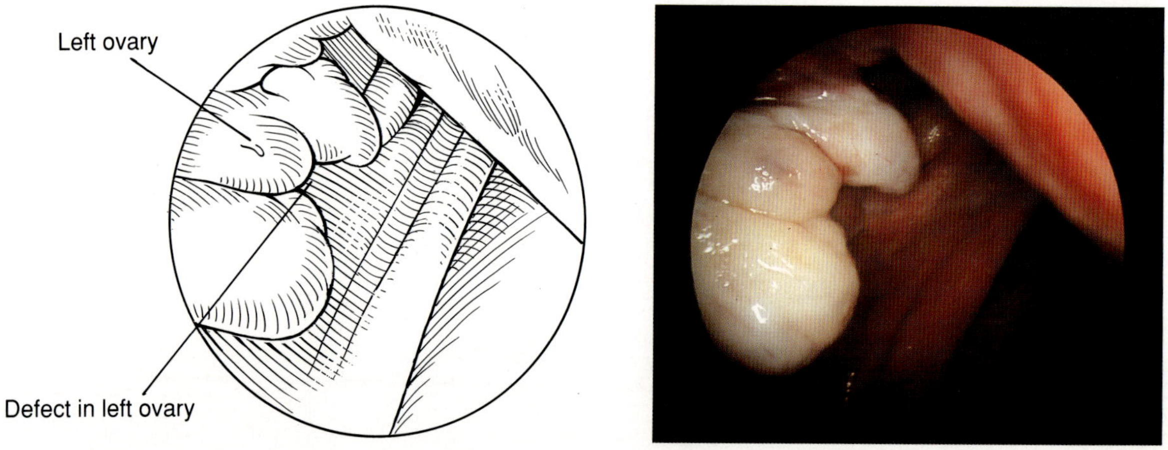

FIG. 5. Second-look laparoscopy in a patient who had a laparoscopic wedge resection for polycystic ovarian syndrome. A defect is noted at the resection, but there were no adhesions.

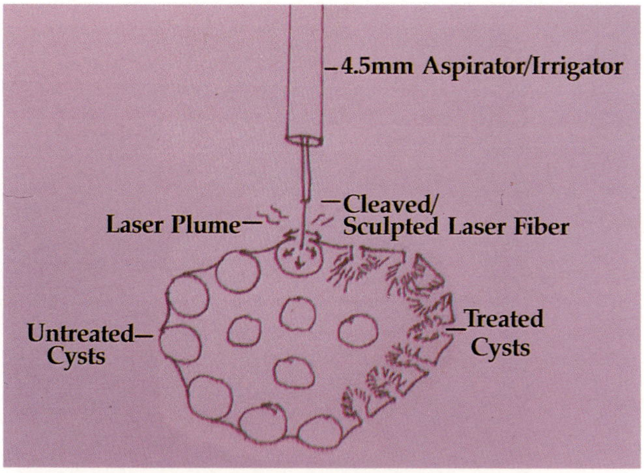

FIG. 6. Cross-section of ovary demonstrating laser oophorotomy.

Laparoscopic surgical techniques without ovarian suturing have been associated with a lower incidence of postoperative adhesion formation. These procedures can be performed on an outpatient basis (27). Laparoscopic wedge resection was the first technique performed in PCOS patients (Fig. 2–5). However, PCOS patients have more recently been treated with various endoscopic ovarian drilling procedures performed with electrosurgery or triple laser system (see Fig. 6).

The technique of electrosurgery for ovarian cystotomy related to PCOS involves the application of a unipolar microcautery tip to penetrate the ovarian cortex. The dimensions of the perforations will vary. "Cutting" power should be utilized to minimize adjacent thermal damage to the ovarian surface. It is important to fix the ovarian position with grasping instruments to prevent injury to adjacent organs. A multiple-puncture pelviscopic approach is required. The instrument tip should be positioned at a right angle to the ovarian surface and repositioned as the contour varies.

The CO_2 laser can be focused on a high-superpulse mode to incise through the ovarian capsule in a similar fashion (Figs. 7 and 8). It is necessary to apply the laser beam at right angles to the ovarian surface to achieve optimal focusing. Excessive amounts of laser plume, which can result from vaporization, and water vapor must be evacuated. The depth of penetration is limited by absorption of the laser energy by the fluid and depends upon both the power and the application time. Each ovary receives 20–30 cystotomy incisions.

Lasers with neodymium:yttrium-aluminum-garnet (Nd:YAG), argon, and potassium-trideuterium-phosphate (KTP-532) as energy sources have the advantage of delivering the high-power output of laser energy to tissue by fine contact fibers. Energy is absorbed diffusely by body tissues, thereby permitting deep penetration within the ovary without significant interruption of the serosal surface (28). The power is not dissipated after absorption of excessive follicular fluid. The fiber tip must be applied at a right angle to the ovarian surface. This should avoid inadvertent damage to adjacent organs (e.g., bowel and ureter vessels).

OUTCOME

Ovulation and pregnancy rates after laparoscopic therapy have been reported by various investigators and range from 70% to 94% and 0 to 80%, respectively (see Table 1). It is important to note that postoperative endocrine changes are rarely long-lived. A return to the previous pathologic state occurs unless pregnancy ensues. Patients who do not ovulate spontaneously postoperatively may prove to be more responsive to ovulation induction agents. Needless to say, therapy should be initiated rapidly to take advantage of this relatively brief improvement in endocrine balance.

HIGHLIGHTS

Laparoscopic oophorocystotomy procedures should *not* be used as the first line of therapy in anovulatory pa-

TABLE 1. *Success of laparoscopic therapy of Polycystic Ovarian Syndrome*

First author and reference	Number of patients	Technique	OR[a] (%)	PR[b] (%)
Daniell (27)	85	KTP and CO_2 laser	99	56
Keckstein (24)	19	CO_2 laser	62	0
Gurgan (29)	10	Nd:YAG laser	70	40
Naether (30)	104	Electrocautery	55	11
Rossmanith (31)	11	Nd:YAG laser	73	36
Armar (32)	21	Electrocautery	81	52
Sakata (33)	9	Electrocautery	89	33

[a] OR, ovulation rate.
[b] PR, pregnancy rate (follow-up periods not provided).

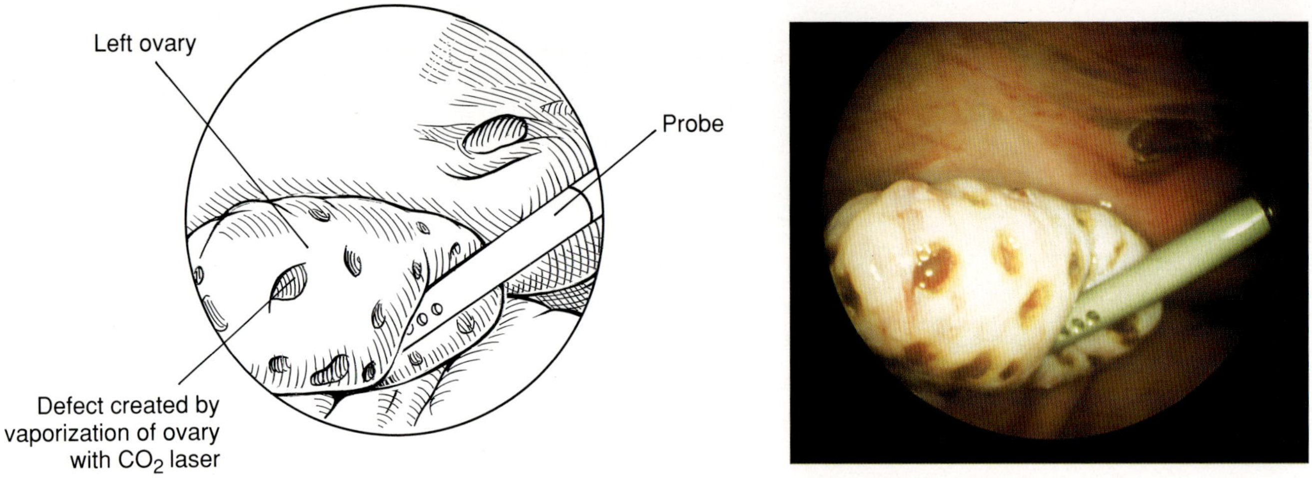

FIG. 7. Appearance of the ovary after drilling with a carbon dioxide laser.

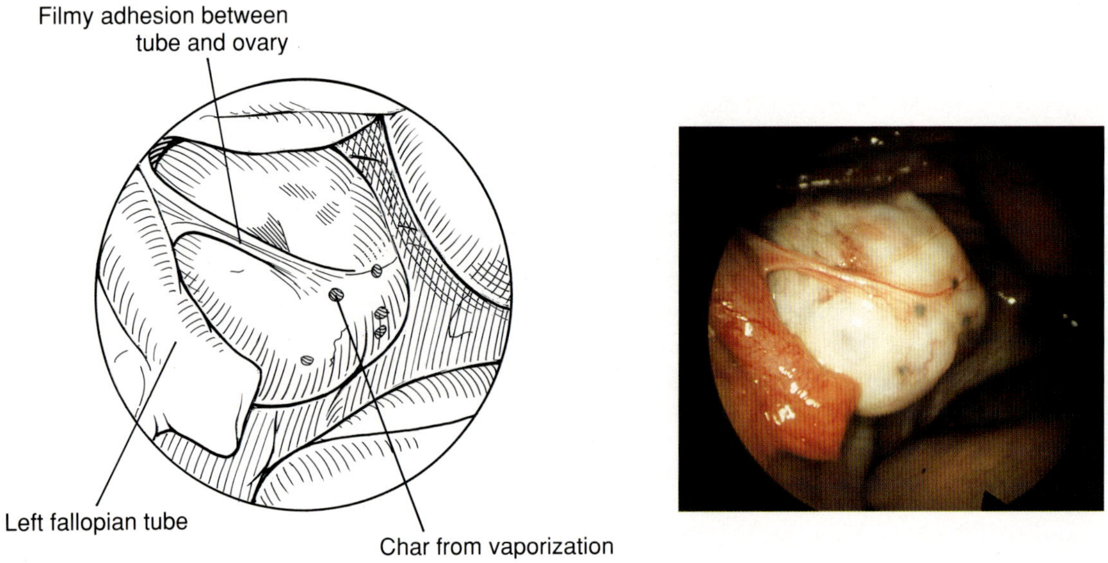

FIG. 8. Ovarian adhesions are uncommon after laparoscopic drilling procedures. When noted, they are generally filmy and easily lysed.

tients with PCOS and who are attempting pregnancy. However, this procedure may represent an effective option for patients refractory to more traditional forms of medical management to achieve a short-term benefit, which lasts until pregnancy can be achieved.

REFERENCES

1. Stein IF, Cohen MR. Surgical treatment of bilateral polycystic ovaries, amenorrhea and sterility. *Am J Obstet Gynecol* 1939;38:465.
2. Yen SSC. The polycystic ovary syndrome. *Clin Endocrinol* 1980;12:177.
3. Franks S. Polycystic ovary syndrome: a changing perspective. *Clin Endocrinol* 1989;31:87.
4. Loy R, Seibel M: Evaluation and therapy of polycystic ovarian syndrome. *Endocr Metab Clin North Am* 1988;17:785.
5. Adashi E. Hypothalamic-pituitary dysfunction in polycystic ovarian disease. *Endocr Metab Clin North Am* 1988;17:649.
6. Dunaif A, Segal KR, Futterweit W, Dobrjansky A. Profound peripheral insulin resistance, independent of obesity, in polycystic ovarian syndrome. *J Clin Endocrinol Metab* 1989;38:1165.
7. Goldzeiher JW, Alexrod LR. Clinical and biochemical features of polycystic ovarian disease. *Fertil Steril* 1978;29:388.
8. Hosseinian AH, Kim MH, Rosenfield RL. Obesity and oligomenorrhea are associated with hyperandrogenism independent of hirsutism. *J Clin Metab* 1976;42:765.
9. Harlass FE, Plymate SR, Fariss BL, et al. Weight loss is associated with correction of gonadotropin and sex steroid abnormalities in the obese anovulatory female. *Fertil Steril* 1984;42:649.
10. Andreyko J, Monroe S, Jaffe R. Treatment of hirsutism with a gonadotropin-releasing hormone agonist (nafarelin). *J Clin Endocrinol Metab* 1986;63:854.

11. Gorlitsky GA, Kase NG, Speroff L. Ovulation and pregnancy rates with clomiphene citrate therapy. *Obstet Gynecol* 1978;51:265.
12. Hammond MG, Halme JK, Talbert LM. Factors affecting the pregnancy rate in clomiphene citrate induction of ovulation. *Obstet Gynecol* 1983;62:196.
13. Fayez JA. Selection of patients for clomiphene citrate therapy. *Obstet Gynecol* 1976;47:671.
14. Wang CF, Gemzell C. The use of human gonadotropins for the induction of ovulation in women with polycystic ovarian disease. *Fertil Steril* 1980;33:479.
15. Schwartz M, Jewlewicz F. The use of gonadotropins for induction of ovulation. *Fertil Steril* 1981;35:3.
16. Armitage M, Wilkin T, Dewbury K. Successful treatment of infertility due to polycystic ovary disease using a combination of luteinizing hormone releasing hormone agonist and low dosage menotrophin. *Br Med J* 1987;295:96.
17. Filicori M, Campaniello E, Michelacci L, et al. Gonadotropin releasing hormone (GnRH) analog suppression renders polycystic ovarian disease patients more susceptible to ovulation induction with pulsatile GnRH. *J Clin Endocrinol Metab* 1988;66:327.
18. Surrey E, deZiegler D, Lu JKH, et al. Effects of gonadotropin releasing hormone (GnRH) agonist on pituitary and ovarian responses to pulsatile GnRH therapy in polycystic ovarian disease. *Fertil Steril* 1989;52:574.
19. Dodson W, Hughes C, Whitesides D, Haney A. The effect of leuprolide acetate on ovulation induction with human menopausal gonadotropins in polycystic ovary syndrome. *J Clin Endocrinol Metab* 1987;65:95.
20. DeVane GW, Guzik DS. Bromocriptine therapy in normoprolactinemic women with unexplained infertility and galactorrhea. *Fertil Steril* 1986;46:1026.
21. Buvat J, Buvat-Herbaut M, Marcolin G, et al. A double blind controlled study of the hormonal and clinical effects of bromocriptine in the polycystic ovary syndrome. *J Clin Endocrinol Metab* 1986;63:119.
22. Stein IF, Cohen MR. Surgical treatment of bilateral polycystic ovaries, amenorrhea and sterility. *Am J Obstet Gynecol* 1939;38:465.
23. Judd H, Rigg L, Anderson D, Yen S. The effects of ovarian wedge resection on circulating gonadotropin and ovarian steroid levels in patients with polycystic ovary syndrome. *J Clin Endocrinol Metab* 1976;43:347.
24. Keckstein J. Laparoscopic treatment of polycystic ovarian syndrome. *Bailliere's Clin Obstet Gynecol* 1989;3:563.
25. Buttram VC Jr, Vaquero C. Post-ovarian wedge resection adhesive disease. *Fertil Steril* 1975;26:874.
26. Surrey M, Friedman S. Second-look laparoscopy after reconstructive pelvic surgery for infertility. *J Reprod Med* 1982;27:658.
27. Daniell JF, Miller W. Polycystic ovaries treated by laparoscopic laser ablation. *Fertil Steril* 1985;51:232.
28. Daniell JF, Miller W, Tosh R, et al. Laparoscopic use of the KTP-532 laser in nonendometriotic pelvic surgery. *Colpo Gyn Laser Surg* 1986;2:107.
29. Gurgan T, Kinisci H, Yarali H, et al. Evaluation of adhesion formation at laparoscopic treatment of polycystic ovarian disease. *Fertil Steril* 1991;56:1176.
30. Naether OGJ, Fischer R, Weise H, et al. Laparoscopic electrocoagulation of the ovarian surface in infertile patients with polycystic ovarian disease. *Fertil Steril* 1993;60:88.
31. Rossmanith W, Keckstein J, Spatzier K, Lauritzen CH. The impact of ovarian laser surgery on the gonadotropin secretion in women with polycystic ovarian disease. *Clin Endocrinol* 1991;34:223.
32. Armar N, McGarrigle H, Honor J. Laparoscopic ovarian diathermy in the management of anovulatory infertility in women with polycystic ovaries: endocrine changes and clinical outcome. *Fertil Steril* 1990;53:45.
33. Sakata M, Tasaka K, Kurachi H, et al. Changes of bioactive luteinizing hormone after laparoscopic ovarian cautery in patients with polycystic ovarian syndrome. *Fertil Steril* 1990;53:610.

Endoscopic Management of Gynecologic Disease,
edited by G.D. Adamson and D.C. Martin.
Lippincott-Raven Publishers, Philadelphia © 1996.

CHAPTER 18

Paratubal and Parovarian Cysts

Barbara Levy

Cystic lesions found in the paratubal area or within the broad ligament are quite common. Often they are encountered as incidental findings at the time of pelvic surgery for unrelated pathology, but on occasion they present as symptomatic or asymptomatic cystic pelvic masses.

Because of its embryonic origin, the paratubal cyst may arise as the distal portion of the fallopian tube is compressed between the pronephros and the mesonephric body (1). Accessory lumina and diverticula develop as a result of this embryologic event. Cystic dilatation of these regions begins at puberty and occurs with secretory activity in the tubal epithelium. In contrast, parovarian cysts are uniformly lined by a bland, single-layer cuboidal or flattened epithelium of mesothelial origin; they do not contain papillary projections.

Hydatids of Morgagni are small, unilocular cysts that dangle from the fimbriated end of the fallopian tube. They are lined by ciliated, secretory epithelium; these are true tubal cysts (2).

OCCURRENCE, PRESENTATION, AND SURGICAL TECHNIQUES

Most paratubal and parovarian cysts are discovered at the time of laparoscopy for other disease. They seem to occur more often in infertile patients, which prompts the speculation that paratubal cysts or hydatids of Morgagni may interfere with tubal motility and ovum pickup. Infrequently, they torse and may necrose, leading to an episode of acute pelvic pain. Large parovarian cysts are indistinguishable from ovarian neoplasms and present as cystic pelvic masses. Ultrasound is helpful in characterizing them as unilocular simple cysts, but ultrasound usually cannot identify the ovary separately (3).

When paratubal cysts are found at the time of laparoscopy for infertility, the surgeon must decide whether they are a factor in the patient's inability to conceive. If so, it is a simple matter to place them on stretch using a grasping forceps and excise them along their stalks with scissors, low-voltage electrocoagulation, or laser. Care must be taken to avoid any damage to the fallopian tube. It is inadvisable to use clips or sutures (Endoloops), as foreign material may impact tubal function.

In general, when paratubal cysts are encountered during laparoscopy for pelvic pain or masses, it is advisable to leave them in situ. The rare exception may be the large cyst on a long stalk which has a high risk for torsion (see Fig. 1).

Small (<2 cm) parovarian cysts, when discovered incidentally, may be documented and ignored. There is a theoretical risk that they will grow and become clinically significant; however, when they are small, their close proximity to the large vessels in the broad ligament makes excision technically difficult. The risk of significant hemorrhage is unacceptable in the removal of an asymptomatic, benign cyst.

Large parovarian cysts (>4 cm) usually present as unilocular pelvic cysts that fail to regress with hormonal suppression. At laparoscopy they are seen as large, thin-walled cystic dilatations of the broad ligament (see Fig. 2), often stretching and compressing the fallopian tube. The anatomy of the affected adnexa may be quite distorted, and care must be taken to identify all vital structures. Although the parovarian cyst is avascular, the vessels of the broad ligament are in close proximity and must not be compromised. It is tempting to puncture the cyst with a sharp needle or trocar, aspirate its clear fluid to deflate it, and do nothing more. However, the epithe-

B. Levy: Department of Obstetrics and Gynecology, University of Washington School of Medicine, Federal Way, Washington 98003.

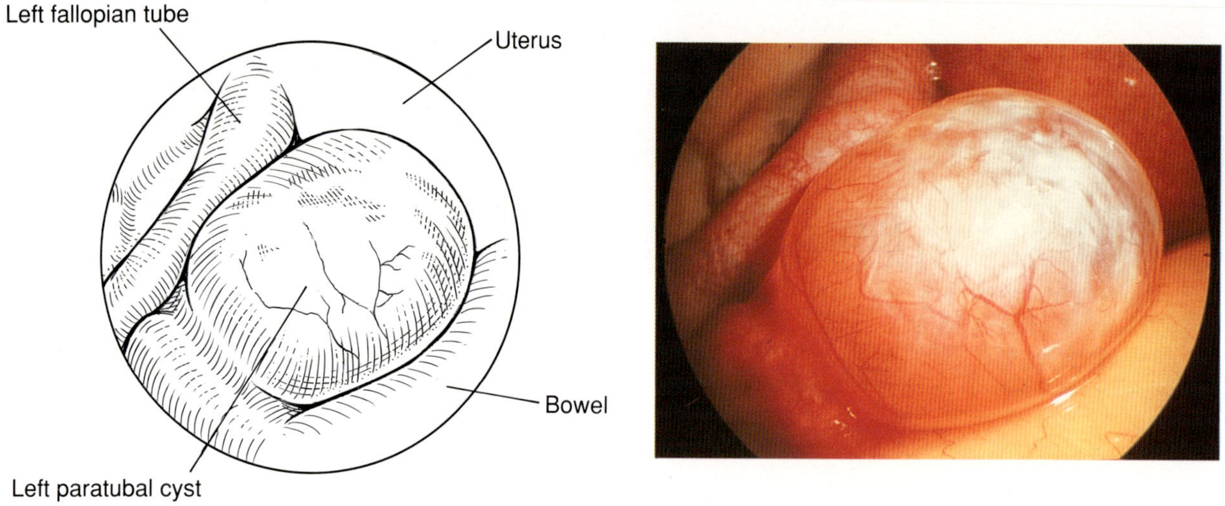

FIG. 1. Large paratubal cyst on narrow stalk.

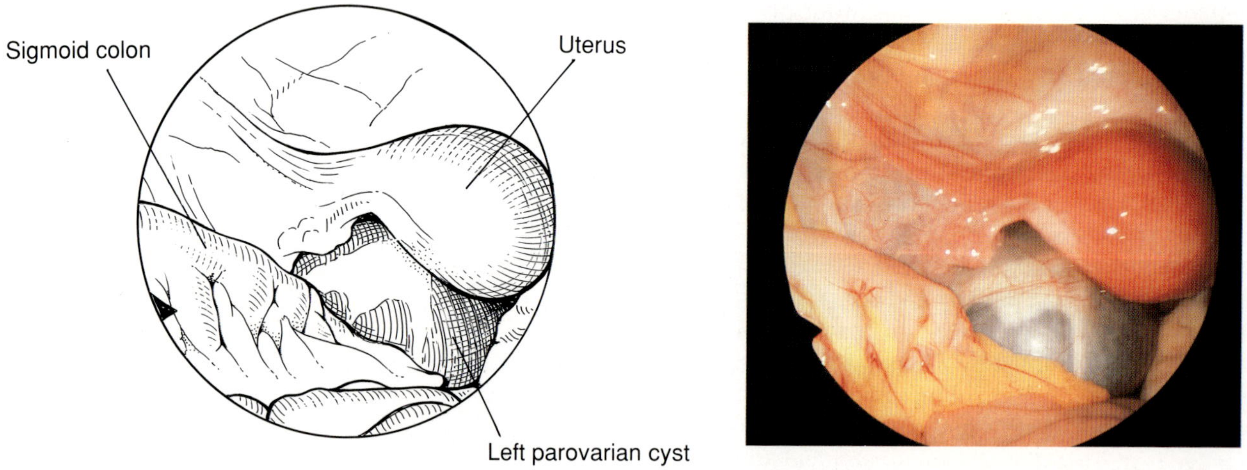

FIG. 2. Large parovarian cyst in left broad ligament.

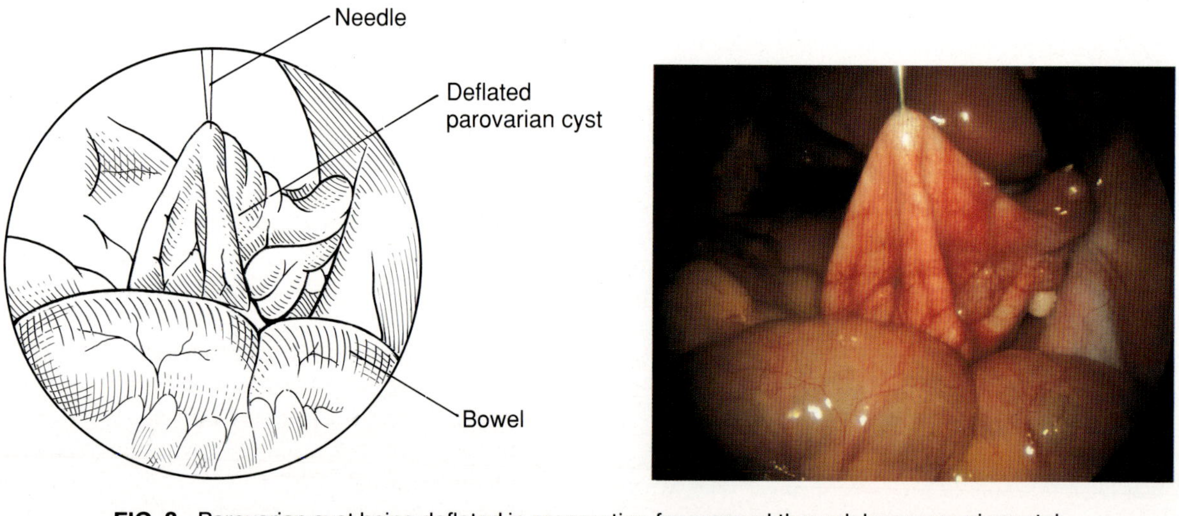

FIG. 3. Parovarian cyst being deflated in preparation for removal through laparoscopic portal.

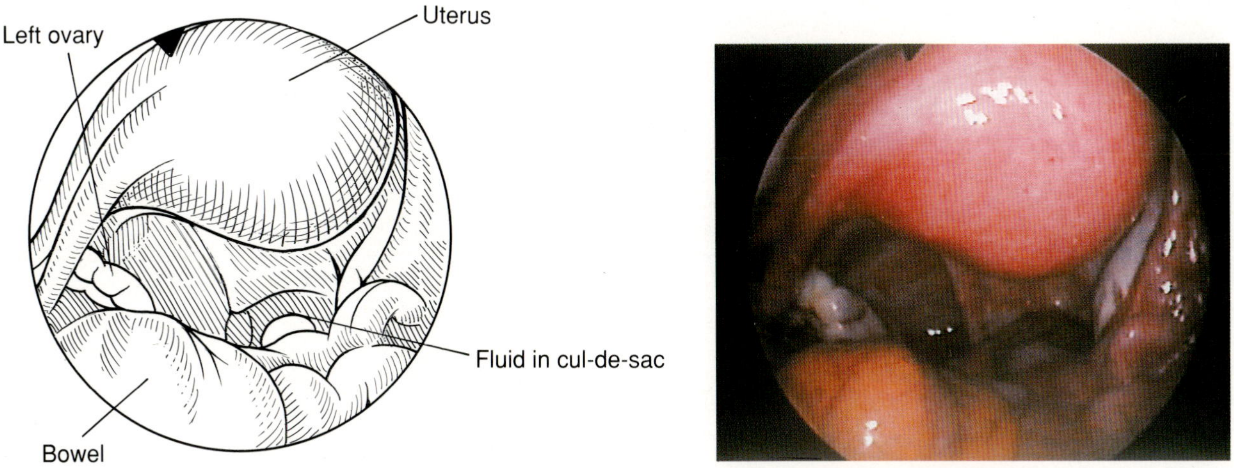

FIG. 4. Postexcision evaluation of cyst bed to ensure complete hemostasis.

lium lining the cyst was clearly secretory at some time and, without excision of at least a portion of the cyst wall, recurrence may be expected. Decompression of the cyst facilitates excision of the wall. Fluid is aspirated through the needle or trocar, which has been placed into the cyst in an avascular region, and sent for cytology. The flaccid cyst wall then may be excised by pulling it through a laparoscope snare, which simultaneously cuts the base and provides hemostasis (see Fig. 3). Alternately, the cyst wall may be placed on traction after which scissors or laser can be used to separate it at the base. It is a simple matter to remove the then-floppy cyst wall from the abdomen through the primary trocar sleeve. The area of excision should be inspected and irrigated to assure hemostasis (see Fig. 4).

COMPLICATIONS

Complications from removal of paratubal or parovarian cysts are minimal. Any damage to the fallopian tube is unacceptable, since the only indication for removal of paratubal cysts may be fertility enhancement. Therefore, great caution must be exercised when using thermal coagulating devices of any type in this procedure. Attempts to remove large parovarian cysts in their entirety may lead the surgeon dangerously close to the ureter or the major vessels within the broad ligament. Since these cysts are benign, total removal is unnecessary.

HIGHLIGHTS

Paratubal and parovarian cysts are benign lesions frequently encountered during laparoscopy. They are recognized commonly as the only abnormality discovered during infertility evaluation and may interfere with tubal mobility and ovum pickup. Their removal can be accomplished endoscopically with minimal difficulty. However, care must be exercised to minimize trauma to the adnexa and adjacent vital structures. Large parovarian cysts require removal en toto or fenestration with removal of at least a portion of the cyst wall to prevent recurrence.

REFERENCES

1. Samaha M, Woodruff JD. Paratubal cysts: frequency, histogenesis and associated clinical features. *Obstet Gynecol* 1985;65:691–694.
2. Kissane JM, ed. *Anderson's pathology*. St. Louis: CV Mosby; 1985: 149.
3. Alpern MB, Sandler MA, Madrazo BL. Sonographic features of parovarian cysts and their complications. *AJR* 1984;143:157–160.

Endoscopic Management of Gynecologic Disease,
edited by G.D. Adamson and D.C. Martin.
Lippincott-Raven Publishers, Philadelphia © 1996.

CHAPTER 19

Laser Uterosacral Nerve Ablation

Joseph R. Feste

Presacral neurectomy and uterosacral nerve ablation have long been used by gynecologists to treat dysmenorrhea in the presence or absence of pelvic pathology (1,2). Although indications and criteria for patient selection are similar for uterosacral nerve ablation and presacral neurectomy, only the former is discussed in this chapter. Presacral neurectomy is described in the following chapter.

Dysmenorrhea is a severe, painful cramping sensation in the lower abdomen often accompanied by other biological symptoms, including sweating, tachycardia, headache, nausea, vomiting, diarrhea, and tremulousness. It is usually characterized by midpelvic pain occurring from a few days to a few hours prior to the menses, and lasting sometimes throughout the menstrual cycle and occasionally for several days after. Primary dysmenorrhea is not associated with any demonstrable pelvic pathology. Secondary dysmenorrhea, on the other hand, is associated with pathologic signs, such as endometriosis, adenomyosis, or uterine leiomyomata. Interestingly, those patients with primary dysmenorrhea are many times the most difficult to treat. It is imperative that appropriate medical therapy be administered before surgical intervention is performed on any patient complaining of dysmenorrhea.

The management of patients with dysmenorrhea has been revolutionized by advances in operative laparoscopy. As operator skills have increased and instrumentation been refined, the laparoscope has been used not only to document pelvic disease and provide histologic diagnosis but to treat extensive endometriosis and adhesions.

The laparoscopic approach to presacral neurectomy and uterosacral nerve ablation is becoming a desirable alternative to laparotomy for performing these procedures since it is associated with minimized trauma, cost, recovery time, and possibility of pelvic adhesions, and it provides similar relief from pain.

J. R. Feste: Department of Obstetrics and Gynecology, Baylor College of Medicine, University Health Science Center, Houston, Texas 77054.

INCIDENCE

The actual incidence of dysmenorrhea is difficult to determine. One of the more comprehensive studies was instituted by Andersch and Milsom from Gothenburg, Sweden in 1982 (3). They found the prevalence of dysmenorrhea in a group of 19-year-old women to be 72%. Fifteen percent suffered dysmenorrhea that limited daily activity and was unimproved by analgesics. Oral contraceptive use as well as smoking was associated with a statistically significant decrease in the incidence of dysmenorrhea. An increased severity of dysmenorrhea was noted in women with an early menarche, in those with an increased amount of menstrual flow, in nulligravidas, and in women who had experienced induced or spontaneous abortion. The authors observed that the severity of dysmenorrhea was not affected by height, weight, or regularity of the menstrual cycle.

ANATOMY

(Refer to the *Anatomy* section of the chapter by Feste and Wilson, "Presacral Neurectomy," for a thorough description.) In a study of 33 cadavers, Campbell identified parasympathetic fibers in the anterior two thirds of the uterosacral ligaments (4). In the area where the ligaments attach directly to the posterior cervix, small ganglia were noted. Therefore, it is theorized that surgical division of the uterosacral ligaments at this point should interrupt the cervical and some uterine sensory fibers, and result in diminished uterine pain.

HISTORY

The procedure from which uterosacral nerve ablation was derived was first described by Ruggi in 1899 (5). In his original article, the procedure was performed through an abdominal incision and gave pelvic pain relief to 11 patients. Later, Doyle designed a vaginal approach as an alternative to interruption of the uterosacral ligaments and nerves (6–8). The procedure he described actually was performed either transabdominally or transvaginally. With respect to the vaginal approach, the attachments of the uterosacral ligaments to the cervix were divided between two Haney clamps, much as in the first steps of a vaginal hysterectomy. To prevent regrowth of the bisected nerve trunks, the surgeon bisects the posterior leaf of the peritoneal incision vertically and the mobilized segments are sutured over the proximal stumps and to the submucosal fascia of the top of the vagina. Doyle's abdominal approach was unique in that he attached the uterosacral ligaments to the back of the cervix about 1 cm higher than the point of their original attachment.

In one of the initial series reported by Doyle, he obtained complete relief of dysmenorrhea in 63 of 73 cases (86%) (7). Thirty had primary dysmenorrhea (85% success) and 33 had secondary dysmenorrhea (86.8% success). Relief was partial in 6 cases, and there were 4 failures. For reasons unknown, this procedure was abandoned for many years. Possible explanations include the fact that the procedure was performed by laparotomy for the most part, even though a vaginal approach was described by Doyle. Interest in Doyle's work was revived in 1981 with the development of surgical lasers that could be used endoscopically to perform the procedure. This laparoscopic technique was first described in 1985 by Feste reporting on 3 years of experience (9).

INDICATIONS AND CONTRAINDICATIONS

Laser uterosacral nerve ablation is indicated primarily in patients who have failed to respond to traditional therapy, which should have included antiprostaglandin therapy, oral contraceptives, or other commonly utilized analgesic therapy. Moreover, until medical therapy has failed and unless the patient's working ability or scholastic activity is affected, a general anesthesia and even a minimally invasive procedure should not be recommended. Even though there have been reports of presacral neurectomy or uterosacral nerve ablation to treat chronic pelvic pain or dyspareunia, this procedure has no place in the treatment of these conditions. It should be used only to treat primary or secondary dysmenorrhea.

Contraindications for uterosacral ablation are very few. One of the most obvious would be the inability to identify the uterosacral ligaments and cervix. In such a situation, attempting to guess the location of the nerve could lead to injury to the uterine vessels or ureter. Under such circumstances, one should be prepared to perform a presacral neurectomy. I find it advantageous to have the patient prepared to undergo either procedure.

SURGICAL TECHNIQUE

With the patient in dorsal lithotomy with a small amount of hip flexion, a deep Trendelenberg position is achieved to remove all the bowel from the cul-de-sac. The uterus is markedly anteflexed allowing easier identification of the uterosacral ligaments. Before the ablation is performed, the cervix and uterosacral ligaments must be identified. On some occasions the ligaments are attenuated and not easily visualized. In such instances, the only way to precisely define the optimal location for uterosacral nerve ligation is first to identify the cervix behind the peritoneum. It is sometimes helpful to place a blunt secondary probe lateral to the ligament and apply gentle pressure medially (Fig. 1). If this can be done, the nerve can be properly destroyed despite poorly developed uterosacral ligaments.

When the uterosacral ligaments are properly identified, a 1 cm hole is drilled into the uterosacral ligament

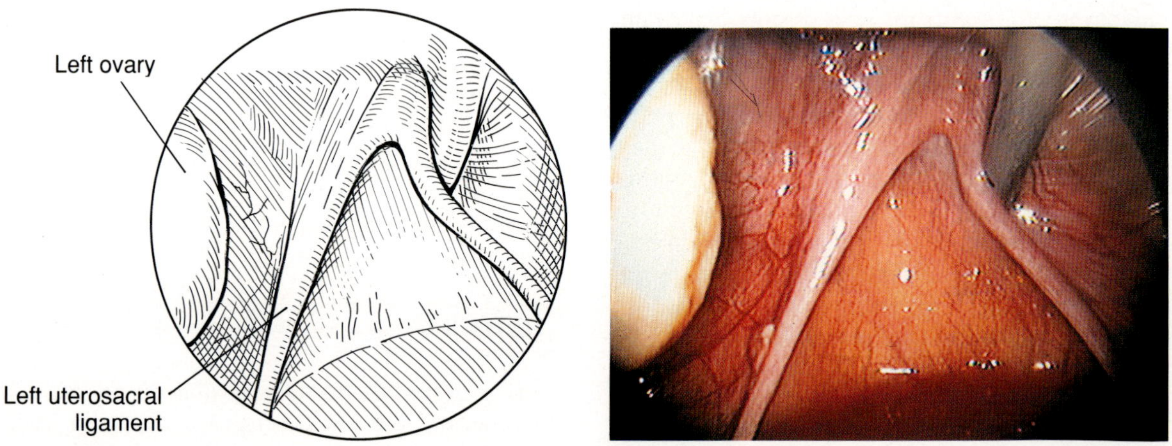

FIG. 1. Location of the uterosacral ligaments, their attachment to the cervix, and proximity to the ureters.

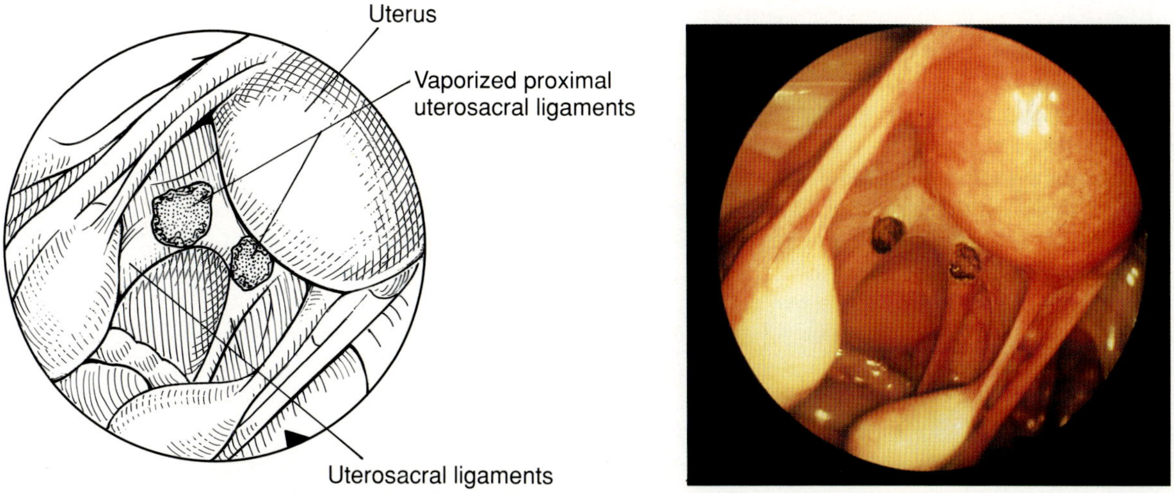

FIG. 2. Location of uterosacral ablation at attachments of uterosacral ligaments.

by CO_2 laser at 15–20 watts (Fig. 2). The usual depth is approximately 1 cm, but the dissection can be carried down the uterosacral ligament another few millimeters if necessary. It is not crucial to vaporize laterally outside of the uterosacral ligament because the uterine vessels and ureters lie only 1–2 cm away. The argon, neodymium: yttrium-aluminum-garnet (Nd:YAG), or potassium-trideuterium-phosphate (KTP) lasers may also be used for this procedure. The wavelengths of these lasers provide more hemostasis than the CO_2 laser. The electrosurgical technique has also been reported to achieve equally good results. Some investigators have advocated destroying tissue between the two ligament attachments on the back of the cervix to destroy further the sensory nerves to the uterus (6).

RESULTS

The literature contains several articles on laparoscopic uterosacral nerve ablation (9–12). Most of these have been reported since the early 1980s. Prior to that time, most surgical procedures for dysmenorrhea were discouraged because of the availability of the nonsteroidal antiinflammatory drugs (13,14). In most cases, the authors have reported separately those patients with primary and secondary dysmenorrhea. Several surgical methods have been used; however, most reports have described use of laser energy (9,12). Pain relief has been recorded in 50–84% of patients both with primary and secondary dysmenorrhea. The first report by Feste described treatment of 42 patients (9). Thirty patients (71%) had complete or significant relief of symptoms. Of 32 who had endometriosis, 72% were cured; of 10 with primary dysmenorrhea, 70% were cured. One review article by Daniell and Feste reported combined results using the carbon dioxide laser in a series of 50 patients (10). Sixty-four percent with endometriosis and 50% with primary dysmenorrhea were cured; 19% and 21%, respectively, were unchanged. After treatment with CO_2 laser, 6% with endometriosis but none with primary dysmenorrhea reported an increase in dysmenorrhea. Feste reported on 146 patients and found a success rate of 78% in patients with endometriosis and a success rate of 82% for patients with primary dysmenorrhea (*unpublished observations*). Sutton reported that of 100 patients with endometriosis, 86% had improvement of dysmenorrhea and 14% had none (12). Of 26 patients with primary dysmenorrhea, 73% had improvement of pain and 27% had none.

One of the more interesting articles in the literature was published by Lichten and Bombard (15). They reported the only double-blind prospective study of the efficacy of uterosacral nerve ablation in 21 patients with primary dysmenorrhea. Eighty-one percent (9 of 11) reported significant relief from menstrual pain. Half of the treated women reported continued relief of menstrual pain at 12 months. No patient in the control group reported relief from dysmenorrhea at 3 and 12 months after surgery. Donnez reported a series of 100 patients followed for more than a year (16). He found complete relief of symptoms in 50% of patients and mild to moderate relief in 41%. There was no change in 9%, and no patient had worsening of her symptoms. Interestingly, both Sutton and Donnez reported some relief of dyspareunia, which has been postulated to be due to relief of taut and well-demarcated uterosacral ligaments (12,16). In Donnez's group, a few of the patients had relief of dysmenorrhea in the absence of obvious endometriosis. However in 10% of patients who showed no laparoscopic evidence of endometriosis, there was evidence of endometriosis in 50% of the biopsies of the uterosacral ligaments.

Several other important issues should be mentioned in connection with uterosacral ablation. First, Daniell reported that some patients may have pain with their first menstrual period after the neurectomy is performed

(11). Sutton suggested that this may be due to a psychological overlay because none of his patients experienced this (12). This phenomenon maybe be due to edema and irritation of the nerve while it is healing. A second concern is the reason for recurrent symptoms. Doyle reported consistently good, lasting results (6–8). The reason may have to do with the fact that Doyle interposed peritoneum between the cut ends of the uterosacral ligaments. This may very well prevent regrowth of the nerves in this area, especially when the two ends of the cut nerve tend to come in close contact with each other when the tension is taken off the ligament and the uterus returns to its original position. Third, I have discussed with Edward Lichten other potential reasons for failure of the LUNA procedure. He measured the intrauterine and intracervical pressure before and after the LUNA procedure. There was a significant difference in the pressure: it decreased in half immediately after the procedure. There was a gradual return to the original pressures 1–2 years following the procedure, coinciding with the times the dysmenorrhea returned in the same patients. These events suggest that the motor nerves are deinervated rather than sensory nerves, resulting in an increase in dysmenorrhea as the pressure within the uterus and cervix returns to the original levels.

COMPLICATIONS

Complications associated with uterosacral nerve ablation have rarely been reported. Sutton reported that of 100 patients, two had immediate postoperative bleeding at the operative site (12). These were controlled by coagulation or with hemostatic clips and the insertion of a redivac drain in the pelvis for 12 hr. In 1985, Feste reported 42 cases of laser neurectomy with no complications except the same minor bleeding reported by Dr. Sutton. Subsequently, Feste has performed over 350 uterosacral nerve ablations with only a few requiring bipolar cautery coagulation of bleeding within the crater of the neurectomy. There have been a few reports of severance of one or both ureters. However, in most instances, these patients had previously undergone laparotomy with a plication of the uterosacral ligaments to obliterate the cul-de-sac. A Kleppenger bipolar forcep was used to cauterize the uterosacral ligament, with the end of the forcep placed across the plicated ligament. Unavoidably, both ligaments are displaced medially with this procedure and therefore the ureters may be pulled in medially as well.

HIGHLIGHTS

Laparoscopic uterosacral ablation has proved to be a valuable procedure for the treatment of primary or secondary dysmenorrhea. The procedure is relatively easy to perform and is associated with very few complications. Yet the long-term results are still somewhat questionable. Whether return of pain is due to regrowth of the severed nerve that could be prevented by superimposing a small piece of Gore-Tex graft in the created defect is yet to be determined. More studies need to be performed regarding the long-term results of the procedure. Certainly, the degree of difficulty is small in the hands of a skilled surgeon. Most notably, the gynecologist has at least one minimally invasive procedure that can aid in the treatment of intractable dysmenorrhea.

REFERENCES

1. Davis A. Intrinsic dysmenorrhea. *Proc R Soc Med* 1936;29:931.
2. Latarjet A, Roget P. Le plexus hypogastrique chez la femme. *Gynecol Obstet* 1922;6:225.
3. Andersch B, Milsom I. An epidemiologic study of young women with dysmenorrhea. *Am J Obstet Gynecol* 1982;144:655.
4. Campbell RM. Anatomy and physiology of sacro-uterine ligaments. *Am J Obstet Gynecol* 1950;59:1.
5. Ruggi G. Della Sympatectamia al collo ed ale adome. *Policlinico* 1899;193.
6. Doyle JB. Paracervical uterine denervation for dysmenorrhea. *Trans N Eng Obstet Gynecol Soc.* 1954;8:143.
7. Doyle JB. Paracervical uterine denervation by transection of the cervical plexus for the relief of dysmenorrhea. *Am J Obstet Gynecol* 1955;70:1.
8. Doyle JB, Des Rosiers JJ. Paracervical uterine denervation for relief of pelvic pain. *Clin Obstet Gynecol* 1963;6:742–753.
9. Feste JR. Laser laparoscopy: a new modality. *J Reprod Med* 1985;30:414.
10. Daniell JF, Feste JR. Laser laparoscopy. In: Keye WR, ed. *Laser surgery in gynecology and obstetrics.* Boston: GK Hall and Co: 1985:147–165.
11. Daniell JF. Fiberoptic laser laparoscopy. In: Sutton C, ed. *Bailliere's Clinical Obstetrics and Gynecology.* London: Bailliere Tindall; 1989.
12. Sutton C. Laser operative laparoscopy and hysteroscopy. Donnez, J, ed. Nauwelpaeats printing - Leaven Belgium. Chapter 3, 1989, p. 43–52.
13. Henzl MR. Dysmenorrhea: achievements and challengds. *Sex Med Today* 1985;9:8.
14. Dawood YM. Dysmenorrhea. *Pain Analg* 1985;1:20.
15. Lichten J. Surgical treatment of dysmenorrhea with laparoscopic uterine nerve ablation. *J Reprod Med* 1987;32:37–42.
16. Donnez J. Carbon-dioxide laser laparoscopy in pelvic pain and infertility in laparoscopy surgery. In: Sutton C, ed. *Bailliere's Clinical Obstetrics and Gynecology.* London: Bailliere Tindall; 1989.

Endoscopic Management of Gynecologic Disease,
edited by G.D. Adamson and D.C. Martin.
Lippincott-Raven Publishers, Philadelphia © 1996.

CHAPTER 20

Presacral Neurectomy

Joseph R. Feste and Ellen E. Wilson

Presacral neurectomy and uterosacral nerve ablation are procedures that have been performed over many decades by gynecologists for the treatment of dysmenorrhea in the presence or absence of pelvic pathology. Dysmenorrhea is one of the most common and perplexing complaints of women presenting for gynecologic consultation. The presence of endometriosis, adenomyosis, or leiomyomata uteri may explain the signs and symptoms of dysmenorrhea in certain patients. However, in many instances no pathology is found. It is important that all patients with dysmenorrhea have adequate medical therapy before surgical intervention is undertaken. In addition, a number of nongynecologic causes of pelvic pain must be considered initially before there is any medical or surgical intervention. Diagnostic laparoscopy is frequently used to document pelvic disease and, on occasion, to provide histologic diagnosis. In recent years, the advent of advanced operative laparoscopy has revolutionized the management of patients with dysmenorrhea or chronic pelvic pain. Patients with extensive endometriosis and adhesions are now treated through the laparoscope (see the chapter by Shamma and Diamond, "Postoperative Adhesion Development After Operative Laparoscopy: Evaluation at Early Second-Look Procedures," and the chapter by Adamson, "Endometriosis").

Formerly performed only by laparotomy, presacral neurectomy and uterosacral nerve ablation are increasingly being performed through the laparoscope. The intention is to minimize trauma, lessen the possibility of pelvic adhesions, and provide relief from pain without resorting to major abdominal surgery.

HISTORY

The first published descriptions of presacral nerve resection in women with severe dysmenorrhea were by Ruggi from Italy and Jaboulay from France in 1899 (1, 2). However, interest in the operation did not gain momentum until Cotte reported his experience with the procedure, beginning in 1925 (3,4). Black reviewed the world literature (72 articles) published between 1936 and 1963, sent out questionnaires to several hundred gynecologists, and evaluated success within his own practice (5). He estimated a 75–80% success rate in 9,937 cases. Since that time, many authors have published numerous reports on their use of presacral neurectomy in the treatment of dysmenorrhea (6–32).

After the introduction of nonsteroidal antiinflammatory agents in the 1970s for the alleviation of dysmenorrhea, fewer surgeries were performed for this condition (33). However, the limited capability of medical therapy together with the widespread use of laparoscopic methods of pelvic denervation led to a resurgence of interest in presacral and uterosacral nerve interruption. One prospective study by Tjaden et al. on the relief of midline dysmenorrhea in patients with stage III–IV endometriosis revealed an 88% success rate when presacral neurectomy was performed in conjunction with resection of endometriosis (29). No patients received relief of midline pain when resection of endometriosis was performed without presacral neurectomy. The majority of retrospective studies on this subject show similar results. Interestingly, the success rate for primary dysmenorrhea is reported to be greater than that for secondary dysmenorrhea (14,16,31). However, since current medical therapy is so successful in ameliorating primary dysmenorrhea, surgery is rarely indicated.

A recent article by Candiani et al. discussed 71 patients with moderate or severe endometriosis and midline dysmenorrhea who were randomized for treatment of endometriosis by laparotomy with and without presacral neurectomy (30). The investigators noted marked reduction in midline component of menstrual pain but no difference in the two groups in the frequency and severity of dysmenorrhea, pelvic pain, and dyspareunia. One would not expect any reduction in the latter three symptoms,

J. R. Feste: Department of Obstetrics and Gynecology, Baylor College of Medicine, Univeristy Health Science Center, Houston, Texas 77054.

E. E. Wilson: Private Practice, Dallas, Texas 75230.

since the presacral neurectomy is to be used only in those patients with midline pain occurring at the time of menses. The variation of technique may also contribute to the differences found in other series where presacral neurectomy provided virtually 90% relief of midline dysmenorrhea.

Thus far, there is scant literature regarding the laparoscopic approach to presacral neurectomy, since this has traditionally been a procedure performed through a large abdominal incision. Perez recently described in detail one technique for performing a presacral neurectomy through the laparoscope and his success rate with 25 patients (23). One patient required exploratory laparotomy for a retroperitoneal bleed and the other 24 experienced significant decrease in their postoperative central pain for a mean follow-up period of 13 months. Subsequently, two patients required repeat laparoscopies for adnexal pain, and two patients required hysterectomies and bilateral salpingo-oophorectomies after failure to respond to conservative management. In my unreported series of 135 patients the overall relief was 89%. These initial results suggest that the laparoscopic approach may be as effective as that by laparotomy, but randomized clinical trials with large patient numbers are required to reach a definitive conclusion.

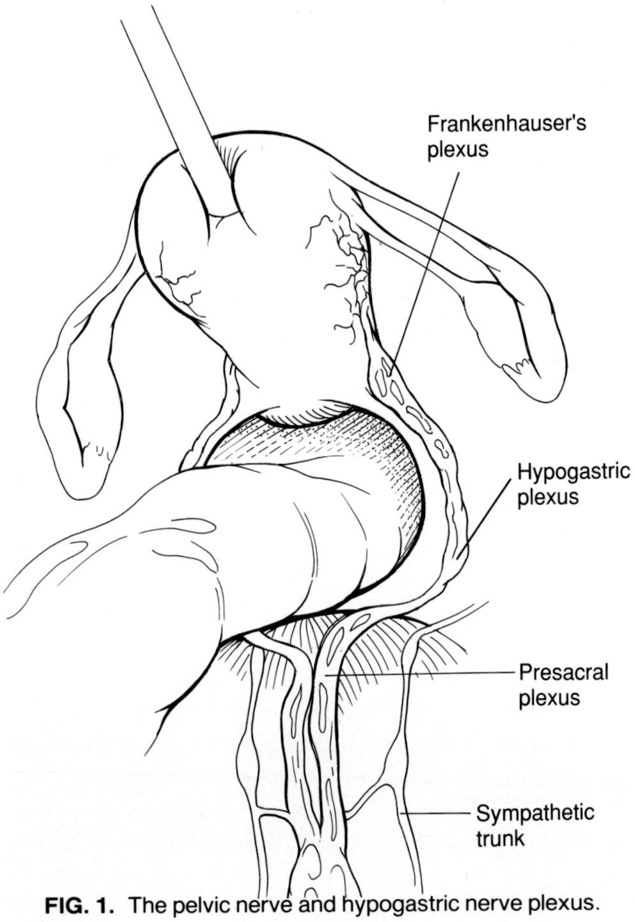

FIG. 1. The pelvic nerve and hypogastric nerve plexus.

ANATOMY

Pain impulses from the cervix, body of the uterus, and proximal fallopian tubes are transmitted through afferent fibers that accompany sympathetic nerves into the spinal cord at the lower thoracic and lumbar levels (21). Specifically, sympathetic nerves emerging from the uterus pass through the uterosacral ligaments along the cardinal ligament to join the pelvic plexus (34). Hemorrhoidal (rectal), vesical (bladder), and uterovaginal plexuses (ganglion of Frankenhauser) contribute fibers to this plexus (35). These afferent fibers course proximally to become the inferior hypogastric plexus, the middle hypogastric plexus, and finally the superior hypogastric plexus—otherwise known as the presacral nerve, at the level of the sacral promontory (Fig. 1). At this point they usually form two or three incompletely fused nerve trunks, which lie in a retroperitoneal position over the bodies of the fourth and fifth lumbar vertebrae. In 20% of cases, the nerve trunks fuse to become a single nerve (34). Superior to the presacral nerve lies the bifurcation of the aorta and inferior is the hollow of the sacrum. The right common iliac artery, vein, and ureter are on the right, and the inferior mesenteric vessels, sigmoid mesocolon, and left ureter are on the left. The middle sacral artery and vein are situated in close proximity to the presacral nerve, and care must be taken during surgery to avoid tramatizing these vessels.

INDICATIONS

Prior to 1960, very broadly defined indications were thought to justify presacral neurectomy (36). In 1949, Cotte's indications for the procedure included not only dysmenorrhea but vaginismus, pelvic neuralgias, resistant vulvar itch, and "genital superexcitement" (4). He reported a 98% success rate in over 1500 patients over a 22-year period. As our knowledge of pelvic anatomy and neural pathways has become more sophisticated, many of these older indications have become obsolete (35). Today, presacral neurectomy is indicated for those patients with dysmenorrhea (primary or secondary) who have failed a trial of medical therapy. Presacral neurectomy is often advocated as an adjunctive procedure to adhesiolysis and conservative therapy for endometriosis (37). The procedure is not indicated for adnexal pain because distal fallopian tubal innervation and ovarian sensory innervation are associated with the inferior mesenteric plexus and not the presacral nerve. In addition, presacral neurectomy is not indicated for pain associated with invasive carcinoma (38).

TECHNIQUE

Presacral neurectomy has traditionally been performed through a midline vertical or lower abdominal

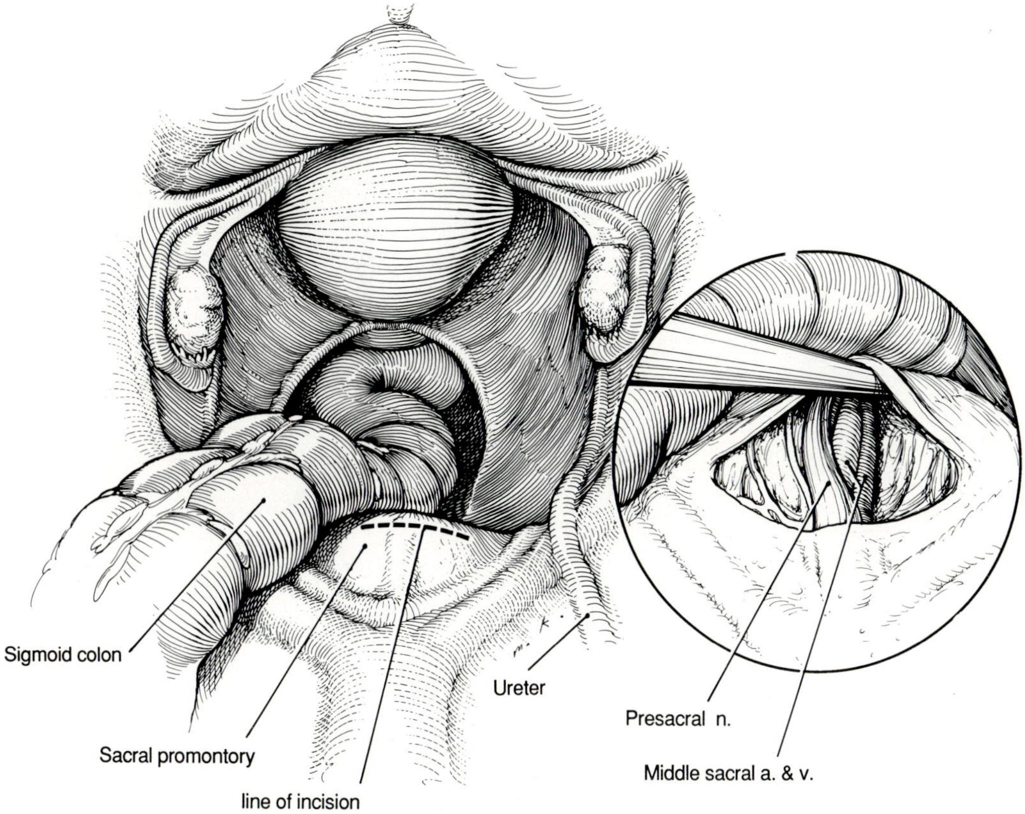

FIG. 2. Panorama view of sacral promontory (*inset*).

transverse incision. With the advent of operative endoscopy for the diagnosis and treatment of various pelvic disorders and with the emphasis on outpatient surgery, a laparoscopic approach to the classic presacral neurectomy has been developed and increasingly used.

The patient is placed in the dorsal lithotomy position with only a small degree of hip flexion. Using a 11-mm umbilical trocar with a 10-mm diagnostic laparoscope and two 5.5-mm suprapubic trocars—one in the midline and the other lateral to the inferior epigastrics—the surgeon is able to perform a thorough investigation of the pelvic and abdominal viscera. Any pelvic adhesions

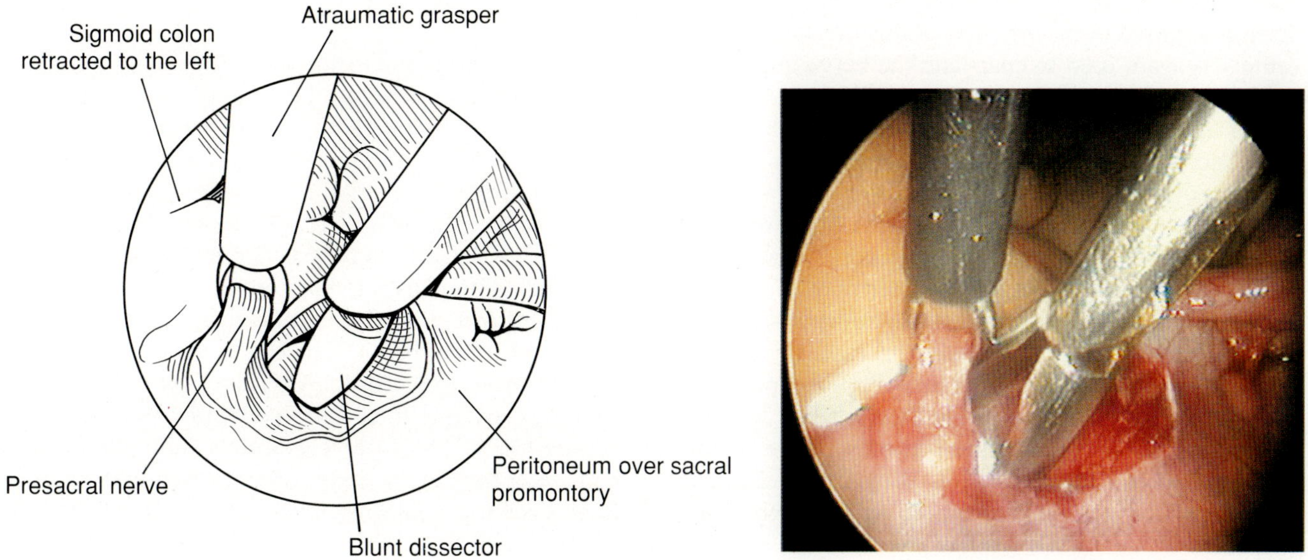

FIG. 3. Blunt dissection used to expose the presacral nerve.

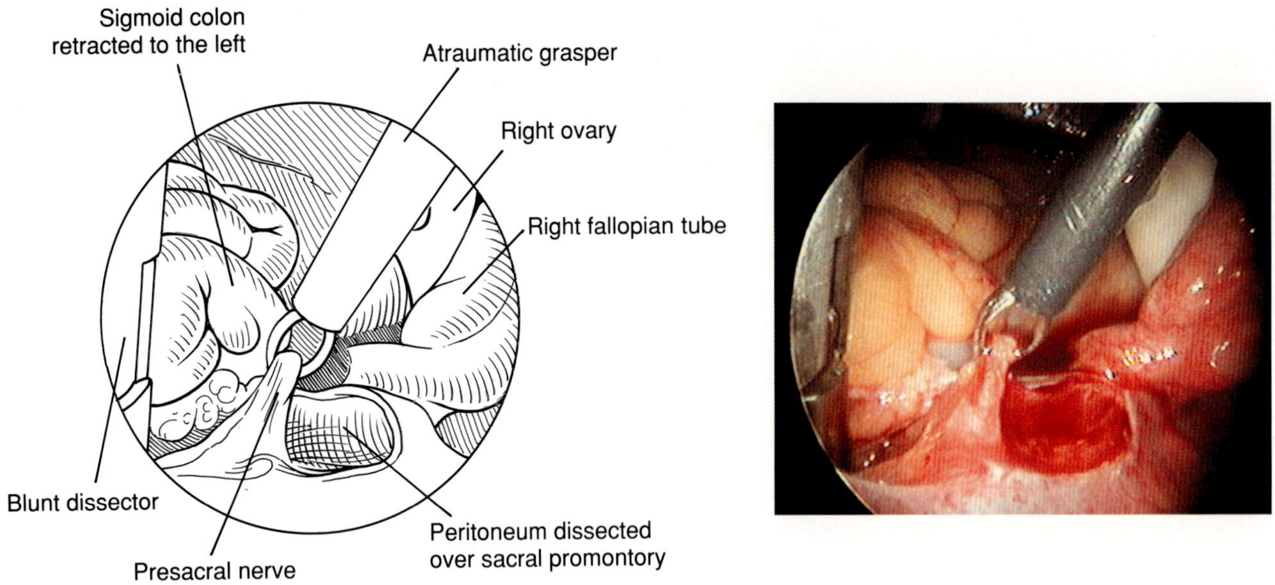

FIG. 4. Isolation of the presacral nerve.

and endometriotic implants are ablated using laser energy. The patient, in full Trendelenburg position, is tilted to the left, and the peritoneum over the sacropromontory is exposed with the bowel displaced to the left and superior (Fig. 2). A 3- to 4-cm incision is made in the peritoneum over the sacropromontory using the CO_2 laser (inset, Fig. 2).

Blunt dissection is used to spread the underlying areolar tissue to expose the presacral nerve and middle sacral vessels (Fig. 3). Any small bleeding vessels are coagulated with a bipolar instrument. A blunt grasping instrument, passed through one of the suprapubic ports, is used to pick up the presacral nerve, and a bipolar instrument is carried down through the operative laparoscope to coagulate the nerve superior to the grasping forceps (Fig. 4). Scissors are used to cut the nerve at this site, and bipolar cautery is again used to coagulate the nerve inferior to the grasping forceps. The 2- to 3-cm segment of nerve within the grasping forceps is then cut, carried from the field, and sent to pathology. It has always been considered important to send a specimen for verification of proper nerve excision in the event that the procedure fails to alleviate dysmenorrhea. Endoscopic clips or the yttrium-aluminum-garnet (YAG) laser may be used in lieu of the bipolar instrument to ligate the nerve. It is recommended that a clip be used on each side of the nerve and that a small segment between the clips be removed. The peritoneal edges are then left free to heal. There is no reason to close the peritoneal space, as the rectosigmoid colon will fall over the incision site and thus protect the incision from exposure to any significant structures.

CONTRAINDICATIONS

Contraindications to laparoscopic presacral neurectomy include those contraindications for laparoscopy alone: extreme obesity and moderate to severe bowel adhesions which limit exposure. Obesity can make the procedure difficult to perform because of retroperitoneal fat formation and increased difficulty in dissection of the sacropromontory area. Moderate to severe bowel adhesions over the area of the sacral promontory may preclude adequate exposure needed for effective performance of the procedure.

COMPLICATIONS

Most notable in the realm of intraoperative complications is excessive bleeding. The middle sacral vessels are located in the midline between the presacral nerve and the periosteum of the sacral promontory. Usually the nerve is dissected anterior to the vessels and ligation is not necessary. However, if bleeding should occur from torn vessels, ligation may be performed without adverse sequelae. Alternatively, hemostasis may be obtained with the use of endocoagulation, argon laser, or thumbtack application (39–41). Dissection must be performed directly over the promontory, and careful attention should be given to the location of both ureters and great vessels. Occasionally one encounters anomalous vessels or a ureter close to the midline, but with careful attention these structures can be avoided. Even though there have been no reported cases, injury to the right ureter would be a more likely complication than injury to the left ureter. A more likely injury would be the common iliac vein or vena cava. An injury to these structures would require immediate attention with an exploratory laparotomy. I have had no complications in 135 patients treated laparoscopically.

With respect to postoperative side effects, there have been a few reports of temporary difficulties in emptying the bladder, continuous leakage of a small amount of urine, and two cases of chronic permanent constipation following presacral neurectomy for central pelvic pain (16,37). It is unknown whether these symptoms resulted from the procedures. In reporting the thousands of cases treated since 1964, few authors have addressed the issue of postoperative complications or disturbing symptoms. Freier reported a 25% incidence (5 of 20 cases) of constipation at follow-up examination (10). He also noted that 6 of 20 patients experienced menorrhagia in the first cycle or two following the operation. This latter finding has also been reported elsewhere, although it does not appear to be a persistent problem (21). No change in sexual function is reported. Of note is that patients who become pregnant following presacral neurectomy may have less discomfort during the first stage of labor. Ingersoll reported that of 24 patients who had undergone presacral neurectomy and subsequently became pregnant, 8 patients, or 33.3%, experienced only mild uterine contraction discomfort and required no medication (14). Two primiparas did not know they were in labor until the vertex appeared at the perineum.

HIGHLIGHTS

Operative endoscopy for the evaluation of pelvic complaints provides a convenient, minimally traumatic way of establishing a diagnosis and treating pelvic pain without recourse to major abdominal surgery. Presacral neurectomy for the treatment of primary or secondary dysmenorrhea has been performed over many decades through a midline or transverse abdominal incision. With the increasing use of operative endoscopy in the management of pelvic pain, several gynecologists have added laparoscopic presacral neurectomy to their armamentarium of procedures for the relief of various types of dysmenorrhea. With a high level of operator skill, laparoscopic presacral neurectomy can be performed safely and effectively. Thus far, evidence suggests good pain relief may be achieved whether the procedure is performed laparoscopically or via a laparotomy incision.

REFERENCES

1. Ruggi G. Della Sympatectamia al collo ed ale adome. *Policlinico* 1899;193.
2. Jaboulay M. Le traitement de la mevralgie pelvienne par la paralysie du sympathique sacre. *Lyon Med* 1899;90:102.
3. Cotte G. Resection of the presacral nerves in the treatment of obstinate dysmenorrhea. *Am J Obstet Gynecol* 1937;33:1034–1040.
4. Cotte G. Technique of presacral neurectomy. *Am J Surg* 1949;78: 50–53.
5. Black WT. Use of presacral sympathectomy in the treatment of dysmenorrhea. *Am J Obstet Gynecol* 1964;89:16–22.
6. Beecham CT. Endometriosis: When is surgical treatment indicated? *Posts Rad Med* 1978;63:221.
7. Browne O. A survey of 113 cases of primary dysmenorrhea treated by neurectomy. *Am J Obstet Gynecol* 1949;57:1053–1068.
8. Counseller VS, Craig W. The treatment of dysmenorrhea by resection of the presacral sympathetic nerves: evaluation and end results. *Am J Obstet Gynecol* 1934;28:161–172.
9. Dawood YM. *Premenstrual syndrome and dysmenorrhea.* Baltimore: Urban and Schwarzenberg; 1985: 99.
10. Freier A. Pelvic neurectomy in gynecology. *Obstet Gynecol* 1965;25:48–55.
11. Garcia CR, David SS. Pelvic endometriosis: Infertility and pelvic pain. *Am J Obstet Gynecol* 1977;129:740–747.
12. Greenhill JP. Sympathectomy for the relief of pelvic pain in women. *J Mt Sinai Hosp* 1947;14:363–368.
13. Henzl MR. Dysmenorrhea: achievements and challenge. *Sex Med Today* 1985;9:8.
14. Ingersoll FM, Meigs JV. Presacral neurectomy for dysmenorrhea. *N Engl J Med* 1948;238:357–360.
15. Keene FE. The treatment of dysmenorrhea by presacral sympathectomy. *Am J Obstet Gynecol* 1935;30:534–543.
16. Lee RB, Stone K, Magelssen D, Belts R, Benson W. Presacral neurectomy for chronic pelvic pain. *Obstet Gynecol* 1986;68:517–521.
17. Mahfoud HK, Hewitt SR. A place for presacral neurectomy. *Ir Med J* 1981;74:198–199.
18. Malinak LR. Operative management of pelvic pain. *Clin Obstet Gynecol* 1980;23:191–200.
19. Malinak LR. Infertility and endometriosis: operative technique, clinical staging, and prognosis. *Clin Obstet Gynecol* 1980;23:925–935.
20. Malinak LR. Pelvic pain—when is surgery indicated? *Contemp Ob Gyn* 1985;26:43–51.
21. Malinak LR. Operative management of pelvic pain. In: Sciarra JJ, ed. *Gynecology and obstetrics.* vol 1. Philadelphia: JB Lippincott; 1988, chap 78.
22. Meigs JV. Excision of the superior hypogastric plexus for primary dysmenorrhea. *SGO* 1939;68:723.
23. Perez JJ. Laparoscopic presacral neurectomy. Results of the first 25 cases. *J Reprod Med* 1990;35:625–630.
24. Phaneuf LE. Presacral neurectomy in intractable dysmenorrhea. *J Mt Sinai Hosp* 1947;14:553–555.
25. Polan M, DeCherney A. Presacral neurectomy for pelvic pain in infertility. *Fertil Steril* 1980;34:557–560.
26. Pratt JH. Discussion section of presacral sympathectomy and dysmenorrhea (Black WT). *Am J Obstet Gynecol* 1964;89:20–22.
27. Puolakka J, Kauppila A, Ronnberg L. Results in the operative treatment of pelvic endometriosis. *Acta Obstet Gynecol Scand* 1980;59:429–431.
28. Taylor PJ, Gomel V: Pelvic pain. *Curr Prob Obstet Gynecol Fertil* 1987;10:9.
29. Tjaden B, Schlaff WD, Kimball A, Rock J. The efficacy of presacral neurectomy for the relief of midline dysmenorrhea. *Obstet Gynecol* 1990;76:89–91.
30. Candiani GB, Fedele L, Vercelini P, Bianchi S, Di Nola G. Presacral neurectomy for the treatment of pelvic pain associated with endometriosis: a controlled study. *Am J Obstet Gynecol* 1992;167: 100–103.
31. Tucker AW. An evaluation of presacral neurectomy in the treatment of dysmenorrhea. *Am J Obstet Gynecol.* 1947;53:226–232.
32. Weed JC, Holland JB. Endometriosis and infertility: an enigma. *Fertil Steril* 1977;28:135.
33. Swartz A, Zor U, Lindner HR, et al. Primary dysmenorrhea: alleviation by an inhibitor of prostaglandin synthesis and action. *Obstet Gynecol* 1974;11:709.
34. Curtis AH, Anson BJ, Ashley FL, Jones T. The anatomy of the

pelvic autonomic nerves in relation to gynecology. *SGO* 1942;73: 743–750.
35. Meyer WR, Diamond MP, Lavy G, DeCherney AH. Presacral neurectomy relieves chronic pelvic pain. *Contemp Ob Gyn* 1989;34:37–44.
36. Ranney BR: Discussion of Black WT: use of presacral sympathectomy in the treatment of dysmenorrhea. *Am J Obstet Gynecol* 1964;89:22.
37. Kistner RW. Management of endometriosis in the infertile patient. *Fertil Steril* 1975;26:1151–1166.
38. Stovall TG, Ling FW. Relieving chronic pelvic pain through surgery. *Contemp Ob Gyn* 1991;36(4):11–22.
39. Patsner B, Orr JW. Intractable venous sacral hemorrhage: use of stainless steel thumbtacks to obtain hemostasis. *Am J Obstet Gynecol* 1990;162:452.
40. Mann WJ. A comment on thumbtacks for hemorrhage control. *Am J Obstet Gynecol* 1990;163:1092–1093.
41. Timmons MC, Kohler MF, Addison WA. Thumbtack use for control of presacral bleeding with description of an instrument for thumbtack application. *Obstet Gynecol* 1991;78:313–315.

Endoscopic Management of Gynecologic Disease,
edited by G.D. Adamson and D.C. Martin.
Lippincott-Raven Publishers, Philadelphia © 1996.

CHAPTER 21

Treatment of Bowel Lesions

David B. Redwine

PREVALENCE

Of all gynecologic laparoscopy procedures possible, treatment of endometriosis is the most commonly performed (1). Although most commonly found on the posterior pelvic peritoneal surfaces (2,3), endometriosis can also involve the bowel and represents the most common gynecologic condition of the intestinal tract. Ovarian remnant syndrome of the anterior sigmoid serosa is a distant second, but the principles of its management are similar to those for endometriosis. In patients with surgically diagnosed endometriosis, the incidence of intestinal involvement may range from less than 1% (4) to 25% (5).

ANATOMY

The gross anatomy of the cecum, ileum, appendix, and sigmoid is straightforward since these structures are not intimately surrounded by other tissues. However, the lower rectosigmoid and rectum are surrounded by tissues that obscure these structures, increasing the risk of unrecognized damage during the treatment of adjacent endometriosis. As the rectosigmoid dives beneath the peritoneal reflection becoming the rectum, small arteries supplying the bowel wall are found on each side of the pelvic floor. These vessels lie medial to the uterosacral ligaments and can potentially be injured during treatment of cul-de-sac disease, particularly if invasive. The rectum is parallel to and separated from the vagina by the fatty rectovaginal septum; this is very important in the treatment of obliteration of the cul-de-sac. Obliteration of the cul-de-sac usually signifies invasive disease of the uterosacral ligaments, posterior cervix, anterior rectal wall, and cul-de-sac. Partial obliteration of the cul-de-sac may draw the bowel wall toward one of the uterosacral ligaments in a subtle way which may be interpreted as simply slight thickening of the ligament and therefore place the bowel in jeopardy. The invasive endometriosis of the rectovaginal septum, which frequently accompanies complete obliteration of the cul-de-sac, rarely extends beyond the upper third of the vaginal length, so development of the normal rectovaginal septum distal to the invasive endometriosis is an important part of the isolation and subsequent treatment of this type of lesion. The rectum is bounded laterally by fibrofatty tissue extending from the lateral pelvic walls, and this tissue must be severed during treatment of the obliterated cul-de-sac, since complete mobilization of the rectum is necessary for safe treatment. Just lateral and distal to the uterosacral ligaments are large vessels ascending from the posterior vaginal wall. These vessels can be obscured by investing fibrosis and the surgeon must anticipate their presence.

D. B. Redwine: St. Charles Medical Center, Bend, Oregon 97701.

PATHOPHYSIOLOGY

The rectosigmoid colon is the bowel site most commonly involved in endometriosis, followed by the ileum, cecum, appendix, and jejunum (5). The layers of the colon include a serosal layer, an outer layer of longitudinal muscularis, an inner layer of circular muscularis, and the mucosa. The serosa does not extend beyond the peritoneal reflection of the cul-de-sac. The ileum is much thinner, consisting of a greatly attenuated serosa, one functional layer of thin muscularis, and the mucosa. Endometriosis of the bowel almost never penetrates through the mucosa of the bowel; therefore in most cases surgical treatment does not involve entering the lumen. Many small lesions can be treated by operating within the layers of the bowel wall and lifting the lesion off the muscularis or mucosa.

The means by which endometriosis causes progressive distortion of the bowel is not clearly known. However, it is clear that cyclic bleeding with the menses is not the likely irritant it was once thought to be, since nonhemorrhagic appearances are frequently found, and both histologic and morphologic studies have shown that endometriosis bleeds unpredictably, noncyclically, or not at all with menses (6,7). Irritation by endometriotic glandular secretions resulting in reactive fibrosis—as well as local invasion—are probably important factors in producing fibrosis, adhesions, and distortion. Since not all bowel lesions ever become invasive, there must exist a predetermined biological potential, which can vary from lesion to lesion even in the same pelvis.

CLINICAL PRESENTATION

At a referral center specializing in the surgical treatment of endometriosis, the mean age of 265 patients with any intestinal disease was 33.46 years, while the mean age of 756 patients without intestinal disease was 30.83 years (8). Many patients with pelvic endometriosis without intestinal involvement can have nonspecific bowel symptoms leading to a diagnosis of irritable bowel syndrome. Presumably the bowel is stimulated by the irritants in the peritoneal fluid of some endometriosis patients. For patients with bowel endometriosis, symptomatology depends highly on the depth of penetration into the bowel wall, as well as the location of the disease. Superficial lesions of the large or small bowel probably cause no symptoms, although their capacity for further invasion is unknown. With further invasion of the bowel wall comes an increase in surrounding fibrotic distortion. With sufficient intramural involvement or fibrotic distortion of the bowel wall, symptoms of partial bowel obstruction occur, including nausea, abdominal bloating, intestinal cramping, and occasional vomiting. Although such obstructive symptoms are to be expected with mechanical distortion of the bowel, a nodule of sufficient size may impede peristaltic waves and result in symptoms even without bowel wall distortion. In addition to obstructive symptoms, partial obstruction of the ileum may bring right lower quadrant pain, whereas large, partially obstructing nodules of the midsigmoid may lead to a sense of rectal fullness and urgency. Rectal nodules with obliteration of the cul-de-sac frequently produce rectal pain, rectal pain with bowel movements throughout the menstrual cycle, backache, and pain with intercourse that seems to be transmitted to the rectum. Of importance, superficial or invasive disease of the uterosacral ligaments or cul-de-sac can also lead to painful bowel movements, although frequently only in association with menses. Although cyclic rectal bleeding with menses is suggestive of intestinal endometriosis, 88% of patients who required full-thickness resections of intestinal lesions at laparotomy did not have rectal bleeding (8). Therefore, the absence of rectal bleeding says nothing about the possible presence of severe intestinal disease.

On pelvic examination, only disease of the rectum and lower sigmoid can be ascertained. Nodularity of the cul-de-sac or uterosacral ligaments suggests the possible presence of intestinal endometriosis, particularly in patients above the age of 30. On rectal examination, the mucosa usually feels like it slides over the nodule.

DIAGNOSIS

Occasionally a patient with intestinal distortion experiences pain during sigmoidoscopy or has a barium enema showing signs of extrinsic compression. However, since intestinal endometriosis almost never penetrates into the bowel lumen, and since most patients do not have significant intestinal distortion, sigmoidoscopy and barium studies are usually negative. Most intestinal studies therefore yield falsely negative results and the patient may receive a diagnosis of neurosis.

Surgery is usually necessary to establish the correct diagnosis of intestinal endometriosis. Methodical attention must be paid to the intestinal sites that are commonly involved in endometriosis. The innate biological potential of each lesion determines its appearance, and one or more lesions of any appearance may be found in any or all bowel sites. During laparoscopy, the use of steep Trendelenberg position helps establish a good field of view and facilitates suctioning of any peritoneal fluid. This exposes the cul-de-sac and distal sigmoid colon. A blunt probe can be used to manipulate the sigmoid and to place it on stretch from the pelvic brim to the cul-de-sac, thus aiding the identification of any surface irregularities. At surgery, the visual appearance of bowel endometriosis is frequently nonhemorrhagic, and the lesion may blend well with the surrounding yellow-white coloration of the large bowel. Colonic lesions usually are located on the antimesenteric surface of the bowel wall, so they are potentially easy to find. Isolated lesions of the mesenteric side of the bowel wall have not been reported, so a clinician need not worry about the bowel wall hidden by mesentery. A ring forceps passed into the rectosigmoid helps to identify any mass effect of the bowel wall. Palpating the bowel with atraumatic graspers often helps, since normal bowel wall can be completely collapsed between the grasper jaws, while even small nodules of endometriosis would snap out of the jaws. Larger nodules can be hidden by hypertrophy of the adjacent appendix epiploica, and even very large nodules can be completely hidden within the loop of bowel that can be gathered in around an irritative bowel nodule. Obliteration of the cul-de-sac is highly predictive of involvement of the uterosacral ligaments and wall of the upper rectum, but the yellowish-white fibrosis may be interpreted only as adhesions or as burned out disease of no consequence, and the diagnosis can be missed. However, invasive endometriosis displays histologic evidence of greater activity (9) and should be thought of as highly active burned in disease. The rectosigmoid colon should be examined methodically at least to the region of the left psoas muscle. Involvement of the descending, transverse, and ascending colon is uncommon. The cecum should be visualized and palpated. A normal appendix can arise from a nodular bed of endometriosis of the cecum. Occasionally endometriosis of the large bowel has associated hemorrhage in addition to some of the features listed above, and this may assist in diagnosis. The sigmoid mesentery also can be involved by usually superficial whitish fibrotic lesions of endometriosis. Endometriosis of the appendix frequently presents as curling and thickening of the tip.

The ileum is usually a slightly darker reddish color than is the colon, and endometriosis frequently appears as multiple or confluent whitish plaques which can be lined up on the antimesenteric surface of the bowel wall, usually within 30 cm of the cecum. Partially obstructing nodules cause rolling and retraction of the bowel wall around the lesion with a resultant mass effect. Rarely two or more obstructing lesions may be present. Occasionally, ileal lesions have adjacent hemorrhage.

INDICATIONS FOR TREATMENT

Physicians treat patients because of the presence of *symptoms* or *signs* of disease. If a patient has sufficient pain, unexplained infertility, or an abnormality on physical examination, such as tenderness, nodularity, or a mass, then surgical diagnosis is indicated. The threshold for surgical action in any patient depends on the patient's subjective evaluation of her pain duration and intensity as well as the degree of suspicion of the clinician. If endometriosis is found, it should be excised at laparoscopy or laparotomy. If it is left behind in the bowel or pelvis, not only may it continue to be the cause of symptoms and signs, but also the patient and her next surgeon will consider residual endometriosis to be the explanation for any symptoms that occur between the diaphragm and the thighs. Although superficial lesions may not be symptomatic, they too should be removed since their potential for causing future symptoms is unknown and they are easily treated. There are no specific contraindications for treatment.

ALTERNATIVE TREATMENT

Medical therapy has been shown not to eradicate endometriosis of any stage or location, resulting in persistence of disease in 78% of patients (10–39). No study has been done to evaluate its use for bowel lesions. The main use of medical suppression is for temporary relief of pain if the patient must wait for excision of her disease. Laser vaporization and electrocoagulation have not been validated as effective in the destruction of invasive disease, which may more frequently cause pain, and neither modality has been sufficiently reviewed for long-term follow-up to illustrate the eventual outcome of patients treated by these modalities. Many clinicians would be understandably hesitant to burn the bowel wall in an effort to destroy endometriosis completely.

SURGICAL TECHNIQUES

If endoscopic bowel surgery is anticipated, the bowel should be cleansed. Four liters of oral colonic lavage (Abbott Laboratories, Chicago) the afternoon before surgery followed by two enemas the evening before surgery usually results in an adequate bowel preparation. The solution can be chilled or flavored with flavor crystals to increase palatability, and some patients may benefit from nose plugs during consumption. Patients with known intolerance to this bowel preparation can substitute either clear liquids for 4 days or magnesium citrate the day before surgery; in either case the patient should have two enemas the evening before surgery. If a patient cannot complete an oral bowel preparation of any type, she can be given tap water enemas until they run clear the morning of surgery. This will result in mechanical cleansing of the colon, which is the most important consideration since the small bowel is considered sterile. If entry into the bowel lumen seems likely, then appropriate prophylactic antibiotics can be given intraoperatively.

Although it is possible to use cutting or coagulation current on the bowel wall, it is preferable to use sharp dissection, since this carries no risk of thermal damage. The techniques outlined below can be used on either the large or the small bowel, although full-thickness penetration of the small bowel is more likely to occur due to its thin wall. These dissections are described for the use of standard 3-mm scissors passed down a 10-mm operating laparoscope, with a suction irrigator passed down a 5.5-mm sheath in the right lower quadrant, and a 3-mm or 5-mm grasper passed through the left lower quadrant. Bipolar coagulation is occasionally useful for hemostasis. Surgeons experienced with monopolar electrosurgery at laparotomy find it extremely versatile in use laparoscopically, as it eliminates the need for lasers, instrument changes, and most bipolar coagulation. Monopolar scissors connected to an electrosurgical generator supplying 70–90 W of pure cutting current or 50 W of coagulation current allow the surgeon the broadest possible range of surgical options. Tissue can be cut by sharp or electrosurgical methods even around a corner; bleeders can be coagulated; large vessels can be coagulated then transected; spot or broad-based coagulation can be applied; blunt dissection can be used; and tissue can be handled, positioned, and retrieved.

Superficial Lesions

Three-millimeter scissors are used to cut perpendicularly into the bowel wall adjacent to the lesion. The depth of the incision should be just enough to arrive at the level of the deepest part of the lesion as determined by visual and tactile cues. The lesion is grasped and undermined with the scissors working in a layer of muscularis. The dissection can quickly proceed beyond the lesion, and care must be taken in deciding when to cut back out of the bowel wall. Although small lesions that are less than 1 cm in diameter and that do not penetrate to the mucosa do not need to be sutured, suture reinforcement of the bowel wall with 3-0 silk is always permissible. Valuable practice can be gained by suturing even small defects in the bowel wall.

Mucosal Skinning

Occasionally, a larger lesion requires dissection down to the mucosa to ensure its complete removal. The mucosa is recognizable by its velvet-red appearance and the absence of overlying whitish fibers of muscularis. If there is no submucosal fibrosis, both layers of muscularis can be peeled off the mucosa by sharp and blunt dissection (Fig. 1). Once the lesion has been completely undermined, the scissors are used to cut back out to the surface of the bowel. Interrupted 3-0 silk suture is used to close the serosa and muscularis in one layer (Figs. 2 and 3). Antibiotic prophylaxis is optional.

Full-Thickness Disk Resection

If submucosal fibrosis is present or if the nodule is large, entry into the lumen of the bowel may be inevitable. Entry into the bowel lumen allows palpation of the lesion through the mucosa as well, so that the point at which the dissection begins to exit the bowel wall can be determined accurately. The bowel can be closed either in one layer of interrupted 3-0 silk suture, or the mucosa can be closed with 3-0 chromic and the serosa/muscularis layer with interrupted 3-0 silk. The pelvis is filled with irrigation fluid, and air can be injected into the sigmoid colon through a sigmoidoscope to check for air leaks. If leakage occurs, it can be stopped with more sutures.

Obliteration of the Cul-de-sac

Many clinicians view obliteration of the cul-de-sac as an adhesive process only: the colon is stuck to the back of the cervix and it must be unstuck. Although this is partly true, the question must be asked, "What is the significance of the rectosigmoid adhering to the back of the cervix and to the uterosacral ligaments in patients with endometriosis?" The answer to this question has two parts. First, since the cul-de-sac and uterosacral ligaments are among the pelvic areas most frequently involved in endometriosis (3), it must be assumed that they are involved in invasive disease. Second, it must be as-

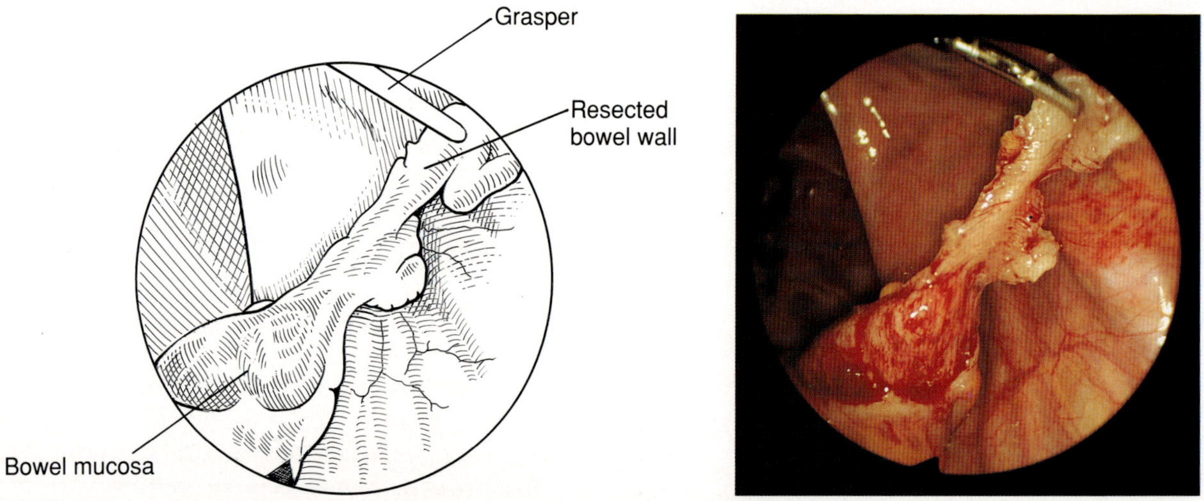

FIG. 1. Endometriosis of the midsigmoid colon being removed by mucosal skinning. The graspers are holding the resected bowel wall containing endometriosis and involving the serosa and muscularis. Notice the linear fibers of the inner circular layer of muscularis. The bowel mucosa is seen below the resected portion and the bowel lumen has not been entered.

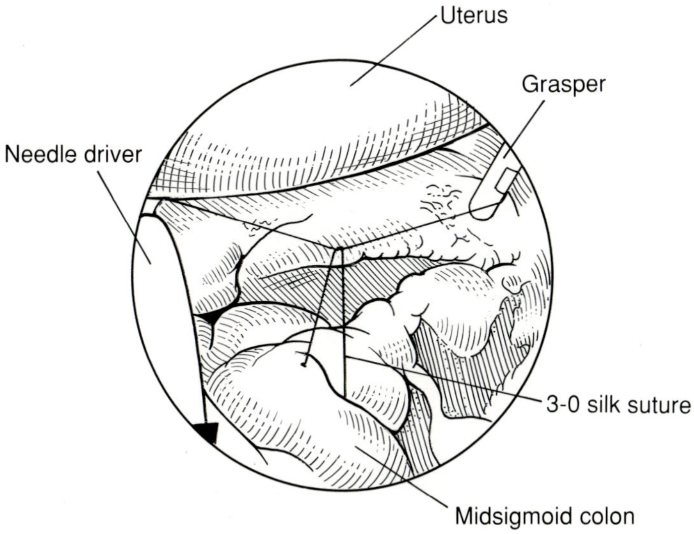

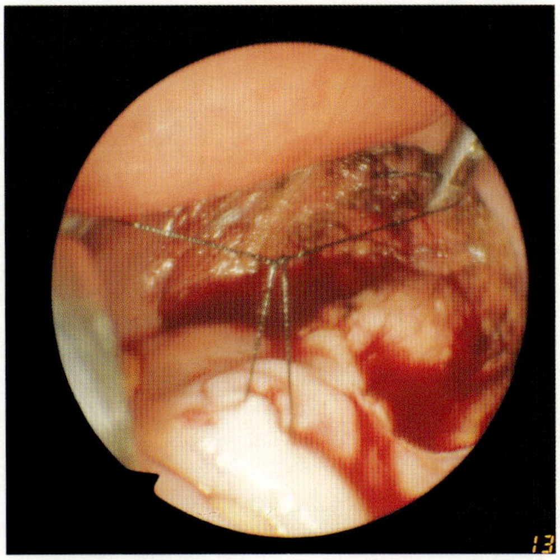

FIG. 2. Interrupted sutures of 3-0 silk are used to close the serosa and muscularis in one layer.

sumed that invasive disease also exists in the wall of the adherent bowel. When these points are recognized, the clinician realizes that the laparoscopic surgical treatment must be expanded to result in complete removal of disease in all of these areas; otherwise most patients will have persistent disease (40). The standard laparoscopic technique that ensures complete removal of all disease is reproducible and straightforward.

Lines of incision are made in normal peritoneum lateral and parallel to the uterosacral ligaments along the length of the ligament to be resected (Fig. 4). This results in automatic retraction of the peritoneum, exposure of the venous structures of the broad ligaments, and isolation of the pathology into the center of the pelvis. A blunt probe can be used to dissect behind the ligaments just below their insertion into the posterior cervix. This isolates the ligaments away from the ureter and uterine vessels. The line of incision in normal peritoneum is then led around the base of each ligament toward the bowel wall, then up and over the bowel wall adjacent to the nodule so that the incisions meet on the anterior wall of the bowel. A transverse incision is made across the cervix just above the point of adherence of the bowel; then a slightly intrafascial dissection is carried down the posterior cervix toward the rectovaginal septum, working between the uterosacral ligaments. Once the cervix has been passed, the surgeon encounters a layer of reddish areolar tissue, which is not the rectovaginal septum. Dissection in this reddish layer will result in excessive bleeding. The yellow fat of the rectovaginal septum is encountered just beyond this layer of reddish tissue. Once the rectovaginal septum has been dissected bluntly, the uterosacral ligaments stand isolated on each side of the rectum. They can be transected at their insertion into the

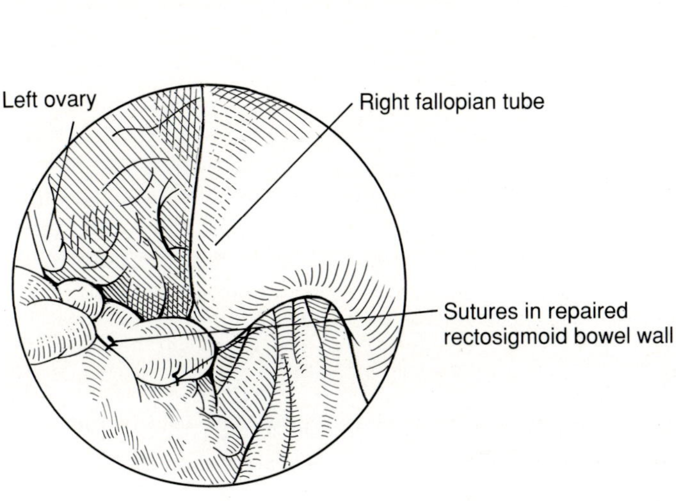

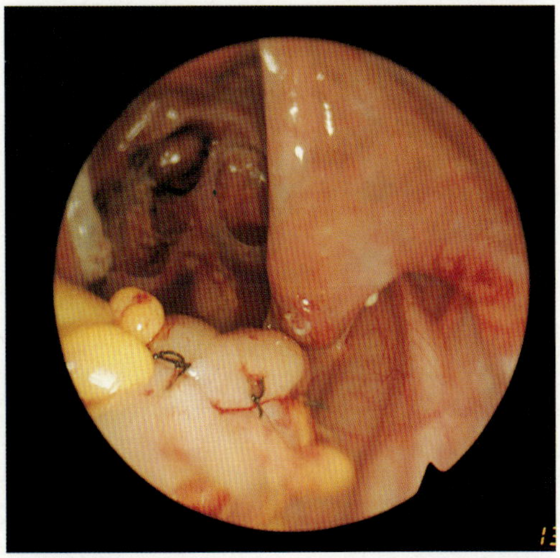

FIG. 3. The repaired bowel wall.

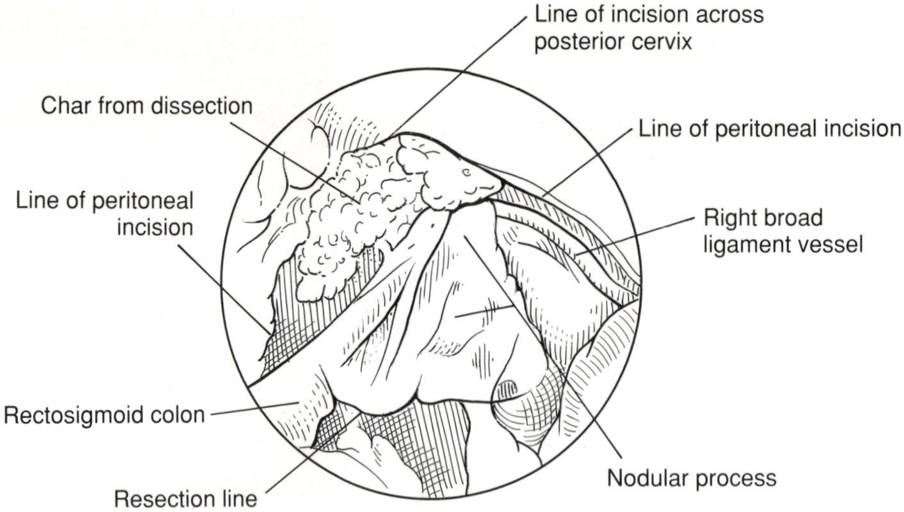

FIG. 4. The rectosigmoid colon is seen as a diagonal structure extending from about 8 o'clock to almost the center of the frame. It was firmly adherent to the posterior cervix, resulting in partial obliteration of the cul-de-sac. Lines of peritoneal incision have been created lateral to each uterosacral ligament. Notice the automatic peritoneal retraction that occurs, exposing the vessels of the broad ligaments. Notice also that the nodular process involving the obliteration of the cul-de-sac and posterior cervix has been isolated into the center of the pelvis. A line of incision has been started across the posterior cervix and, when this has been taken down to the rectovaginal septum, this will allow the nodular mass to fall away from the cervix to the center of the pelvis.

posterior cervix by bipolar coagulation and sharp division or with monopolar scissors. The uterosacral ligaments are then dissected off the pelvic floor, working from the cervix posteriorly toward the previous line of peritoneal incision adjacent to the sacrum. This exposes the fibrous attachments of the rectum to the lateral pelvic walls. These are progressively severed until sufficient mobility of the bowel has been achieved. All nodular disease of the cul-de-sac, uterosacral ligaments, and rectal wall is now isolated in the center of the pelvis attached to the anterior wall of the rectum. The fatty tissue of the rectovaginal septum is stripped off the bowel to expose the longitudinal layer of outer muscularis distal to the mass. At this point, the decision is made to perform either a partial (Fig. 5) or full-thickness disk resection, as discussed above, or a segmental resection with end-to-end anastomosis (5). With full-thickness resections, the surgical specimen can be retrieved transanally. After bowel closure or anastomosis, the bowel is checked for leaks as described above. With an adequate bowel preparation and antibiotic prophylaxis, no complications have been reported following laparoscopic repair of full-thickness bowel resections (5,40,41).

Segmental Colonic Resection with End-to-End Anastomosis (5)

When the bowel lesion is large (>3 cm) or when multiple bowel nodules are present, full-thickness disk

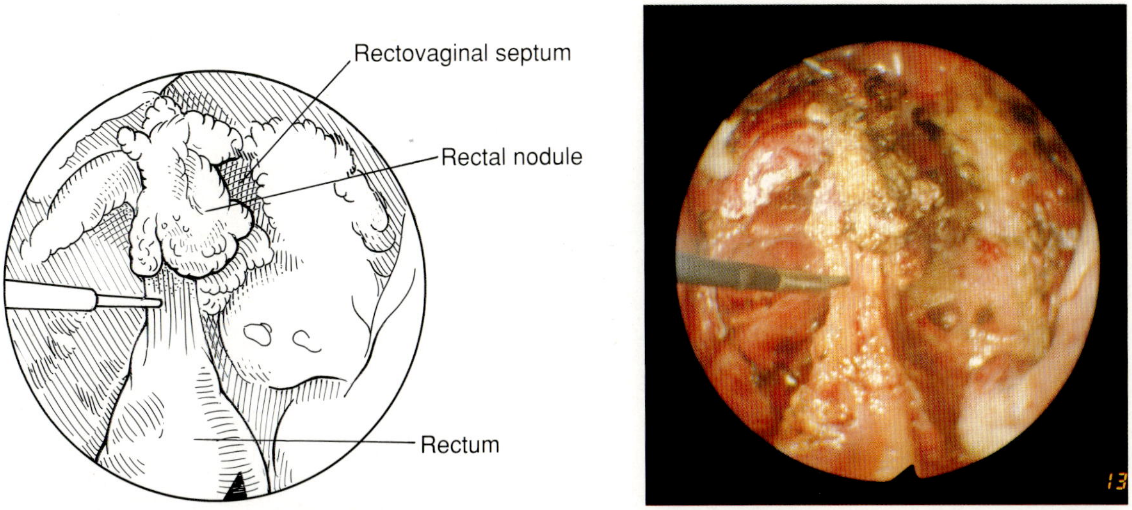

FIG. 5. The rectal nodule has been isolated onto the anterior bowel wall. It is being dissected off the wall of the rectum in a partial thickness resection. Notice the rectovaginal septum in the background. This has been completely dissected with consequent isolation of the distal margin of the rectal nodule.

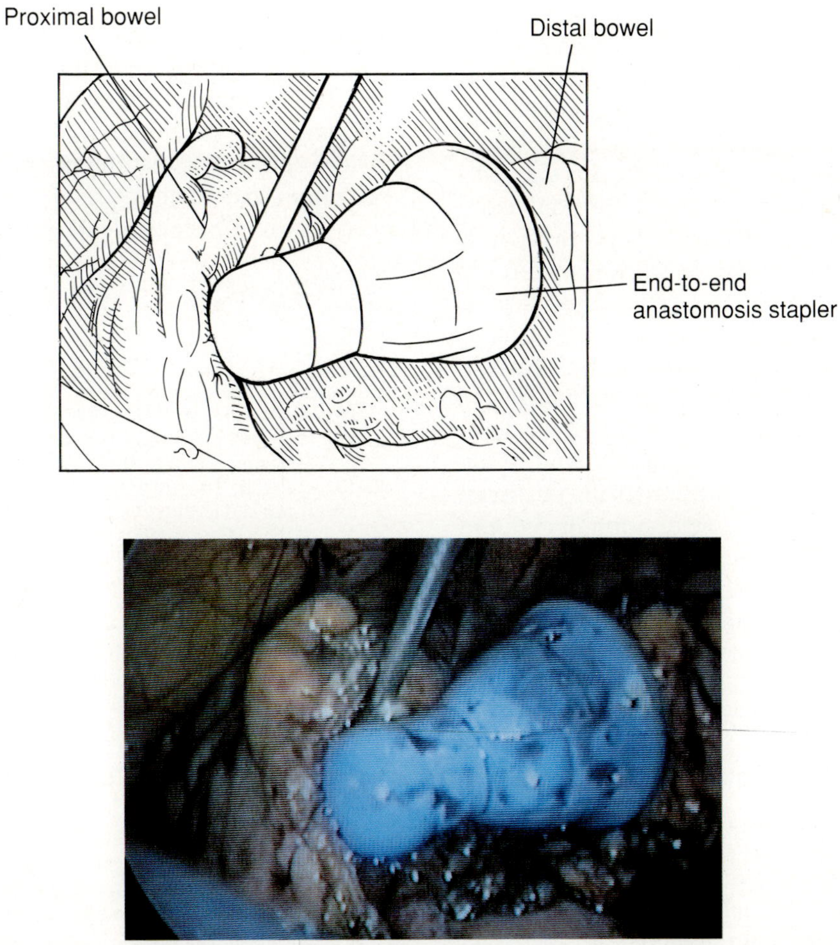

FIG. 6. The end-to-end anastomosis stapler is visible as it passes out of the distal bowel during laparoscopic segmental bowel resection.

resection and repair may result in unacceptable bowel wall distortion. In such a case, resection of a segment of bowel may be necessary. Stay sutures are used to control the bowel segment, and the bowel is transected proximally with electrosurgery. The mesentery is separated from the bowel wall by electrosurgery with the surgeon operating down the axis of the bowel. Once the segment has been sufficiently isolated, the bowel is transected distally and the segment retrieved transanally. An end-to-end anastomosis is performed with a stapler (Fig. 6) after placement of proximal and distal pursestring sutures using either endoloops or traditional pursestring sutures.

DISCUSSION

Laparoscopic bowel surgery is not for every surgeon. Patients with intestinal disease have more pelvic areas involved in endometriosis than patients without intestinal disease. Of 97 patients undergoing laparoscopic excision of intestinal endometriosis, the median number of other pelvic areas involved in endometriosis was 5. Therefore, surgery on the bowel usually follows surgery done elsewhere in the pelvis, potentially resulting in a lengthy surgery requiring mental and physical stamina. This is particularly true if the patient has bilateral large endometrioma cysts adherent to the pelvic sidewalls over invasive disease. Each surgeon must decide how long a laparoscopic procedure should last and open the abdomen to complete the surgery if that time limit is exceeded. An exhausted surgeon is more likely to do harm than one who is merely tired but has help at laparotomy.

It is the official position of the American College of Obstetricians and Gynecologists that excision of endometriosis is equivalent to laser vaporization or fulguration when performed at laparoscopy, although this equivalence disappears at laparotomy (42). No evidence has been offered in support of this unusual stand. While robust follow-up exists for long-term results of disease destruction following laparoscopic excision of endometriosis (43), no such follow-up exists for laser vaporization or fulguration. Most clinicians would probably be hesitant to attempt to treat intestinal endometriosis by burning the bowel with laser or electricity, and the complete destruction of deeply invasive disease would always remain in doubt. Indeed, failure of symptom relief with electrocoagulation is more likely to occur when the uterosacral ligaments are involved by possibly deeply invasive disease (44). Only if each method of disease destruction has been shown to be equally effective by long-term outcome analysis should the various methods be considered equivalent. The lack of long-term follow-up of laser vaporization or fulguration should not be accepted as evidence that there is no demonstrated difference between these methods and excision, since this would be an instance of using lack of scientific data to support a positive conclusion. Instead, this lack of follow-up simply means that laser vaporization and fulguration remain unvalidated as being effective treatment for endometriosis. Studies focusing on the response of symptoms, such as infertility or pain, do not necessarily say anything about the response of the disease to treatment.

COMPLICATIONS

Of 260 patients having biopsy-proven bowel endometriosis in the author's private practice, 97 have undergone laparoscopic treatment of bowel lesions without any complications. This includes 10 patients with full-thickness resections and 3 with segmental resections with end-to-end anastomosis. One patient had an aborted laparoscopic segmental resection due to technical difficulty with the stapler and required a laparotomy to complete the procedure.

HIGHLIGHTS

Major and minor bowel surgery can be safely performed laparoscopically using excisional methods, which successfully treat even deeply invasive endometriosis. Obliteration of the cul-de-sac usually signifies the presence of a rectal nodule of endometriosis as well as invasive disease of the uterosacral ligaments. Laser vaporization and fulguration of endometriosis have not been shown to be equivalent to excision.

REFERENCES

1. Peterson HB, Hulka JF, Phillips JM. American Association of Gynecologic Laparoscopists' 1988 membership survey on operative laparoscopy. *J Reprod Med* 1990;35:587–589.
2. Fallon J. Endometriosis. Evidence of tubal origin in the distribution of lesions. *Arch Surg* 1951;62:412–418.
3. Redwine DB. The distribution of endometriosis in the pelvis by age groups and fertility. *Fertil Steril* 1987;47:173–175.
4. Henriksen E. Endometriosis. *Am J Surg* 1955;90:331–336.
5. Redwine DB, Sharpe DR. Laparoscopic segmental resection of the sigmoid colon for endometriosis. *J Laparoendosc Surg* 1991;1:217–220.
6. Metzger DA, Olive DL, Haney AF. Limited hormonal responsiveness of ectopic endometrium: histologic correlation with intrauterine endometrium. *Hum Pathol* 1988;19:1417–1424.
7. Koninckx PR, Meuleman C, Demeyere S, Lesaffre E, Cornillie FJ. Suggestive evidence that pelvic endometriosis is a progressive disease, whereas deeply infiltrating endometriosis is associated with pelvic pain. *Fertil Steril* 1991;55:759–765.
8. Redwine DB. Laparoscopic en bloc resection for treatment of the obliterated cul-de-sac in endometriosis. *J Reprod Med* 1992;37:695–698.
9. Cornillie FJ, Oosterlynck D, Lauweryns JM, Koninckx PR. Deeply infiltrating pelvic endometriosis: histology and clinical significance. *Fertil Steril* 1990;53:978–983.
10. Creadick RN. The non-surgical treatment of endometriosis. *NC Med J* 1950;11:576–577.
11. Kistner RW. The use of newer progestins in the treatment of endometriosis. *Am J Obstet Gynecol* 1958;75:264–278.
12. Kistner RW. The treatment of endometriosis by inducing pseudo-

pregnancy with ovarian hormones. A report of 58 cases. *Fertil Steril* 1959;10:539–556.
13. Andrews MC, Andrews WC, Strauss AF. Effects of progestin-induced pseudopregnancy on endometriosis: clinical and microscopic studies. *Am J Obstet Gynecol* 1959;78:776–783.
14. Kourides IA, Kistner RW. Three new synthetic progestins in the treatment of endometriosis. *Obstet Gynecol* 1968;31:821–828.
15. Chalmers JA: Conservative management of endometriosis. *Proc R Soc Med* 1968;61:14–16.
16. Dmowski WP, Kapetanakis E, Scommegna A. Variable effects of danazol on endometriosis at 4 low-dose levels. *Obstet Gynecol* 1982;59:408–415.
17. Barbieri RL, Evans S, Kistner RW. Danazol in the treatment of endometriosis: analysis of 100 cases with a 4-year follow-up. *Fertil Steril* 1982;37:737–746.
18. Schweppe K-W, Wynn RM, Beller FK. Ultrastructural comparison of endometriotic implants and eutopic endometrium. *Am J Obstet Gynecol* 1984;148:1024–1037.
19. Brosens IA, Verleyen A, Cornillie F. The morphologic effect of short-term medical therapy of endometriosis. *Am J Obstet Gynecol* 1987;157:1215–1221.
20. Dmowski WP. Visual assessment of peritoneal implants for staging endometriosis: do number and cumulative size of lesions reflect the severity of a systemic disease? *Fertil Steril* 1987;47:382–384.
21. Dmowski WP. Visual assessment of peritoneal implants for staging endometriosis: do number and cumulative size of lesions reflect the severity of a systemic disease? *Fertil Steril* 1987;47:382–384.
22. Evers JLH. The second-look laparoscopy for evaluation of the result of medical treatment of endometriosis should not be performed during ovarian suppression. *Fertil Steril* 1987;47:502–504.
23. Steingold KA, Cedars M, Lu JKH, Randle D, Judd HL, Meldrum DR. Treatment of endometriosis with a long-acting gonadotropin-releasing hormone agonist. *Obstet Gynecol* 1987;69:403–411.
24. Fayez JA, Collazo LM, Vernon C. Comparison of different modalities of treatment for minimal and mild endometriosis. *Am J Obstet Gynecol* 1988;159:927–932.
25. Henzl MR, Corson SL, Moghissi K, et al. Administration of nafarelin as compared with oral danazol for endometriosis. A multicenter double-blind comparative clinical trial. *N Engl J Med* 1988;318:485–489.
26. Fedele L, Arcaini L, Bianchi S, Baglioni A, Vercellini P. Comparison of cyproterone acetate and danazol in the treatment of pelvic pain associated with endometriosis. *Obstet Gynecol* 1989;73:1000–1004.
27. Dmowski WP, Radwanska E, Binor Z, Tummon I, Pepping P. Ovarian suppression induced with Buserelin or danazol in the management of endometriosis: a randomized, comparative study. *Fertil Steril* 1989;51:395–400.
28. Franssen AMHW, Kauer FM, Chada DR, Zijlstra JA, Rolland R. Endometriosis: treatment with gonadotropin-releasing hormone agonist Buserelin. *Fertil Steril* 1989;51:401–408.
29. Fedele L, Bianchi S, Viessoli T, Arcaini L, Candiani GB: Gestrinone versus danazol in the treatment of endometriosis. *Fertil Steril* 1989;51:781–785.
30. Kennedy SH, Williams IA, Brodribb J, Barlow DH, Shaw RW. A comparison of nafarelin acetate and danazol in the treatment of endometriosis. *Fertil Steril* 1990;53:998–1003.
31. Cedars MI, Lu JKH, Meldrum DR, Judd HL. Treatment of endometriosis with a long-acting gonadotropin-releasing hormone agonist plus medroxyprogesterone acetate. *Obstet Gynecol* 1990;75:641–645.
31. Lemay A, Maheux R, Faure N, Jean C, Fazekas ATA. Reversible hypogonadism induced by a luteinizing hormone-releasing hormone (LH-RH) agonist (Buserelin) as a new therapeutic approach for endometriosis. *Fertil Steril* 1984;41:863–871.
32. Lemay A, Sandow J, Bureau M, Maheux R, Fontaine J-Y, Merat P. Prevention of follicular maturation in endometriosis by subcutaneous infusion of luteinizing hormone-releasing hormone agonist started in the luteal phase. *Fertil Steril* 1988;49:410–417.
33. Moore EE, Harger JH, Rock JA, Archer DF. Management of pelvic endometriosis with low-dose danazol. *Fertil Steril* 1981;36:15–19.
34. Haber GM, Behelak YF. Preliminary report on the use of tamoxifen in the treatment of endometriosis. *Am J Obstet Gynecol* 1987;156:582–586.
35. Tummon IS, Pepping ME, Binor Z, et al. A randomized, prospective comparison of endocrine changes induced with intranasal leuprolide or danazol for treatment of endometriosis. *Fertil Steril* 1989;51:390–394.
36. Surrey ES, Gambone JC, Lu JKH, Judd HL. The effects of combining norethindrone with a gonadotropin-releasing hormone agonist in the treatment of symptomatic endometriosis. *Fertil Steril* 1990;53:620–626.
37. Venturini PL, Bertolini S, Brunenghi MC, et al. Endocrine, metabolic, and clinical effects of gestrinone in women with endometriosis. *Fertil Steril* 1989;52:589–595.
38. Venturini PL, Fasce V, Costantini S, Anserini P, Cucuccio S, de Cecco L. Treatment of endometriosis with goserelin depot, a long-acting gonadotropin-releasing hormone agonist analog: endocrine and clinical results. *Fertil Steril* 1990;54:1021–1027.
39. Zorn J-R, Mathieson J, Risquez F, Comaru-Schally AM, Schally AV. Treatment of endometriosis with a delayed release preparation of the agonist D-Trp6-luteinizing hormone-releasing hormone: long-term follow-up in a series of 50 patients. *Fertil Steril* 1990;53:401–406.
40. Reich H, McGlynn F, Salvat J. Laparoscopic treatment of cul-de-sac obliteration secondary to retrocervical deep fibrotic endometriosis. *J Reprod Med* 1991;36:516–522.
41. Nezhat C, Silfen S, Nezhat F, Martin D. Surgery for endometriosis. *Curr Opin Obstet Gynecol* 1991;3:385–393.
42. Griffin L, Kaminetzky H, Noller K, Pearse W. Personal communications.
43. Redwine DB. Conservative laparoscopic excision of endometriosis by sharp dissection: Life table analysis of reoperation and persistant or recurrent disease. *Fertil Steril* 1991;56:628–634.
44. Hasson HM. Electrocoagulation of pelvic endometriotic lesions with laparoscopic control. *Am J Obstet Gynecol* 135:115–119.

Endoscopic Management of Gynecologic Disease,
edited by G.D. Adamson and D.C. Martin.
Lippincott-Raven Publishers, Philadelphia © 1996.

CHAPTER 22

Laparoscopic Urologic Procedures

Thierry G. Vancaillie

Laparoscopic bladder neck suspension is a misnomer, but the term has been in use for so long that it would be difficult to eliminate it from our jargon. The term "suspension" ensues from the fact that the majority of the patients with genuine stress incontinence do indeed have an anatomic defect consisting of a detachment of the urethral attachments from their pelvic support. It is said that the bladder neck "has come down." The natural surgical cure would then be to replace the urethra in its natural position by "suspending" it to the pelvic wall. However, there is more and more evidence that the true etiology for incontinence is hypermobility of the bladder neck. The logical surgical procedure to cure the condition is then one that causes reduction in mobility of the bladder neck. This in turn allows the patient to control her bladder. This difference is not of mere academic interest because when a "suspension" is performed the surgeon intuitively tries to elevate the bladder neck as high as possible, whereas when reduction of mobility is the purpose of the surgery, elevation is less critical and the surgeon therefore does not exert as much traction to the suture. As is emphasized in the section on anatomy, the aim of the surgery is immobilization of the bladder neck or, better, the urethra, by fixation with minimal traction of the endopelvic fascia and pubourethral ligaments to a strong ligamentary structure, such as Cooper's ligament.

In 1947 a retropubic urethrovesical suspension operation was first described by Williams. Sutures were placed between the bladder wall and the periosteum of the symphysis pubis. Over subsequent years there have been a number of changes and modifications. Marshall et al. (1) in 1949 changed the procedure to involve approximation of the vaginal wall, rather than the bladder wall, and cartilage of the symphysis pubis. Burch (2) devised a colposuspension operation in 1961, in which sutures were placed into the ileopectineal line or Cooper's ligament, which was more secure. There have been a number of other modifications along the way, such as the number and type of sutures involved; these will not be detailed here. The most recent issue has been the viability of performing these procedures under laparoscopic control, thus reducing postoperative pain and recovery and hopefully without compromising the success of treatment and without increased complication rate or operative time.

High success rates (3,4) have been described for transabdominal retropubic urethropexy, ranging from 60% to 98% for Marshall–Marchetti–Kranz (MMK) procedures and 80% to 100% for Burch procedures. This is superior to results reported for the Stamey and modified Pereyra procedures.

The author has been the first to report successful use of laparoscopic (5) techniques to perform an MMK- or Burch-type procedure without the morbidity of a large skin incision. The two chief advantages of laparoscopy in performing incontinence surgery are that the anatomy is clearly defined due to the optical characteristics of the method and that laparoscopy provides access to the cul-de-sac, thus allowing evaluation and possibly cure of an enterocele during the same surgical session.

PREVALENCE

Urinary incontinence is one of the most common problems for women in general and postmenopausal women in particular. The incidence of stress, urgency, and other urinary incontinence syndromes in the general population is unknown. Of women over 60, 38% experience some degree of urinary incontinence, stress, or other bladder dysfunction. Women residing in nursing homes (6) or other institutions show a significantly higher (55%) incidence of incontinence. A breakdown of these figures according to the type of incontinence is not available. Most likely, because of the complexity of in-

T. G. Vancaillie: Center for Gynecologic Endosurgery, San Antonio, Texas 78229.

continence, such figures may never become available. The rising number of elderly people in our society puts incontinence and other symptoms derived from pelvic floor relaxation on the forefront in many ways. The main issue is that physicians will be confronted more and more with elderly patients demanding treatment of their condition to achieve a better quality of life. Moreover, incontinence in elderly patients presents rarely as straightforward stress or urgency. One needs to become familiar with a number of new therapeutic approaches besides surgery, such as electrostimulation, biofeedback, physiotherapy, and behavioral intervention.

ANATOMY

There are no well-defined ligamentary suspensory structures that hold the bladder in place. This gives the bladder its characteristic distensibility. Fibrous attachments run from the posterior rectus muscle to the anterior wall of the bladder. The so-called bladder "pillars" are extensions of the endopelvic fascia covering the anterior vagina. They provide some support for the base of the bladder, although most rigidity is provided by the vagina itself. The base of the bladder, resting on the upper half of the vagina, is in actuality the weak spot of the pelvic floor. Defects in that region are the most difficult to repair due to the lack of muscular or ligamentary tissue in that area.

The urethra runs above the endopelvic fascia of the middle third of the vagina and can be dissected from the vagina at that level with relative ease. When the urethra reaches the lower third of the vagina, it becomes incorporated into the vaginal wall and surrounding fascial and muscular tissue. Dissection of the urethra at that level is not feasible. It is at the same level where one can identify the so-called pubourethral ligaments. These ligaments enclose the urethra and anterior vaginal wall and then project toward the pubic bone anteriorly and toward the obturator muscle laterally. The dominance of the pubic component vs. the obturator component varies from one patient to another. Whether the configuration of the ligament plays a role in the development of incontinence is unknown.

The knowledge of how the force transmission occurs within the abdominal cavity is important when surgical correction of the relaxed pelvic floor is undertaken. The relationship between the cul-de-sac and the anterior vaginal wall is critical in maintaining a pressure transmission that will add to urethral closure. Resecting an enterocele, for instance, may dramatically change the forces that were transmitted to the urethra through the vagina (provided there is no concomitant vault prolapse). In the presence of hypermobility of the urethra without stress incontinence in a patient undergoing repair of an enterocele, reduction of this hypermobility to prevent occurrence of postoperative stress incontinence is indicated. A preoperative cystometrogram is in many cases completely normal and does not provide indications that incontinence may become problematic.

PATHOPHYSIOLOGY

Genuine stress incontinence occurs when there is insufficient force counteracting an increase in intraabdominal pressure. This lack of force is due to a combination of weak muscular support and an anatomic defect in the relationship between the bladder outlet and the surrounding pelvic structures.

In the upright position, the intraabdominal force presents its main vector toward the promontory and hollow of the sacrum, the bony structures of which are quite solid and can absorb the pressure. However, by virtue of the fact that the abdomen is a fluid-filled cavity, the force vectors reflect and transmit pressure to all sides. Under normal anatomic circumstances, this pressure maintains good closure of the urethra. When urethral detachment occurs, the force vector that helped close the urethra becomes less and less important. Compensatory contraction of the sphincters is sufficient in some cases to prevent incontinence, especially if the patient can anticipate the intraabdominal pressure increase.

The occurrence and frequency of stress incontinence is the result of an equilibrium, or lack of it, between the intraabdominal pressure, the intravesical pressure, and the closing pressure. The intravesical pressure depends on the amount of urine in the bladder and the transmission of force from the abdomen. The intravesical volume is in itself not a major contributor to intravesical pressure. However, a distended bladder has to absorb more force, which is transmitted from the abdomen. The degree to which the bladder is full significantly affects the ability of an individual to withstand increased pressures.

CLINICAL PRESENTATION

The clinical presentation of genuine stress incontinence is simple: involuntary loss of urine upon increase of intraabdominal pressure by activities such as coughing, sneezing, or jumping. Less straightforward is the clinical evaluation of the severity of the symptoms. Environmental factors, such as the patient's occupation and access to a bathroom, affect the impact that the stress incontinence may have on a person's well-being.

In our society, stress urinary incontinence is perceived as normal by many individuals, especially by menopausal patients. Stress incontinence often is interpreted as a necessary evil that one needs to live with once menopause is reached. Therefore, quite often, the patient does not seek help and in many cases does not even mention the problem when presenting for a routine annual physical. Frankly, this belief is reinforced by many physicians who tend to minimize the importance of incontinence in older women. Intervention is considered too risky for this group of individuals. Nonetheless quality of life continues to be important after menopause or retirement, and treatment should not be withheld from these individuals on the basis of a subjective assessment of the risk-vs.-benefit equation. Electrostimulation and physical reeducation programs achieve marked improvement in the quality of life in those individuals.

Stress incontinence, which is the result of a mechanical failure to counter increased intraabdominal pressure, may be complicated by the presence of additional nonstress symptoms. The presence of urgency symptoms complicates treatment of stress incontinence, but they do not preclude surgical correction of the condition. Stress incontinence may be considered a mechanical defect, which can be corrected by mechanical means, i.e., surgery. However, concomitant pathology, such as hypersensitivity of the bladder, needs to be addressed. It must be emphasized that treatment of urinary incontinence is an ongoing process rather than a one-time intervention and, ideally, the patient is informed of this.

On physical examination, prolapse and hypermobility of the urethra and bladder neck are readily observed. Tests such as the "Q-tip" test and vaginal ultrasonography are useful to quantify the anatomic defect. The absence of an anatomic defect in the presence of stress incontinence symptoms is a challenge. The objective of a colposuspension operation is correction of a mechanical defect. In the absence of such a defect, it is unlikely that the surgery will be of any benefit to the patient.

During physical examination of the patient, other features of pelvic floor relaxation are evaluated. These include the presence of an enterocele or a rectocele. This evaluation determines the extent of the surgical correction that is indicated in a particular patient. An enterocele is almost invariably present in those patients who are menopausal and have undergone hysterectomy. In the presence of a large enterocele combined with a cystocele, stress urinary incontinence may be masked. Under these anatomic conditions, the upper urethra is kinked, which leads to continence by compression of the upper urethra by the base of the bladder during increased intraabdominal pressure. Correction of the enterocele may then present the "hidden" incontinence. Only careful evaluation of the anatomy with or without vaginal ultrasonography provides the examiner with the necessary information to prevent postoperative incontinence.

DIAGNOSIS

The diagnosis of genuine stress incontinence is made chiefly by taking a careful history of the patient. Further clinical evaluation is necessary for planning adequate treatment. Again it is stressed that only the patient is able to determine the impact of the incontinence on quality of life. It is true that not all patients with genuine stress incontinence should be operated on, especially because electrostimulation procedures have proven to be effective alternative procedures in selected cases. On the other hand, the physician's approval or disapproval regarding adequacy of treatment should not be judgmental.

Certain tests are helpful in confirming the presence of stress incontinence and are aimed at reproducing or arresting hypermobility of the bladder neck. These tests have predictive value inasmuch as they mimic the mechanical impact of the corrective surgical procedure.

The Q-tip test is administered to reproduce and quantify the hypermobility of the bladder neck. There is no clear correlation between the severity of the hypermobility and the occurrence of incontinence. Muscle tone and estrogen depletion are among the confounding variables that help determine the severity of the condition. However, the surgeon cannot correct stress incontinence with a simple colposuspension operation in the absence of hypermobility. The Bennett test reproduces the effect of surgical immobilization of the bladder neck on the occurrence of stress incontinence. In combination, these two simple tests are quite effective in predicting a positive outcome of the procedure.

In the presence of atypical symptomatology and inconclusive physical examination, a cystometrogram and, possibly, cystoscopy are indicated. These are aimed at detecting concomitant pathologies, which complicate the clinical presentation. In addition, patients who have been operated on previously for incontinence are also subjected to a complete urodynamic evaluation. The principal objective of a cystometrogram is detection of detrusor instability and urethral pathology. Neurologic disorders secondary to spine injuries, multiple sclerosis, diabetes, and other systemic conditions will not be considered in this chapter.

INDICATIONS

The indication for laparoscopic bladder neck suspension is the presence of genuine stress incontinence. The use of laparoscopy is only aimed at eliminating the need for a large skin incision. Another basic difference between the laparoscopic approach and the classical suprapubic approach is the fact that access to the space of Retzius is achieved transperitoneally in the laparoscopic procedure. The immobilization of the bladder neck also is indicated in some patients with pelvic prolapse, who do not complain of urinary incontinence but in whom correction of the prolapse may result in incontinence.

The author defends two issues in the treatment of genuine stress incontinence. First of all, genuine stress urinary incontinence (GSUI) is a symptom of pelvic floor relaxation. The ideal treatment is the one that addresses all aspects of pelvic floor weakness in a particular patient. Rare is the case in which only a bladder neck immobilization is required. Examination of the patient with this in mind results in much better treatment of her condition. In addition, one must convince the patient that the condition with which she is afflicted cannot be treated with surgery alone. Treatment requires effort from the patient. She must actively participate in the reeducation process of training the muscles of the pelvic floor. The second point is that a combined abdominal and vaginal approach for surgical correction of the pelvic floor is not necessarily a fundamental mistake or illogical, as some may argue. The best surgical approach is the one that provides the surgeon with the best exposure and access to the anatomic element he or she wants to reach. In addition, the best surgical approach should not be given up because the procedure has been initiated by a particular route. On the other hand, I am certainly not opposed to learning techniques that may obviate the change of approach, if these techniques are equivalent to the ones that I know are effective in achieving the desired anatomic correction. These theoretical considerations, which cannot be supported by hard scientific data, have resulted in the introduction of laparoscopy in surgical correction of the pelvic floor. The procedures that I consider optimal for particular aspects of the correction of pelvic floor relaxation, such as the Burch and enterocele repair, are performed through the abdominal route. Laparoscopy can be substituted to avoid the morbidity of dissection of the abdominal wall. The reduction in postoperative morbidity for the patient contributes significantly to the applicability of abdominal procedures in pelvic floor reconstruction.

CONTRAINDICATIONS

Contraindications to laparoscopy are first those related to surgery, namely, systemic conditions that would jeopardize the patient's life, such as low cardiac output, severe emphysema, etc. Contraindications more specific to laparoscopy are the ones related to insufflation of CO_2 and positioning of the patient. Carbon dioxide gas is more readily absorbed by the body if the peritoneal surface is transgressed for the simple reason that more capillaries are opened. Patients with normal lungs and acid–base metabolism readily exhale the excess CO_2. However, in patients with impaired lung function, for instance, one must pay attention to the occurrence of hypercarbia. The use of a capnograph, which measures carbon dioxide in the expiratory air of the patient, is indicated. There are no hard data on the degree of reduction in lung function that would preclude the use of laparoscopy. Patients who cannot be placed in Trendelenburg are not candidates for laparoscopy.

Other reasons for avoiding laparoscopy are related to access of the abdominal cavity. When excess adhesions are suspected, the surgeon may opt to avoid the transperitoneal approach. Alternatives are preperitoneal surgery by a classical Burch procedure or preperitoneal endoscopy.

Contraindications related to the correction of incontinence are related to intrinsic urethral pathology. These patients have stress incontinence, but immobilization of the urethra does not result in cure. Patients presenting with intrinsic urethral pathology are best treated with a sling procedure, if surgery is indicated at all.

ALTERNATIVE TREATMENT

A colposuspension operation can be performed in different ways, resulting in an approximately identical outcome. These are the classical suprapubic preperitoneal access (Burch and Marshall-Marchetti-Kranz), the endoscopic preperitoneal access, and the endoscopic transperitoneal access. In addition to these there are a myriad of transvaginal needle suspension procedures, which in essence aim at reproducing a similar surgical intervention through vaginal access.

My subjective evaluation of the differences among those procedures is summarized in Table 1. As indicated in Table 1, the preperitoneal procedures exclude enterocele repair at least from the abdominal route. This is the main reason why the author does not perform preperitoneal procedures if at all possible. My bias is toward the transperitoneal approach. Objective factors are reduced postoperative morbidity of a laparoscopic procedure as

TABLE 1. *Evaluation of different approaches to colposuspension in primary patients*

Factor	Preperitoneal open	Preperitoneal closed	Transvaginal	Transperitoneal
Anatomic detail	Fair	Good	Fair	Excellent
Technical skill required	Low	High	Moderate	High
Morbidity or pain	Moderate	Low	Moderate to severe	Low
Complication rate	Low	Unknown	Low	Acceptable
Simultaneous enterocele repair	Not possible	Not possible	Good access	Excellent access

compared to an abdominal incision and simultaneous access to the cul-de-sac for treatment of the enterocele.

It would appear that the vaginal procedures and the transperitoneal approach are the most favorable. This results from the fact that these procedures appear to be patient-friendly. However, the bulk of the literature supports the position that the Burch-type procedure is superior to the transvaginal one in terms of long-term results. The only remaining argument against the laparoscopic approach is the level of surgical skill required to perform the transperitoneal intervention.

SURGICAL TECHNIQUE

The pelvic reconstruction may include a vaginal hysterectomy and anterior and posterior repair. Once these interventions are done, the legs of the patient are repositioned. The patient should be supine with the upper leg in continuity with the trunk. The knees are flexed to provide stability when the patient is lowered in Trendelenburg position. The legs are in abduction to provide access to the vagina. In some way this position is similar to what is sometimes referred to as the frog position. A roll of towels is placed underneath the patient's buttocks to optimize access to the cul-de-sac in preparation for the enterocele repair.

If right-handed, the surgeon stands on the left side of the patient. The following descriptions are given for a right-handed operator; a mirror image should be envisioned for a left-handed person.

A total of four trocars are used for the completion of enterocele repair and bladder neck suspension. The umbilical trocar provides access for the laparoscope; three additional trocars allow manipulation. A 10-mm suprapubic trocar is used to introduce the suture material. Two 5-mm lateral trocars are placed at the level of the iliac crests, some 3–4 cm inward.

Pneumoperitoneum is established with CO_2 insufflation through the umbilicus with a Veress needle. If there has been previous pelvic surgery, except for cesarean section, insufflation is performed through a left paramedial incision. Once pneumoperitoneum is established, the umbilical trocar is inserted and visualization is set. Alternatively, the umbilical trocar can be directly inserted without prior insufflation. Adhesiolysis and enterolysis may be required to access the cul-de-sac. The enterocele repair is performed first because access to the cul-de-sac is difficult after a bladder neck suspension. The anatomic landmarks are the cul-de-sac, the sacrouterine ligaments, the ureters, and the vagina. A forceps introduced into the vagina and pushed upward stretches the sacrouterine ligaments and highlights the edge of the "hernia," which then replaces the cul-de-sac.

A brief description of the enterocele repair follows. First the hernia sac is completely resected (Fig. 1). The first stitch is applied posteriorly in front of the dorsal insertion of the sacrouterine ligaments. The needle first is driven through the right ligament and then several times through the edge of the peritoneal resection at the level of the anterior wall of the rectum. Finally the needle is passed through the left sacrouterine ligament and the suture tied with an extracorporeal knot. Care is taken not to strangle the rectum. Once the suture is tied, the position of the ureters is checked. Invariably there is some degree of medial displacement. Should this be judged excessive, an incision to release tension can be made into the peritoneum between the ligament and the ureter. Once the posterior border of the hernia has been closed, the large defect in the pelvic floor becomes apparent between the sacrouterine ligaments, the anterior wall of the rectum, and the vagina. Forceps are introduced into the vagina and are used to gently push the vaginal cuff upward to evaluate how far it reaches without excess force. The needle is passed through the right sacrouterine ligament at the level where the vaginal cuff reaches. Then

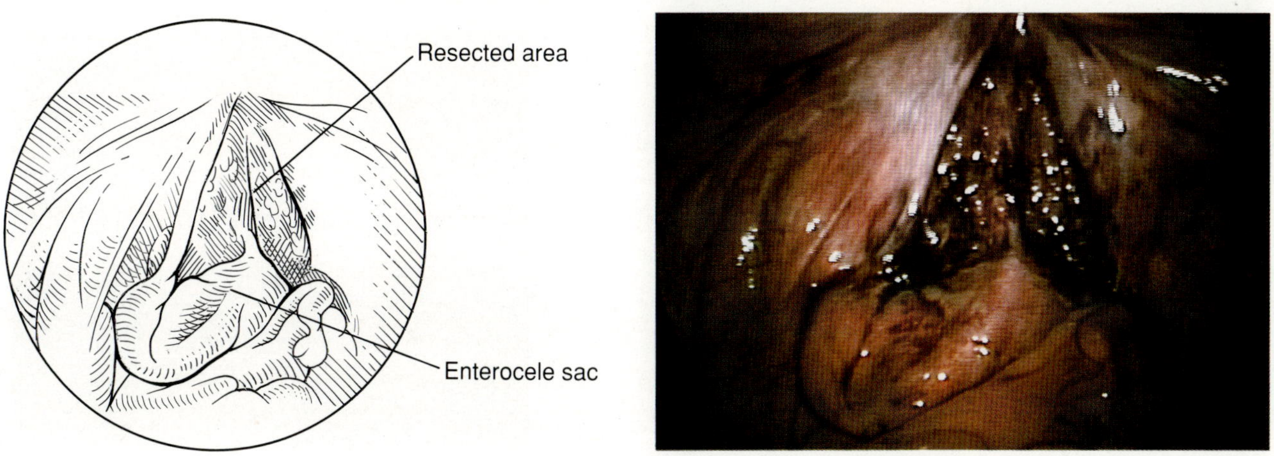

FIG. 1. The enterocele sac has been completely resected.

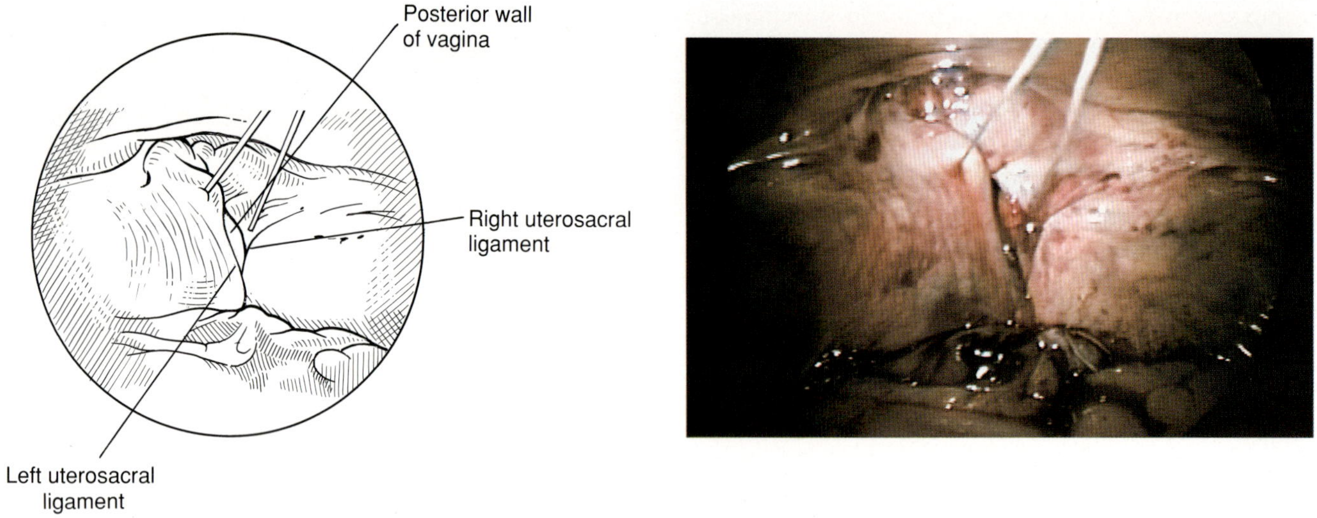

FIG. 2. The second suture approximating the two sacrouterine ligaments incorporates the posterior wall of the vagina, thus creating a vaginal suspension.

the needle catches the vaginal wall and the left ligament. When this suture is tied, the vagina becomes suspended to the sacrouterine ligaments and occupies the space previously taken by the enterocele (Fig. 2). This surgical procedure reconstructs the rectovaginal septum because it reestablishes the anatomic relationship between the vagina and the rectum. Some degree of overcorrection is unavoidable. Two or three more sutures are applied to close the defect completely (Fig. 3). One or two of these additional stitches are placed in front of the new position of the vaginal cuff and provide some support for the bottom of the bladder. It may be required to dissect the bladder off the anterior wall of the vagina prior to closing the enterocele. This is the case in patients who have had a hysterectomy and in whom the bladder bulges over the vaginal vault.

After completion of the enterocele repair, the surgeon begins the colposuspension. The landmarks are the left umbilical ligament, which delineates the lateral border of the dissection, the pubic bone, and the lateral edge of the bladder on the left. The Foley catheter is commonly easily visible and helps in locating the bladder during the first procedures. Filling the bladder is sometimes helpful in a patient with multiple previous surgeries. The pubic bone is located by gentle probing with an ancillary instrument. The pubic bone establishes the inferior border of the initial incision (Fig. 4) into the peritoneum because it acts as a guide for the surgeon to avoid the superior vesical pedicle, which runs anterior to the round ligament but slightly below the level of the pubic bone. The superior vesical pedicle is not easily recognized. However, the venous plexus is significant and bleeds profusely if accidently incised. Avoiding this vascular structure is important because its bleeding would obscure the tissue planes and increase the degree of difficulty of the procedure from the start.

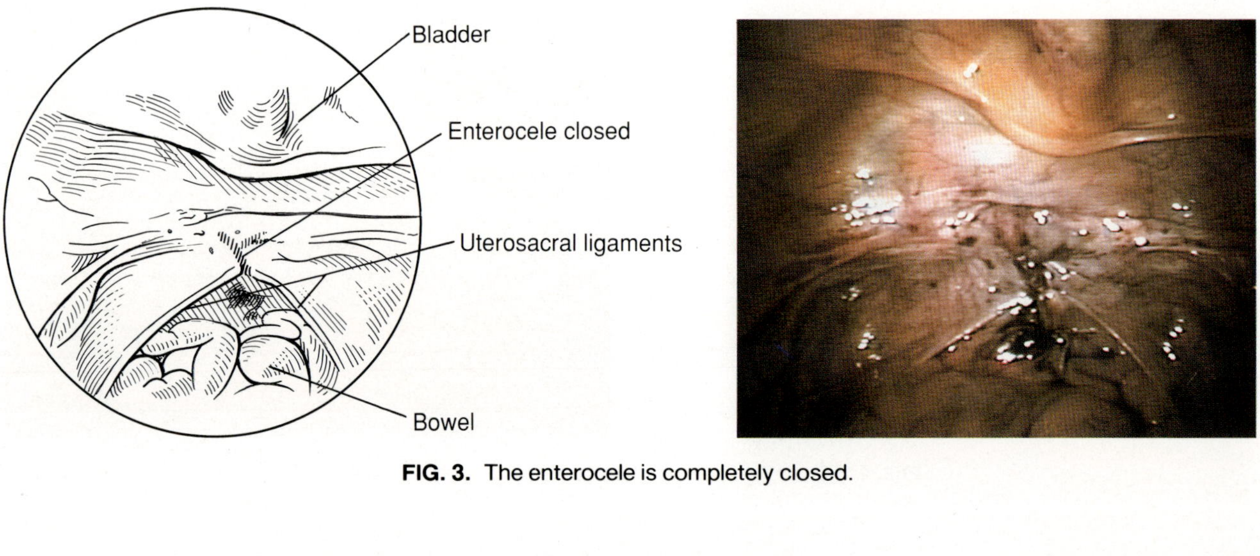

FIG. 3. The enterocele is completely closed.

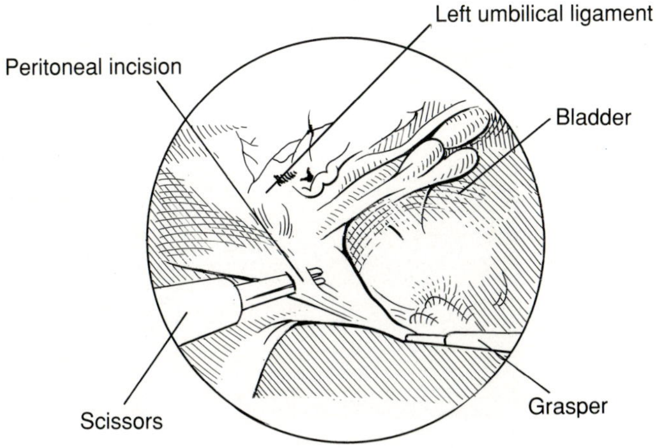

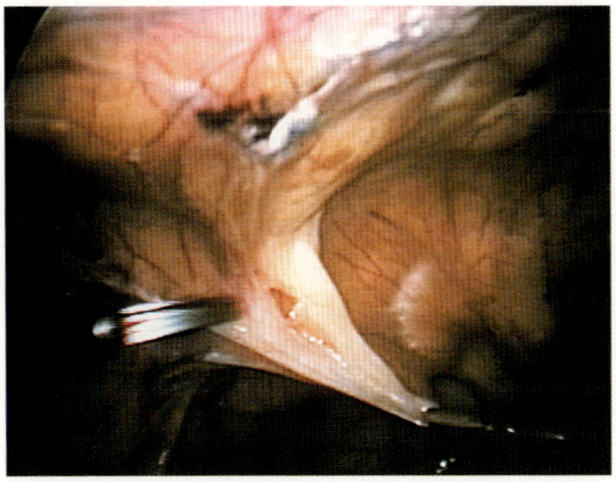

FIG. 4. Peritoneal incision preceding the Burch procedure. The incision is made on the left of the bladder, medially from the left umbilical ligament at the level of the upper border of the pubic bone.

The initial peritoneal incision is made immediately medial to the left umbilical ligament and above the pubic bone. A left-handed surgeon may choose to approach the space of Retzius from the right. The surgeon tries to gain access to and expose the pubic bone as quickly as possible (Fig. 5). The distance between the peritoneum and the pubic bone is short, even in the obese patient. The surgeon must remain in a plane perpendicular to the pubic bone. There is a tendency to shift toward the midline too early, leading to bladder injury. Once the pubic bone is reached, the assistant inserts a blunt instrument into the incision and retracts the bladder to the right. The space of Retzius is easily opened with minimal traction and some blunt dissection (Fig. 6). The dissection is continued until the entire space is opened and all anatomic structures can be identified on both sides. The urachus is seldom an obstacle to complete dissection of the field. The identifiable anatomic structures are the urethra, the bladder neck, the anterior wall of the bladder, the vaginal wall, the obturator muscles, the pubourethral ligaments, and the pubic bone with its symphysis and ligaments (Fig. 7). Identification of Cooper's ligament is a challenge; a wide dissection of the pubic bone facilitates identification of the ligament. Either of the techniques described by Kranz or by Burch can be performed. Other surgical procedures for correction of stress incontinence may be technically feasible, but our experience in performing them is lacking. The placement of the suture into the vaginal wall is identical for both the Burch and the MMK. The operator places his or her left hand in the patient's vagina, thereby displacing the bladder neck toward the left of the patient for application of the right-sided suture. The vaginal wall is only minimally elevated because otherwise the space between the vagina and the pubic bone is reduced to the extent that it becomes difficult to introduce the needle in the right position.

The needle (Ethibond 2/0, 36 in.) is introduced through either the suprapubic or paramedial 10-mm trocar. The needle holder is passed through the left lateral trocar, allowing optimum access to the space of Retzius. The needle is grasped and then guided into the space of Retzius. The right-sided stitch is placed first. The needle

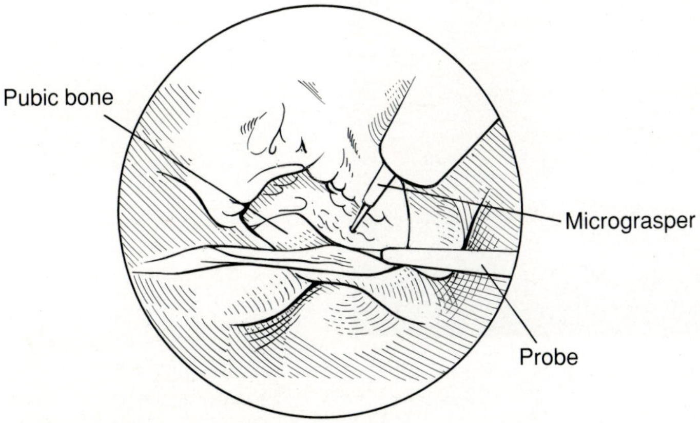

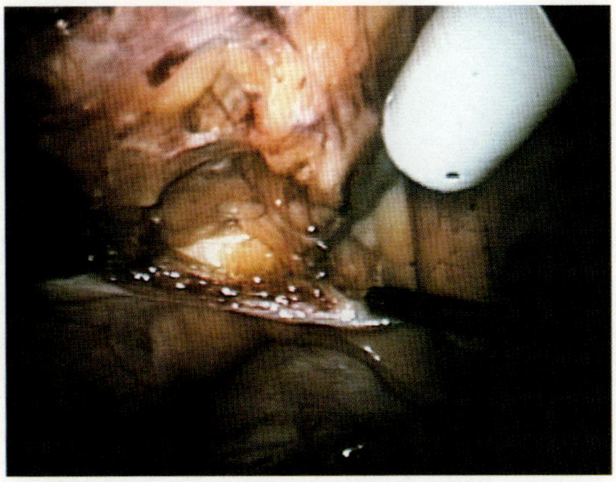

FIG. 5. As soon as possible after initial incision of the peritoneum, the operator needs to gain access to and expose the pubic bone.

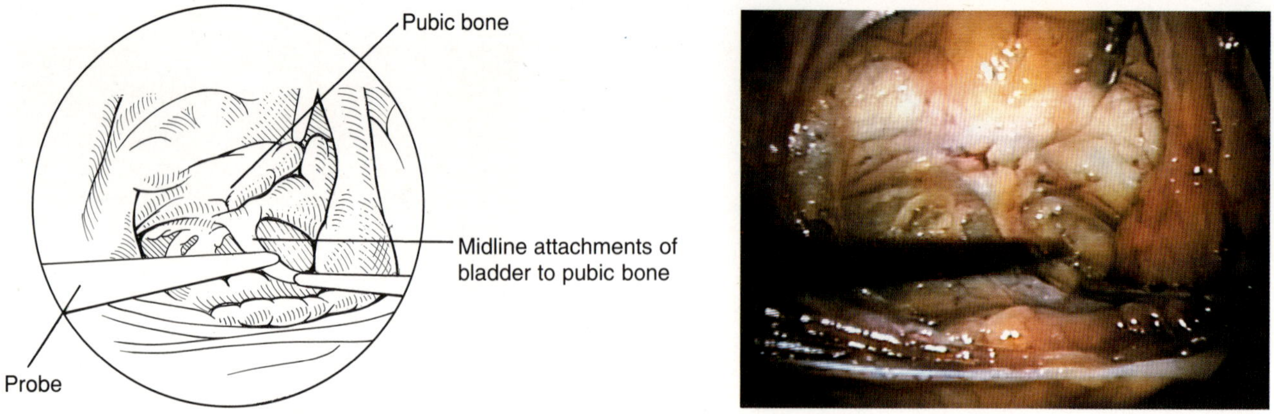

FIG. 6. Further dissection of the space of Retzius is mainly done bluntly. The midline attachments of the urethra to the pubic bone are left intact.

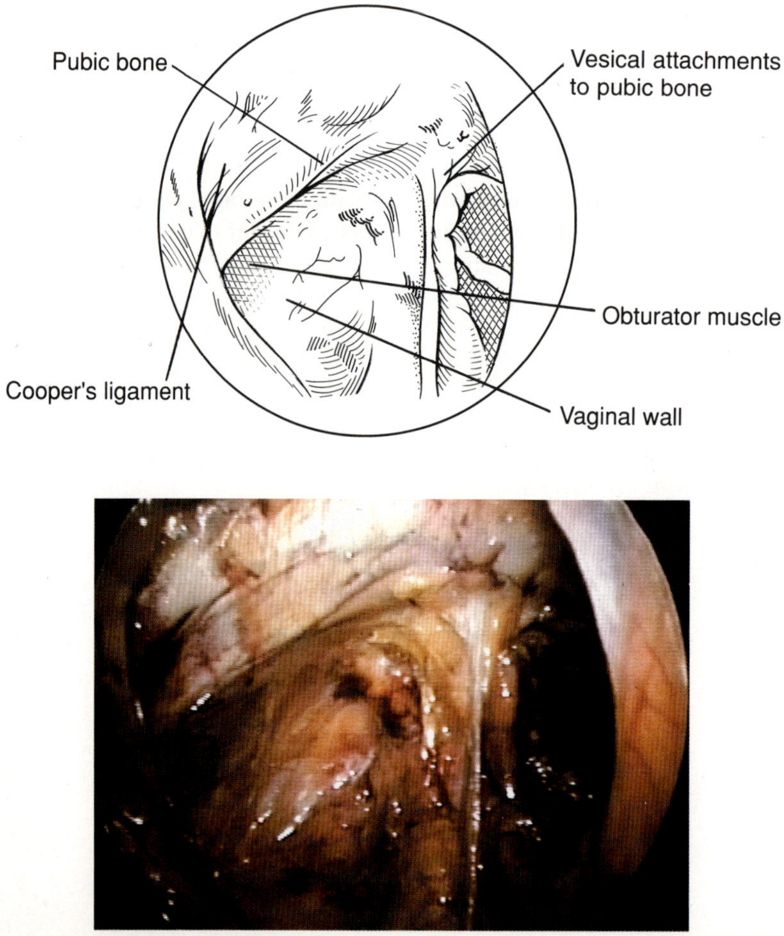

FIG. 7. End stage of the dissection. It is possible to identify all anatomic structures in great detail: the urethra with its attachments to the pubic bone, the vaginal wall, the obturator muscle, and the pubic bone with Cooper's ligament.

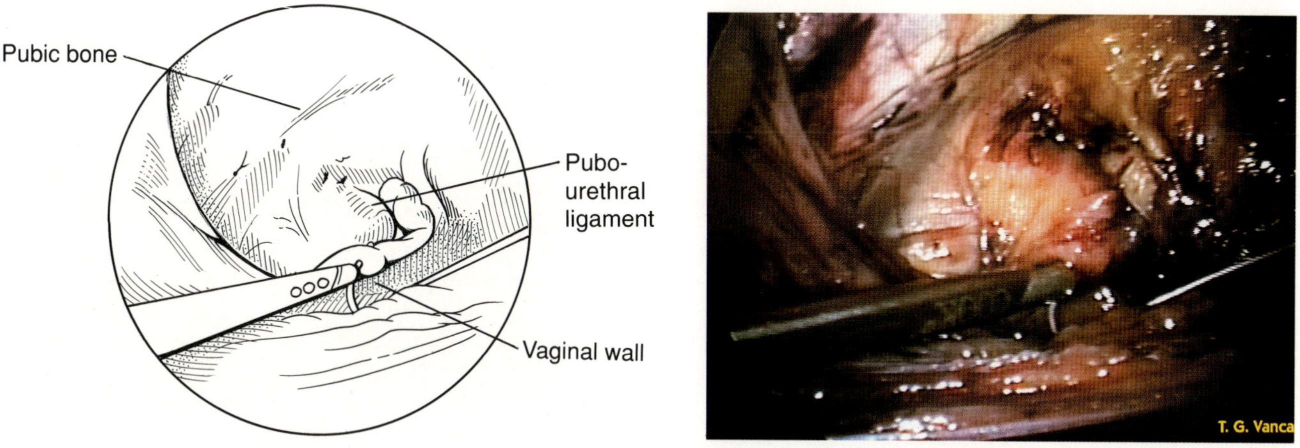

FIG. 8. The needle is passed through the vaginal wall on the left of the urethra, incorporating the pubourethral ligament.

is passed through the fascia of the vaginal wall, alongside the urethra. An effort is made to incorporate the pubourethral ligament into the suture (Fig. 8). Because the laparoscope is situated close to the bladder neck, the visualization of the anatomic detail is excellent.

In all cases I initially attempt to attach the suture to Cooper's ligament (Fig. 9). If this fails, then I attempt to use the symphysis. Failure to suture to Cooper's ligament may occur in patients who have been operated on and where the dissection along the pubic bone is difficult. Manipulation of the bladder neck with the left hand in the patient's vagina allows the surgeon to evaluate the degree of elevation of the bladder neck. It is recommended that the surgeon perform a manual evaluation of the bladder neck at least for diagnostic purposes. Elevation of the bladder neck during actual suturing then can be performed by the assistant if needed.

Knotting is best performed using the extracorporeal technique, and one or two extra throws secures the knot. Tension on the suture is minimized by elevating the vaginal wall during tightening of the knot. The right-sided stitch is placed and tightened before insertion of the left-sided one. When performing the Burch procedure, it is important not to tighten the first knot excessively because this leads to a gap on the other side of the bladder neck.

One stitch is placed on each side (Fig. 10). In patients with moderate cystocele, two stitches are placed on each side in order to correct the cystocele while achieving elevation of the bladder neck. In the presence of a large cystocele, repair is best performed from below. It is possible to apply one suture after another and to wait until all stitches are placed before tightening the knots. Each surgeon's preference in applying the sutures can be accommodated at laparoscopy. The number of supporting stitches is not a limitation of the methodology as some

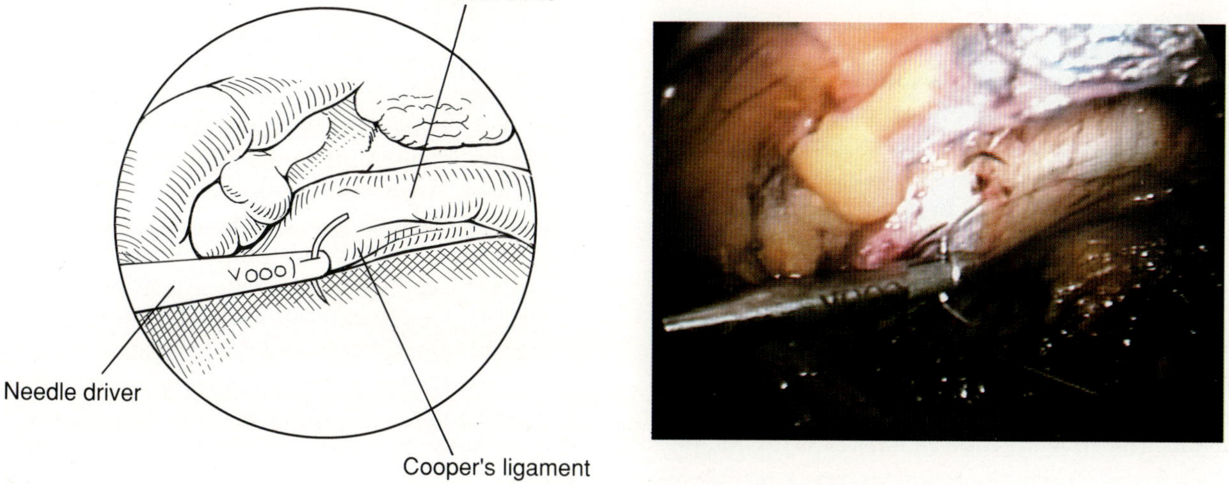

FIG. 9. The needle is passed through Cooper's ligament on the left.

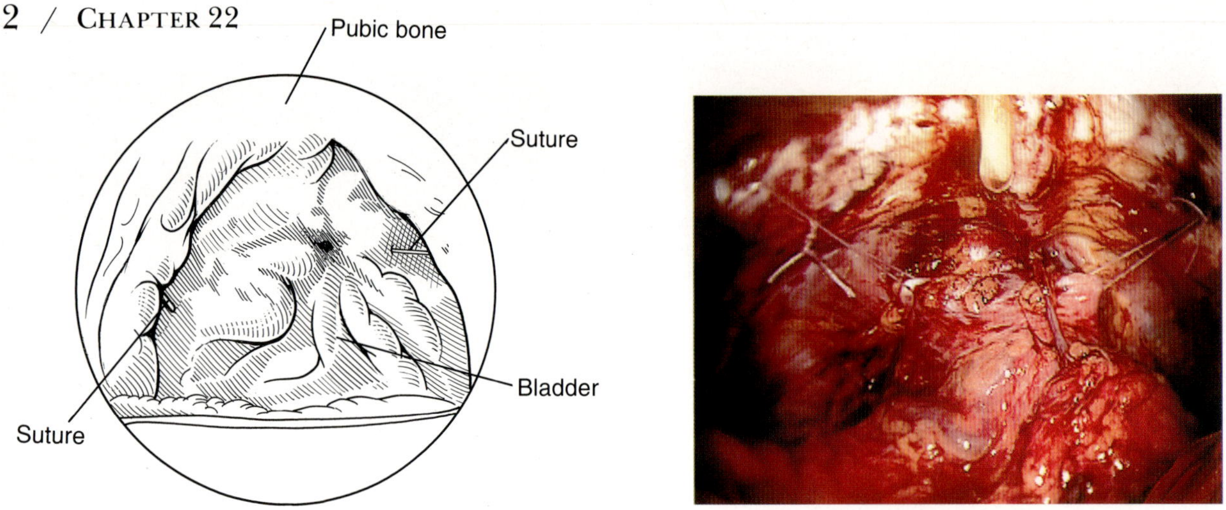

FIG. 10. End result of the colposuspension. The two sutures have elevated the vaginal wall, which now forms a "hammock" underneath the upper half of the urethra.

detractors of the method state. Closing the peritoneal defect can be achieved by applying one or two additional sutures.

OUTCOME

The author has performed more than 80 transperitoneal colposuspension procedures, either according to the MMK technique or according to the Burch technique. A group of 42 patients was prospectively studied from June 1991 to December 1992. Two had previous surgery for incontinence and both were vaginal procedures. The follow-up period was 6–24 months with a median of 16 months at the time of this writing. In summary, one patient was lost to follow-up and another presented with recurrence of her symptoms less than 3 months after the procedure, and the outcome was therefore considered a failure. She staunchly refused to submit to objective testing. The remaining 40 patients are satisfied. Eight of them present with residual symptoms of stress, urgency, or a combination of both. In some cases the residual urgency was predicted following the preoperative cystometrogram.

Definite comments about the validity of the procedure await the 5-year follow-up evaluation. Thus far the results are in line with what would be expected after a classical intervention. This is not surprising because the procedure performed is a copy in many aspects of the one described by Burch. The main difference is in the mode of access.

COMPLICATIONS

During the 80 procedures, some complications occurred which can be ascribed to the use of laparoscopy. Bladder injury during dissection occurred in four instances, two early on in our experience and two later. The latter cases were repeat interventions in which the dissection of the space of Retzius was expectedly difficult. Three of these bladder lacerations were repaired under laparoscopic control. The first one, which occurred in the second patient undergoing the procedure, was repaired at laparotomy because of additional difficulty in completing the actual procedure.

Inability to complete the procedure under laparoscopic control occurred in two instances, expectedly among the very first cases attempted. Further complications, such as bleeding, infection, injury to bowel or urinary structures other than the bladder, did not occur but are a real possibility. Whether the incidence of these types of complications is higher in patients treated with the laparoscopic approach vs. the alternative routes remains to be seen.

The last type of complication which can occur, is iatrogenic. Bladder dysfunction can result from the manipulation involved in the surgical correction. The most common complications are overcorrection, which may require long-term catheterization or continuous self-catheterization, and de novo bladder symptomatology. Overcorrection occurred in one patient who underwent a procedure of the MMK type. After approximately 3 months, the patient was able to void without help of a catheter. Tallying urgency symptoms that occur de novo is difficult because of their subjective nature. Many patients with preoperative mixed incontinence have difficulty understanding that the surgery did not cure them completely. This may lead to increased incapacitation by the urgency component, which in actuality remained unchanged or even improved. Nonetheless, de novo symptomatology is real and therefore an integral part of treatment of urinary incontinence. The incidence of such symptoms was at 24% in the group of 42 patients. This incidence is comparable to the numbers reported in the literature for the classical procedures according to MMK or Burch.

HIGHLIGHTS

Laparoscopy is a valuable surgical technique for the performance of reconstructive surgery of the pelvic floor. Although preliminary, the results in the author's series indicate that equivalence between the classical procedures and the laparoscopic interventions is likely.

REFERENCES

1. Marshall VF, Marchetti AA, Krantz KE. The correction of stress incontinence by simple vesico-urethral suspension. *Surg Gynecol Obstet* 1949;88:509.
2. Burch JC. Urethro-vaginal fixation to Cooper's ligament for correction of stress incontinence, cystocele, and prolapse. *Am J Obstet Gynecol* 1961;81:281.
3. Bergman A, Ballard CA, Koonings PP. Comparison of three different surgical procedures for genuine stress incontinence: prospective randomized study. *Am J Obstet Gynecol* 1989;160:1102.
4. Bergman A, Koonings PP, Ballard CA. Primary stress urinary incontinence and pelvic relaxation: prospective randomized comparison of three different operations. *Am J Obstet Gynecol* 1989;161:91.
5. Vancaillie TG, Schuessler W. Laparoscopic bladder neck suspension. *J Laparoendosc Surg* 1991;1:169.
6. Herzog AR, Fultz NH. Prevalence and incidence of urinary incontinence in community-dwelling populations. *J Am Geriatr Soc* 1990;38:273.

Endoscopic Management of Gynecologic Disease,
edited by G.D. Adamson and D.C. Martin.
Lippincott-Raven Publishers, Philadelphia © 1996.

CHAPTER 23

Pelvic and Paraaortic Lymphadenectomy

Joel M. Childers

DEFINITION AND PREVALENCE

Currently, vulvar, endometrial, and ovarian carcinomas are surgically staged. Part of the surgical staging in malignancies of these sites includes evaluation of the regional lymph nodes. Laparoscopic lymphadenectomy potentially can be used in the surgical staging of patients with endometrial and ovarian carcinomas. Although cervical cancer is a clinically staged malignancy, the usefulness of laparoscopic lymphadenectomy in the management of this disease was recently evaluated (1–5).

Lymph nodes from the abdominal aorta to the pelvic floor can be the primary sites of metastases in cervical, endometrial, and ovarian carcinoma. Reported cases of these cancers in the United States in 1993 were as follows: invasive cervical carcinoma, 13,000; endometrial carcinoma, 33,000; and ovarian carcinoma, 19,000 (6). Most gynecologic oncologists perform selective lymphadenectomy or a lymph node sampling for endometrial and ovarian carcinomas. Patients with early carcinoma of the cervix undergo complete or therapeutic pelvic lymphadenectomy. During a lymph node sampling procedure, most of the regional lymph nodes are removed; however, emphasis is not placed on extracting nodal tissue behind the external iliac artery and vein in the pelvis nor beneath the aorta and vena cava in the paraaortic region. A therapeutic or complete lymphadenectomy requires removal of all lymphatic tissue in the targeted area. For practical purposes, the definition of lymphadenectomy in this chapter is the procedure referred to by most gynecologic oncologists as selective lymphadenectomy.

J. M. Childers: Department of Obstetrics and Gynecology, University Medical Center, Tucson, Arizona 85712.

INDICATIONS

Indications for laparoscopic lymphadenectomy in gynecologic oncology are listed in Table 1.

Cervical Cancer

Laparoscopic lymphadenectomy may be utilized in two categories of patients with cervical cancer. The first consists of patients with early cervical cancer who are considered candidates for radical hysterectomy. These patients generally undergo a lymph node sampling, and frozen section is performed for evaluation of metastatic disease. Depending on the philosophies of the surgeon, the radical hysterectomy would be aborted if the lymph nodes contain metastatic disease. If laparotomy is to be avoided, then the radical hysterectomy can be accomplished laparoscopically or vaginally, and a therapeutic pelvic lymphadenectomy is performed laparoscopically.

The second category of patients includes those with early or late cervical cancer who are to be treated primarily with radiotherapy. Since these patients are to receive standard whole-pelvis radiotherapy, they require only sampling of the lymph nodes high (cephalad) in the radiation field and just outside the radiation field. This would include the proximal common and low paraaortic lymph nodes bilaterally. The surgeon should carry out a thorough inspection for intraperitoneal disease in these patients as well. Albeit a rare phenomenon, intraperitoneal disease would certainly change the treatment plans. This laparoscopic approach in patients scheduled for radiotherapy is controversial because of the higher incidence of postirradiation, regional enteric complications associated with extended field radiotherapy in patients who undergo transperitoneal paraaortic lymphadenectomy (7). The second group of candidates in this category in-

TABLE 1. *Indications for laparoscopic lymphadenectomy in gynecologic oncology*

- I. Cervical cancer
  - A. Radical hysterectomy candidate
    - 1. Prior to laparotomy to rule out positive nodes
    - 2. To convert abdominal procedure to
      - a. Laparoscopic radical hysterectomy
      - b. Laparoscopic-assisted radical hysterectomy
      - c. Radical vaginal hysterectomy
  - B. Radiotherapy candidate
    - 1. Before standard pelvic radiotherapy
    - 2. During transperitoneal interstitial needle placement
- II. Ovarian cancer
  - A. Staging early carcinoma
  - B. Second-look laparoscopy
- III. Endometrial cancer
  - A. With laparoscopic-assisted hysterectomy for clinical stage I carcinoma
  - B. Following hysterectomy in the nonstaged patient

cludes those patients who are to receive transperitoneal interstitial radiation following external irradiation. These patients may have laparoscopic-assisted needle placement, sampling of the lymph nodes outside the pelvic radiotherapy field, and placement of an omental carpet in the pelvis.

Ovarian Carcinoma

Laparoscopic lymphadenectomy is used in patients with ovarian carcinoma in two situations. First are those patients with presumed early (stage I or II) ovarian carcinoma who require surgical staging. In these instances, unilateral or bilateral lymphadenectomy from the renal vessels to the pelvis is required. This includes sampling the obturator lymph nodes; the external, internal, and common iliac lymph nodes; as well as the paraaortic nodes both above and below the inferior mesenteric artery.

The second category of patients eligible for laparoscopic lymphadenectomy includes those with advanced ovarian carcinoma who have undergone surgical debulking and platinum-based chemotherapy and who have no evidence of disease following treatment. A thorough evaluation of the entire intraperitoneal cavity and sites of disease remaining after the surgical debulking should be done first, as the lymphadenectomy should be the final step of a laparoscopic second-look procedure and performed only if no other evidence of disease is found. Second-look operations for ovarian cancer should be performed only in an investigational setting.

Endometrial Carcinoma

Patients with clinical stage I adenocarcinoma of the endometrium can be managed with a combined laparoscopic and vaginal surgery approach. If a laparoscopically assisted surgical staging procedure (LASS) is to be performed, a thorough inspection of the intraperitoneal cavity, procurement of intraperitoneal washings, and a lymphadenectomy should be performed in addition to the vaginal hysterectomy. Laparoscopic-assisted surgical staging can also be used in the patient who was not surgically staged at the time of hysterectomy. For staging of endometrial cancer, it is particularly important to sample the pelvic lymph nodes, including the obturator, external, internal, and common iliac lymph nodes. Removal of the paraaortic lymph nodes is left to the discretion of the individual surgeon; but, when it is performed, only the lymph nodes below the inferior mesenteric artery are removed.

CONTRAINDICATIONS

It is imperative that the survival of patients with pelvic malignancies not be compromised by employing laparoscopic lymphadenectomy. This procedure should not be performed by surgeons not experienced in oncologic surgery, laparotomy, lymphadenectomy, and laparoscopic surgery. Currently, survival data for patients with pelvic malignancies who have been managed with laparoscopy are lacking. The learning curve associated with this surgical procedure is significant and is unlikely to be overcome by the surgeon with no experience in abdominal pelvic and paraaortic lymphadenectomy or by the experienced oncologic surgeon who performs this laparoscopic procedure only occasionally. Only the experienced, committed oncologic surgeon will master laparoscopic pelvic and paraaortic lymphadenectomy. Future clinical trials with experienced surgeons and long-term survival data will help determine the role of laparoscopic lymphadenectomy in oncology.

SURGICAL TECHNIQUES

It was an extraperitoneal approach that ushered modern operative laparoscopy into the world of gynecologic oncology. This technique originated in France and was first popularized by Daniell Dargent (1). Dargent et al. reported a series of patients with early cervical carcinoma in whom pelvic lymph nodes were sampled laparoscopically prior to radical hysterectomy (1). An average of 13 nodes were obtained with his technique.

The first transperitoneal lymphadenectomies were reported in 1991 by Querleu et al. (2). Like Dargent, these authors used this technique for staging patients with early cervical cancer prior to radical hysterectomy. Subsequent reports were published on laparoscopic low paraaortic lymphadenectomy in patients with cervical, endometrial, and ovarian cancer (3,8,9). The final phase of development of laparoscopic lymphadenectomy came with the ability to perform high paraaortic lymphadenectomies (10–12). These infrarenal lymphadenectomies have been performed on patients with ovarian cancer and represent what some investigators believe to be the final hurdle in complete laparoscopic staging of ovarian carcinoma.

This chapter outlines the transperitoneal technique of pelvic and paraaortic lymphadenectomy that was begun at the University of Arizona in 1990.

PREOPERATIVE CONSIDERATIONS

Bowel Preparation

Evacuation of the large and small bowel facilitates the laparoscopic approach to the paraaortic nodes. This is easily accomplished by having the patient on a liquid diet for 2 days prior to the procedure and administering one bottle (240 cm^3) of magnesium citrate on each of the two days prior to the procedure. An enema on the morning of admission aids in the evacuation of the lower bowel. This is routinely performed on our patients prior to laparoscopic surgery. In general, we do not use oral erythromycin- and/or neomycin-based antibiotics.

Anesthesia Considerations

General anesthesia is used. Use and placement of endotracheal tube, nasogastric or oral gastric tube, pulse oximeter, and Foley catheter as well as detailed anesthetic considerations are discussed in the chapter by Collins and Jackson. Positioning of the lymphadenectomy patient is important. The supine position is preferred except for patients with stage I endometrial cancer in whom the dorsal lithotomy position is used (13).

Since the patient's arms are tucked by her sides to facilitate mobility of the surgeon, the anesthesiologist may prefer to place an arterial line and/or a central line. A heating blanket is placed beneath the patient and body temperature is monitored. Sequential compression stockings are currently used.

Operating Room Considerations and Instrumentation

Abdominal preparation of the patient is performed in the usual fashion. Vaginal preparation is necessary for patients with stage I endometrial cancer.

Although adequate training is obviously necessary to perform this procedure, even the trained physician will not be able to accomplish these tasks without proper instrumentation. In general, the procedure can be accomplished with the instruments available on a laparoscopic cholecystectomy tray. It is absolutely necessary, however, to have (a) *sharp scissors* with monopolar electrosurgery capabilities, (b) a large forceps (spoon-shaped, toothed, or tripronged) that fits through a 10-mm laparoscopic sleeve, and (c) an irrigation-suction apparatus. I prefer disposable scissors because they are always sharp. The large forceps is necessary for extirpation of the lymphatic tissue. A 10-mm laparoscopic telescope with a 0° lens is preferable for most cases.

Special instruments, such as needle drivers, knot pushers, pretied slip-knots, and stapling devices, are not absolutely necessary for the lymphadenectomy, but they are very helpful if a laparoscopically assisted vaginal hysterectomy is to be performed. On occasion, the laparoscopic clip applier may be needed. This is most commonly used for perforating veins over the vena cava.

OPERATIVE TECHNIQUE

Instrument Insertion

Gaining of access to the intraperitoneal cavity is a procedure well known to most gynecologists. We prefer the technique of direct trocar insertion without the prior establishment of a pneumoperitoneum. This is accomplished by placing a 10-mm or larger laparoscopic trocar and sleeve through an incision made in the umbilicus. Upward traction on the anterior abdominal wall with the aid of towel clips placed on either side of the umbilicus is important. This technique is safe, saves time, and decreases the incidence of annoying preperitoneal emphysema (14).

In patients with previous abdominal incisions extending through the umbilicus or in patients with umbilical hernias, I use the left upper quadrant (15). The Veress needle is placed in the ninth or tenth intercostal space in the left upper quadrant. Once the pneumoperitoneum is established, the primary trocar is placed in the midclavicular line just below the left costal margin. A 5-mm trocar and sleeve should be used to minimize resistance and downward tenting of the anterior abdominal wall. The telescope is then used to assess the intraperitoneal cavity for adhesions and optimal sites for placement of ancillary trocars for adhesiolysis. If the surgeon prefers, open laparoscopy can be performed with the use of a Hasson cannula (16). However, the left upper quadrant technique allows access to the intraperitoneal cavity lateral to the midline adhesions and offers better visualization during adhesiolysis. I would recommend using a lateral site even if open laparoscopy is used. The operative laparoscopist should be familiar with more than one technique for obtaining access to the intraperitoneal cavity.

Four laparoscopic ports are needed to perform this procedure. The primary port is placed in the umbilicus and should be 10 mm for use with a 10-mm telescope and camera. The three ancillary ports are placed under direct laparoscopic visualization. Two 5-mm trocars and sleeves are placed lateral to the inferior epigastric vessels and the rectus muscle bilaterally. The third ancillary port is placed in the midline above the symphysis and should be 10–12 mm to allow removal of the nodal tissue, which at times can contain sizable specimens.

Inspection of the Intraperitoneal Cavity

After the laparoscopic ports are in place and before the patient is placed in Trendelenburg position, it is important to explore the entire intraperitoneal cavity. This should be done in a systematic fashion. The cecum and appendix should be visualized as should the right paracolic gutter. The gallbladder, the surface of the right lobe of the liver, the right hemidiaphragm, the falciform ligament, the greater curvature of the stomach, the anterior wall of the stomach, the left hemidiaphragm with its left ventricular pulsations, the supracolic omentum, the transverse colon, and the infracolic omentum should be carefully inspected. This systematic clockwise inspection continues with evaluation of the descending colon and left paracolic gutter, which leads the surgeon to the pelvis. The pelvis is evaluated after the establishment of Trendelenburg position. It is helpful, when evaluating the pelvic side walls, to grasp the uteroovarian ligament and lift the ovary in order to adequately visualize the ovarian fossa. If pelvic washings are to be taken, they should be obtained before any operative procedures are undertaken.

In examining the paraaortic area, the root of the small bowel mesentery can be lifted and often the transverse duodenum can be seen. The area from the third part of the duodenum to the lower pelvis should be inspected for obvious adenopathy. A peritoneal incision over the aorta between the mesentery of the small bowel and the common iliac arteries allows access to the paraaortic nodal tissue from the renal vessels to the proximal common iliac arteries bilaterally.

On the left side, the nodal tissue over the distal common iliac vessels and their bifurcation can be obtained only through a peritoneal incision in the pelvis. However, on the right side, these nodes may be removed through the peritoneal incision over the aorta and right common iliac artery.

Laparoscopic Pelvic Lymphadenectomy

Dissection of the obturator, external iliac, hypogastric, or low common iliac nodes can be performed in the following fashion. The surgeon stands on the side opposite the nodes to be dissected. The telescope is placed through the umbilical port and is held by the assistant. The assistant also uses a grasper placed through the ipsilateral lateral port. The surgeon uses a grasper through the lower midline port and scissors with monopolar capability through the contralateral lateral port.

The peritoneum is incised over the external iliac artery and vein, between the round ligament and the infundibulopelvic ligament. The round ligament is left intact unless a hysterectomy is to be performed. The peritoneum is opened and the paravesical/obturator space opened. This is aided by isolating the obliterated umbilical artery and retracting it medially (Fig. 1). It can be easily identified in the pelvis by pushing on it at the anterior abdominal wall and watching for its movement in

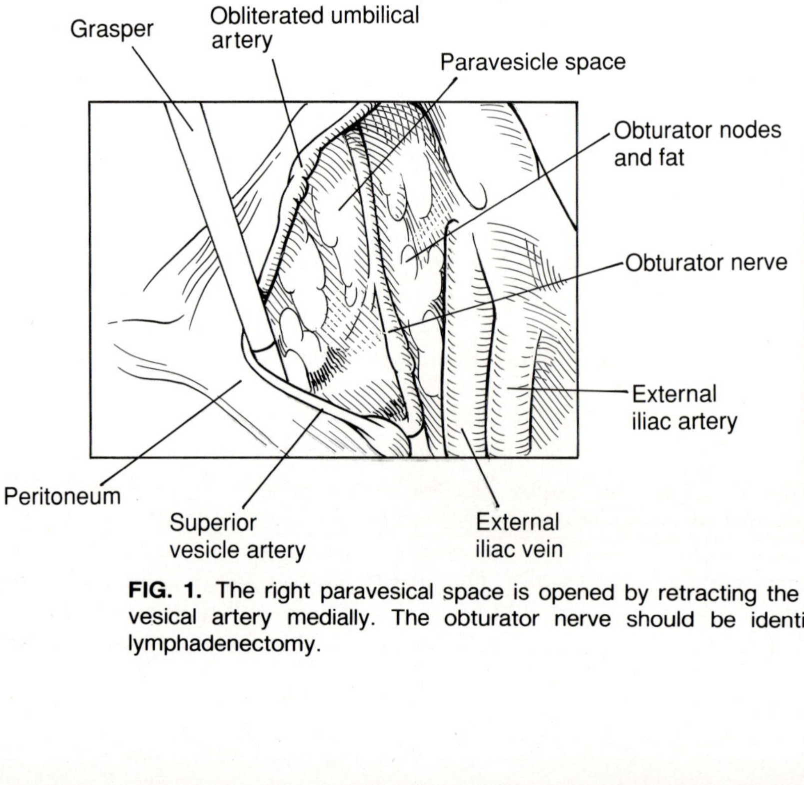

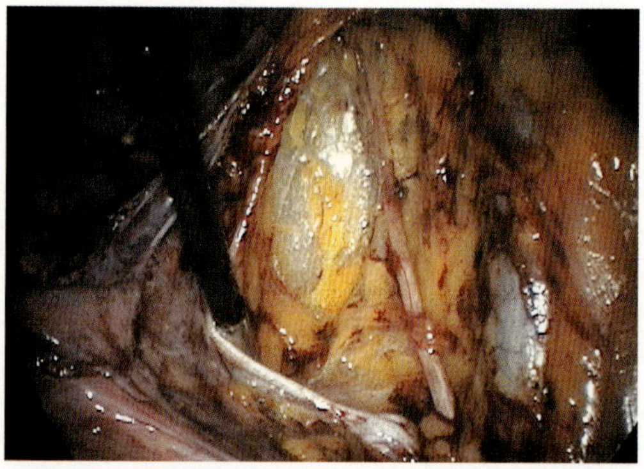

FIG. 1. The right paravesical space is opened by retracting the obliterated umbilical artery/superior vesical artery medially. The obturator nerve should be identified prior to proceeding with the lymphadenectomy.

the pelvis. It is always near the external iliac vein. The space between this obliterated umbilical artery and the external iliac vein is easily opened.

We perform the obturator lymphadenectomy first because blood, lymph fluid, or irrigation fluid can accumulate in this dependent area and may obscure visualization somewhat if these nodes are not removed first. The obturator nerve is identified and the nodal tissue anteriorly is separated from the nerve by blunt and sharp dissection.

The nodal tissue along the medial aspect of the external iliac vein then is dissected off along the length of the vein. In performing this dissection, the surgeon should take care not to damage any aberrant or accessory veins emptying into the external iliac vein.

It is my preference then to follow the nodal bundle distally to the pelvic wall and to coagulate and cut the nodal package at the pelvic wall. Once this is completed, the only remaining attachment of the obturator nodal package is at the junction of the hypogastric and external iliac arteries. This is usually the most difficult part of removing the obturator nodes. Adequate visualization can be difficult to obtain as the nodal bundle starts to course laterally. Care also should be taken in this area to avoid ureteral damage. The nodal bundle is removed intact through the lower 10- to 12-mm port using large forceps.

Attention is then drawn to the external iliac nodes. This dissection is accomplished by creating a plane in the adventitia of the external iliac artery and dissecting it up to the circumflex iliac artery. I find it to be easily and simply performed with sharp scissors and monopolar electricity. Effort should be made to avoid damaging the genitofemoral nerve laterally (Fig. 2). The dissection can be extended proximally to the point where the ovarian vessels and/or the ureter cross the iliac vessels. Through this same peritoneal incision, the assistant can retract the ureter in a cephalad direction and the nodal dissection can be continued up the distal common iliac artery.

When the pelvic lymphadenectomy is performed on the left side, the rectosigmoid generally needs to be taken down from the left pelvic side wall. This can be accomplished by incising the peritoneum in this area along the

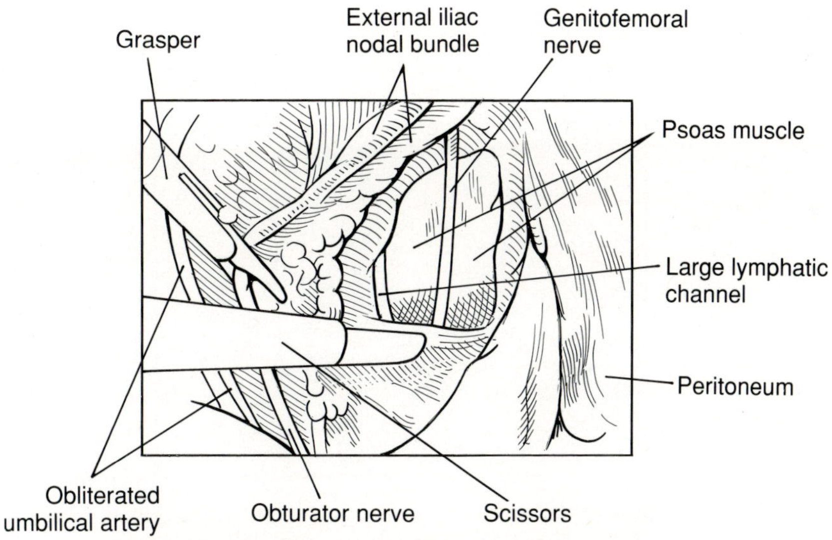

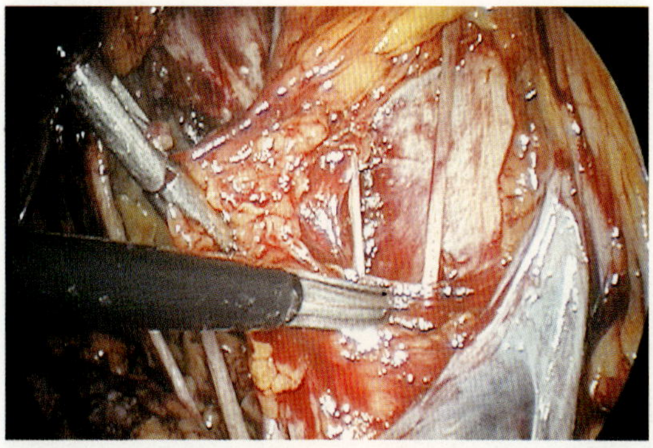

FIG. 2. The right genitofemoral nerve is identified by retracting the external iliac nodal bundle medially. It lies on the psoas muscle and at times, under the magnification of the laparoscope, may be confused for large lymphatic channels.

white line of Toldt, which will give access to the retroperitoneal space. If mobilization of the rectosigmoid is not required, the same incision, as described, is made between the round ligament and the ovarian vessels. The surgeon stands on the right side of the patient and operates through the midline port and the lateral port and uses scissors and graspers.

At the end of the procedure, the operative site is irrigated and carefully inspected to ensure that hemostasis is adequate. The peritoneum is left open and no drains are used (Fig. 3).

Laparoscopic Paraaortic Lymphadenectomy

Key to the successful removal of the paraaortic nodes is proper placement of the small bowel into the upper abdomen. The mesentery of the small bowel should be identified, flipped in a cephalad direction, and splayed out across the abdomen. This places the small bowel into the upper abdomen and exposes the paraaortic area. Trendelenburg position, a good bowel preparation, and—occasionally—lateral tilt of the operating table assist in keeping the bowel in the upper abdomen. It is during this process that the small bowel can be inspected for metastatic disease. This packing of the bowel is extremely important and time should be taken to accomplish this correctly, lest time be lost later. Occasionally, the use of additional ports to keep the bowel in the upper abdomen may be required to accomplish a paraaortic lymphadenectomy, especially in heavier patients. Depending on its location, the transverse duodenum often can be visualized as it crosses the vena cava and aorta. Lifting the mesentery of the small bowel as it crosses the aorta aids the surgeon in visualizing the third portion of the duodenum. The aorta, right common iliac artery, and the ureter as it crosses the right iliac vessels are landmarks that should be identified prior to beginning the dissection.

Right-Side, Paraaortic Lymphadenectomy

The surgeon, while on the left side of the patient, performs the procedure with graspers in the lower midline

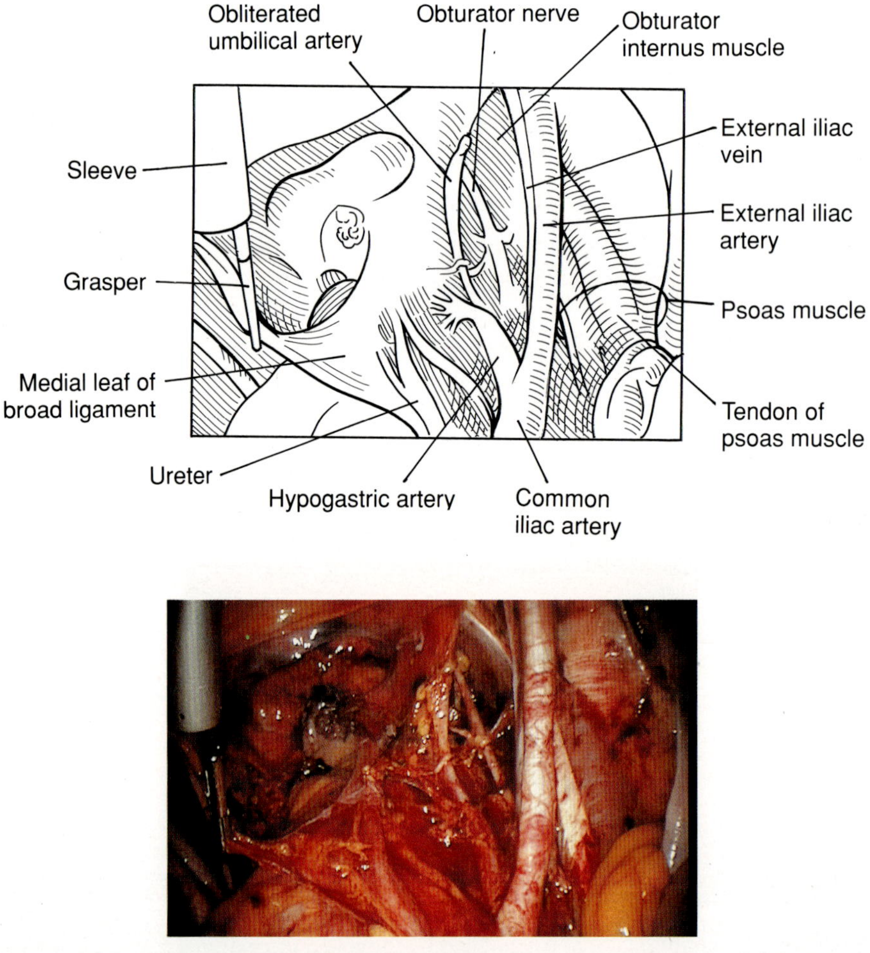

FIG. 3. After the right pelvic lymphadenectomy is completed, the broad ligament is retracted medially and the entire operative site is inspected for hemostasis.

port and scissors in the left lateral port. The assistant holds the camera in the umbilical port and uses graspers in the right lateral port. It is helpful to rotate the camera so that the aorta and vena cava are horizontal on the color monitor, with the patient's head to the right of the monitor.

An incision is made in the peritoneum over the aorta. This incision is extended down the right common iliac artery to where the ureter crosses the iliac vessels and up the aorta to the mesentery of the small bowel or the transverse duodenum. The peritoneum is lifted with graspers and blunt dissection is performed laterally toward the right psoas muscle. The right ureter is identified and lifted away from the underlying areolar tissue. The grasper in the midline port then is used to retract the ureter anteriorly and laterally. The right psoas and tendon of the psoas should be easily seen.

The assistant then places his or her grasper, which is in the right lateral port, underneath the ureter to retract it anteriorly and laterally out of the operative field. This also creates a small tent, which helps prevent small bowel from falling into the operative field.

The surgeon then dissects the nodal and fatty tissue off the aorta by sharply developing the adventitial plane of the aorta. This arterial dissection is continued in a cephalad and caudad direction, up the aorta and down the common iliac artery, with the surgeon using the scissors and electrosurgery as needed. Lateral dissection then is performed toward the psoas muscle so that a portion of the vena cava is unroofed. Care should be taken to avoid lacerating perforating vessels when unroofing the aorta. It is uncommon to encounter a perforating vein from the vena cava that cannot be controlled with monopolar electricity.

Dissection is continued up and down the vena cava. Small vessels and lymphatic channels are easily coagulated with the scissors. Large perforating vessels from the vena cava or aorta should be clipped.

One end of the nodal bundle then is transected. This can be performed easily and quickly using short bursts of monopolar electricity. Once the nodal package is transected at one end, it is easy to peel the bundle off the vena cava toward the opposite end. Transection of the remaining end again is accomplished by monopolar elec-

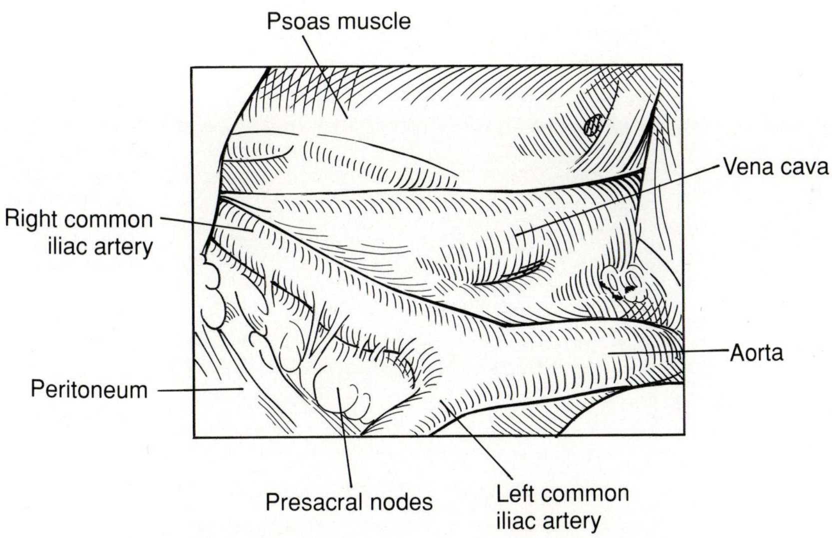

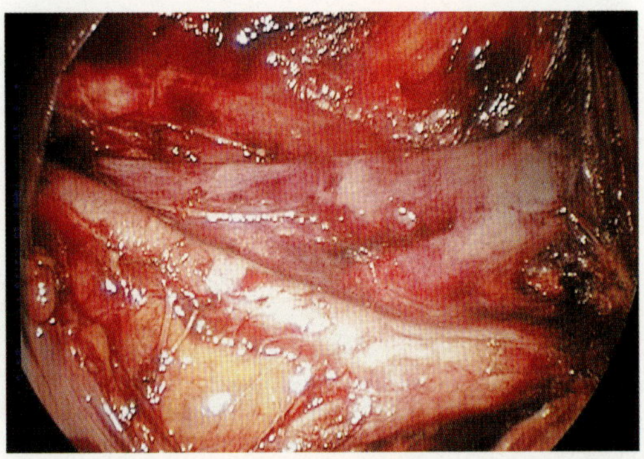

FIG. 4. After completion of a low right paraaortic lymphadenectomy, the ureter and the ovarian vessels are retracted upward (out of the picture), and the entire field is inspected for adequate hemostasis.

trosurgery. The nodal tissue is extracted using the large forceps through the lower midline port. The operative field is irrigated and hemostasis is secured (Fig. 4).

If the nodal tissue over the right common iliac artery is to be removed as well, it can be accomplished through the same peritoneal incision. The assistant uses the grasper to retract the ureter atraumatically in a caudad direction. This exposes the nodal tissue over this artery and beyond its bifurcation. The nodal dissection is continued down the common iliac to the proximal internal and external iliac vessels (Fig. 5).

This maneuver cannot be used to remove obturator or external iliac nodes. In addition, because of the location of the mesentery of the rectosigmoid, this maneuver has limited applicability for the left-side pelvic nodes.

Left-side Paraaortic Lymphadenectomy

The surgeon, while standing on the right side of the patient, performs this procedure using instruments placed through the lower midline and right lateral ports. The assistant holds the telescope and camera through the umbilical port. The camera is rotated so that the aorta and the vena cava are horizontal on the color monitor and the patient's head to the left. The image on the monitor is upside down in orientation for the assistant.

If the peritoneal incision has not already been made, an incision is made similar to that used for the right-side paraaortic lymphadenectomy. This incision over the aorta is extended in the cephalad direction as far as possible. The mesentery of the small bowel or the third portion of the duodenum limits the cephalad extent. The incision is extended in a caudad direction over the proximal left common iliac artery.

The surgeon dissects in the adventitial plane of the aorta in a cephalad and caudad direction. It is important to extend this adventitial dissection as far as possible in both directions to allow ample room to perform the lymphadenectomy safely. On the left side, the cephalad extent is limited by the inferior mesenteric artery. Care should be taken to avoid injuring this artery, as its origin

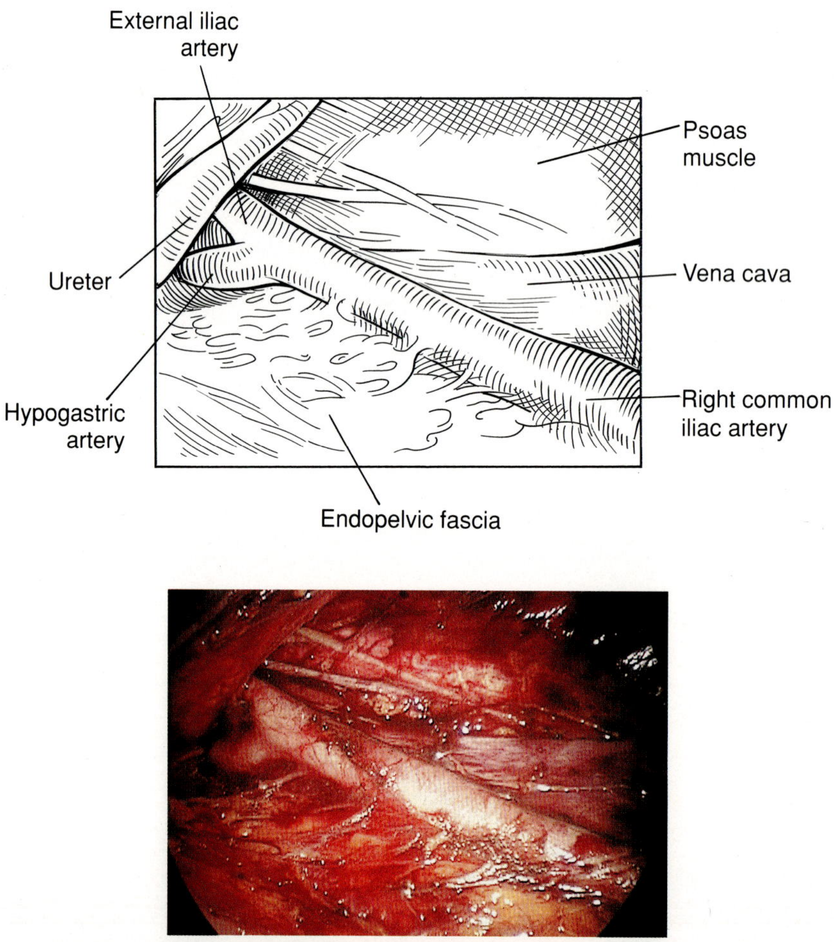

FIG. 5. A right pelvic lymphadenectomy can be performed through the paraaortic peritoneal incision. Lymph nodes distal to the bifurcation of the common iliac artery can be obtained through this incision by retraction of the ureter in a caudad direction.

on the abdominal aorta is often difficult to identify. The more the aorta and left common iliac are separated from the endopelvic fascia, the more space and visibility the surgeon will have.

Only after the adventitia over the aorta has been adequately dissected free should lateral dissection toward the left psoas muscle be carried out. The surgeon can safely dissect beneath the left ureter and mesentery of the rectosigmoid using this plane (Fig. 6). This differs from the right-side paraaortic lymphadenectomy, where lateral dissection is carried out after making the peritoneal incision but before dissecting the aortic adventitia.

Lateral dissection continues until the psoas muscle and its tendon are identified. The assistant now places the grasper or irrigator/aspirator into the dissected space beneath the mesentery of the rectosigmoid and the left ureter. This retraction is critically important for adequate exposure, which is mandatory since the left-side paraaortic lymph nodes in this area are lateral to the aorta.

Once there is adequate exposure, the surgeon grasps the nodal bundle near the bifurcation of the aorta and lifts anteriorly while simultaneously pushing down on the aorta with another instrument. This frees the loose attachments between these two structures and assists in the dissection beneath the nodal chain (Fig. 7). A window is created beneath the nodal chain at its caudad end by blunt dissection. I prefer transecting the chain with scissors and monopolar electricity. The dissection is then extended in a cephalad direction using blunt and sharp dissection and electrosurgery with the scissors as needed. Then the nodal chain is transected at the cephalad end near the inferior mesenteric artery. The specimen is removed through the lower midline 10-mm port, and the operative field is irrigated and inspected for hemostasis (Fig. 8).

Infrarenal Paraaortic Lymphadenectomy

The transverse duodenum is separated from the vena cava and the aorta by blunt and sharp dissection (Fig. 9). This dissection is continued in a cephalad direction, but lateral dissection is also accomplished by sweeping the

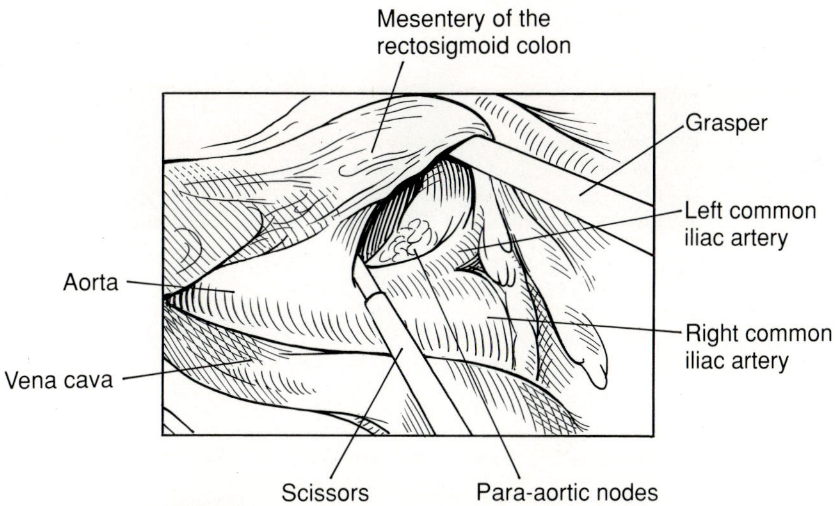

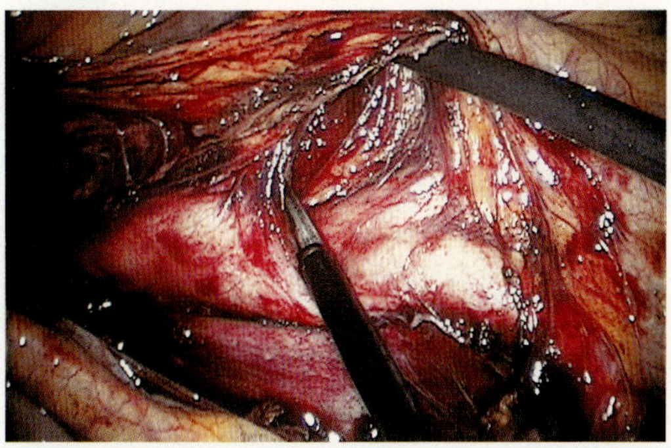

FIG. 6. The mesentery of the rectosigmoid, which contains the inferior mesenteric artery, is lifted off the aorta by blunt dissection. Lateral dissection is then continued until the left ureter, ovarian vessels, and psoas muscle have been identified.

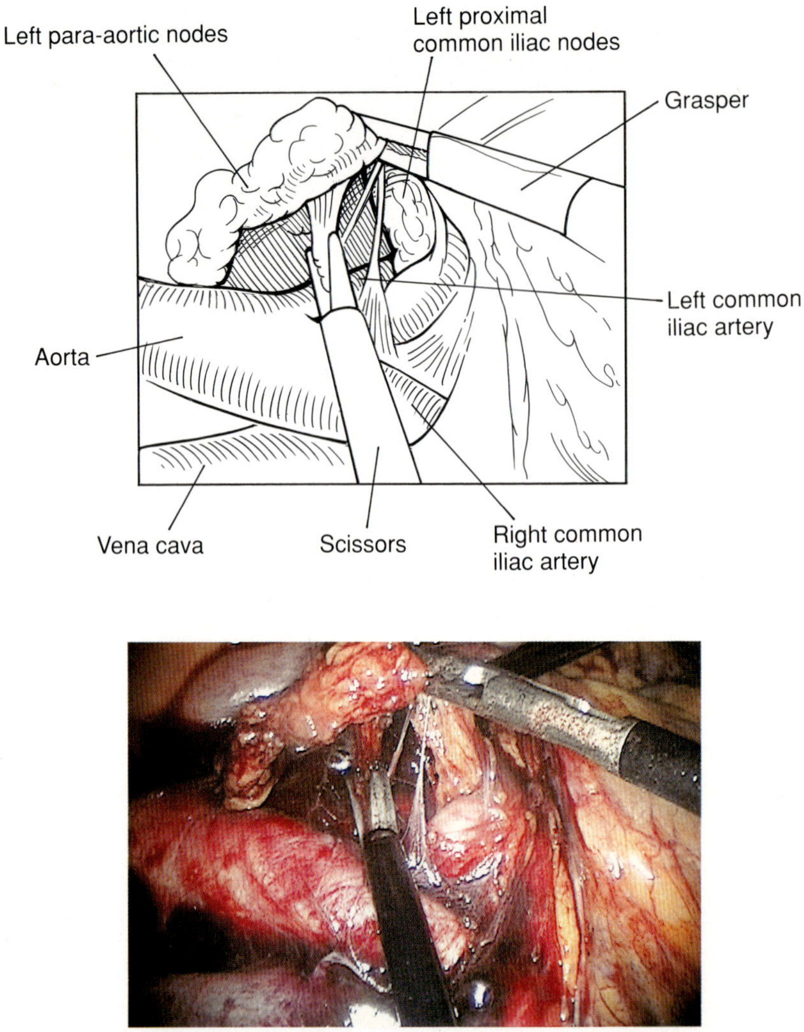

FIG. 7. The low left paraaortic nodal bundle is grasped, and sharp dissection with monopolar electrosurgery transects the underlying lymphatic and vascular vessels.

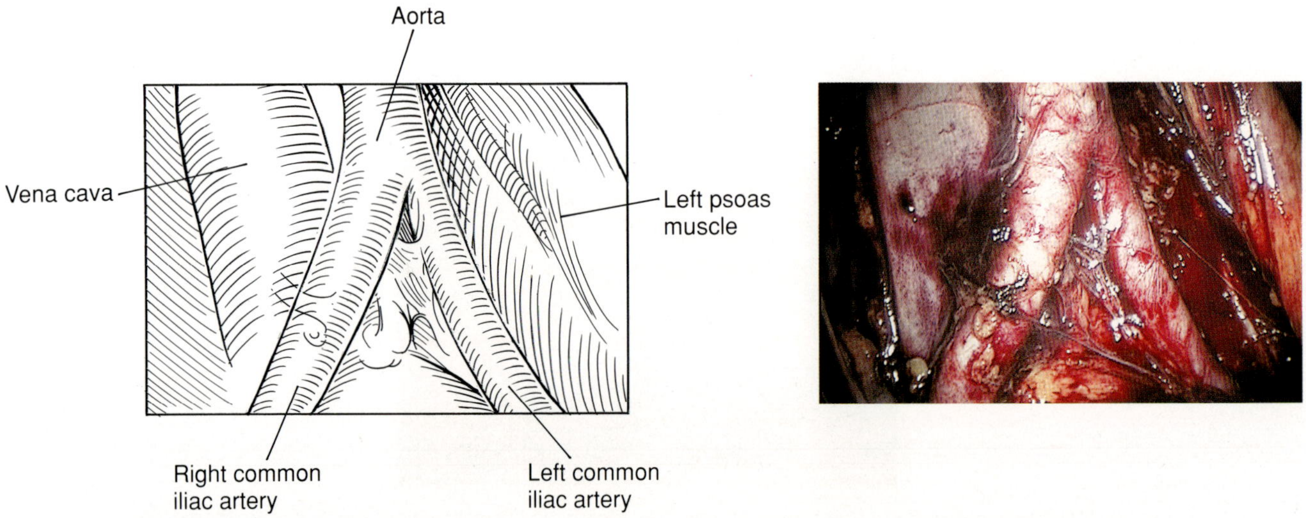

FIG. 8. After a low bilateral paraaortic lymphadenectomy, the operative site should be irrigated and inspected for hemostasis.

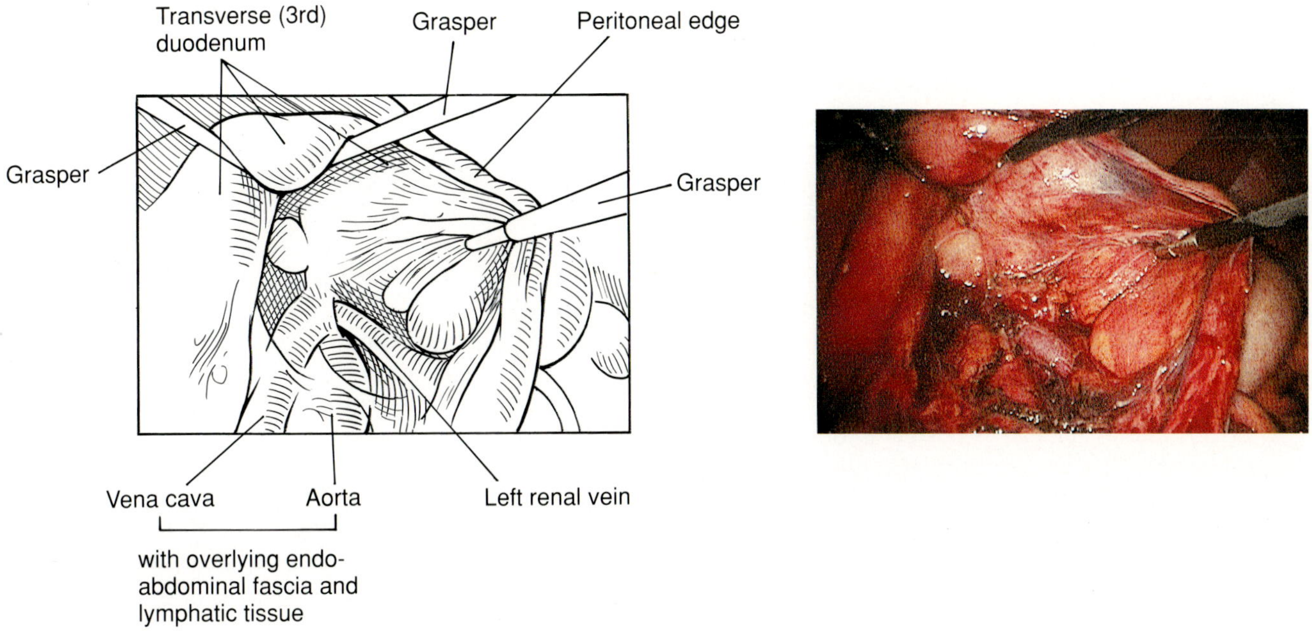

FIG. 9. The transverse (third) duodenum is elevated, exposing the retroperitoneal structures. It is important to gain adequate exposure prior to beginning the lymphadenectomy. Note how difficult it is to appreciate important vascular structures when the endoabdominal fascia and lymphatic tissue have not been removed.

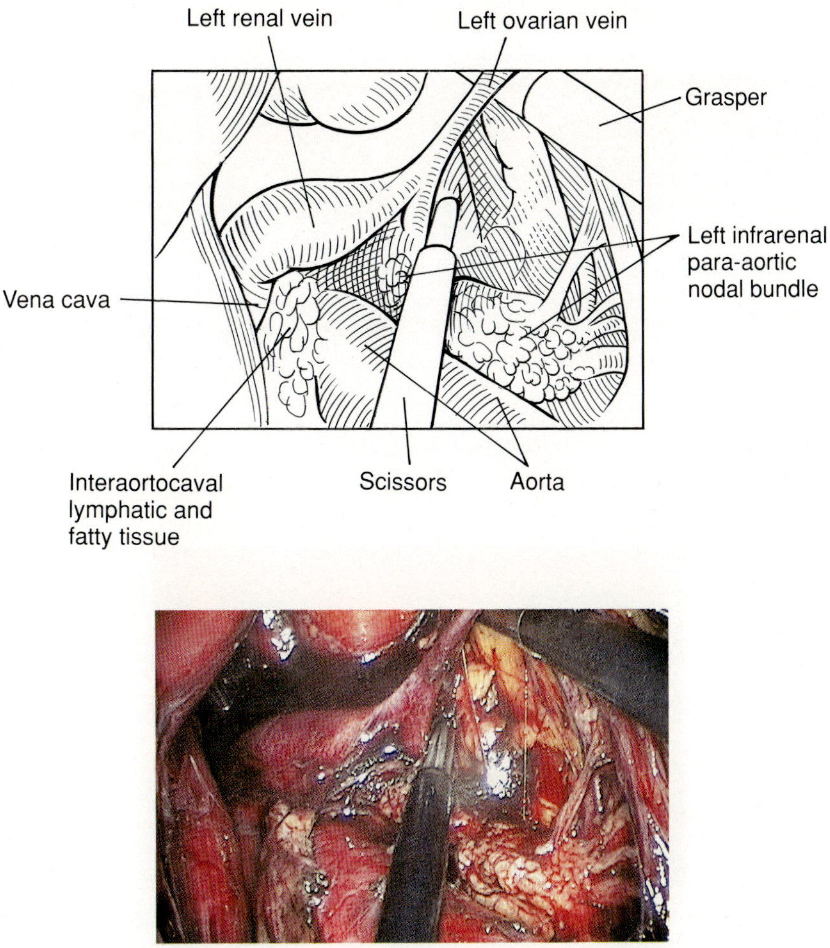

FIG. 10. The left ovarian vein is dissected off the underlying nodal tissue prior to removal of the nodal bundle.

laparoscopic instruments bluntly toward the psoas muscles. The assistant provides exposure to the vena cava and aorta by maintaining upward retraction on the transverse duodenum. It is helpful to place a fifth port in the mid- to upper abdomen to help elevate the duodenum, but this usually is not necessary. With anterior retraction on the transverse duodenum, the surgeon and assistant surgeon now face cephalad, with monitors moved toward the patient's head. As with the pelvic and lower paraaortic procedures, I perform this standing on the contralateral side of the nodes to be removed; however, these higher nodes can be removed by my standing on the right or left side of the patient.

After adequate cephalad exposure is obtained, the nodal dissection begins. On the right, this is simply a matter of continuing the previously performed lymphadenectomy up to the origin of the ovarian vein, which may enter the vena cava distal to or very near the left renal vein. On the left, the surgeon is faced with the lateral location of the nodal chain and must work around the inferior mesenteric artery. It is extremely important to identify the left renal vein as soon as possible. It is often disguised in the endoabdominal fascia and can be damaged easily (Fig. 9). Likewise, rapid identification of the right ovarian vein is important to prevent its transection during the removal of these high paraaortic nodes. Once these vessels are located, dissection in the adventitia of the aorta should be carried out. With generous use of monopolar electricity, annoying small bleeders are minimized. The ovarian artery may need to be sacrificed; this can be done with bipolar or monopolar electricity. The nodal bundle is transected near the left renal vein and the right ovarian vein as they enter the vena cava (Fig. 10). This entire dissection can be performed with monopolar electricity (Fig. 11).

The peritoneum is not closed and no retroperitoneal drains are placed. The mesentery of the small bowel is repositioned over the paraaortic incision site at the com-

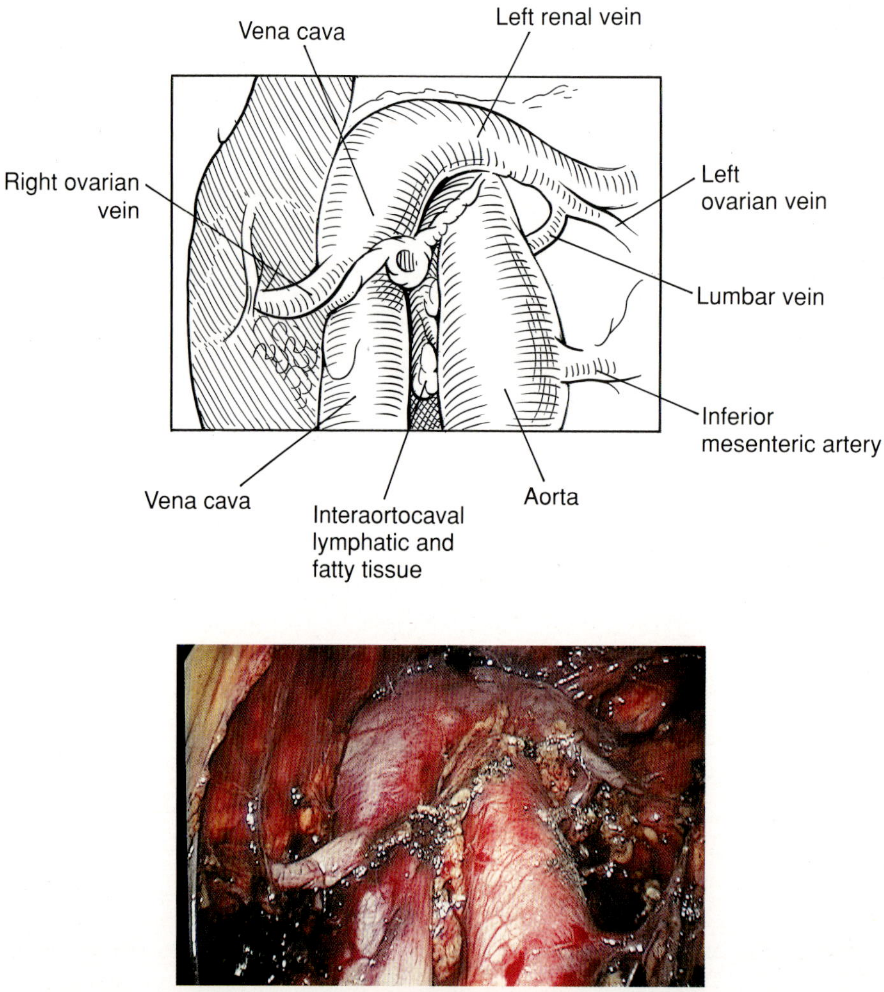

FIG. 11. At completion of the infrarenal paraaortic lymphadenectomy, vascular structures are easily identified. The surgeon removes any remaining nodal tissue as desired and adequate hemostasis is assured.

pletion of the dissection. Patients undergoing only laparoscopic surgery are given a regular diet on the day of the procedure.

COMPLICATIONS

Complications of laparoscopic lymphadenectomy include not only the potential complications of surgical removal of lymph nodes but the complications inherent to laparoscopy. Reports detailing these complications in patients with gynecologic malignancies are few; however, by including reports on pelvic lymphadenectomy done for urologic indications, a better understanding of the complications of laparoscopic lymphadenectomy can be gained.

Complications resulting in laparotomy have been related to damage to the ureter, bladder, bowel, and vascular system. Kavoussi et al. reported a 4% (13 of 372) incidence of laparotomy related to laparoscopic pelvic lymphadenectomy (17). Complications were recognized in seven patients during their laparoscopic procedures, and six patients required secondary laparotomy. Reasons for laparotomy included ureteral transection (two patients), bowel injuries or obstruction (four patients), bladder perforation (two patients), vascular injury (four patients), and wound dehiscence (one patient).

Burney et al. reported an 8% (4 of 54) laparotomy rate for their patients who underwent laparoscopic pelvic lymphadenectomy for urologic reasons (18). Only one of their four patients had the laparotomy at the time of the laparoscopic procedure. Indications for laparotomy in this group included ureteral damage (one patient), small bowel obstruction (two patients), and mesenteric hematoma (one patient). Including two patients with bladder perforations, one patient with a large extrafascial hematoma, and two patients who required blood transfusions, Burney et al. reported an overall major complication rate of 16.7% (9 of 54).

Laparotomy was required in 10% (3 of 29) of the series by Boitke et al. of patients undergoing laparoscopic lymphadenectomy for endometrial carcinoma (19). Two patients underwent secondary operations because of small bowel obstruction, and one patient had uncontrolled bleeding from a small vessel off the aorta, which was recognized intraoperatively and did not result in transfusion. Both patients with small bowel obstructions in their series were related to small bowel herniation through trocar sites. All trocar sites were ≥ 10 mm. These authors reported no complications from the pelvic lymphadenectomy; however, 9% (2 of 22) of their patients undergoing paraaortic lymphadenectomy had major complications. In addition to the above-mentioned bleeding during a right-side paraaortic lymph node dissection, which required immediate laparotomy, a second patient required percutaneous nephrostomy 3 weeks postoperatively because of a leak in the left lumbar ureter. These authors attributed this delayed leak to thermal injury from monopolar electrosurgery that occurred during the left paraaortic lymphadenectomy.

Other authors report a much lower incidence of laparotomy consequent to laparoscopic lymphadenectomy. None of the 39 patients who underwent laparoscopic lymphadenectomy for cervical cancer in a series by Querleu et al. required laparotomy (2). Childers et al. reported a 1.7% (1 of 60) laparotomy rate for patients undergoing paraaortic lymphadenectomy for cervical, endometrial, and ovarian carcinoma (11). One patient required laparotomy for a hole in the vena cava, which was created during a right-side paraaortic lymphadenectomy. She required 4 U of blood and developed a deep venous thrombosis postoperatively.

Vascular injuries related to laparoscopic lymphadenectomy vary significantly. The majority of reported major vascular complications are secondary to injury of anterior abdominal wall vessels. Sixty percent (6 of 10) of the vascular injuries reported by Kavoussi et al. resulted from trocar injury to these vessels (17). This is a relatively common complication related to any pelvic operative laparoscopic procedure (20,21). Reported vascular complications related to pelvic and paraaortic lymphadenectomies include injury to the medial umbilical ligament, the obturator vein, the external iliac artery, the aorta, and the vena cava (11,17,19). Potential injuries during this procedure include damage to aberrant obturator veins; the obturator artery; the internal, external, and common iliac veins; the inferior mesenteric artery; the ovarian artery; the lumbar veins; and the renal vein. It is likely that these as yet unreported complications will occur as more cases are performed by an increasing number of surgeons.

Injury related to unspecified vessels resulting in postoperative hematomas has also been reported. Querleu et al. reported one patient with a spontaneous resolving pelvic hematoma (2). Additional reports include patients who have presented postoperatively with infected pelvic hematomas or hematomas that became infected after percutaneous drainage (17,18). Additional sequelae to postoperative pelvic hematoma include an increased likelihood of blood transfusion (17).

Miscellaneous complications reported in association with laparoscopic lymphadenectomy include lymphedema, lymphocele, prolonged ileus, deep venous thrombosis, pulmonary embolism, damage to the obturator nerve, and diarrhea related to *Clostridium difficile* (17,18). These complications also have been reported following lymphadenectomies performed via laparotomy (22). Thus far, there have been no deaths reported related to laparoscopic lymphadenectomy.

Most authors reporting their initial experiences with laparoscopic lymphadenectomy have commented on the learning curve involved with this procedure (11,17,18).

Early experience is associated with higher complication rates and longer operating times. A reduction in both of these variables is seen with increasing experience. Eighty-eight percent (14 of 16) of the aborted laparoscopic lymphadenectomies in the report by Kavoussi et al. occurred during the initial eight dissections at each contributing institution (17). The adequacy of the procedure increases with increasing experience as well. Inadequate procedures result in inadequate staging and mismanagement of the patient. Fowler et al. reported 12 patients with stage Ib cervical carcinoma who underwent laparoscopic transperitoneal lymphadenectomy followed immediately by laparotomy (23). A clear improvement in yield was evident as the operators gained experience with the technique. The percentage of lymph nodes removed through the laparoscope increased from 63% in the first six patients to 85% in the last six.

HIGHLIGHTS

Laparoscopic lymphadenectomy is in its infancy. The role that this technique will play in managing patients with pelvic malignancies is yet to be determined. Initial reports indicate that laparoscopic lymphadenectomy—both pelvic and paraaortic—is feasible, adequate, and safe. Utilization of this technique allows conversion of abdominal procedures to vaginal procedures for patients with cervical and endometrial cancer. Patients with early endometrial and ovarian malignancies who were incompletely surgically staged with their primary procedures may also avoid laparotomy by being staged laparoscopically (11,12,24).

REFERENCES

1. Dargent D, Salvat J. *Envahissenent ganglionnaire pelvien: Place de la pelviscopie retroperitoneale.* Medsi, Paris: McGraw-Hill, 1989.
2. Querleu D, LeBlanc E, Castelain B. Laparoscopic pelvic lymphadenectomy in the staging of early carcinoma of the cervix. *Am J Obstet Gynecol* 1991;164:579–581.
3. Childers J, Hatch K, Surwit E. The role of laparoscopic lymphadenectomy in the management of cervical cancer. *Gynecol Oncol* 1992;47:38–43.
4. Childers JM, Brainard P, Rogoff EE, Surwit EA. Laparoscopic-assisted transperineal interstitial irradiation and surgical staging for advanced cervical carcinoma: a case report. *Endocurietherapy/Hyperthermia Oncol* 1994;10.
5. Querleu D. Laparoscopically assisted radical vaginal hysterectomy. *Gynecol Oncol* 1993;51:248–254.
6. *Ca—A Cancer Journal for Clinicians.* Annual statistics issue. 1994;vol 42, no 1.
7. Weiser ET, Bundy BN, Hoskins WJ, et al. Extraperitoneal versus transperitoneal selective para-aortic lymphadenectomy in the pretreatment surgical staging of advanced cervical cancer (a G.O.G. study). *Gynecol Oncol* 1989;33:283–289.
8. Childers J, Surwit E. A combined laparoscopic vaginal approach in the management of stage I endometrial cancer. *Gynecol Oncol* 1991;45:46–51.
9. Nezhat C, Burrell M, Nezhat F. Laparoscopic radical hysterectomy with para-aortic and pelvic node dissection. *Am J Obstet Gynecol* 1992;166:864–865.
10. Querleu D. Laparoscopic para-aortic node sampling in gynecologic oncology: a preliminary experience. *Gynecol Oncol* 1993;49:24–29.
11. Childers JM, Hatch KD, Surwit EA. Laparoscopic para-aortic lymphadenectomy in gynecologic malignancies. *Obstet Gynecol* 1993;82:741–747.
12. Querleu D, LeBlanc E. Laparoscopic infrarenal paraaortic node dissection in the restaging of carcinomas of the ovary and fallopian tube. *Cancer* 1994;73:1467–1471.
13. Childers JM, Brzechffa PR, Hatch KD, Surwit EA. Laparoscopic assisted surgical staging (LASS) of endometrial carcinoma. *Gynecol Oncol* 1993;52:33–38.
14. Byron JW, Markenson G. A randomized comparison of Verres needle and direct trocar insertion for laparoscopy. *Surg Gynecol Obstet* 1993;177:259–262.
15. Childers JM, Brzechffa PR, Surwit EA. Laparoscopy using the left upper quadrant as the primary trocar site. *Gynecol Oncol* 1993;50:221–225.
16. Hasson H. A modified instrument and method for laparoscopy. *Am J Obstet Gynecol* 1971;110:886–887.
17. Kavoussi LR, Sosa E, Chandhoke P, et al. Complications of laparoscopic pelvic node dissection. *J Urol* 1993;149:322–325.
18. Burney TL, Campbell EC, Naslund MJ, Jacobs SC. Complications of staging laparoscopic pelvic lymphadenectomy. *Surg Lap Endosc* 1993;3:184–190.
19. Boitke GM, Lurain JR, Burke JJ. A comparison of laparoscopic management of endometrial cancer with traditional laparotomy. Twenty-fifth annual meeting, Society of Gynecologic Oncologists, Orlando, FL, February 1994.
20. Hill D, Maher PJ, Wood CE, et al. Complications of laparoscopic hysterectomy. *J Am Assoc Gynecol Laparoscop* 1994;1:159–162.
21. Vasquez JM, Demarque AM, Diamond MP. Vascular complications of laparoscopic surgery. *J Am Assoc Gynecol Laparoscop* 1994;1:163–167.
22. Benedetti-Panici PB, Scambia G, Baiocchi G, Greggi S, Mancuso S. Technique and feasibility of radical para-aortic and pelvic lymphadenectomy for gynecologic malignancies: a prospective study. *Int J Gynecol Cancer* 1991;1:133–140.
23. Fowler JM, Carter J, Carlson J, et al. Lymph-node yield from laparoscopic lymphadenectomy in cervical cancer: a comparative study. *Gynecol Oncol* 1993;51:187–192.
24. Childers JM, Spirtos NM, Brainard P, Surwit EA. Laparoscopic staging of the patient with incompletely staged early adenocarcinoma of the endometrium. *Obstet Gynecol* 1994;83(4):597–600.

Endoscopic Management of Gynecologic Disease,
edited by G.D. Adamson and D.C. Martin.
Lippincott-Raven Publishers, Philadelphia © 1996.

CHAPTER 24

Appendectomy

Bryan R. Kurtz and James F. Daniell

Appendectomy is one of the most common operations performed by general surgeons, primarily for acute appendicitis. Gynecologists often are called on to assess a patient with pelvic pain, and frequently the differential diagnosis includes acute appendicitis. Indeed, acute inflammation of the appendix often extends into the right adnexa. A correct diagnosis is often critical, and a delay can be fatal to the patient.

Although the incidence of appendicitis is higher in teenagers, the incidence in women in reproductive years remains significant. The overall lifetime risk of females developing appendicitis is about 1 in 6 at birth and 1 in 50 at 50 years of age (1). The risk of females developing appendicitis in the 15- to 19-year old group is about 1 in 99. The overall death rate from appendicitis for women up to 80 years old is 1 in 1100.

In the evaluation of nonacute chronic pelvic pain, especially with right-sided involvement, disease of the appendix should be considered. Periappendiceal adhesions or endometriosis of the tip may exist and are indications for its removal. Incidental appendectomy at the time of pelvic surgery is more controversial. Whereas many authors recommend routine appendectomy when the appendix is conveniently available, surveys of gynecologists indicate its infrequency (2).

EMBRYOLOGY AND ANATOMY

The cecal diverticulum, which is the primordium of the cecum and appendix, appears in the sixth week as a conical pouch on the antemesenteric border of the caudal limb of the midgut loop (3). The apex of this blind sac does not grow very rapidly and results in the formation of the appendix. Because of the unequal growth of the right wall of the cecum, the appendix is displaced toward its medial surface. As the proximal part of the colon elongates, the appendix may pass posterior to the cecum (retrocecal) or the colon (retrocolic), or it may descend over the brim of the pelvis (pelvic, or descending). Sixty-four percent of the time the appendix is retrocecal. The root of the appendix is the only fixed point. It is located about 3 cm below the ileocecal valve. The tip of the appendix may be directed anywhere in a large semicircle between the root of the mesentery and the peritoneal fixation of the ascending colon. When hidden, the appendix can be located by following the anterior tinea of the cecum down to its root.

The mesoappendix is derived from the left leaf of the peritoneum and is continuous with the mesentery. Triangular in form, it is attached to the whole length of the appendix. The appendicular artery descends behind the terminal part of the ileum, enters the mesoappendix, and runs along its free margin. The appendix normally has a complete but narrow lumen. Occasionally, and especially later in life, the lumen may become obliterated, leaving only a fibrous cord.

In approximately 6% of fetuses, more commonly in males, there is a failure of the proximal part of the colon to elongate, resulting in the cecum remaining near the liver as the abdomen enlarges (3). In this case, the cecum and appendix are located in the subcostal region near the inferior surface of the liver. However, since there continues to be some elongation of the colon during childhood, a subhepatic cecum is not so common in adults.

In about 10% of patients, the cecum may have an unusual amount of freedom (1). This is due to incomplete fixation of the ascending colon. As a result, there may be significant variation in the position of the appendix, and it may even become herniated to the right inguinal canal. Rarely, volvulus of the cecum may occur in these patients.

B. R. Kurtz and J. F. Daniell: Department of Obstetrics and Gynecology, Centennial Medical Center, Nashville, Tennessee 37203.

PATHOPHYSIOLOGY

Acute appendicitis is usually initiated by obstruction of the appendiceal lumen. This can be due to hyperplasia; stricture of the lumen; or presence of submucosal follicles, fecalith, a foreign body, or tumor. Mucus accumulates and causes distention of the lumen. Bacterial contamination converts the mucus to pus. With the increased luminal pressure, the lymphatics become obstructed, with resultant edema and mucosal ulceration. As the process worsens, there is venous obstruction and thrombosis, with edema and tissue ischemia. Bacteria invade the appendiceal wall and the serosa becomes inflamed. Because of the compromised circulation, the appendiceal wall infarcts, resulting in leakage of bacterial contaminants into the peritoneal cavity. With continued high intraluminal pressure, the gangrenous wall perforates, with resultant bacterial peritonitis. As the process worsens, the mortality rate increases from 0.1% in acute suppurative appendicitis to 5% with a perforative appendicitis (1).

An association exists between disease of the appendix and infertility. Pittaway reported a 13% appendiceal involvement in patients with endometriosis (4). In certain cases, mechanical infertility may be related to periappendiceal and pelvic adhesions especially if there is perforation and/or pelvic abscess formation. Wiig et al. reported that 19% of women under the age of 25 years who develop appendicitis with perforation subsequently became infertile (5). Also, 31% of patients with pelvic abscess were subsequently infertile. Powley found a similar relationship between appendicitis and subsequent fertility (6).

It should be remembered that the appendix is the most common site for carcinoid tumors, the incidence of which is 0.03% of all appendices removed (1). Most of these carcinoids are benign. Sanders and Axtell reported only a 2.9% rate of metastases in their series of patients with appendiceal carcinoid tumors (7). The carcinoid syndrome is rare.

INDICATIONS

Laparoscopic appendectomy can be performed either for indicated reasons or incidentally during laparoscopy. Disease of the appendix is often found during evaluation for acute or chronic right lower quadrant or pelvic pain. Often the differential diagnosis for acute right lower quadrant pain with fever and leukocytosis in women, especially of reproductive years, comes down to acute appendicitis vs. pelvic inflammatory disease. Treatment of these two processes differs significantly, and a delay in diagnosis can be catastrophic. Many authors recommend laparoscopy to confirm the diagnosis. Patients found to have appendicitis often can be managed laparoscopically, obviating laparotomy.

Laparoscopic appendectomy should also be considered in a variety of other circumstances. Endometriosis involving the appendix, adhesions between the appendix and pelvic viscera, or periappendiceal scarring that may be secondary to subclinical endometriosis or chronic inflammation should be considered indications for laparoscopic appendectomy. Also, a patient who has a history of chronic right lower quadrant pain with no discernable pathology on laparoscopic examination of the pelvis should be considered for laparoscopic appendectomy, both as a therapeutic trial and to eliminate appendicitis from the differential diagnosis in the future.

The merits of incidental appendectomy at laparotomy, although not universally accepted, have been well summarized (1). Many general surgeons offer incidental appendectomy at the time of laparoscopic cholecystectomy. In gynecology, there are several circumstances under which the surgeon may offer the procedure to patients. Laparoscopically assisted vaginal hysterectomy, tubal ligation, laparoscopy for pelvic pain in noninfertility patients, and infertility surgery in which the right side is irreparably damaged or removed are all opportunities for laparoscopic appendectomy.

CONTRAINDICATIONS

Laparoscopic appendectomy should be performed only in the hands of an experienced and confident surgeon. More significantly, the surgeon must be able to recognize his or her limitations. As the inflammatory process progresses, and especially in the case of appendicitis complicated by abscess formation, patients may be better served by laparotomy. Significant peritonitis, especially with evidence of ileus or bowel obstruction, should be considered a contraindication to laparoscopy.

Incidental appendectomy in the absence of visible disease of the appendix should not be considered if the patient has undergone extensive pelvic dissection, such as extensive adhesiolysis treatment, treatment of ovarian endometriosis, or tubal surgery for infertility. Especially if the right side affords the patient the best opportunity for future fertility, the effect of postoperative adhesion or abscess formation could be devastating to the future fertility of such patients.

SURGICAL TECHNIQUES

Laparoscopic appendectomy was first reported by Kurt Semm in 1983 (8). Since then, several authors have reported their techniques in a series of patient groups ranging from 4 to 388. The first reports of laparoscopic surgery for acute appendicitis were published in 1987 (9,10). Gotz et al. reported a series of 388 patients who

TABLE 1. *Complications of laparoscopic appendectomy*

Author (Date)	Laparoscopic Procedures	Subsequent Laparotomies	Infection
Schreiber (9) (1987)	70	None	1
Gotz et al. (11) (1990)	388	12	2
Leahy (12) (1989)	4	None	None
McKernan and Saye (13) (1990)	32	None	None
Schreiber (14) (1990)	6	None	None
Daniell et al. (15) (1991)	10	None	None
O'Regan (16) (1991)	12	None	None

underwent laparoscopic appendectomy (11). Acute appendicitis was confirmed in 72% of the patients and chronic inflammation in 14% by histology. Only 12 patients required open laparotomy because of complications or dense adhesion formation. Normal appendices were removed in fewer than 12% of the patients. Fourteen patients had postoperative wound infections limited to areas of cellulitis surrounding the umbilical puncture site. Two patients developed postoperative abscesses, which required interval laparotomy. Other authors confirm low complication rates (9,11–16) (see Table 1).

Most authors describe methods involving the use of laparoscopic pretied loops. Semm describes ducking the appendiceal stump with a pursestring suture, similar to those techniques used in laparotomy (8). We recently described the use of a laparoscopic automatic stapling system for appendectomy (15). The device allows simpler, more rapid removal of the appendix at laparoscopy compared to other techniques.

After visualization of the appendix through the intraumbilically placed telescope, the procedure requires placement of two or three ancillary trocars in various sites. These sites include the suprapubic midline, right or left lower quadrants, and, occasionally, the right midabdominal region.

The procedure involves ligation of the vessels in the mesoappendix, followed by the occlusion of the appendiceal lumen. The mesoappendix can be bluntly dissected and the vessels controlled using either chromic ligatures or endoscopically applied hemoclips. Alternately, thermocoagulation or bipolar cautery can be used to occlude the vascular supply (Fig. 1). After the base of the appendix is exposed, it is doubly ligated with pretied chromic Roeder loops and incised between these two proximal ligatures, and a third Roeder loop is placed approximately 1 cm distally (Figs. 2 and 3). If the appendix is not too large and does not have an excessive mesoappendix attached, it can be brought through the intraumbilical trocar, either with the aid of an operative laparoscope or with the use of graspers aided by visualization through a 5-mm laparoscope at an alternate trocar site. The mucosa of the appendiceal stump may be treated lightly with laser or electrocautery for dessication (Fig. 4). The pelvis is copiously irrigated. We prefer to use a gastrourologic (GU) irrigant solution containing dilute antibiotics: two ampules of polymyxin-neomycin-bacitracin per 1000 cm^3 solution.

An automatic stapling device has been developed for laparoscopic procedures (15). The device simultaneously occludes the lumen with two triple-staggered lines of ti-

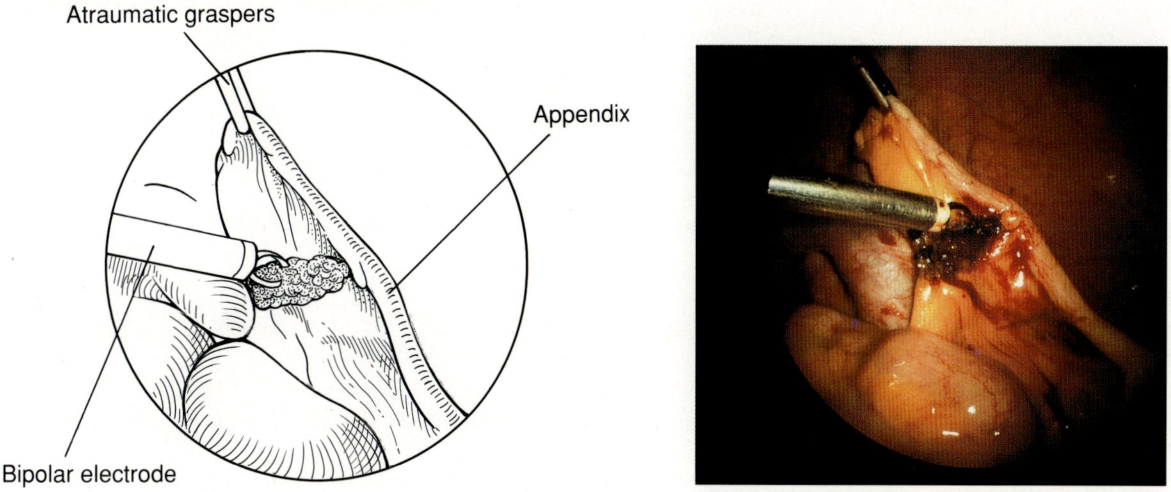

FIG. 1. Coagulation of the mesoappendiceal vessels carefully with bipolar cautery.

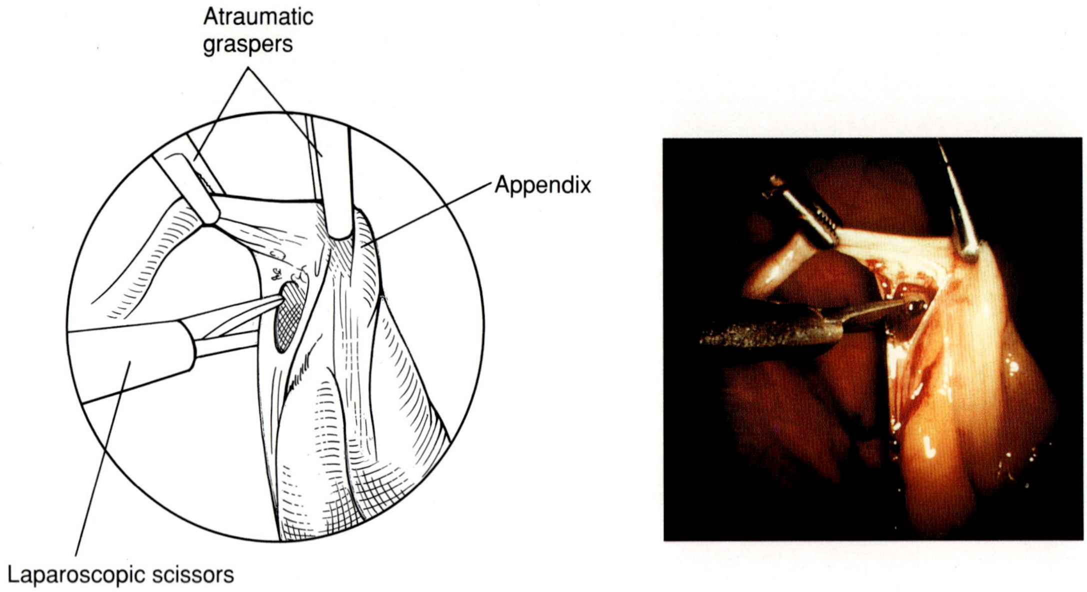

FIG. 2. Incision of the mesoappendix with scissors after bipolar coagulation.

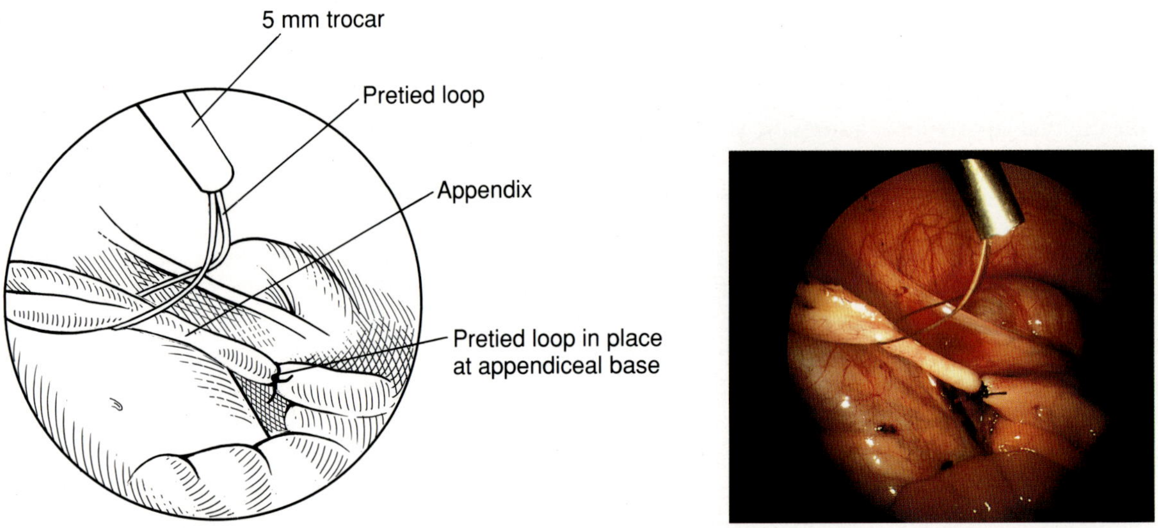

FIG. 3. Placement of pretied suture loops at the appendiceal base. Two sutures are placed at the appendiceal base followed by a third suture placed approximately 1 cm distally.

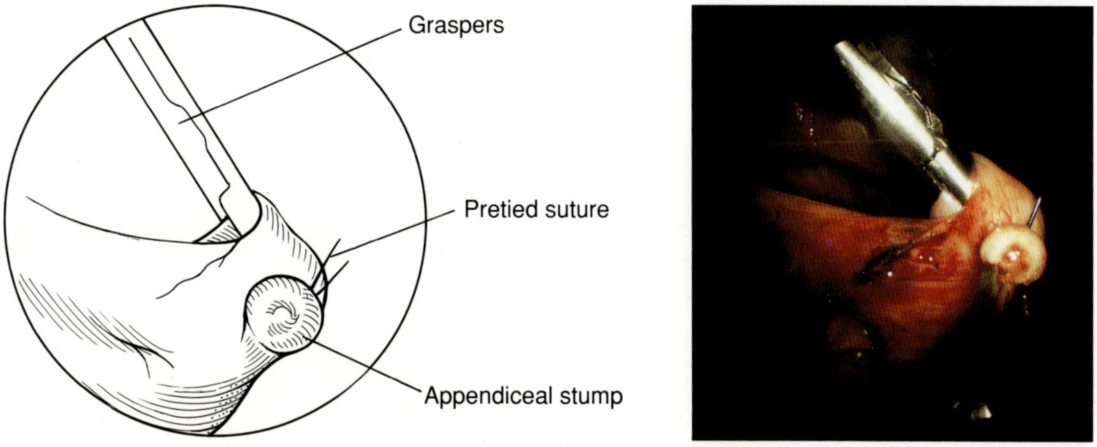

FIG. 4. Appendiceal stump after transection.

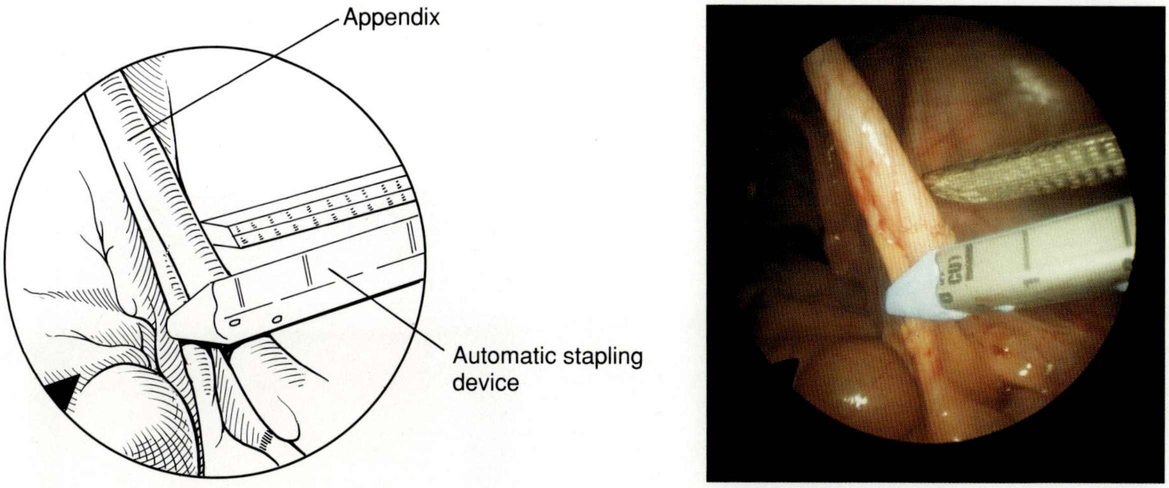

FIG. 5. Placement of the automatic stapling device at the appendiceal base.

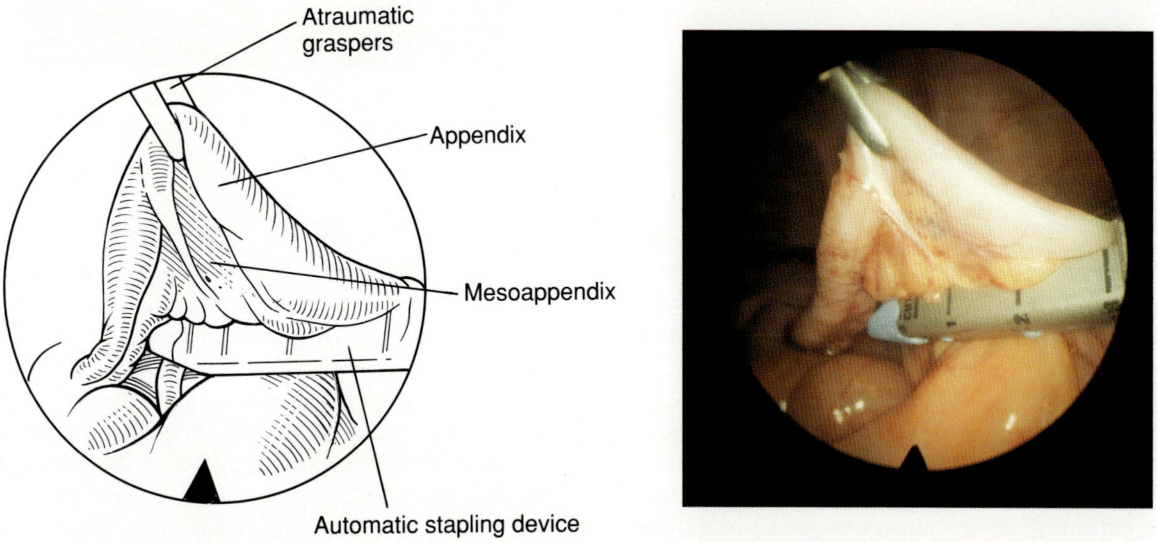

FIG. 6. Automatic stapling device placed across the appendiceal base and fired to occlude and transect the appendiceal lumen.

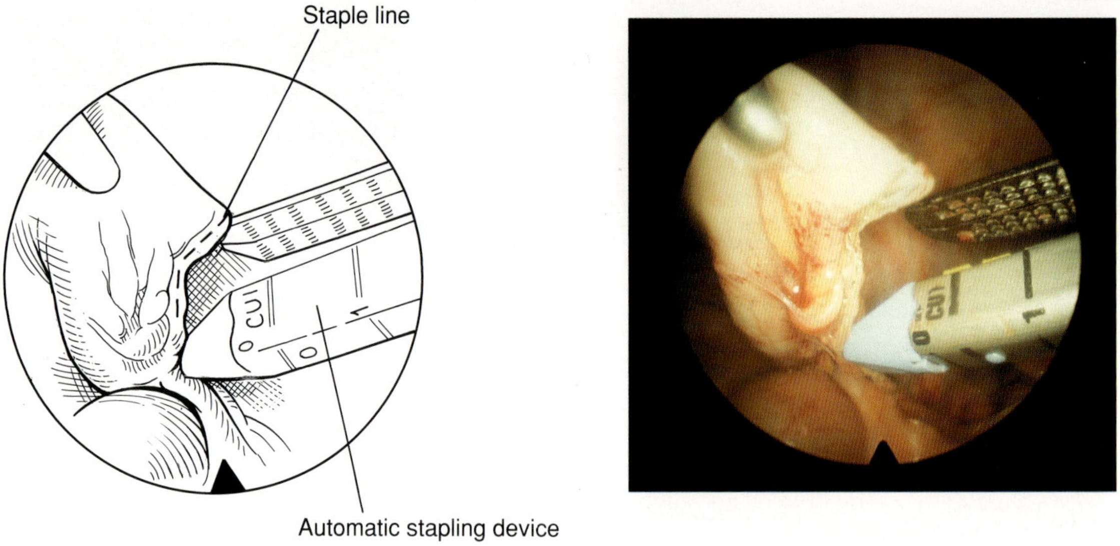

FIG. 7. View after firing of automatic stapling device. Note two triple-staggered lines of titanium staples on the proximal distal appendiceal stump.

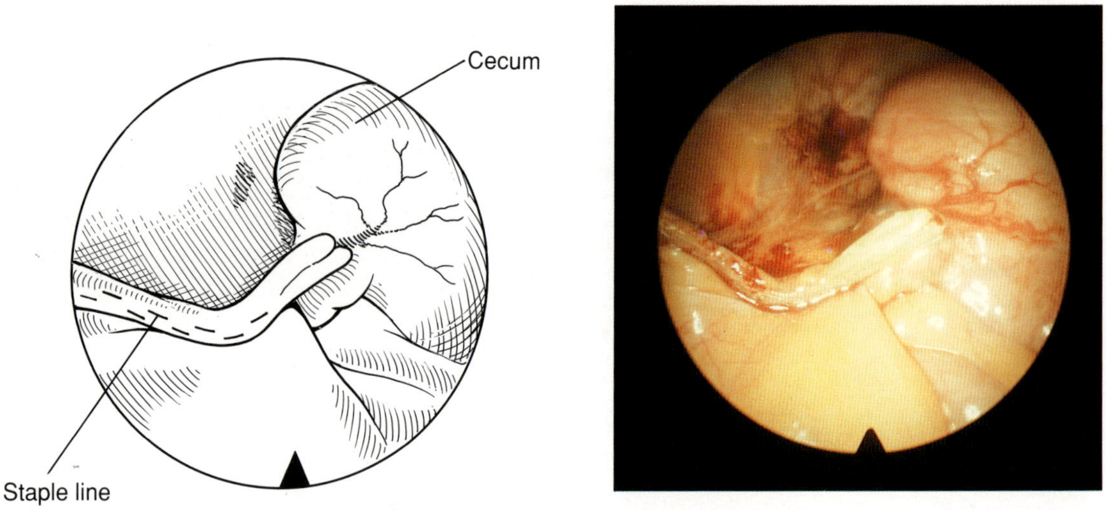

FIG. 8. Staple line at the cecum and mesoappendix.

tanium staples while it incises between the two staple lines (Figs. 5–8). Our initial experience substantiates its advantage in reducing the time required for the procedure. Additionally, the close approximation of the two staple lines to the cutting blade in the cartridge head eliminates the risk of the contents of the appendiceal lumen spilling into the peritoneal cavity. A special larger trocar is required for the passage of the stapling device into the peritoneal cavity. However, the 12-mm diameter of this trocar facilitates removal of the excised appendix from the peritoneal cavity. A cartridge designed specifically for occlusion of blood vessels also is available. This can be used to clamp and incise the mesoappendix. After dissection of the mesoappendix with either this device, laparoscopic clips, or cautery, the base of the appendix is clamped and transected. Alternately, the appendiceal base can be initially occluded and transected, followed by ligation and incision of the mesoappendix with a Roeder loop and scissors. Occasionally, if the mesoappendix is redundant and mobile, it can be simply transected along the length of the appendix with the stapling device.

OUTCOME

Several authors have demonstrated the utility of laparoscopic appendectomy with minimal risks for complication (8). We recently published an article in which the automatic laparoscopic stapling system was evaluated in 10 patients (15). Indications for appendectomy included endometriosis of the appendix, fixation to the right tube or ovary, early acute appendicitis, and elective removal. Our preliminary experience suggested that laparoscopy provides a safe, easy, and rapid method of removing the appendix. We subsequently reviewed the use of the device in 13 patients who underwent incidental appendectomy. One patient developed significant postoperative anemia, requiring transfusion, but not reexploration. This patient also underwent a right salpingo-oophorectomy via the laparoscope.

COMPLICATIONS

When possible, all patients must be counseled preoperatively regarding the potential complications of laparoscopic appendectomy. Consenting patients must be informed that the procedure includes the possibility for a laparotomy. Circumstances encountered unexpectedly during the laparoscopic procedure may require intraoperative discussion with a family member.

The most significant postoperative complications include bleeding and infection. Laparoscopic appendectomy should not be attempted unless several backup methods of hemostasis are available. Pretied ligatures, hemoclips, or cautery alone may be inadequate to obtain hemostasis in every instance. Bleeding from a mesoappendix that is in close proximity to the cecum or underlying peritoneum is best controlled with hemoclips to avoid the risk of thermal injury from laser energy or electrocautery. It is important to apply the pretied Roeder loops to the base of the appendix correctly by exerting firm, continuous pressure against the knot for a period of about 10 sec and taking care to avoid repetitive pulls.

When using the automatic stapling devices, we have found that there may be bleeding at the junction of the mesoappendix to the appendiceal serosa. This is probably due to the staple line including both the thicker appendiceal tissue and the thinner mesoappendiceal tissue and vessels. This often can be controlled by grasping the area with atraumatic graspers and applying pressure to the staple line. Alternatively, laparoscopic clips or careful electrocautery can be used to achieve hemostasis.

When transecting the appendix, it is possible for a small amount of appendiceal contents to leak into the peritoneal cavity, possibly resulting in postoperative infection. This can be minimized by milking the contents of the appendix distally prior to placing the third distal Roeder loop. The risk of spilling of appendiceal contents with the automatic stapling device is minimal, as the distance between the staple line and the area of transection is minute. To reduce the possibility of postoperative infection, we irrigate the area extensively with GU irrigant. Prophylactic antibiotics are not generally thought to be necessary unless there is evidence of inflammation of the appendix or suspicion of spill of intraluminal contents. In these cases, the patient should be treated with one to three doses of broad-spectrum antibiotic. It is prudent to avoid appendectomy in patients with simultaneous extensive pelvic surgery involving large residual areas of denuded peritoneum.

HIGHLIGHTS

Laparoscopic appendectomy is becoming more common, as evidenced by the increased interest by both general surgeons and gynecologists in minimally invasive surgery. Especially with the development of newer techniques and devices and in the right hands, the procedure is easily and safely performed. Incidental appendectomy at the time of laparoscopy is a viable option under the right circumstance. However, no advanced form of instrumentation can ever take the place of the surgeon's knowledge of anatomy, ability to perform systematic tissue dissection, and experience with multiple techniques of hemostasis. We therefore feel strongly that working with a preceptor prior to attempting laparoscopic appendectomy is essential and should be required by each hospital's credentialing committee.

REFERENCES

1. Te Linde RW. In: Mattingly RF, Thompson JD, eds. *Operative gynecology, 6th ed.* Philadelphia: JB Lippincott; 1985.
2. Hays RJ. Incidental appendectomy: current teaching. *JAMA* 1977;238:31.
3. Moore KW. *The developing human.* Philadelphia: WB Saunders; 1982.
4. Pittaway DE. Appendectomy in the surgical treatment of endometriosis. *Obstet Gynecol* 1983;61:421.
5. Wiig JN, Janssen CW Jr, Fuglesang P, et al. Infertility as a complication of perforated appendicitis. *Acta Chir Scand* 1979;145:409.
6. Powley PH. Infertility due to pelvic abscess and pelvic peritonitis in appendicitis. *Lancet* 1965;1:27.
7. Sanders RJ, Axtell K. Carcinoids of the gastrointestinal tract. *Surg Obstet Gynecol* 1964;119:369.
8. Semm K. Endoscopic appendectomy. *Endoscopy* 1964;15:15.
9. Schreiber JH. Early experience with laparoscopic appendectomy in women. *Surg Endosc* 1990;4:6.
10. Gangal HT, Gangal MH. Laparoscopic appendectomy. *Endoscopy* 1987;19:127.
11. Gotz F, Pier A, Bacher C. Modified laparoscopic appendicectomy in surgery. *Surg Endosc* 1990;4:6.
12. Leahy PF. Technique of laparoscopic appendicectomy. *Br J Surg* 1989;76:616.
13. McKernan JB, Saye WB. Laparoscopic techniques and appendectomy with argon laser. *South Med J* 1990;83:1019.
14. Schreiber JH. Laparoscopic appendectomy in pregnancy. *Surg Endosc* 1990;4:100.
15. Daniell JF, Gurley LD, Kurtz BR, Chambers JF. The use of an automatic stapling device for laparoscopic appendectomy. *Obstet Gynecol* 1991;4:721.
16. O'Regan P. Laparoscopic appendectomy. *Can J Surg* 1991;3:256.

Endoscopic Management of Gynecologic Disease,
edited by G.D. Adamson and D.C. Martin.
Lippincott-Raven Publishers, Philadelphia © 1996.

CHAPTER 25

Laparoscopic Hysterectomy

Harry Reich

Laparoscopic hysterectomy has become a high-profile procedure in the United States due to media attention, consumer interest, and the incidence of hysterectomy (600,000/year). Most hysterectomies (75%) are done abdominally (1).

Laparoscopic hysterectomy, defined as the laparoscopic ligation of the uterine vessels, was first done in January 1988 (2). It is a substitute for abdominal hysterectomy and involves more attention to ureteral identification (3–5). The indications include benign pathology usually requiring the selection of an abdominal approach to hysterectomy: endometriosis, fibroids, adnexal masses, and adhesions from previous surgery. Laparoscopic hysterectomy may also be considered for stage I endometrial, ovarian, and cervical cancer (6–8).

Most hysterectomies currently requiring an abdominal approach may be performed with laparoscopic dissection of part or all of the abdominal portion followed by vaginal removal. There are many surgical advantages, in particular magnification of anatomy and pathology, easy access to the vagina and rectum, and the ability to achieve complete hemostasis and clot evacuation during underwater examination. Patient advantages are multiple and are related to avoidance of a painful abdominal incision. They also include a reduced period of hospitalization and recuperation and an extremely low rate of cuff infection and ileus.

There are a variety of situations whereby the laparoscope is used as an aid to hysterectomy (Table 1). It is important that these different procedures be clearly delineated:

Diagnostic laparoscopy with vaginal hysterectomy indicates that the laparoscope is used for *diagnostic* purposes, when indications for a vaginal approach are equivocal, to determine if *vaginal hysterectomy* is possible (9). It also assures that vaginal cuff and pedicle hemostasis is complete and allows clot evacuation.

Laparoscopic vault suspension (LVS) after vaginal hysterectomy is useful when vaginal hysterectomy alone cannot accomplish appropriate repair for prolapse. Ureteral dissection before vaginal hysterectomy aids in high uterosacral ligament plication.

Laparoscopic-assisted vaginal hysterectomy (LAVH) is a vaginal hysterectomy after laparoscopic adhesiolysis, endometriosis excision, or oophorectomy (10–12).

Laparoscopic hysterectomy (LH) denotes laparoscopic ligation of the uterine arteries by electrosurgery desiccation, suture ligature, or staples. All maneuvers after uterine vessel ligation can be done vaginally or laparoscopically; these include anterior and posterior vaginal entry, cardinal and uterosacral ligaments division, uterine removal intact or by morcellation, and vertical or transverse vaginal closure. Laparoscopic ligation of the uterine vessels is the sine qua non for laparoscopic hysterectomy. Ureteral isolation has always been advised.

Total laparoscopic hysterectomy (TLH) is a laparoscopic-assisted abdominal hysterectomy. Laparoscopic dissection continues until the uterus lies free of all attachments in the peritoneal cavity. The uterus is removed through the vagina with morcellation if necessary. The vagina is closed with laparoscopically placed sutures.

Laparoscopic supracervical hysterectomy (LSH) has recently regained advocates (13). The uterus is removed by morcellation from above or below. Kurt Semm's version of supracervical hysterectomy is called the CASH procedure (classical abdominal Semm hysterectomy). It leaves the cardinal ligaments intact while eliminating the columnar cells of the endocervical canal. After perforation of the uterine fundus with a long sound dilator, a calibrated uterine resection tool (CURT), which fits around this instrument, is used to

H. Reich: New Rochelle Hospital, New Rochelle, New York 10802, and Wyoming Valley Health Care System, Wilkes-Barre, Pennsylvania 18704.

TABLE 1. *Classification of laparoscopic procedures with hysterectomy*

1. Diagnostic laparoscopy with vaginal hysterectomy
2. Vaginal hysterectomy with laparoscopic vault suspension (LVS)
3. Laparoscopic-assisted vaginal hysterectomy (LAVH)
   With or without morcellation
   With or without laparoscopic vault suspension (LVS)
4. Laparoscopic hysterectomy (LH)
   With or without morcellation
   With or without LVS
5. Total laparoscopic hysterectomy (TLH)
   With or without morcellation
   With or without LVS
6. Laparoscopic supracervical hysterectomy (LSH)
   Including classical abdominal Semm hysterectomy (CASH)
7. Laparoscopic hysterectomy with lymphadenectomy
8. Laparoscopic hysterectomy with lymphadenectomy and omentectomy
9. Laparoscopic radical hysterectomy with lymphadenectomy

core out the endocervical canal. Thereafter, at laparoscopy, suture techniques are used to ligate the utero-ovarian ligaments. An endoloop is placed around the uterine fundus to the level of the internal os of the cervix and is tied. The uterus is divided at its junction with the cervix and is removed by laparoscopic morcellation.

Laparoscopic extrafascial hysterectomy with lymphadenectomy is performed for endometrial cancer.

Laparoscopic hysterectomy with lymphadenectomy and omentectomy is done for ovarian cancer.

Laparoscopic radical hysterectomy with lymphadenectomy is required for cervical cancer.

INDICATIONS AND CONTRAINDICATIONS

Indications for laparoscopic hysterectomy presently include benign pathology, such as endometriosis, fibroids, adhesions, and adnexal masses. All of these conditions traditionally required an abdominal incision.

The most common indication for laparoscopic hysterectomy is a symptomatic fibroid uterus. Morcellation is often necessary. Cystocele repair may be accomplished from above, but rectocele repair usually requires a perineal approach.

Uterine size and weight measurements are important to document the appropriateness of laparoscopic hysterectomies as most small uteri can be removed vaginally. The normal uterus weighs 70–125 g. A 12-week gestational age uterus weighs 280–320 g, and a 24-week one weighs 580–620 g.

Laparoscopic hysterectomy also is indicated when vaginal hysterectomy is contraindicated, such as in cases of a narrow pubic arch, a narrow vagina with no prolapse, or severe arthritis that prohibits placement of the patient in sufficient lithotomy position for vaginal exposure. Fibroids fixed in the pelvis or abdomen without descent are easier to mobilize at laparoscopy than at laparotomy. Laparoscopic procedures in obese women allow the surgeon to make an incision above the panniculus and operate below it.

Hysterectomy should not be done for stage IV endometriosis with extensive cul-de-sac involvement unless the surgeon has the capability and time to resect all deep fibrotic endometriosis from the posterior vagina, uterosacral ligaments, and anterior rectum. Excision of the uterus using an intrafascial technique leaves the deep fibrotic endometriosis behind to cause future problems. It is much more difficult to remove deep fibrotic endometriosis when there is no uterus between the anterior rectum and the bladder; after hysterectomy, the endometriosis left in the anterior rectum and vaginal cuff frequently becomes densely adherent or invades the bladder and one or both ureters. In most cases, stage IV endometriosis with extensive cul-de-sac obliteration is a reason to preserve the uterus to prevent future vaginal cuff, bladder, and ureteral problems (14). Obviously, this approach will not be effective when uterine adenomyosis is present. In these cases, after excision of cul-de-sac endometriosis, persistent pain will lead ultimately to hysterectomy. Oophorectomy is not necessary at hysterectomy; if the endometriosis is removed, it should not recur. Bilateral oophorectomy is rarely indicated in women under age 40 undergoing hysterectomy for endometriosis.

Hysterectomy is performed for abnormal uterine bleeding in women of reproductive age. Abnormal uterine bleeding is defined as excessive uterine bleeding or irregular uterine bleeding for more than 8 days during more than a single cycle or as profuse bleeding requiring additional protection (large clots, gushes, or limitations on activity). There should be no history of a bleeding diathesis or use of medication that may cause bleeding. A negative effect on quality of life should be documented. Physical examination, laboratory data, ultrasound, and, if necessary, hysteroscopy and/or D&C are frequently negative. Prior to hysterectomy, hormone treatment is attempted and its failure, contraindication, or refusal is documented. The presence of anemia is recorded and correction is attempted. If hysterectomy is chosen, a vaginal approach may be appropriate. Laparoscopic hysterectomy is done when vaginal hysterectomy is not possible, including history of previous surgery, lack of prolapse (nulliparous or multiparous), or inexperience of the surgeon with the vaginal approach.

Abdominal hysterectomy is almost never indicated except when an ovarian cyst is too large to remove without spill or when stage III ovarian cancer is present. We have not found uterine or patient size to be a contraindication. Age should rarely be a deterrent. Absolute contraindications include inexperience of the surgeon and cesarean hysterectomy. Peripartum hysterectomy for placenta accreta, uterine atony, unspecified uterine bleeding, and uterine rupture are relative contraindications at present. Laparoscopic hysterectomy may be considered for patients needing a postpartum hysterectomy.

The place of endometrial ablation as an alternative method to hysterectomy is controversial. This author believes that endometrial ablation causes symptomatic adenomyosis in many patients similar to the fibrotic uterosacral ligament nodules seen with endometriosis. A recent report indicated that 20% of women required hysterectomy for pelvic pain 2 years after the ablation procedure (15). In the future, rollerball ablation may be replaced by supracervical hysterectomy in patients with hypermenorrhea from a small uterus without prolapse.

EQUIPMENT

High-flow CO_2 insufflation up to 10–15 L/min is necessary to compensate for the rapid loss of CO_2 during suctioning. The ability to maintain a relatively constant intraabdominal pressure between 10 and 15 mm Hg during laparoscopic hysterectomy is essential.

Operating room tables capable of 30° Trendelenburg position are extremely valuable for laparoscopic hysterectomy. Unfortunately, these tables are rare, and this author has much difficulty when operating in other institutions where there is a limited degree of body tilt that can be obtained. For the past 16 years steep Trendelenburg position (20–40°), with shoulder braces and the arms at the patient's sides, has been used without adverse effects.

A Valtchev uterine mobilizer (Conkin Surgical Instruments, Toronto, Canada) is the best available single instrument to antevert the uterus and delineate the posterior vagina. The uterus can be anteverted to about 120° and moved in an arc about 45° to the left or right by turning the mobilizer around its longitudinal axis. The obturator—either 100 mm long and 10 mm thick or 80 mm long and 8 mm thick—is used for uterine manipulation during hysterectomy (16). When this device is in the anteverted position, the cervix sits on a wide acorn making the cervicovaginal junction readily visible between the uterosacral ligaments when the cul-de-sac is inspected laparoscopically.

If a Valtchev uterine mobilizer is not available, a sponge on a ring forceps is inserted into the posterior vaginal fornix, and a no. 81 French rectal probe (Reznik Instruments, Skokie, IL) is placed in the rectum to define the rectum and posterior vagina to excise endometriosis or to open the posterior vagina (culdotomy). In addition, a no. 3 or no. 4 Sims curette or Hulka uterine elevator is placed in the endometrial cavity to antevert the uterus markedly and stretch out the cul-de-sac. The rectal probe and intraoperative rectovaginal examinations remain important techniques even when the Valtchev is available. Whenever rectal location is in doubt, it is identified by placing a probe.

Trocar sleeves are available in many sizes and shapes. For most cases, 5.5-mm cannulas are adequate. Newer electrosurgical electrodes that eliminate capacitance and insulation failures (Electroshield from Electroscope, Boulder, CO), require 7- to 8-mm sleeves. Laparoscopic stapling is performed through 12- to 13-mm Surgiports (U.S. Surgical Corporation, Norwalk, CT).

A short, trapless, 5-mm trocar sleeve with a retention screw grid around its external surface (Richard Wolf Medical Instruments, Vernon Hills, IL; Apple Medical, Bolton, MA) is used on the left to facilitate efficient instrument exchanges and evacuation of tissue while allowing unlimited freedom during extracorporeal suture tying (17). With practice, a good laparoscopic surgical team makes instrument exchanges so fast that little pneumoperitoneum is lost.

The high-frequency, low-voltage cutting current (20–50 W) of bipolar forceps coagulates vessels as large as the ovarian and uterine arteries. The Kleppinger bipolar forceps (Richard Wolf) are excellent for large vessel hemostasis. Specially insulated bipolar forceps (Apple Medical) are available and allow current to pass only through their tips, so that precise hemostasis can be obtained. Microbipolar forceps contain a channel for irrigation and provide a fixed distance between the electrodes. They are used to irrigate bleeding sites so as to identify vessels before coagulation and to prevent sticking of the electrode to the eschar created. Irrigation is used during underwater examination to identify the bleeding vessel before coagulation by removing surrounding blood products.

Disposable stapling instruments are rarely used for large vessel hemostasis during laparoscopic hysterectomy because of their expense and propensity for hematoma formation. Most laparoscopic staplers place six rows of titanium staples through a 12-mm cannula and simultaneously divide the clamped tissue. The disposable handle is designed to fire up to six staple cartridges.

PREOPERATIVE PREPARATION

The preoperative use of gonadotropin-releasing hormone (GnRH) analogs for at least 2 months before hysterectomy for large myomas should be encouraged as it may reduce the total uterine volume and may shrink the leiomyoma, thereby making laparoscopic or vaginal hysterectomy easier (18,19). During treatment with depoleuprolide (Lupron Depot) at a dose of 3.75 mg IM once a month for 3–6 months, anemia secondary to hypermenorrhea resolves, and autologous blood donation can be considered prior to laparoscopic hysterectomy. Packed red blood cells obtained in this manner have a shelf life of 35 days if stored at 1–6°C. In addition, depo-leuprolide is often administered after ovulation in the cycle preceding surgery to avoid operating on ovaries containing a corpus luteum.

Patients are encouraged to hydrate and eat lightly for 24 hours before admission on the day of surgery. When extensive cul-de-sac involvement with endometriosis is suspected, either clinically or from another doctor's operative record, a mechanical bowel prep is ordered (polyethylene glycol-based isosmotic solution: GoLytely or Colyte). Lower abdominal, pubic, and perineal hair is *not* shaved. A Foley catheter is inserted during surgery to distend the bladder with 50-cm^3 indigo-carmine solution aiding in its identification, and the catheter is removed the next morning. Antibiotics (usually cefoxitin) are administered in all cases lasting over 2 hr, at the 2-hr mark.

POSITIONING OF PATIENT

All laparoscopic surgical procedures are done under general anesthesia with endotracheal intubation and an orogastric tube. The routine use of an orogastric tube is recommended to diminish the possibility of a trocar injury to the stomach and to reduce small bowel distension. The patient is flat (0°) until after the umbilical trocar sleeve has been inserted and then is placed in steep Trendelenburg position (20–30°). Lithotomy position with the hip extended (thigh parallel to abdomen) is obtained with Allan stirrups (Edgewater Medical Systems, Mayfield Heights, OH) or knee braces, which are adjusted to each individual patient before she is anesthetized. Anesthesia examination is always performed prior to prepping the patient.

Laparoscopy was never thought to be a sterile procedure before the incorporation of video with the laparoscope, as the surgeon operated with his head in the surgical field, attached to the laparoscopic optic. Since 1983, this author has maintained a policy of not sterilizing or draping the camera or laser arm. Infection has been rare: less than 1 per 200 cases. The umbilical incision is closed with a single 4-0 vicryl suture opposing deep fascia and skin dermis, with the knot buried beneath the fascia to prevent the suture from acting like a wick to transmit bacteria into the soft tissue or peritoneal cavity.

HYSTERECTOMY TECHNIQUE

The technique described is for total laparoscopic hysterectomy. Visual documentation of several steps in this procedure in a 48-year-old woman with persistent left adnexal cystic mass and a 12-week size fibroid uterus is provided in Figs. 1–8.

1. Incisions. Three laparoscopic puncture sites including the umbilicus are used: 10 or 12 mm umbilical, 5 mm right, and 5 mm left lower quadrant. The left lower quadrant puncture is the major portal for operative manipulation. The right trocar sleeve is used for retraction with atraumatic grasping forceps. When the laparoscopic stapler is used, it is inserted through the umbilical incision and the procedure is viewed through a 5-mm laparoscope in one of the 5-mm lower quadrant sites.

Placement of the lower quadrant trocar sleeves just above the pubic hairline and lateral to the deep epigastric vessels (and thus the rectus abdominis muscle) is preferred. These vessels—an artery flanked by two veins (venae comitantes)—are located lateral to the umbilical ligaments (obliterated umbilical artery) by direct laparoscopic inspection of the anterior abdominal wall. The deep epigastric vessels arise near the junction of the external iliac vessels with the femoral vessels and make up the medial border of the internal inguinal ring. The round ligament curls around these vessels to enter the inguinal canal. When the anterior abdominal wall pari-

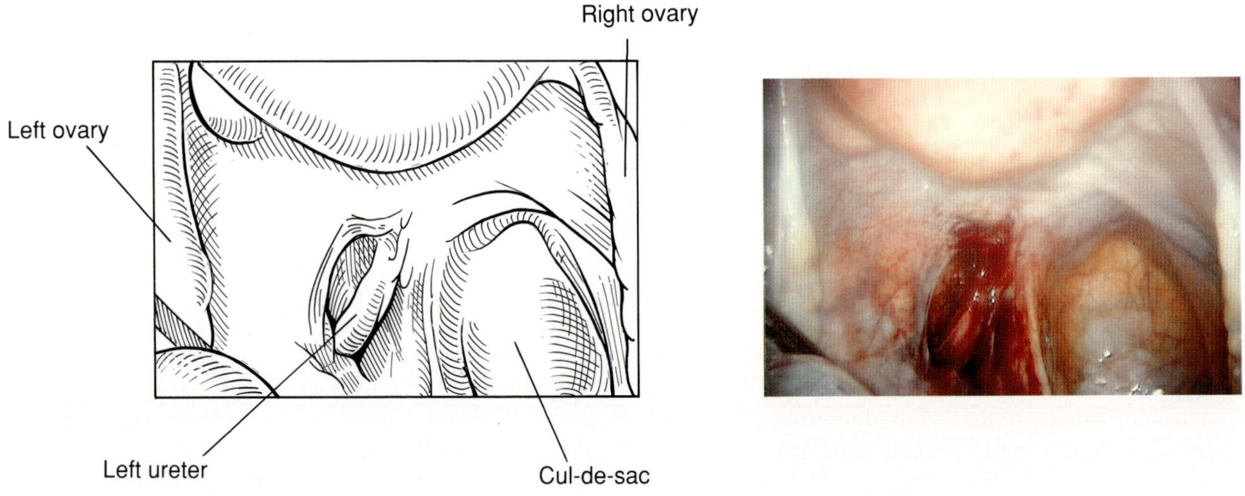

FIG. 1. Left ureter is isolated using scissors dissection.

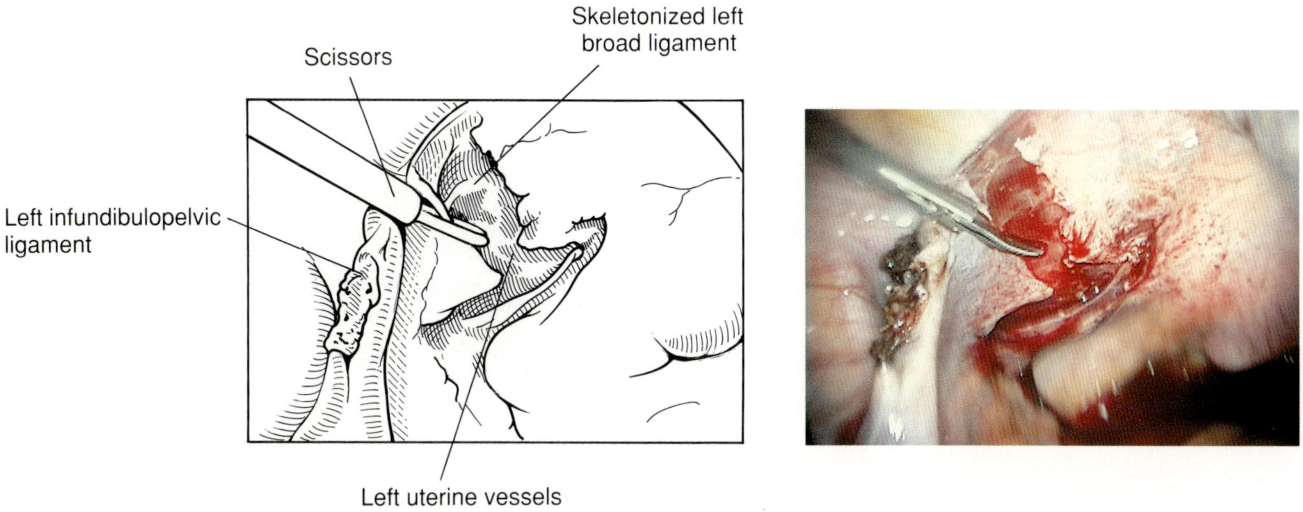

FIG. 2. Left broad ligament is skeletonized down to uterine vessels using scissors. Note previously desiccated left infundibulopelvic ligament on left pelvic side wall.

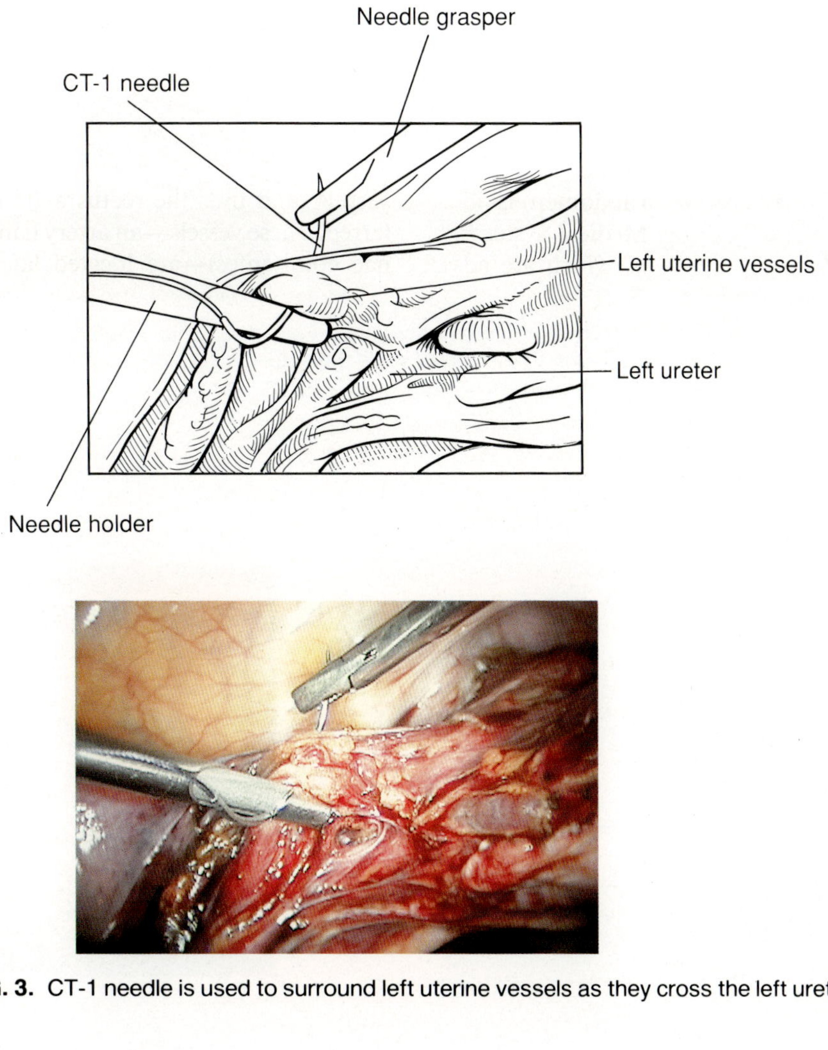

FIG. 3. CT-1 needle is used to surround left uterine vessels as they cross the left ureter.

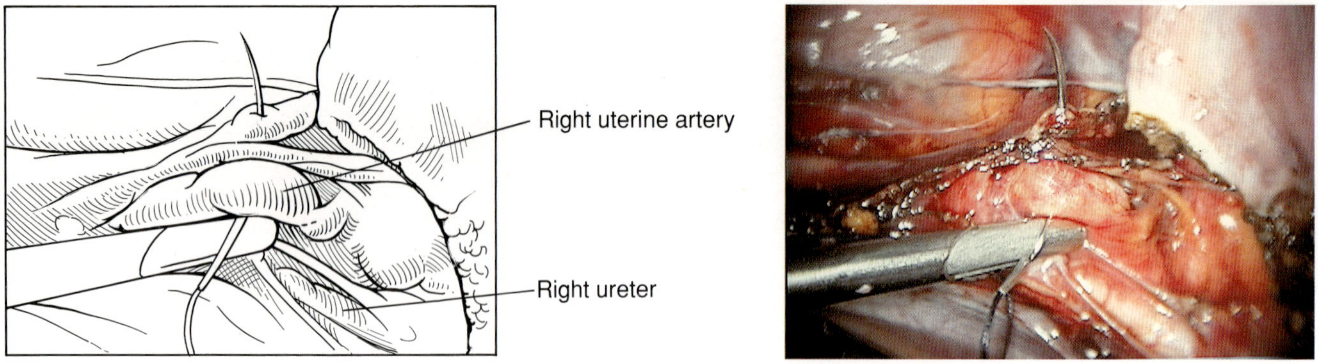

FIG. 4. Right uterine artery is ligated with CT-1 needle on Cook oblique-curved needle holder. Note right ureter below the needle.

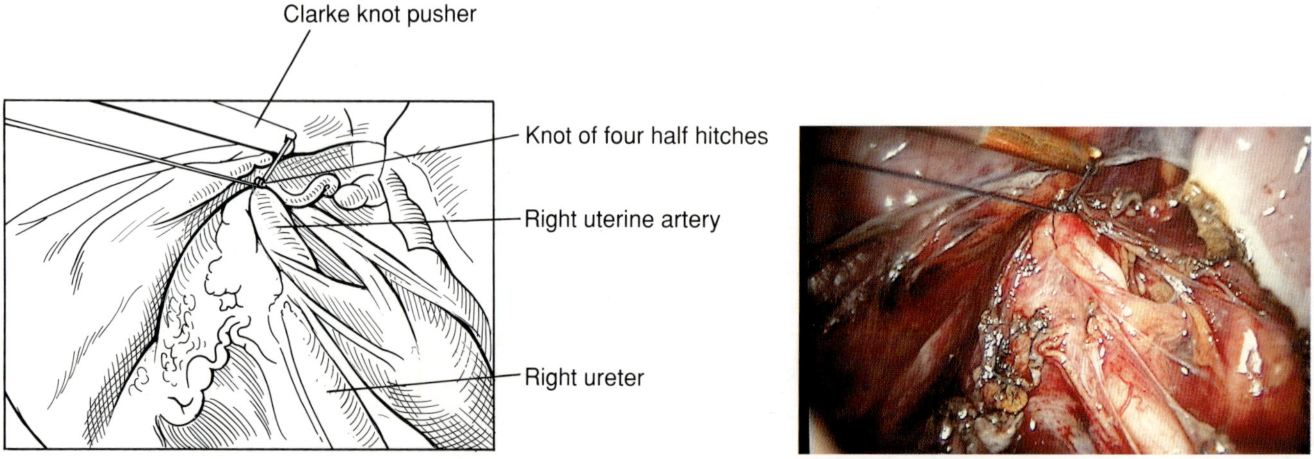

FIG. 5. Right uterine artery ligated with Clarke knot pusher. Four simple half hitches are made outside the peritoneal cavity and pushed down to the vessel while the suture is kept on tension.

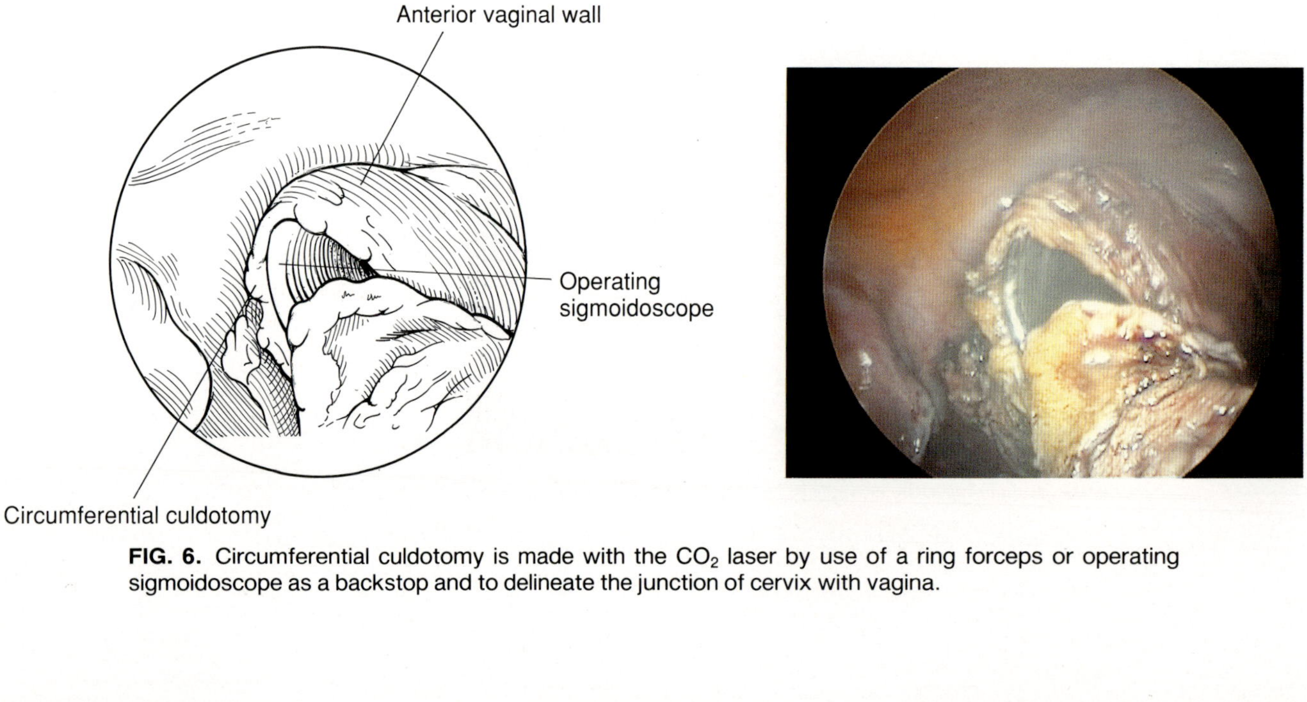

FIG. 6. Circumferential culdotomy is made with the CO_2 laser by use of a ring forceps or operating sigmoidoscope as a backstop and to delineate the junction of cervix with vagina.

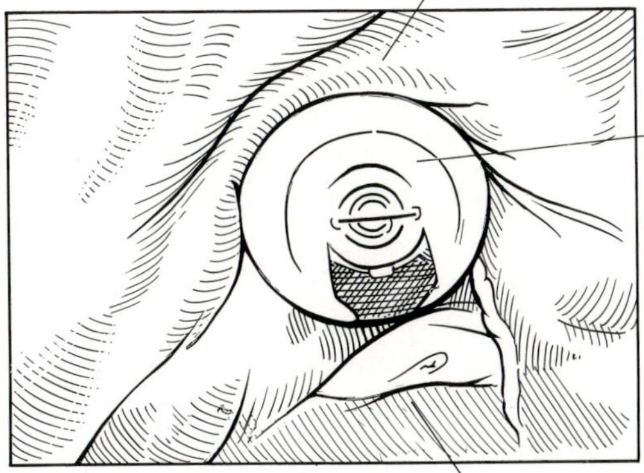

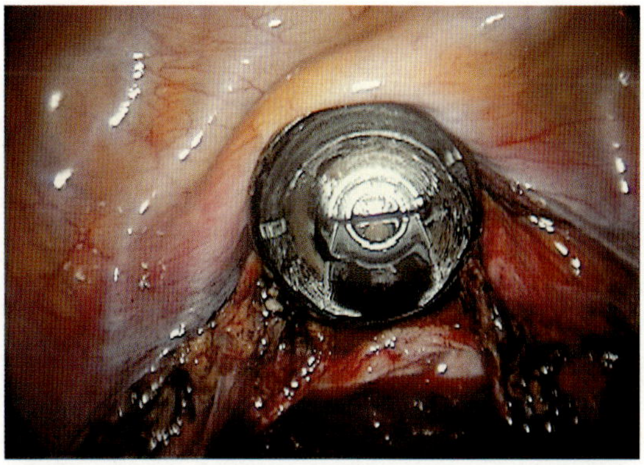

FIG. 7. View of operating sigmoidoscope after uterus is severed from the vagina.

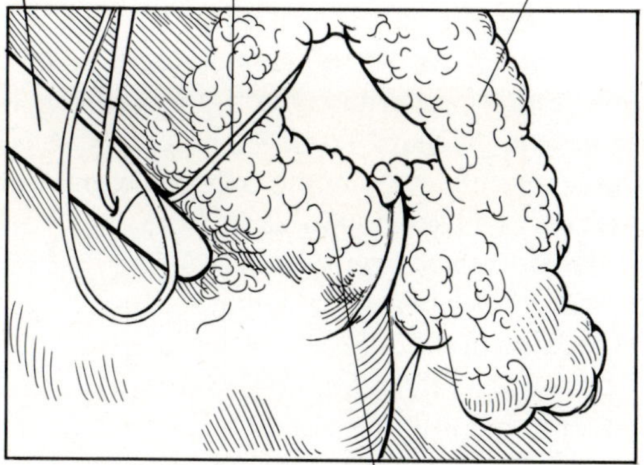

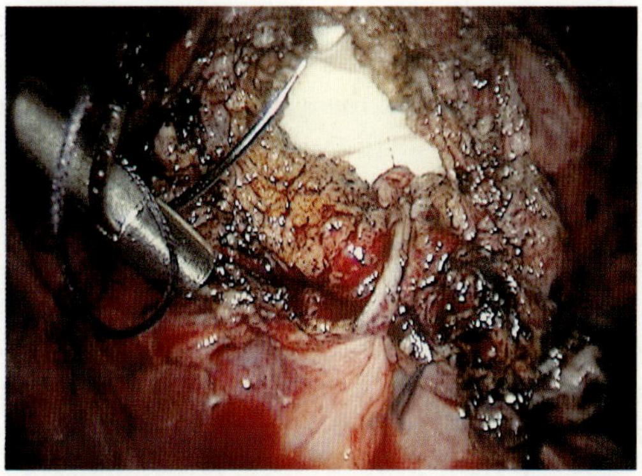

FIG. 8. Uterosacral ligaments are together. The second and final suture is being negotiated: a figure of 8 apposing pubocervicovesicular fascia and vagina across the midline.

etal peritoneum is thickened from previous surgery or obesity, the position of these vessels is judged by palpating and depressing the anterior abdominal wall with the back of the scalpel; the wall appears thicker where rectus muscle is enclosed, and the incision site should be chosen lateral to this area near the anterior superior iliac spine.

2. *Vaginal preparation.* Hysteroscopy with CO_2 is performed during insufflation of pneumoperitoneum. This is especially useful for myoma hysterectomies to identify the location of the fibroids. Following hysteroscopy, the endocervical canal is dilated to Pratt no. 25 and the Valtchev uterine mobilizer (Conkin Surgical Instruments) is inserted to antevert the uterus and delineate the posterior vagina. When this device is in the anteverted position, the cervix sits on a wide pedestal thereby making the cervicovaginal junction readily visible between the uterosacral ligaments when the cul-de-sac is viewed laparoscopically.

3. *Exploration.* The upper abdomen and pelvis are inspected and the appendix is identified. If appendiceal pathology is present, i.e., dilatation, adhesions, or endometriosis, appendectomy is performed after ureteral isolation by mobilizing the appendix, desiccating its blood supply, and placing three endoloops at the appendiceal–

cecal junction after desiccating the appendix just above this juncture. The appendix is left attached to the cecum and its stump divided later in the procedure after opening of the cul-de-sac, so that removal from the peritoneal cavity is accomplished immediately after separation.

4. Ureteral dissection. Immediately after exploration of the upper abdomen and pelvis, each ureter is isolated deep in the pelvis, if possible. This is done early in the operation before the pelvic side wall peritoneum becomes edematous and/or opaque from irritation by the CO_2 pneumoperitoneum or aquadissection and before ureteral peristalsis is inhibited by surgical stress, pressure, or the Trendelenburg position. The ureter and its overlying peritoneum are grasped deep in the pelvis on the left to avoid division of the lateral rectosigmoid attachments whose clear identification is requisite. An atraumatic grasping forceps is used from a right-sided cannula to grasp the ureter and its overlying peritoneum on the left pelvic side wall below and caudad to the left ovary, lateral to the left uterosacral ligament. Scissors are used to divide the peritoneum overlying the ureter; they are then inserted into the created defect and are spread (Fig. 1). Thereafter one blade of the scissors is placed on top of the ureter, the buried scissors blade visualized through the peritoneum, and the peritoneum divided. This is continued into the deep pelvis where the uterine vessels cross the ureter and lateral to the cardinal ligament insertion into the cervix. Connective tissue between the ureter and the vessels is separated with scissors. Bleeding is controlled with microbipolar forceps.

5. Bladder mobilization. The left round ligament is divided at its midportion with minimal bleeding using a spoon electrode (Electroscope, Boulder, CO) at 150-W cutting current. Persistent bleeding is controlled with monopolar fulguration at 80-W coagulation current or bipolar desiccation at 30-W cutting current. Thereafter scissors are used to divide the vesicouterine peritoneal fold starting at the left side and continuing across the midline to the right round ligament. The right round ligament is divided, as was the left, with unipolar electrosurgery. The bladder is mobilized off the uterus and upper vagina using scissors.

6. Upper uterine vascular ligation. When ovarian preservation is desired, the uteroovarian ligament and fallopian tube are divided adjacent to the uterus with the laparoscopic stapler. For this portion of the procedure, a 5-mm laparoscope is inserted through the left 5-mm cannula. The stapler is then inserted through the umbilical incision either through a 12-mm cannula or directly with no cannula. The stapler is applied to the pedicle and fired. Often two staplers are necessary on each side for this part of the procedure. When ovarian preservation is not desired, the infundibulopelvic ligaments and broad ligaments are coagulated until desiccated and then divided.

7. Uterine vessel ligation. The broad ligament on each side is skeletonized down to the uterine vessels (Fig. 2). Each uterine vessel pedicle is suture-ligated with 0-Vicryl on a CT-1 needle (27 in.). The needles are introduced into the peritoneal cavity by being pulled through a 5-mm incision. The curved needle is inserted on top of the unroofed ureter where it turns medially toward the previously mobilized bladder (Fig. 3). A short rotary movement of the Cook oblique curved needle holder brings the needle around the uterine vessel pedicle (Fig. 4). Sutures are tied extracorporeally using a Clarke knot pusher (Fig. 5) (20). A single suture placed in this manner on each side serves as a sentinel stitch, identifying and watching over the ureter for the rest of the case.

8. Circumferential culdotomy (division of cervicovaginal attachments). The cardinal ligaments on each side are divided with the CO_2 laser at high power or the spoon electrode at 150-W cutting current (Fig. 6). Often bleeding control is necessary using bipolar forceps. The vagina is entered posteriorly over the Valtchev retractor, which identifies the junction of cervix and vagina. A ring forceps inserted into the anterior vagina above the tenaculum on the anterior cervical lip identifies the anterior cervicovaginal junction, which is entered using the laser. With the ring forceps or the aquapurator tip as a backstop, the lateral vaginal fornices are divided. The uterus is then morcellated when necessary and pulled from the vagina (Fig. 7). Alternately, a 4-cm-diameter operative colonoscope (Richard Wolf, Vernon Hills, IL) is used to outline circumferentially the cervicovaginal junction; it also serves as a backstop for laser work.

9. Laparoscopic vaginal vault closure and suspension with McCall culdoplasty. Vaginal repair is accomplished after packing of the vagina. The left uterosacral ligament and posterolateral vagina are first elevated. A suture is placed through this uterosacral ligament and into the vagina, exits the vagina including posterior vaginal tissue near the midline on the left, and reenters just adjacent to this spot on the right. Finally, an opposite-sided oblique Cook needle holder is used to fixate the right posterolateral vagina to the right uterosacral ligament. This suture is tied extracorporeally and gives excellent support to the vaginal cuff apex, elevating it superiorly and back toward the hollow of the sacrum. The rest of the vagina and overlying pubocervical fascia is closed vertically with a figure of 8 suture (Fig. 8).

10. Underwater examination. At the close of each operation, an underwater examination is used to detect bleeding from vessels and viscera tamponaded during the procedure by the increased intraperitoneal pressure of the CO_2 pneumoperitoneum. The CO_2 pneumoperitoneum is displaced with 2–5 L of Ringer's lactate solution, and the peritoneal cavity is vigorously irrigated and suctioned until the effluent is clear of blood products. Any further bleeding is controlled underwater using microbipolar forceps to coagulate through the electrolyte solution, and at least 2 L of lactated Ringer's solution is left in the peritoneal cavity.

OUTCOME

In our experience, estimated blood loss averaged 150 ml. Length of stay ranged from 1 to 5 days with an average of 2 days. In more than 200 cases, laparotomy was not needed regardless of the size of uterine fibroids or the extent of endometriosis. One woman with extensive pelvic adhesions and endometrial cancer had laparotomy to complete the hysterectomy and to reinforce enterotomy repair.

COMPLICATIONS

Complications of laparoscopic hysterectomy are the same as with hysterectomy in general: anesthetic accidents; postoperative pulmonary emboli; hemorrhage; injury to ureters, bladder, and rectum; and infections especially of the vaginal cuff (21). Since the introduction of prophylactic antibiotics, vaginal cuff abscess, pelvic thrombophlebitis, septicemia, pelvic cellulitis, and adnexal abscesses are rare. Abdominal wound infection is rare, but the incidence of incisional hernias after operative laparoscopy is greatly increased if 10-mm or larger trocars are placed at extraumbilical sites.

Febrile morbidity with a vaginal approach is about half that of abdominal hysterectomy. Laparoscopic treatment with evacuation of all blood clots and the sealing of all blood vessels after the uterus is out should reduce the infection rate further. Morcellation during laparoscopic or vaginal hysterectomy results in a slightly increased risk of fever, especially if prophylactic antibiotics are not used.

HIGHLIGHTS

The laparoscope can be used in combination with hysterectomy in a variety of ways with significant surgical and patient advantages. With few exceptions, laparoscopic hysterectomy can replace abdominal hysterectomy. Surgical outcome is the same. In experienced hands, the complication rate is low. Patient benefits are related to avoidance of an abdominal incision and include improved cosmetics and more rapid recovery.

REFERENCES

1. Bachmann GA. Hysterectomy: a critical review. *J Reprod Med* 1990;35:839–862.
2. Reich H, DeCaprio J, McGlynn F. Laparoscopic hysterectomy. *J Gynecol Surg* 1989;5:213–216.
3. Reich H. Laparoscopic hysterectomy. *Surg Laparosc Endosc* 1992;2:85–88.
4. Liu CY. Laparoscopic hysterectomy: a review of 72 cases. *J Reprod Med* 1992;37:351–354.
5. Liu CY. Laparoscopic hysterectomy. Report of 215 cases. *Gynaecol Endosc* 1992;1:73–77.
6. Reich H. Laparoscopic extrafascial hysterectomy with bilateral salpingo-oophorectomy using stapling techniques for endometrial adenocarcinoma. AAGL 19th Annual Meeting Orlando Florida, November 14–18, 1990.
7. Reich H, McGlynn F, Wilkie W. Laparoscopic management of stage I ovarian cancer. *J Reprod Med* 1990;35:601–605.
8. Canis M, Mage G, Wattiez A, Pouly JL, et al. Does endoscopic surgery have a role in radical surgery of cancer of the cervix uteri? *J Gynecol Obstet Biol Reprod* 1990;19:921.
9. Kovac SR, Cruikshank SH, Retto HF. Laparoscopy-assisted vaginal hysterectomy. *J Gynecol Surg* 1990;6:185–189.
10. Summit RL, Stovall TG, Lipscomb GH, Ling FW. Randomized comparison of laparoscopy-assisted vaginal hysterectomy with standard vaginal hysterectomy in an outpatient setting. *Obstet Gynecol* 1992;80:895–901.
11. Minelli L, Angiolillo M, Caione C, Palmara V. Laparoscopically-assisted vaginal hysterectomy. *Endoscopy* 1991;23:64–66.
12. Maher PJ, Wood EC, Hill DJ, Lolatgis NA. Laparoscopically assisted hysterectomy. *Med J Aust* 1992;156:316–318.
13. Lyons TL. Laparoscopic supracervical hysterectomy. In: Hunt RB, Martin DC, eds. *Endoscopy in gynecology.* Proceedings of the World Congress of Gynecologic Endoscopy. AAGL 20th Annual Meeting, Las Vegas. Baltimore: Port City Press; 1993:129–131.
14. Reich H, McGlynn F, Salvat J. Laparoscopic treatment of cul-de-sac obliteration secondary to retrocervical deep fibrotic endometriosis. *J Reprod Med* 1991;36:516–522.
15. McDonald R, Phipps J, Singer A. Endometrial ablation: a safe procedure. *Gynaecol Endosc* 1992;1:7–9.
16. Valtchev KL, Papsin FR. A new uterine mobilizer for laparoscopy: its use in 518 patients. *Am J Obstet Gynecol* 1977;127:738–740.
17. Reich H, McGlynn F. Short self-retaining trocar sleeves. *Am J Obstet Gynecol* 1990;162:453–454.
18. Schlaff WD, Zerhouni EA, Huth JA, Chen J, Damewood MD, Rock JA. A placebo-controlled trial of a depot gonadotropin-releasing hormone analogue (leuprolide) in the treatment of uterine leiomyomata. *Obstet Gynecol* 1989;74:856–862.
19. Freidman AJ, Hoffman DI, Comite F, Browneller RW, Miller JD (Leuprolide Study Group). Treatment of leiomyomata uteri with leuprolide acetate depot: a double-blind, placebo-controlled, multicenter study. *Obstet Gynecol* 1991;77:720–725.
20. Reich H, Clarke HC, Sekel L. A simple method for ligating in operative laparoscopy with straight and curved needles. *Obstet Gynecol* 1992;79:143–147.
21. Woodland MB. Ureter injury during laparoscopy-assisted vaginal hysterectomy with the endoscopic linear stapler. *Am J Obstet Gynecol* 1992;167:756–757.

Endoscopic Management of Gynecologic Disease,
edited by G.D. Adamson and D.C. Martin.
Lippincott-Raven Publishers, Philadelphia © 1996.

CHAPTER 26

Sterilization

H. Preston Nelson

HISTORY AND GENERAL CONSIDERATIONS

Laparoscopic tubal sterilization was first performed in the late 1930s using unipolar electrocoagulation (1). For several reasons, the decade of the 1970s saw laparoscopy and elective female sterilization become commonplace (2):

Hazards of oral contraceptives and intrauterine devices were defined and publicized.
Social acceptability of voluntary sterilization increased markedly.
Traditional institutionalized restriction of sterilization to women with medical indications, advanced age, or high parity was abandoned.
Safe, effective, relatively simple outpatient techniques for laparoscopic sterilization were developed.

Outpatient female sterilization under local anesthesia was introduced in 57 countries from 1970 to 1975 (3). By 1982, sterilization had become the most common contraceptive practice among American women aged 15–44 years (2).

The initial laparoscopic technique, midtubal unipolar electrocoagulation using available high-voltage generators, provided very low failure rates. However, reports of occasional serious bowel or abdominal wall injury prompted refinement of the unipolar technique as well as development of alternative electrical and mechanical systems for tubal occlusion. The most widely used techniques, unipolar or bipolar coagulation, silastic clip, and spring-loaded clip, are discussed at length below. Less frequently used laparoscopic methods include thermal coagulation ("endocoagulation") (4), shielded low-voltage cautery hook (5), unipolar wire snare (6), endoloop suture (7), and salpingectomy.

Tubal ligation is best performed in the preovulatory period to avoid luteal phase pregnancy. If preoperative history or findings raise any suspicion of pregnancy, a sensitive pregnancy test should be obtained. Perioperative prophylactic antibiotic administration is indicated if pregnancy termination or intrauterine device removal is performed at the time of tubal sterilization. It is recommended that patients avoid sexual activity for at least a week following surgery.

INDICATIONS AND CONTRAINDICATIONS

Most indications for sterilization are elective because absolute medical contraindications to pregnancy are rare. Contraindications to tubal sterilization include inability to tolerate anesthesia, gynecologic pathology requiring major surgical procedure in the near future, and possibly massive peritubal adhesions. Indications should be clearly documented with appropriate consultation if there are medical (e.g., heart disease) or psychiatric reasons. Informed consent should emphasize that sterilization is intended to be permanent; that no guarantee of sterility can be given; that rare complications of surgery include hemorrhage, infection, injury to the gastrointestinal or genitourinary tracts, and anesthetic complications; and that accompanying laparotomy occasionally is necessary (3).

OUTCOME

Large follow-up series of the common laparoscopic techniques performed by experienced surgeons show subsequent pregnancy rates of 0.5–1.0% (8,9). Initially higher failure rates decline with operator experience (10). Pregnancy following tubal sterilization can result from failure to occlude both tubes, recanalization of a tube, or tuboperitoneal fistula formation at the proximal tubal

H. P. Nelson: Department of Obstetrics and Gynecology, University of California, San Francisco, California 94143; and Fertility Physicians of Northern California, Palo Alto, California 94301.

stump. In the event of pregnancy following tubal ligation, ectopic implantation is common, especially following electrocoagulation (11). Maximum safety and efficacy require careful adherence to technique.

There is no long-term difference in menstrual pattern or pelvic pain between sterilized and nonsterilized women who are not taking oral contraceptives. Increased bleeding and dysmenorrhea observed following sterilization usually results from discontinuation of oral contraceptives rather than from tubal sterilization per se. The low but increased rate of hysterectomy following sterilization may be related to a higher patient acceptance rate of hysterectomy as a treatment option once a woman has been sterilized (12).

Pregnancy following microsurgical tubal anastomosis is related to the amount of remaining normal tube and the site of anastomosis (13). Mechanical methods usually injure less tube than electrocoagulation and have higher rates of successful reversal. Women sterilized before age 30 are more likely than women in older age groups to request subsequent reversal; therefore some gynecologists favor use of mechanical methods in younger women (14).

UNIPOLAR COAGULATION

Although unipolar electrocoagulation initially set the standard for efficacy of laparoscopic sterilization, associated serious abdominal wall and bowel injuries occasionally occurred and required investigation. Abdominal wall burns were probably caused by high-voltage current arcing from the active electrode to the laparoscope and discharging through the metal trocar sheath into the abdominal wall. When low-voltage generators and nonconductive fiberglass trocar sleeves were employed, abdominal wall injury became rare but the frequency of bowel injury remained constant (15). It was then learned that the metal laparoscope—when insulated from the abdominal wall and from unidirectional electrical current running down its center—is a potent capacitor, storing electrical energy that discharges upon contact of the laparoscope to any grounded surface including bowel. Use of metal trocar sleeves and restriction of electrogenerator power to less than 100 W and 600 V peak voltage is now recommended; this reduces capacitance to a level allowing safe flow through the abdominal wall without risk of thermal injury to the abdominal wall or viscera (16).

In 1981 the Centers for Disease Control (CDC) attributed three deaths from bowel perforation and sepsis to the use of unipolar coagulation for sterilization. These conclusions were subsequently challenged when histologic methods to differentiate electric from nonelectric bowel injuries showed that many cases assumed to be electrical burns were instead traumatic bowel injuries (17). Today laparoscopic unipolar electrocoagulation for sterilization is recognized as effective and safe when appropriate careful technique is employed.

Technique (3,15)

After laparoscope placement, initial careful inspection of the entire pelvis defines anatomy and any abnormalities. Intestines are moved to the upper abdomen. Anterolateral positioning of the uterus facilitates tracing the fallopian tube from cornu to fimbriated end.

The fallopian tube is grasped approximately 4 cm from the cornu with a bite that includes the entire tube and a small portion of mesosalpinx (Fig. 1). The laparoscope must usually then be withdrawn slightly to establish a panoramic view of all pelvic structures. One must confirm extension of the insulated portion of the forceps beyond the end of the laparoscope or sheath and elevation of the tube away from bowel and bladder before attaching the generator electrode to the forceps. Visualization of the forceps is maintained whenever the surgeon activates coagulation by foot switch.

As current flows from the forceps to the ground plate, tissue in the grasper blanches, swells, and collapses. These changes spread radially, and tissue injury extends beyond the extent of visual change. At least 3 cm of tube must be destroyed—pregnancy failures have occurred at less than 3 cm—so that more than one application of the coagulation forceps is usually necessary. Because tissue desiccated by coagulation possesses increased electrical resistance, it is recommended that sites of repeated coagulation occur progressively closer to the uterus. Current flows along the path of least resistance and is thus directed toward the uterus rather than possibly out the distal tube to adjacent bowel. Coagulation of the uterotubal junction is avoided because it may be associated with increased rates of fistula formation and subsequent pregnancy (18).

Avulsion or resection of a segment of fallopian tube can provide a specimen to prove tubal interruption, although the coagulated tissue often is not definitively identifiable as tube by the pathologist. Tubal transection does not reduce failure rates. It does allow inspection of the coagulated tubal cross-section as well as secondary coagulation of the proximal, but not distal, stump of the tube (3). However, tubal transection frequently causes troublesome bleeding from the mesosalpinx that requires further coagulation.

Serious bowel burns are often unrecognized at the time of surgery and can present with peritonitis 5–15 days later (19). Unipolar electrical injury extends wide and deep, so that excision of bowel at least 5 cm beyond the visible edge of thermal damage is recommended.

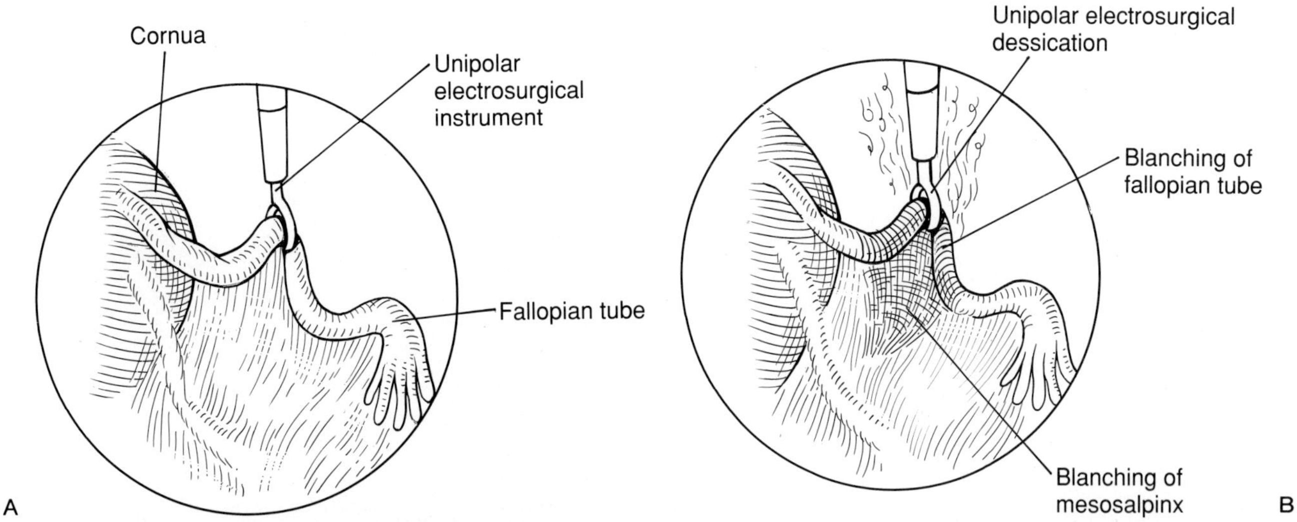

FIG. 1. Unipolar electrocoagulation. **A:** The fallopian tube is grasped approximately 4 cm from the cornu and elevated away from the bowel and bladder. Extension of insulation beyond the end of the laparoscope is confirmed. **B:** Tissue injury extends beyond visible blanching and desiccation. Coagulation is repeated progressively closer to the uterus so that current is directed medially and a 3-cm segment of tube is destroyed (not shown). (From ref. 24, with permission.)

BIPOLAR COAGULATION

In bipolar coagulation, electricity flows between the jaws of the forceps so that only the jaws and intervening tissue are heated. Equal bidirectional current flow through the laparoscope prevents any capacitance effect.

Bipolar injury is more superficial with less lateral spread than is associated with unipolar coagulation. When bipolar coagulation produces tubal appearance like that after unipolar coagulation, deep tissue destruction is often inadequate. Histologic studies have shown that consistent tubal destruction can be achieved with cutting waveform—not coagulating or blend—adjusted to 25 W of power output. Current is applied until an in-line ammeter shows no further electrical flow (18).

Technique (3,15)

The surgeon inspects the pelvis, positions the bowel, identifies the fallopian tubes, and establishes a panoramic view. The midportion of the tube is grasped so that the bipolar jaws enclose the entire tubal width and extend onto the mesosalpinx. With the tube elevated away from neighboring structures, the jaws are kept in view while the foot switch triggers coagulation (Fig. 2).

As with unipolar coagulation, 3 cm of proximal tube should be destroyed with obliteration of the underlying mesosalpingeal vessels. Care is taken when moving the grasper because the jaws can remain hot for several seconds after coagulation. Usually three adjacent sites are completely coagulated to assure destruction of an adequate length of tube. Some authors recommend tubal transection and coagulation of the stumps, but significant mesosalpingeal bleeding can result (3).

SILASTIC RING

The silastic ring for tubal sterilization was developed to eliminate the risk of electrical burns. Known as the Falope ring or Yoon band, it is a silicone elastic band containing a small amount of barium for identification and has an internal diameter of 1.0 mm. The ring applicator consists of two concentric cylinders around a retractable grasping forceps. A dilating device is used to stretch rings onto the outside of the inner cylinder. After a fold of proximal tube is drawn into the applicator barrel, advancement of the outer cylinder applies a band over the fold, creating a loop of strangulated tube. There are different applicator designs for endoscopic single puncture, double puncture, or minilaparotomy use (20).

The proximal tube must have normal diameter and mobility so that it can be drawn into the end of the cylindrical applicator. Equipment for bipolar coagulation should be available for hemostasis and as an alternative for sterilization (21).

Technique (22)

After pelvic inspection and identification of both fallopian tubes by their fimbriated ends, the applicator is loaded. The grasper is opened under laparoscopic visual-

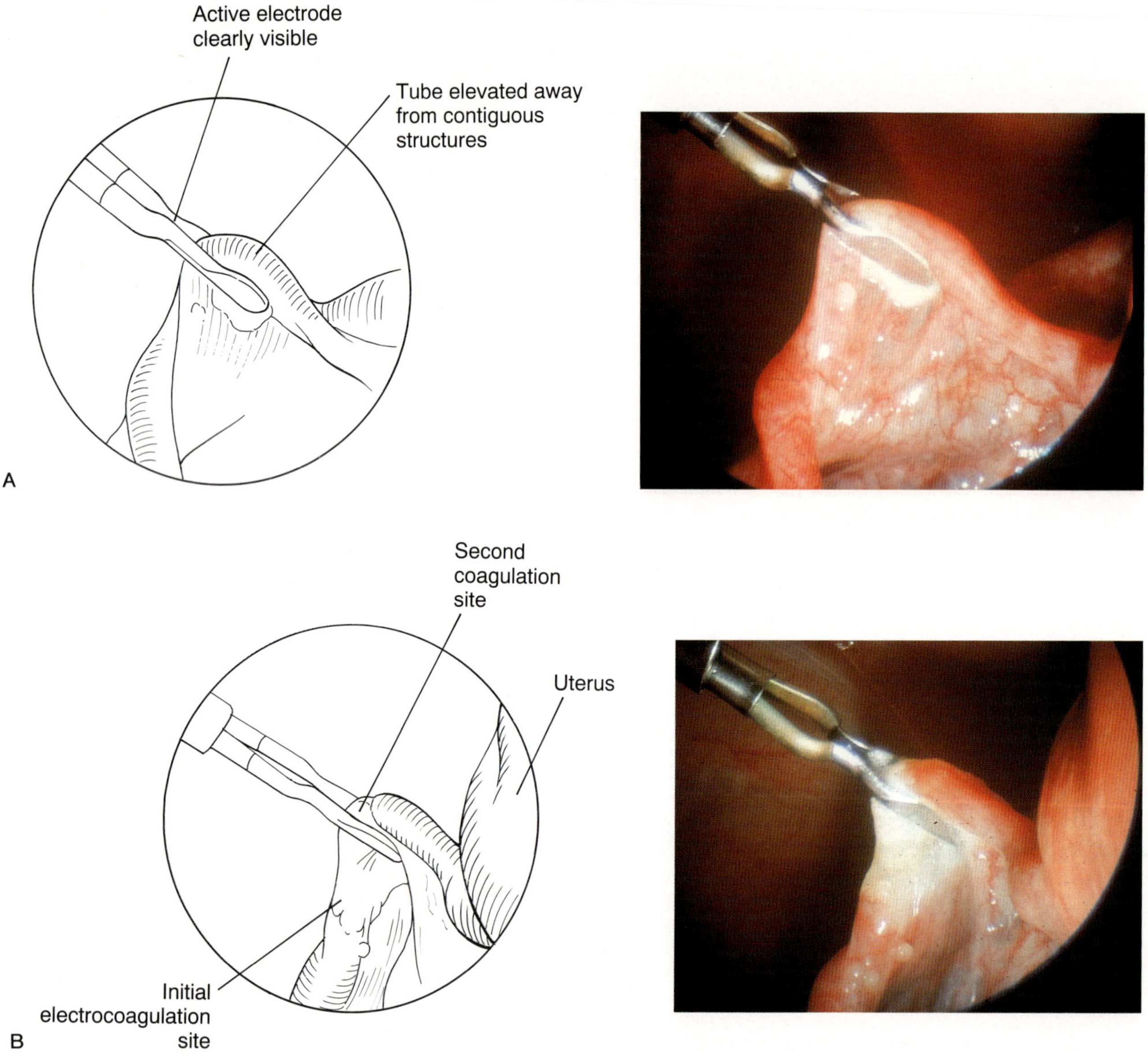

FIG. 2. **A:** Bipolar electrosurgical paddles initially grasping fallopian tube and mesosalpinx while elevating tube away from bowel and other structures. **B:** Electrosurgical heating of fallopian tube and mesosalpinx at second site more proximal to the uterus from the first site.

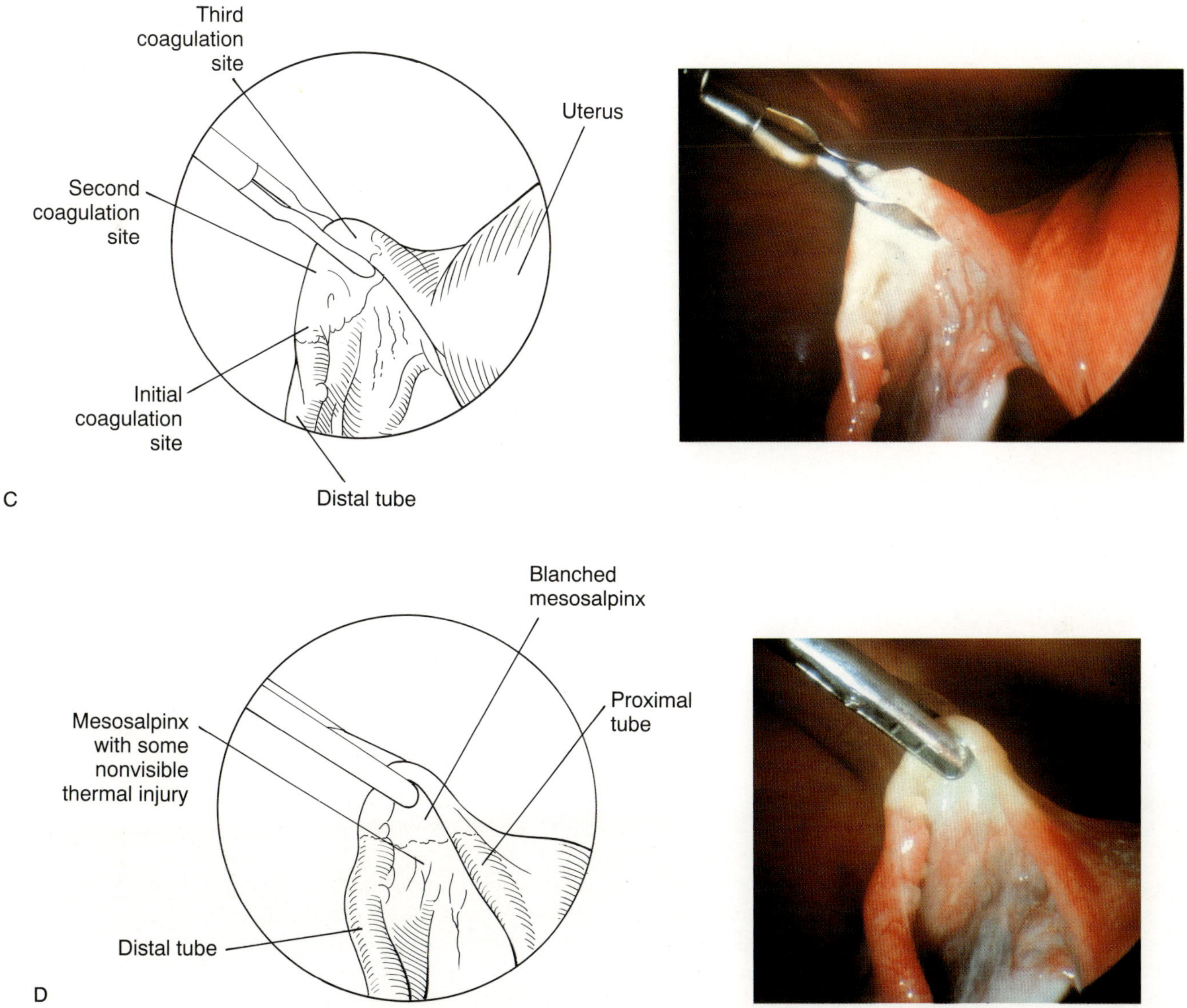

FIG. 2. (*Continued.*) **C:** Electrosurgical heating of fallopian tube and mesosalpinx at the third most proximal site. **D:** Tubal and mesosalpingeal blanching as a result of complete electrosurgical dessication. (Courtesy of Richard K. Kleppinger.)

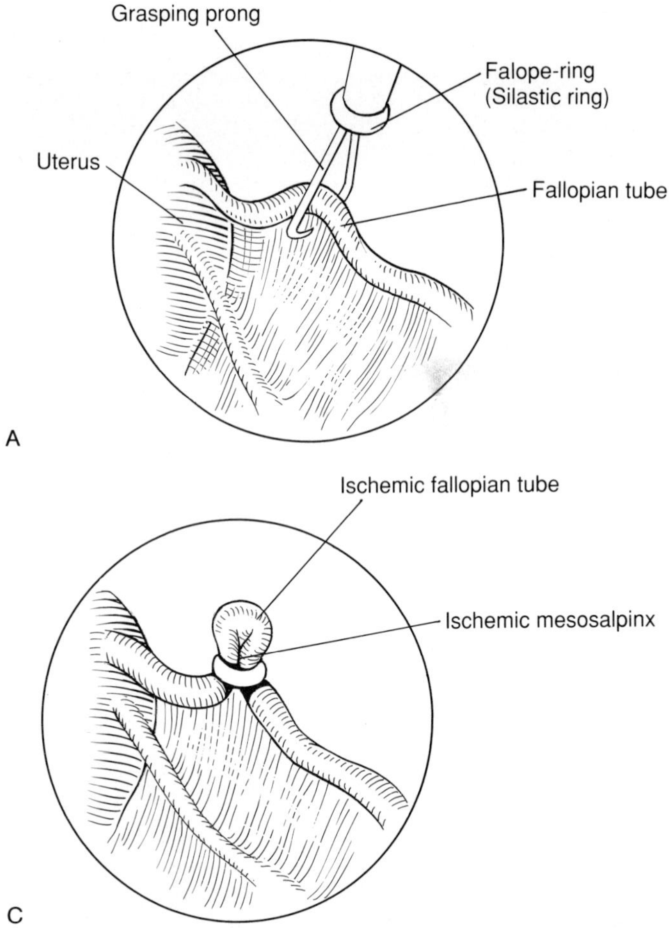

FIG. 3. Silastic ring application. **A:** The proximal tube is carefully grasped at least 2 cm from the cornu. **B:** A ring is applied over the knuckle of tube when it is fully retracted into the barrel. **C:** Ischemic mesosalpinx within the loop of tube created by the ring should be 1 cm in height. (From ref. 24, with permission.)

ization. The slender proximal half of the tube is grasped at least 2 cm from the uterine cornu, minimizing the chance of inadequate loop formation (Fig. 3). The tube must be handled very carefully to avoid unintended tubal transection or mesosalpingeal bleeding, which could require coagulation, salpingectomy, or laparotomy. As the tube is retracted into the barrel, the applicator is moved toward the tube to minimize tension. After full retraction, a ring is applied over the knuckle of tube. Ischemic mesosalpinx 1.0 cm in height should be visible within the loop of tube created by the ring. If the loop of tube is inadequate, a second ring can be used. If a ring is dropped into the abdomen and cannot be found, it may be left in place without danger.

Postoperative pain from nerves in the strangulated tubal segment can be minimized by injecting or spraying local anesthetic solution (e.g., Marcaine) around the loop as well as the adjacent tube and mesosalpinx. Anesthetic jelly should not be used because it can cause a ring to slip off.

SPRING-LOADED CLIP

The Hulka spring-loaded clip was developed to avoid the risks of electrical burns and mesosalpingeal bleeding. The hinged, tooth-bearing plastic clip is locked shut by advancement of a C-shaped metal spring. Because the clip destroys only a small portion of the tubal isthmus, occlusion by this method offers a maximal chance of successful microsurgical reversal (23).

Effective clip placement requires essentially normal pelvic anatomy and considerable coordination to accomplish precise positioning of the clip. Second-puncture application is less difficult to master than single-puncture technique. Although one clip correctly applied across the isthmus of each tube is effective, it has been recommended that a surgeon's first dozen procedures include application of two clips on each tube to build expertise and reduce the number of initial failures (14).

Technique (14)

The tube is identified by its fimbriated end and put on tension using the uterine manipulator or, if necessary, a grasper through the laparoscope's operating channel. A clip is carefully applied at a right angle to the tubal isthmus and closed (Fig. 4). Tubal muscularis should fill the clip all the way up to the hinge, and the clip should extend onto the mesosalpinx. The spring is then advanced

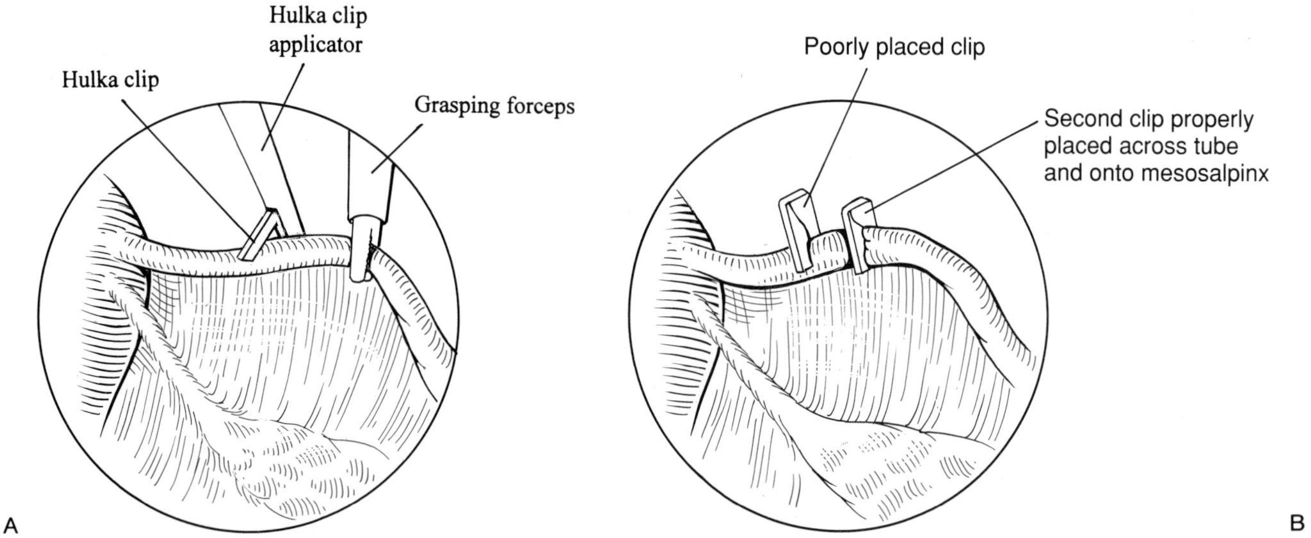

FIG. 4. Clip application. **A:** The applicator with open clip approaches the left mesosalpinx. **B:** A second clip is applied if the first does not extend beyond the tubal muscularis onto the mesosalpinx. (From ref. 14, with permission.)

to lock the jaws closed. Care is taken not to tear tissues when releasing the clip from the applicator. Inspection confirms correct placement. An open clip dropped in the abdomen should be retrieved if possible, although there have been no reports of complications in patients in whom an open clip was not retrieved.

HIGHLIGHTS

Several electrical and mechanical systems have been developed to accomplish laparoscopic tubal sterilization. Maximum safety and efficacy require careful adherence to technique. This chapter reviews the principles, hazards, and techniques of the most common methods including unipolar and bipolar electrocoagulation, silastic ring, and spring-loaded clip.

REFERENCES

1. Powers FH, Barnes AC. Sterilization by means of perineoscope tubal fulguration. *Am J Obstet Gynecol* 1941;4:1038.
2. Chatman DL, Cohen MR. History of endoscopy. In: Martin DC, ed. *Manual of endoscopy.* Santa Fe Springs, CA: American Association of Gynecologic Laparoscopists; 1990.
3. Wheeless CR Jr. Tubal sterilization. In: Thompson JD, Rock JA, eds. *Te Linde's operative gynecology.* 7th ed. Philadelphia: JB Lippincott; 1992.
4. Semm K. Endocoagulation. In: Phillips JM, ed. *Endoscopic female sterilization.* Downey, CA: American Association of Gynecologic Laparoscopists; 1983.
5. Valle RF. Laparoscopic tubal sterilization by shielded thermocautery. In: Phillips JM, ed. *Endoscopic female sterilization.* Downey, CA: American Association of Gynecologic Laparoscopists; 1983.
6. Soderstrom RM, Smith MR, Hayden GE. The snare method of laparoscopic sterilization: an analysis of 1,000 cases with four failures. *J Reprod Med* 1977;18:246.
7. Murray JE, Hibbert ML, Heth SR, Letterie GS. A technique for laparoscopic Pomeroy tubal ligation with endoloop sutures. *Obstet Gynecol* 1992;80:1053.
8. Koetsawang S, Gates DS, Suwanichati S, et al. Long-term follow-up of laparoscopic sterilizations by electrocoagulation, the Hulka clip and the tubal ring. *Contraception* 1990;41:9.
9. Bhiwandiwala PP, Mumford SD, Feldblum PJ. Comparison of different laparoscopic sterilization occlusion techniques in 24,439 procedures. *Am J Obstet Gynecol* 1982;144:319.
10. Hulka JF. Complications of laparoscopy. *Curr Probl Obstet Gynecol* 1980;4:23.
11. Kleppinger RK. Analysis of 7,000 laparoscopic sterilizations: unipolar, bipolar, and mechanical occlusive. In: Philips JM, ed. *Endoscopic female sterilization.* Downey, CA: American Association of Gynecologic Laparoscopists; 1983.
12. Rulin MC, Davidson AR, Philliber SG, et al. Long-term effect of tubal sterilization on menstrual indices and pelvic pain. *Obstet Gynecol* 1993;82:118.
13. Silber SJ, Cohen R. Microsurgical reversal of female sterilization: the role of tubal length. *Fertil Steril* 1980;33:598.
14. Hulka JF. Clip technique of sterilization. In Martin DC, ed: *Manual of endoscopy.* Santa Fe Springs, CA, American Association of Gynecologic Laparoscopists, 1990.
15. Levy BS, Soderstrom RM. Electrical techniques of sterilization. In: Martin DC, ed. *Manual of endoscopy.* Santa Fe Springs, CA: American Association of Gynecologic Laparoscopists; 1990.
16. Soderstrom RM. Electrical safety in laparoscopy. In: Phillips JM, ed. *Endoscopy in gynecology.* Downey, CA: American Association of Gynecologic Laparoscopists; 1978.
17. Levy BS, Soderstrom RM, Dail DH. Bowel injuries during laparoscopy: gross anatomy and histology. *J Reprod Med* 1985;30:168.
18. Soderstrom RM, Levy BS, Engel T. Reducing bipolar sterilization failures. *Obstet Gynecol* 1989;74:60.
19. Soderstrom RM. Bowel injury litigation after laparoscopy. *J Am Assoc Gynecol Laparoscop* 1993;1:74.
20. Yoon IB. The Yoon ring as compared with other sterilization methods. In: Phillips JM, ed. *Endoscopic female sterilization.* Downey, CA: American Association of Gynecologic Laparoscopists; 1983.
21. Levinson CJ. Falope ring complications. In: Phillips JM, ed. *Endoscopic female sterilization.* Downey, CA: American Association of Gynecologic Laparoscopists; 1983.
22. Yoon IB. Yoon Falope ring technique of sterilization. In: Martin DC, ed. *Manual of endoscopy.* Santa Fe Springs, CA: American Association of Gynecologic Laparoscopists; 1990.
23. Hulka JF, Noble AD, Letchworth AT, et al. Reversibility of clip sterilizations. *Lancet* 1982;2:927.
24. Wheeless CR Jr. *Atlas of pelvic surgery.* 2nd ed. Philadelphia: Lea and Febiger; 1988.

PART IV

Preparation for Hysteroscopy

Endoscopic Management of Gynecologic Disease,
edited by G.D. Adamson and D.C. Martin.
Lippincott-Raven Publishers, Philadelphia © 1996.

CHAPTER 27

Operating Room Setup

Charles M. March

Although the hallmark of hysteroscopy is simplicity, including simplicity in instrumentation, careful planning in the operating room is essential to prevent unnecessary prolongation of surgery and anesthesia, to assure that all indicated surgery is completed, to avoid complications, and to facilitate patient comfort. Pressure points should be padded well to reduce the risk of nerve injury. Surgeon comfort and convenience is also important. This last goal is not a frivolous one. Endoscopic procedures can be long, complex, and tedious. Patient risk increases if the location or paucity of equipment leads to frustration and/or increased operating time.

If uterine pathology had been suggested by the hysterogram, those x-rays should be reviewed prior to the surgery. They also should be in the operating room if correlation with the hysteroscopic findings is necessary during surgery.

EQUIPMENT AND OPERATING ROOM CONFIGURATION

Obtaining and assembling all equipment as well as properly configuring the patient, the anesthetist, the surgeon(s), the equipment, and the monitor(s) assures a smooth operative course even if the procedure is prolonged and/or complicated. The equipment necessary for all hysteroscopic/resectoscopic procedures is listed in Table 1. If the diagnosis is known with a fair degree of certainty prior to surgery, only those items that are likely to be needed should be opened prior to commencement of the procedure. Because the ancillary equipment, such as scissors, grasping forceps, and biopsy forceps, tends to be fragile, more than one of each should be available in the event that a key piece of equipment malfunctions during surgery.

Figure 1 demonstrates the operating room setup for a right-handed surgeon. The surgical technician is to the surgeon's left. This person passes instruments to the surgeon and may infuse uterine-distending medium, e.g., if dextran 70 is infused via hand-held syringes. Irrespective of which medium is used, it should be to the left of the surgeon on the same side as the surgical technician who can monitor infusion pressures and assure that the flow of medium is not interrupted during changeover from one bag to another. With the surgical technician positioned away from the surgeon's dominant hand, he or she may pass instruments conveniently and prevent the inflow and outflow tubing from becoming intertwined with the light and camera cables.

The console for the monitor, camera, light source, cassette recorder, and printer is to the surgeon's right, close to the head of the patient. This location allows the surgeon to keep the screen in the same axis with the patient and the endoscope. This is a much more natural viewing position than if the monitor were closer to the foot of the operating table and off to the side, thereby forcing the surgeon to turn his head away from the patient and the instruments. If the monitor is placed close to the patient's feet, the surgeon may become fatigued, especially during long procedures. The ideal location also allows the surgical technician and anesthetist to view the procedure. If regional or local anesthesia is used, this location allows the patient to see the screen, if she desires, and permits the surgeon to explain the nature of the pathology and procedure as it is being performed.

Placement of a sterile basin to the right of the surgeon provides a convenient location for instruments that he or she may wish to use repetitively. The other instruments are located on the back table for use by the surgical

C. M. March: Department of Obstetrics and Gynecology, University of Southern California School of Medicine, Los Angeles, California 90033.

TABLE 1. *Equipment needed for hysteroscopic/resectoscopic procedures*

Miscellaneous
Bivalve speculum
Vaginal wall retractors
Tenacula
Dilators up to at least 30 french
Polyp forceps
Suture scissors
Sponge forceps
Uterine sound
Small and medium sharp curettes
Kevorkian curette
Long needle driver
Long forceps with teeth
Panoramic Hysteroscope
0° and 30° telescopes
Diagnostic/operating sheaths
Large-diameter tubing
Scissors (2)
Grasping forceps (2)
Biopsy forceps (2)
Aspirating catheters (2)
Tubal cannulation catheters (2)
Resectoscope
Continuous-flow resectoscope
12° telescope
Loop electrodes
Roller electrodes
Inflow tubing
Outflow tubing
Media stand with warming element and infusion pump
Multiple container suction collection apparatus
Video Cart
Halogen light source
Light cable
Video camera
Video monitor
VCR
Printer
Laparoscopy Set
Laparoscope
Trocars
Accessory instruments
Light source and cable
Video camera
Video monitor
VCR
Printer

technician and are arranged according to that person's specifications.

MONITORING FLUID INFUSION AND OUTPUT

During complex and prolonged surgical procedures, it is possible that large volumes of uterine-distending media may be utilized. If excessive amounts of media are infused, fluid overload, electrolyte imbalance, coagulation defects, and hypothermia may occur. Thus it is mandatory that operating room personnel monitor carefully the total volume infused as well as the output. The total input combines both the intravenous infusion and the fluid that cannot be recovered from the peritoneal cavity or from sponges, drapes, etc. The safest interpretation for all such fluid is that it was absorbed intravenously.

If a low-viscosity fluid is used, the outflow tubing is connected to suction which carriers the effluent to a multiple-container collection apparatus, which is placed to the right of the surgeon. This location permits the surgeon, the anesthetist, and the circulating nurse a clear view of the uterine effluent. Fluid balance, including that which was infused intravenously, should be monitored at 15-min intervals. Responsibility for assessing the intake and output is a joint one, but rests primarily with the anesthetist and the circulating nurse, whose attention to this important detail will allow the surgeon to concentrate on the surgery. Thus, it is critical that the same circulating nurse be present for the entire procedure. Experience has shown that whenever too many persons are responsible for recording the fluid balance, none does and complications ensue. If the absorption of large amounts of fluid is detected early during the surgical procedure, furosemide may be administered to reduce the risk of acute fluid overload and to permit continuation of the surgical procedure. Guidelines for fluid overload vary depending on the individual patient, but after 3 L of a low-viscosity fluid or 300 mL of dextran 70 have been absorbed, consideration should be given to terminating the procedure or administering a potent diuretic. Special consideration should be given to the use of dextran 70. Absorption of 200–300 mL has been associated with clotting defects in healthy volunteers (1,2). Thus if major surgery, such as an abdominal myomectomy, is planned to follow immediately after the hysteroscopic examination, extra caution is necessary to reduce the risk of excessive blood loss during the laparotomy.

LAPAROSCOPIC EQUIPMENT

If simultaneous laparoscopy is performed, the monitor for that surgeon is placed at the foot of the table behind the hysteroscopist. This location affords the laparoscopist a more natural viewing angle than if other sites are utilized, thereby facilitating his assisting the hysteroscopist during combined procedures.

HIGHLIGHTS

Hysteroscopy has come a long way over the past two decades. Brief diagnostic studies have now been comple-

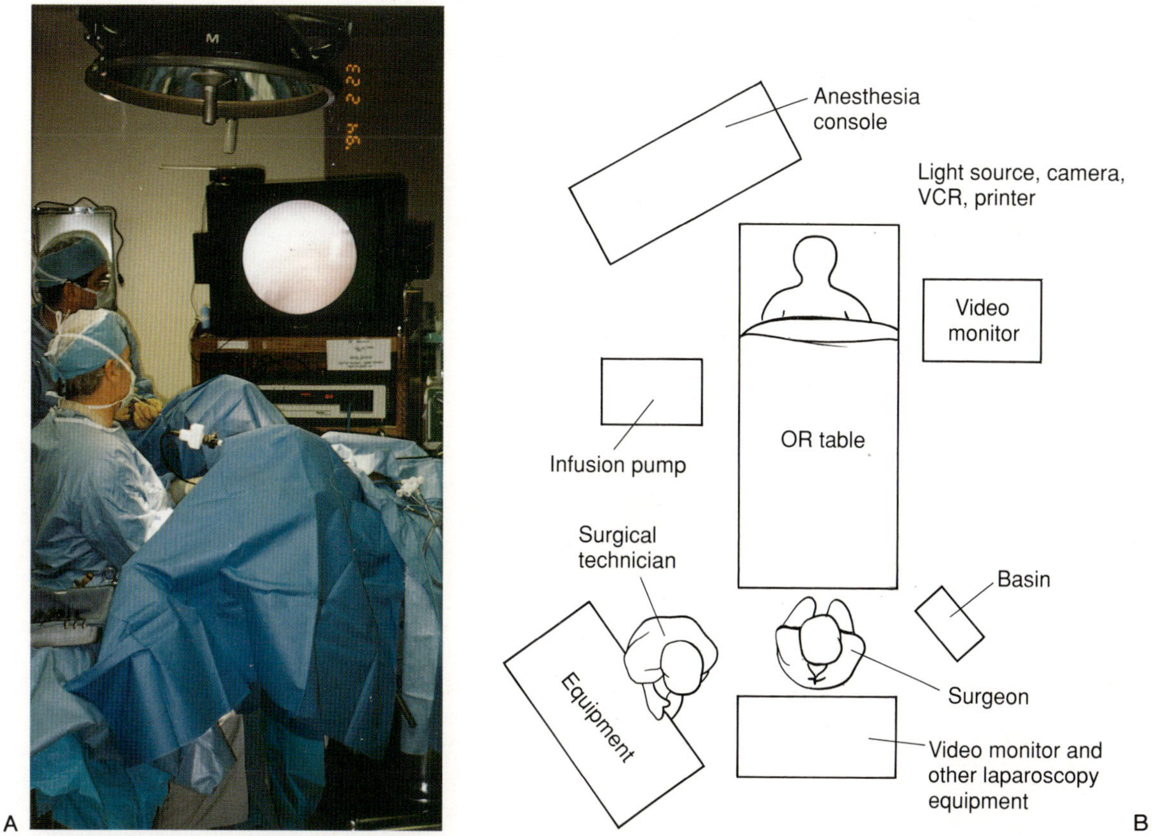

FIG. 1. A: Operating room setup for hysteroscopy with laparoscopy. **B:** Ideal hysteroscopy operating room setup for a right-handed surgeon.

mented by complex and time-consuming operative procedures. Their safe and expeditious completion requires careful preoperative planning, including the proper arrangement of personnel and equipment in the operating room.

REFERENCES

1. Jedeikin R, Olsfanger D. Disseminated intravascular coagulopathy and adult respiratory distress syndrome: life-threatening complications of hysteroscopy. *Am J Obstet Gynecol* 1990;162:44–45.
2. Cronberg S, Robertson B, Nilsson IM, et al. Supressive effect of dextran on platelet adhesiveness. *Thromb Diath Haemorrh* 1966;16:384–392.

Endoscopic Management of Gynecologic Disease,
edited by G.D. Adamson and D.C. Martin.
Lippincott-Raven Publishers, Philadelphia © 1996.

CHAPTER 28

Preoperative Patient Preparation, Clinical Investigation, and Diagnostic Imaging for Hysteroscopy

Brian M. Cohen, Stephen A. Agatson, and Cynthia Sherry

PATIENT SELECTION

Indications for hysteroscopy—both diagnostic and operative—are listed in Table 1. These diagnostic indications occasionally apply on an emergency basis.

Where operative hysteroscopy is contemplated, it is preferable to commence and complete the procedure in the operating room where the necessary equipment is available, thereby affording the patient a single operative procedure.

CONTRAINDICATIONS TO HYSTEROSCOPY

Contraindications to hysteroscopy are few but include the possibility of active infection and heavy bleeding where technical difficulties preclude completion of the procedure in a clinically effective manner. In the case of gross cervical hypoplasia and stenosis, it may not be possible to dilate the cervix adequately to complete an operative hysteroscopy procedure. In these patients, diagnostic hysteroscopy with a smaller diameter hysteroscope is often accomplished. It may not be possible to dilate the cervix adequately without incurring the risk of cervicoisthmic rupture. The therapeutic procedure therefore may require laparotomy and hysterotomy.

In the case of extensive intrauterine pathology necessitating major dissection, particularly large fibroids or thickened, ischemic uterine adhesions, monitoring the procedure by laparoscopy is essential to prevent and diagnose possible uterine perforation. Where endometrial ablation is contemplated, prior diagnostic hysteroscopy, curettage, and adequate endometrial sampling together with confirmed negative Pap smears are all essential to minimize the theoretical risk of burying pathologic tissue within the healing fibrotic layer of the endometrial cavity.

CONDITIONS TO BE FULFILLED PRIOR TO HYSTEROSCOPY

The patient should be in excellent medical health and free of any infection or possible carcinomatous condi-

TABLE 1. *Indications for hysteroscopy*

1. Assessment of possible congenital uterine anomalies
2. Uterine synechiae
3. Hypomenorrhea
4. Abnormal uterine bleeding, including menorrhagia and irregular vaginal bleeding
5. Uterine enlargement and possible tumor formation, including polyps, fibroids, adenomyosis, possible uterine endometrial hyperplasia and carcinoma
6. Possible intrauterine foreign bodies: primarily intrauterine devices, but also retained foreign objects, e.g., cotton buds or catheters.

B. M. Cohen: Department of Obstetrics and Gynecology, The University of Texas Southwestern Medical School, National Fertility Center of Texas, Dallas, Texas 75230.

S. A. Agatson and C. Sherry: Department of Radiology, Presbyterian Hospital of Dallas, Dallas, Texas 75231.

tion, and there should be no extensive vaginal bleeding. Preoperative assessment includes confirmation of a negative Pap smear, an afebrile patient, and one in whom chlamydial and gonococcal cultures are negative and endometrial biopsy is free of carcinoma. A normal, complete blood count and sedimentation rate are reassuring. When hysteroscopy is carried out for infertility, the procedure should be undertaken in the midproliferative phase at about day 8 in a 28-day menstrual cycle. This affords definition of the total endometrial cavity when the endometrium is relatively thin, permits easy visualization of the tubal cornu with minimal enlarged endometrial cushioning of this area and facilitates tubal cannulation in a simple fashion. Such cannulation may be diagnostic or therapeutic as the salpingoscope can be introduced and/or various catheter dilatation of cornual isthmic obstructions can be completed.

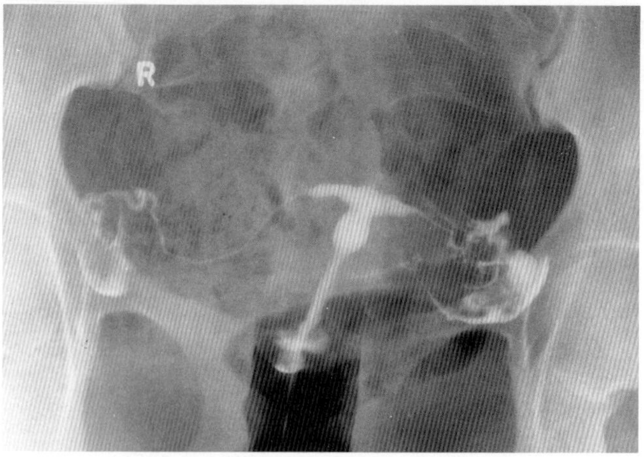

FIG. 1. T-shaped uterus. Diethylstilbestrol exposure frequently results in a narrowed lower segment, flared cornua, and small cavity.

A 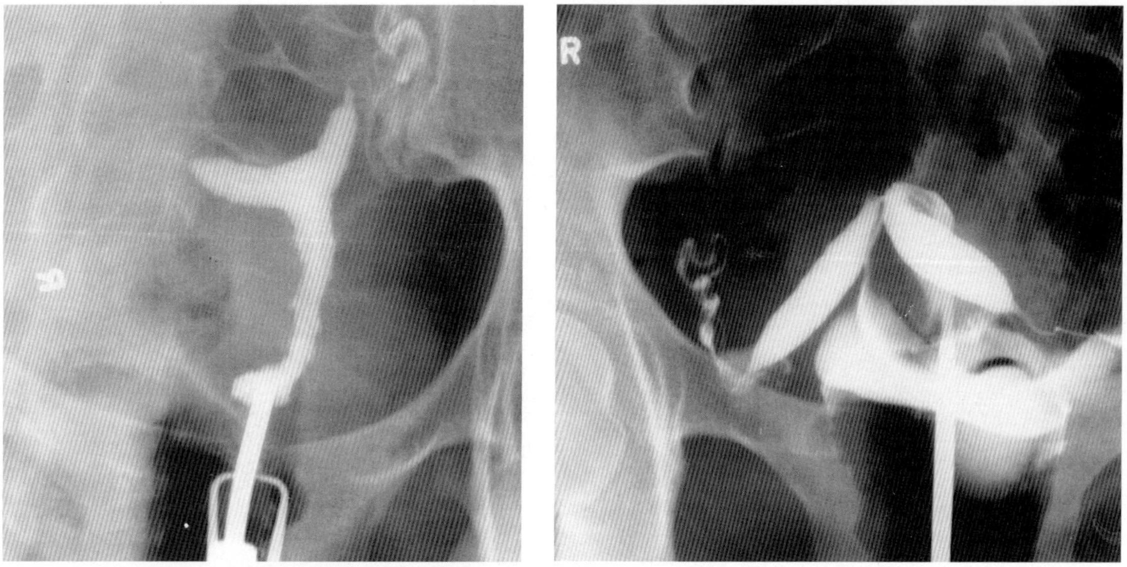 B

C 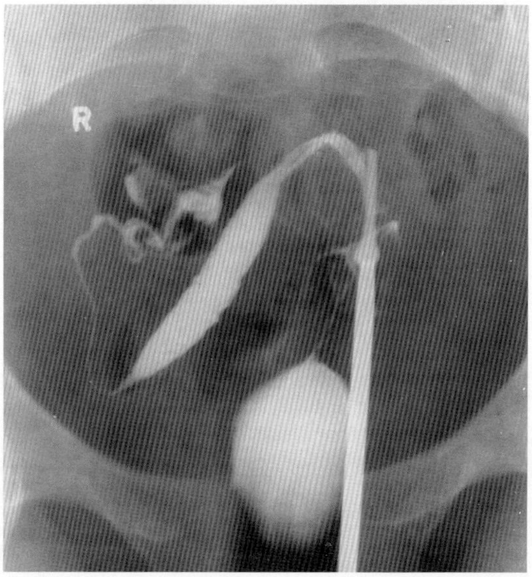

FIG. 2. A: Subseptate uterus. A V-shaped deformity of the fundal aspect of the uterine cavity is indicative of an incomplete uterine septum. **B:** Bicornuate uterus. Two separate uterine horns converge to join at the cervix. **C:** Unicornuate uterus. This rare anomaly results from faulty development of the contralateral müllerian system.

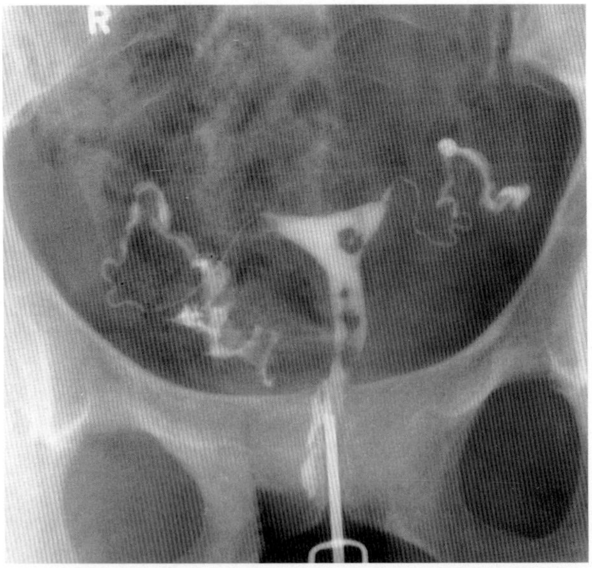

FIG. 3. Uterine synechiae. Irregular filling defects caused by adhesions are usually multiple and represent areas where the uterine cavity has been obliterated by scars.

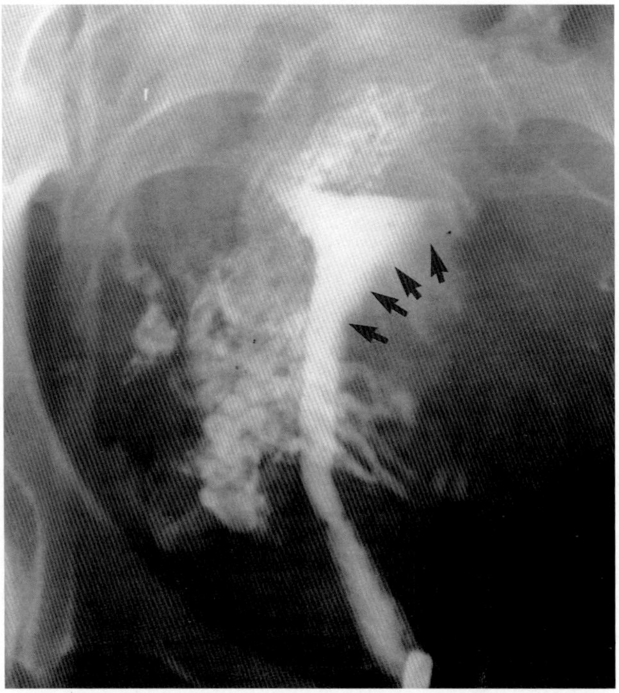

FIG. 5. Intramural fibroid. A large intramural fibroid deforms the left lateral contour of this uterine cavity. Although the pressure of injection results in intravasation, the left cornu cannot be fully opacified because of the extrinsic mass.

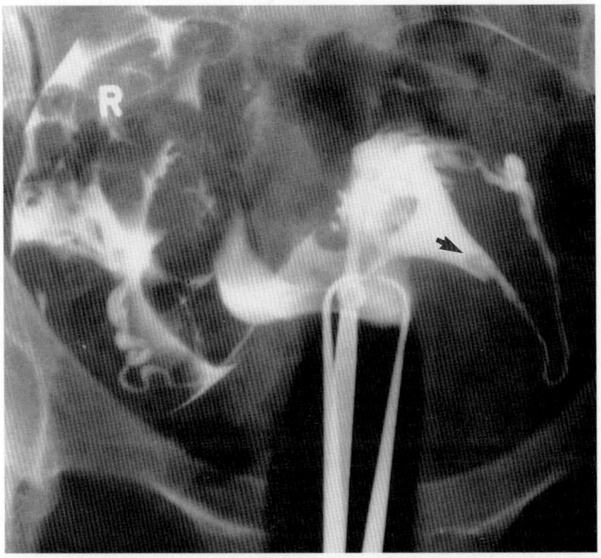

FIG. 4. Endometrial polyps. Polyps are well circumscribed, rounded, filling defects. Because of their small size, they are easily obscured by moderate amounts of contrast.

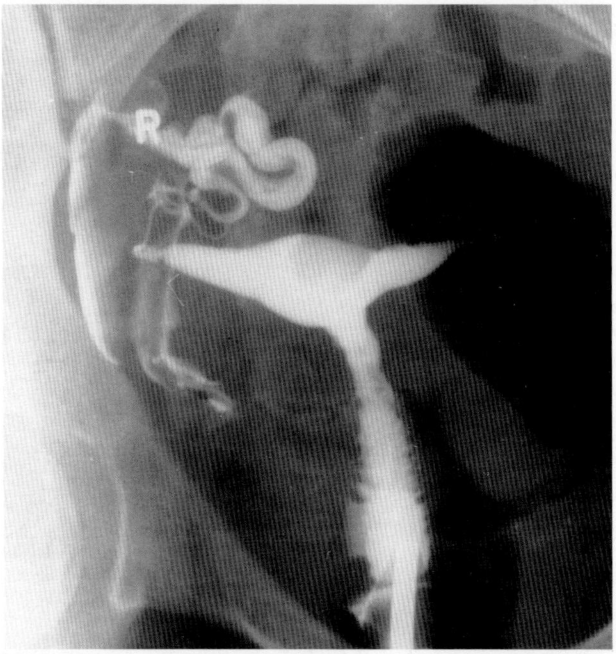

FIG. 6. Submucosal fibroid. Myoma arising from the left fundal wall produces a rounded, filling defect. The uterine cavity is slightly enlarged.

DIAGNOSTIC IMAGING PRIOR TO HYSTEROSCOPY

The diagnosis of intrauterine pathology, which provides indications for diagnostic and operative hysteroscopy, usually are obtained at hysterosalpingography or vaginosonography.

THE HYSTEROSALPINGOGRAM

Detailed assessment of the uterine cavity is accomplished by use of a cannula placed at the entrance of the cervix such that the total cervical canal, uterine isthmus, and fundus can all be visualized. Placement of intrauterine catheters for hysterosalpingography usually excludes a significant segment of the lower uterus and/or one of the uterine cornual areas, so that catheter placement is not considered a favorable technique when total uterine cavity assessment is necessary. A minimal amount of contrast material (2–4 ml) should be injected slowly. If a cavity defect is noted and there is difficulty visualizing detail, oil contrast medium should be used and/or some

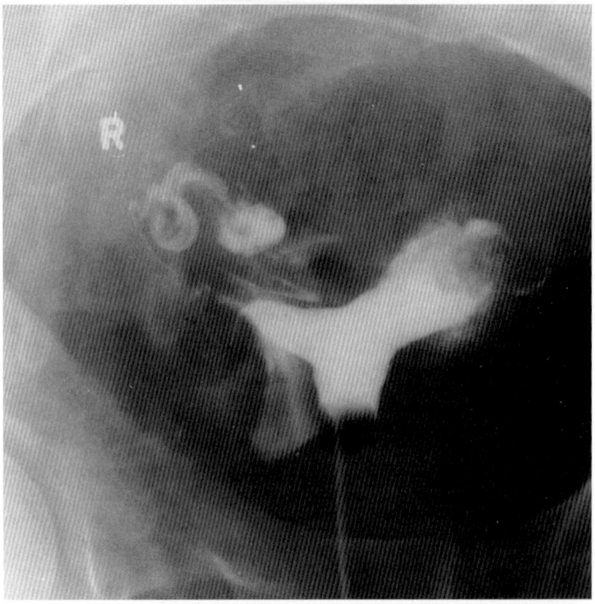

FIG. 7. Uterine vascular malformation. There is mass-like enlargement of the left cornu with several serpiginous filling defects. A halo of intravasation surrounds the hemangioma.

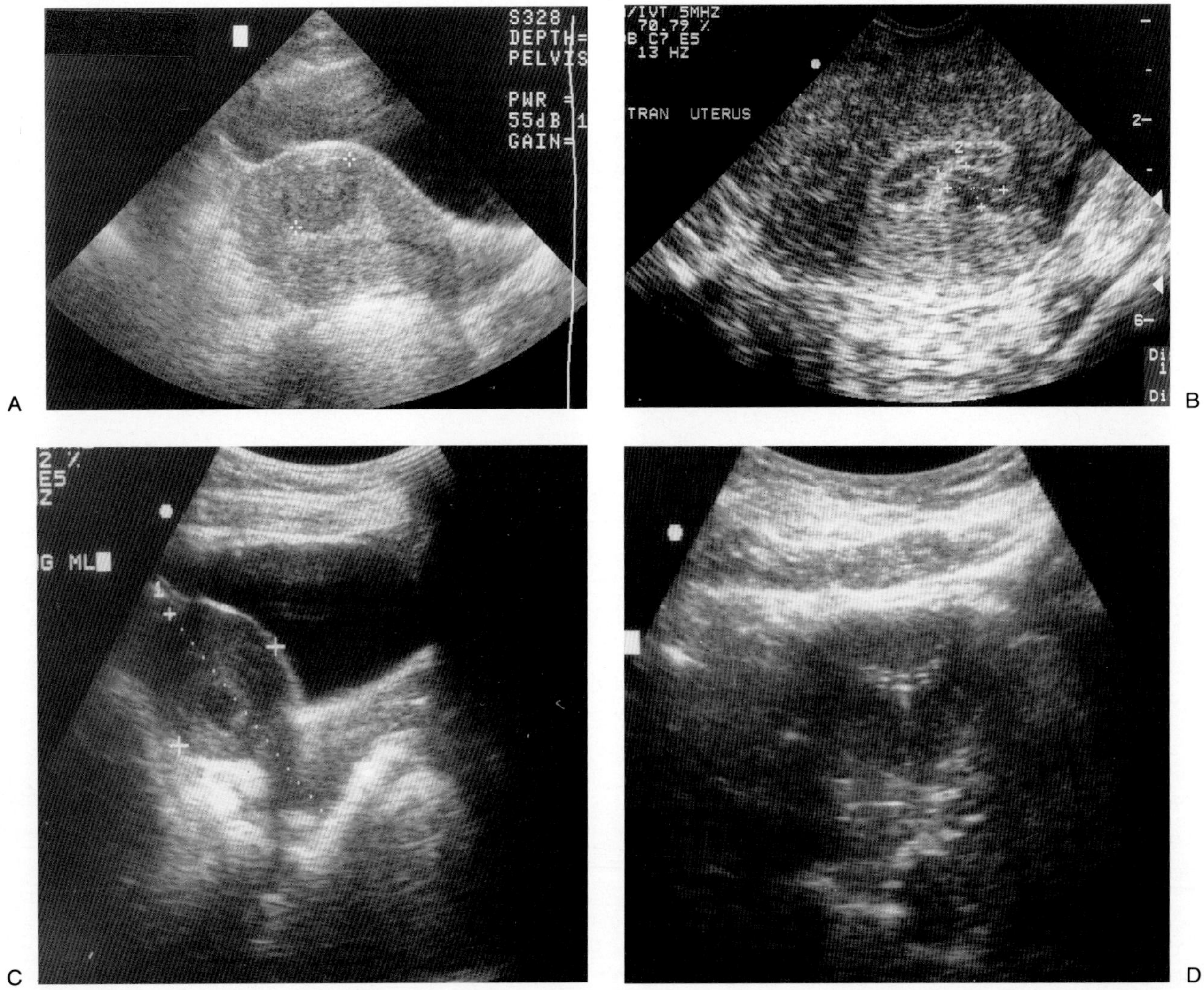

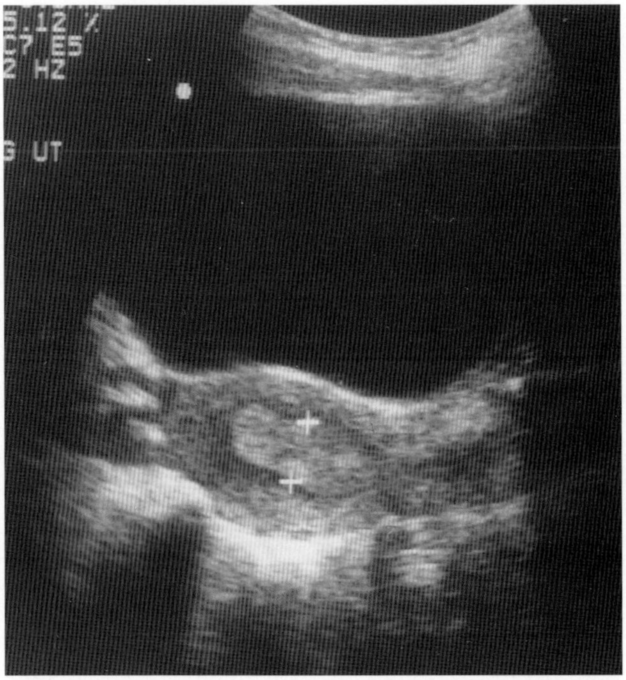

FIG. 9. Hyperplasia. The endometrium is hyperechoic and thick.

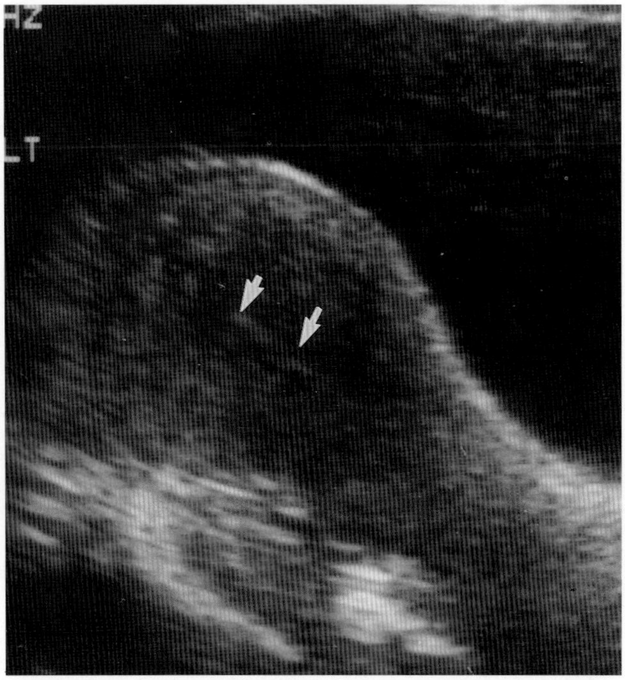

FIG. 10. Hypoplasia. The endometrial stripe is thin and nearly isoechoic with the myometrium.

carbon dioxide added to provide a double-contrast assessment of the uterine cavity. The classical diethylstilbestrol (DES)–exposed uterus may have many configurations but is classically T-shaped (Fig. 1).

The subseptate and/or bicornuate uterus (Figs. 2A and 2B, respectively) may have a very similar appearance. In such cases the need for laparoscopy at the time of operative hysteroscopy is essential to ensure that the uterine fundus is compatible with a uterine septum and not a bicornuate uterus. The unicornuate anomaly is easily diagnosed on a hysterogram (Fig. 2C).

Intrauterine synechiae present as partial or near total obliteration of the uterine cavity (Fig. 3). Intrauterine polyps present as small space-occupying masses within the uterine cavity (Fig. 4). Common locations are cervical and pericornual. Uterine fibroids present as gross distortions of the uterine cavity when intramural (Fig. 5) and as space-occupying masses when submucosal or intracavitary (Fig. 6).

Uterine carcinoma and other neoplasms can be seen as space-occupying masses within the cavity or associated with obvious intravasation resulting from neovascularization (Fig. 7). Foreign bodies, such as intrauterine devices (IUDs), present with their typical shadowing as assessed on the x-ray.

ASSESSMENT AT SONOGRAPHY

Sagittal and transverse scans of the uterus and detailed examination of the endometrial cavity may reveal myometrial fibroids and polyps, foreign bodies, and space-occupying masses (Fig. 8A–D). The presence of abundant echogenic endometrium in the postmenopausal patient (Fig. 9) suggests endometrial hyperplasia and indicates hysteroscopy and dilatation and curettage, especially if it is focal or irregular.

The absence of endometrial growth and a transcavity diameter of less than 4 mm throughout the endometrium usually excludes significant uterine pathology (Fig. 10), such as endometrial carcinoma. Detailed examination of the pelvis, including fluid in the cul-de-sac, and/or presence or absence of ovarian cystic masses (Fig. 11A,B) can contribute to the diagnosis of endometriosis and benign and malignant ovarian tumors where the intrauterine pathology may be of a secondary nature. The use of serum CA-125 to assess the possible nature of the lesion is always helpful and essential in alerting one to the possibility of carcinoma particularly in the nonendometriosis, postmenopausal patient.

FIG. 8. A: Intramural fibroid. Rounded mass in the anterior corpus is hypoechoic compared with the myometrium. Although slightly inhomogeneous, there is no calcification or necrosis. The endometrium is displaced. **B:** Submucosal fibroid. A large portion of this leiomyoma protrudes into the endometrial cavity. **C:** Adenofibroma. This hypoechoic polypoid tumor expands the endometrial cavity. **D:** Intrauterine device (IUD). The echogenic limbs of this T-shaped device are easily recognized.

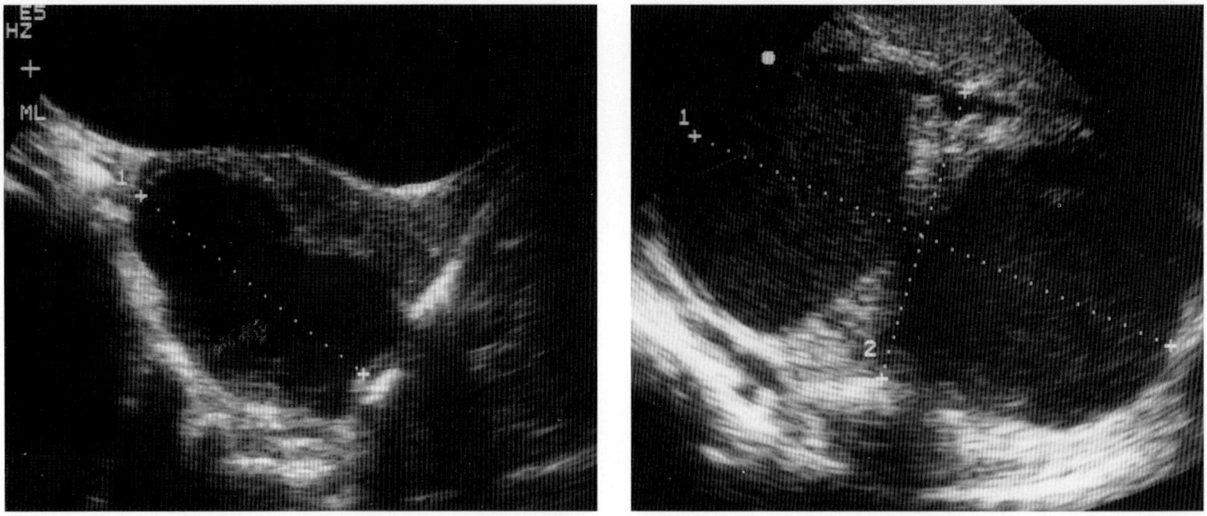

A B

FIG. 11. A: Endometrioma. Transvesicle sonography shows a lobulated adnexal mass that appears to be a simple cyst. **B:** Endovaginal sonography of the same mass reveals low-level homogeneous echoes incompatible with a simple cyst and more suggestive of the true diagnosis, endometrioma.

HIGHLIGHTS

Indications for hysteroscopy are based on the clinical history, examination, and diagnostic imaging that define lesions of a congenital, postinflammatory, or postadhesive nature. Tumors that may be benign or malignant together with the possibility of a foreign body in the uterine cavity may all be defined. These diagnoses are arrived at by detailed history, thorough examination, and the use of vaginosonography and hysterography. The use of serum assays, CA-125, and assessment of normal blood count and sedimentation rates, together with the exclusion of any infection, such as chlamydia, are all important preoperative requisites.

The ability to visualize the cervical canal, isthmus, and inner uterus at hysteroscopy provides detail and accuracy of the morphologic changes present. Selective biopsy, excision, or curettage allows one to obtain the pathology specimen for histologic confirmation.

PART V

Surgical Technique: Hysteroscopy

Endoscopic Management of Gynecologic Disease,
edited by G.D. Adamson and D.C. Martin.
Lippincott-Raven Publishers, Philadelphia © 1996.

CHAPTER 29

Intrauterine Adhesions

Charles M. March

DEFINITION, PREVALENCE, AND PATHOPHYSIOLOGY

Intrauterine adhesions (IUAs) are avascular bands that fuse the anterior and posterior uterine walls together. They may be isolated bands or broad confluent bridges. Although intrauterine adhesions were described initially by Fritsch in 1894, this condition received widespread attention only after the reports by Asherman of the syndrome that bears his name (1,2). Unfortunately, even after these reports, most physicians did not consider the condition to be a common one. This philosophy persists today despite many reports to the contrary (Table 1).

There are three common etiologies for the development of IUAs. The most common antecedent factor is curettage of the pregnant or recently pregnant uterus. Almost 40% of the patients with IUAs and who have been referred to this medical center have had an elective termination of pregnancy (3). Patients may also develop synechiae following curettage performed because of spontaneous abortion. It appears that those women who have had missed abortions are at greatest risk among all patients in the abortion category. In one study, the frequency of IUAs was 6.4% among those who had undergone curettage because of an incomplete abortion, but the rate rose to 30.9% if the precurettage diagnosis was a missed abortion (4).

Another common etiology for the subsequent development of IUAs is the presence of endometritis. Endometritis may be the sole cause of IUAs in patients who have tuberculous infection of the endometrium. However, the presence of other types of bacterial infection increases the risk for the development of adhesive disease in patients who have had either endometrial curettage or uterine surgery. Despite the opinion of Rabau and David that infection is present in all cases of traumatic amenorrhea, few of the more than 300 patients we have treated had any clinical evidence of infection and none of these women had only a curettage (5). Claims that subclinical infection is present can be neither supported nor refuted. The same is true for lower uterine or cervical reflexes leading to poor vascular perfusion and amenorrhea.

A final antecedent factor for IUAs is previous uterine surgery. Adhesions have been noted following cesarean sections, hysterotomies, myomectomies, metroplasties, and diagnostic curettages. The routine dilation and curettage performed at the time of laparoscopy for the infertile woman serves no purpose and may be harmful. Thus, it should be abandoned unless clinically indicated. An endometrial biopsy provides an adequate sample for assessing the endometrial response to estradiol and progesterone.

The common denominator for the development of IUAs in all of these conditions is endometrial trauma, which includes damage to the basalis layer. Additive factors in the patient who has been pregnant are tetanic uterine contractions, which maintain the anterior and posterior walls in close apposition, and the low levels of estradiol that are present immediately following pregnancy. Because the levels of estradiol are low, the stimulus to endometrial regeneration is reduced markedly. Lactation maintains hypoestrogenism for a longer period and increases the risk of IUA development following a postpartum hemorrhage and curettage. The uterus is most vulnerable to injury between the second and fourth weeks after delivery (6). Perhaps estrogen therapy and placement of a splint would reduce the frequency of IUA formation after a curettage following delayed postpartum hemorrhage, but no data are available.

The adhesive bands bridge the anterior and posterior uterine walls. Following curettage, white blood cells infiltrate the endometrial surface and are replaced by fi-

C. M. March: Department of Obstetrics and Gynecology, University of Southern California School of Medicine, Los Angeles, California 90033.

TABLE 1. *Frequency of intrauterine adhesions in various conditions*

Condition	%	Ref.
Amenorrhea	1.7	14
Infertility	4	15
Incomplete abortion	6.4	4
Recurrent abortion	39	13
Elective abortion	13	16
Any postpartum hemorrhage	3.7	17
Late postpartum hemorrhage	23.4	6
Missed abortion	30.9	4

broblasts. Hamoù et al. performed microhysteroscopy in patients who developed IUAs after postpartum curettage (7). Adhesions were thin, vascular strands initially. As they matured, the adhesions became thicker and more fibrous. The final product is an avascular, fibrous bridge of variable width and length that maintains the uterine walls in apposition (Fig. 1). In some patients, endometrial trauma is followed by amenorrhea, but adhesions do not form. Patients with this problem (endometrial sclerosis) have had extensive endometrial necrosis, which has left only rare isolated islands of basal cells clinging to the myometrium. In these women, the diagnosis cannot be made by hysterosalpingography (HSG), because the cavity is normal and only hysteroscopy can demonstrate the marked atrophy.

CLINICAL PRESENTATION AND DIAGNOSIS

The key to establishing the diagnosis is a high index of suspicion. All women who have menstrual complaints

TABLE 2. *Symptoms, signs, and tests used to diagnose intrauterine adhesions*

Amenorrhea despite luteal phase activity
Amenorrhea after estrogen-progestin therapy
Difficulty in sounding uterine cavity
Ultrasound
Hysterosalpingography
Hysteroscopy

and/or infertility and who have a history of prior endometrial trauma should be investigated for the presence of IUAs. The following five diagnostic techniques have been used to establish the presence of intrauterine adhesions (Table 2).

Amenorrhea with evidence of luteal phase activity, such as a biphasic basal body temperature graph or an elevated level of serum progesterone is evidence of end-organ failure. However, the same symptoms may occur in patients with cervical stenosis even in the absence of cyclic abdominal pain. Absence of withdrawal uterine bleeding following combined or sequential estrogen-progestin treatment is also evidence of endometrial insufficiency. If this hormone withdrawal test is used, sequential estrogen-progestin therapy is preferable to the use of oral contraceptives because the latter may cause hypomenorrhea or amenorrhea. However, because IUAs may exist in patients with normal menses, neither regimen may be used to rule out the presence of intrauterine synechiae. Difficulty in sounding the endometrial cavity or the impression of an irregular or small cavity also suggests the presence of adhesions. Ultrasound may demonstrate a normal endometrial echo complex in an amenorrheic patient, suggesting cervical stenosis or no endometrial echoes in an amenorrheic pa-

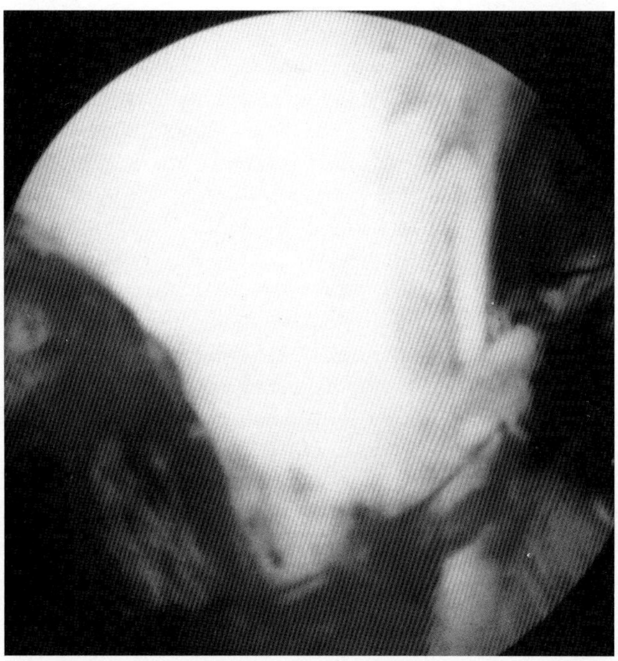

FIG. 1. Hysteroscopic appearance of an intrauterine scar.

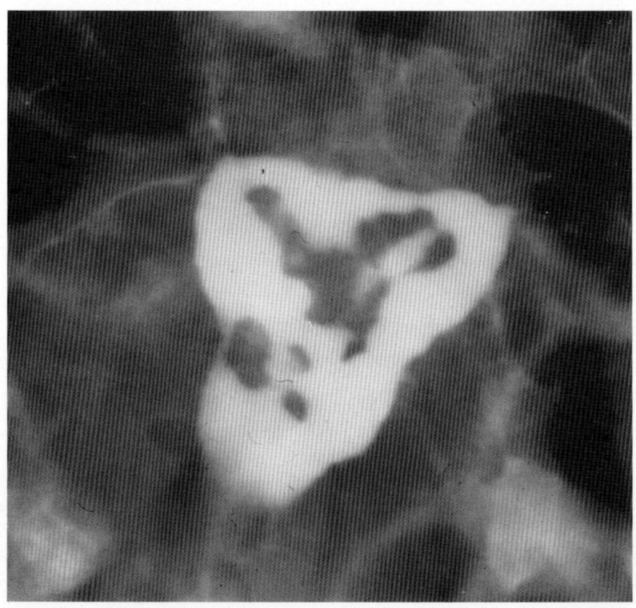

FIG. 2. Characteristic hysterogram in patient with intrauterine adhesions.

Patient's Name ______________________ Date __________ Chart # __________

Age ______ G ______ P ______ Sp Ab ______ VTP ______ Ectopic ______ Infertile Yes ______ No ______

Other Significant History (i.e. surgery, infection, etc.) ______________________

____

HSG ________ Sonography ________ Photography ________ Laparoscopy ________ Laparotomy ________

Extent of Cavity Involved	<1/3	1/3 - 2/3	>2/3
	1	2	4
Type of Adhesions	Filmy	Filmy & Dense	Dense
	1	2	4
Menstrual Pattern	Normal	Hypomenorrhea	Amenorrhea
	0	2	4

Prognostic Classification		HSG* Score	Hysteroscopy Score
Stage I (Mild)	1-4	______	______
Stage II (Moderate)	5-8	______	______
Stage III (Severe)	9-12	______	______

*All adhesions should be considered dense

Treatment (Surgical Procedures): ______________________

____

Prognosis for Conception & Subsequent Viable Infant*

______ Excellent (> 75%)

______ Good (50-75%)

______ Fair (25%-50%)

______ Poor (< 25%)

*Physician's judgment based upon tubal patency.

Recommended Followup Treatment: ______________________

____

Property of
The American Fertility Society

Additional Findings: ______________________

____

DRAWING

HSG Findings

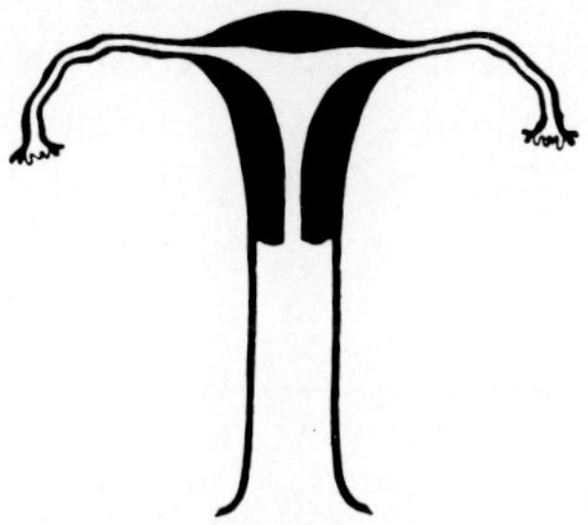

Hysteroscopy Findings

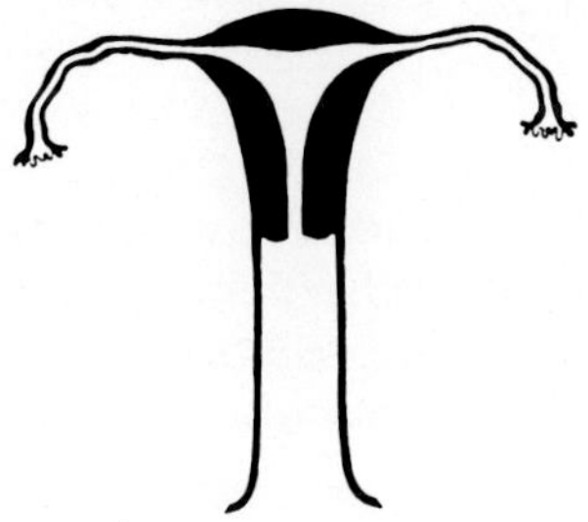

For additional supply write to:
The American Fertility Society
2140 11th Avenue, South
Suite 200
Birmingham, Alabama 35205

FIG. 3. American Fertility Society (now the American Society for Reproductive Medicine) Classification of Intrauterine Adhesions. (From Ref. 9, with permission.)

TABLE 3. *Hysteroscopic classification: Asherman's syndrome*

Severe:	>75% of uterine cavity involved; agglutination of walls and thick bands; ostial areas and upper cavity occluded
Moderate:	25%–75% of uterine cavity involved; walls not agglutinated—adhesions only; ostial areas and upper fundus partially occluded
Minimal:	<25% of uterine cavity involved; filmy adhesions; ostial areas and upper fundus minimally involved or clear

Modified from ref. 10.

tient who has normal ovarian function, suggesting endometrial sclerosis. Hysterosalpingography under fluoroscopic control is the study used most often to establish the presence of adhesions. The finding of lacunar-shaped defects irregularly throughout the cavity strongly supports the impression of IUAs (Fig. 2). Unfortunately, false-positive studies occur and neither the extent nor the exact location of the adhesions can be determined with certainty. Ultrasound with an endovaginal transducer has been used to document the presence of adhesions by visualizing the uterine cavity outlined by saline, which is instilled via a narrow gauge catheter. False-positive studies are common and this technique adds little. However, patients with normal hysterosalpingograms do not have adhesions (8). The definitive diagnostic study is hysteroscopy. Under direct vision the extent and location of the adhesions can be determined with accuracy. These factors together with the density of the adhesions permit the disease to be classified (Table 3, Fig. 3) (9,10).

Patients with IUAs may complain of amenorrhea or hypomenorrhea, infertility, or recurrent abortion. Others conceive and deliver without difficulty but have problems with removal of the placenta. Despite even extensive adhesions, a woman may have painless, spontaneous menses of normal flow and duration. The relation between recurrent abortion and adhesions is difficult to assess. Women with recurrent abortion are frequently diagnosed to have IUAs. However, such a diagnosis might be made only after multiple curettages have been performed; the adhesions, therefore, may be the sequelae to treatment for each loss rather than the cause of recurrent abortion. Moreover, these adhesions may have developed only after the last curettage.

TABLE 4. *Therapeutic principles of managing intrauterine adhesions*

Ends	Means
Restore normal architecture	Hysteroscopic lysis
Prevent readherence	Splint
Promote endometrial overgrowth	High-dose estrogen treatment
Verify cavity normalcy	Hysterosalpingography; hysteroscopy

TREATMENT

Therapy of IUAs is directed to four goals (Table 4). These are restoration of normal uterine architecture, prevention of readherence, stimulation of endometrial regeneration, and verification that the uterus is normal before conception is attempted. To prevent possible complicated pregnancies, treatment should be instituted as soon as the diagnosis is established whether or not the patient wishes to conceive at that time. However, there is no information to suggest that the condition is progressive. If the patient does not wish to conceive she must be cautioned that IUAs cannot be used as a method of contraception, even if she is amenorrheic and has a hysterosalpingogram that suggests total obliteration of the cavity. Contraindications to treatment of IUA are the same as for any hysteroscopy: pelvic infection, pregnancy, and cervical cancer.

The treatment of choice is hysteroscopic lysis of adhesions. This method of therapy is safer and easier than blind disruption of adhesions using a uterine sound or a curette or by hysterotomy. Under direct vision, the surgeon can lyse all the adhesions and not traumatize normal endometrium. A 7-mm or 8-mm panoramic hysteroscope with one or two operating channels is used to inspect the cavity (Fig. 4). The medium used to distend the uterine cavity during hysteroscopy is the viscous 32% solution of dextran with an average molecular weight of 70,000 in 10% glucose in water (Hyskon hysteroscopy fluid). This medium is not miscible with blood and permits the surgeon a clear view of the cavity even after extensive surgery has been performed. Hysteroscopy may be performed under local anesthesia using either meperidine or diazepam for sedation and paracervical block anesthesia. If the dissection is unusually difficult or prolonged, general anesthesia should be used.

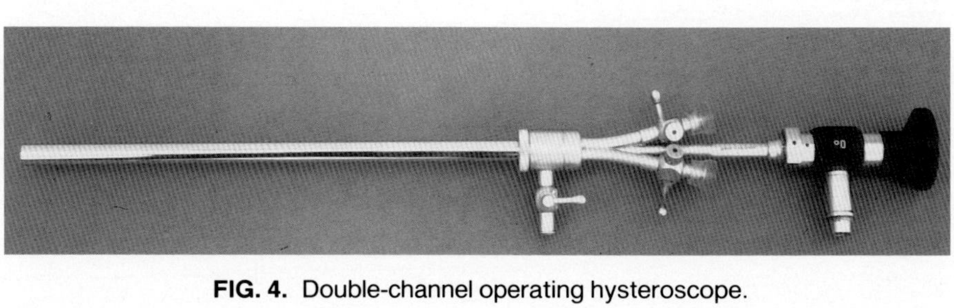

FIG. 4. Double-channel operating hysteroscope.

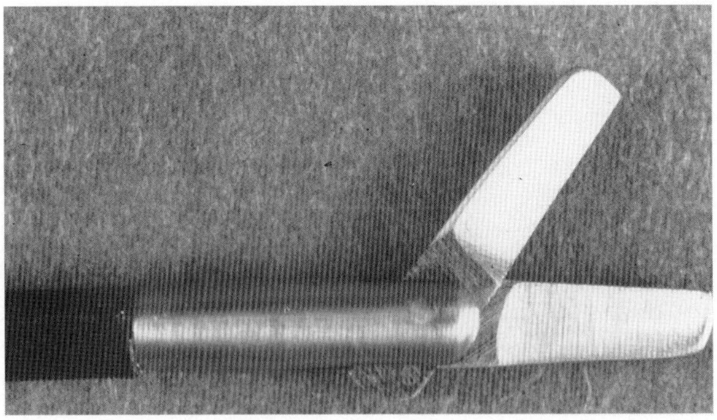

FIG. 5. Flexible scissors used to lyse intrauterine adhesions.

IUAs may be diagnosed definitively and their extent classified (9,10). Prior to beginning adhesiolysis, the surgeon should classify the extent of the disease. Classification of IUAs allows different treatment regimens to be compared. Miniature scissors are used to incise the adhesions (Fig. 5). Scissors produce less trauma than either a laser or electrosurgical knife and are the preferred method of lysing adhesions. In some patients referred to this center, more extensive adhesions have formed after prior treatment with a neodymium:yttrium-aluminum-garnet (Nd:YAG) laser or a resectoscope. Both instruments can cause thermal injury ≥3 mm deep, making them effective for endometrial ablation. However, thermal injury is not desired for intrauterine adhesiolysis, and since these instruments have no advantage over scissor dissection, they have no place in the management of IUAs. Under hysteroscopic guidance, only scar tissue is incised and adjacent normal endometrium is not traumatized (Fig. 6). This tissue becomes a source for endometrial regrowth over the freshly dissected surfaces. Each adhesive band is identified and divided. Restoration of uterine architecture to normal can be achieved even where there is complete uterine obliteration. However, women who have very extensive disease should undergo simultaneous laparoscopy. The laparoscopist guides the hysteroscopist to reduce the risk of uterine perforation. If the intensity of the light source for the laparoscope is reduced markedly, the laparoscopist can detect dissection into the myometrium sooner because the light of the hysteroscope begins to shine through the uterine serosa at a single point. In contrast, after the cavity's configuration has been restored, the uterus has a uniform glow.

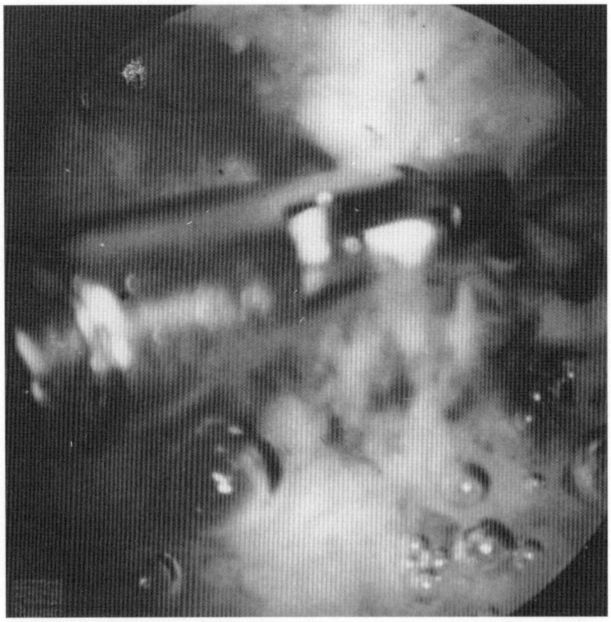

FIG. 6. Adhesion being lysed under hysteroscopic guidance.

Following adhesiolysis as large a loop intrauterine device (IUD) as possible is placed in the cavity and retained for 2 months. Postoperative use of an IUD may reduce the chances that the raw, dissected surfaces readhere. Copper-bearing IUDs or the Progestasert (Alza, Palo Alto, CA) IUD may have too small a surface area to prevent adhesion reformation, and those that contain copper may induce an excessive inflammatory reaction. Therefore their use is not advised. If a loop IUD is not available, an 8-French Foley catheter with a 3-ml balloon can be used. The balloon is inflated, the catheter remains for 1 week, and a broad-spectrum antibiotic is prescribed during that time period. Special silastic uterine splints are also available to maintain separation of the uterine walls (Fig. 7).

Conjugated equine estrogens, 5 mg/day, are given to all patients for 60 days, and medroxyprogesterone acetate, 10 mg, is added during the last 5 days of estrogen therapy. This high-dose steroid regimen stimulates the endometrium maximally to promote reepithelialization of the previously scarred surfaces. The adequacy of therapy should be assessed accurately by repeat hysteroscopy or by hysterosalpingogram following withdrawal bleeding. If the hysterosalpingogram is normal, complete res-

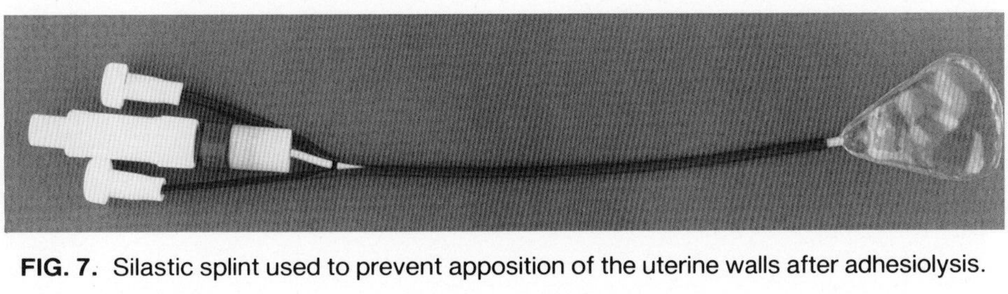

FIG. 7. Silastic splint used to prevent apposition of the uterine walls after adhesiolysis.

olution may be presumed. An abnormal hysterosalpingogram, however, does not definitively indicate persistent adhesions, and hysteroscopy should be repeated.

COMPLICATIONS AND OUTCOME

Complications of this protocol include reactions to the media utilized or to the hormonal agents or anesthetics. Specific complications of the surgery are uterine perforation, hemorrhage, and infection. Simultaneous laparoscopy greatly reduces the risk of perforation or hemorrhage secondary to complete or partial myometrial dissection for the reason described earlier. Infection is a very rare sequela to operative hysteroscopy. Prophylactic antibiotics have not been proven to be efficacious. After one hysteroscopic treatment, 90% of our patients have had normal follow-up hysteroscopies or hysterosalpingograms. Although most of the others have needed only a second procedure to restore normal uterine architecture, a few women have needed three to six operations. Ninety-eight percent of those who had amenorrhea or hypomenorrhea now have normal menses. Therefore, our approach to patients with IUAs is a four-pronged one. The importance of a postoperative study to verify normalcy of the cavity prior to permitting conception cannot be overemphasized. Severe obstetric complications have been reported in patients who conceived prior to having postoperative studies performed to document complete resolution of the adhesions (11). It is likely that these women had persistent disease causing the subsequent obstetric problems.

The pregnancy results are excellent and surpass other types of therapy (12,13). Seventy-five percent of our patients who wished to conceive and who had no other known infertility factors have done so and more than 85% of the pregnancies have been successful. Two patients have had placenta previa and two required manual removal of the placenta. One patient had retained placental fragments, which were detected when a curettage was performed to stop hemorrhage 3 weeks after delivery. Her follow-up hysterosalpingogram had been abnormal, but she conceived before another hysteroscopic procedure was performed. These results are superior to those achieved by outdated treatment modalities, such as blind disruption of adhesions using a uterine sound or a curette.

HIGHLIGHTS

The hysteroscopic approach to IUAs offers complete management: diagnosis, treatment, and follow-up. For each step, the hysteroscopic approach surpasses any and all alternatives. A return to the past cannot be justified.

REFERENCES

1. Asherman JG. Amenorrhoea traumatica (atretica). *J Obstet Gynaecol Br Emp* 1948;55:23.
2. Fritsch H. Ein Fall von volligen Schwund der Gebarmutterhohle nach. Auskratzung. *Zentralbl Gynaekol* 1894;18:1337.
3. March CM, Israel R. Intrauterine adhesions secondary to elective abortion. *Obstet Gynecol* 1976;48:422.
4. Adoni A, Palti Z, Milwidsky A, et al. The incidence of intrauterine adhesions following spontaneous abortion. *Int J Fertil* 1982;27:117.
5. Rabau E, David A. Intrauterine adhesions: etiology, prevention and treatment. *Obstet Gynecol* 1963;22:626.
6. Eriksen J, Kaestel C. The incidence of uterine atresia after postpartum curettage: a follow-up examination of 141 patients. *Dan Med Bull* 1960;7:50.
7. Hamou J, Salat-Baroux J, Siegler AM. Diagnosis and treatment of intrauterine adhesions by microsurgery. *Fertil Steril* 1983;39:321.
8. Fayez JA, Mutie G, Schneider PJ. The diagnostic value of hysterosalpingography and hysteroscopy in infertility investigation. *Am J Obstet Gynecol* 1987;156:558.
9. American Fertility Society. The American Fertility Society classification of adnexal adhesions, distal tubal occlusion, tubal occlusion secondary to tubal ligation, tubal pregnancies, müllerian anomalies and intrauterine adhesions. *Fertil Steril* 1988;49:944.
10. March CM, Israel R, March AD. The hysteroscopic management of intrauterine adhesions. *Am J Obstet Gynecol* 1978;130:653.
11. Jewelewicz R, Khalaf S, Neuwirth RS, Vande Wiele RL. Obstetric complications after treatment of intrauterine synechiae (Asherman's syndrome). *Obstet Gynecol* 1976;47:701.
12. March CM, Israel R: Gestational outcome following hysteroscopic lysis of adhesions. *Fertil Steril* 1981;36:455.
13. Valle RF, Sciarra JJ. Intrauterine adhesions: Hysteroscopic diagnosis, classification, treatment, and reproductive outcome. *Am J Obstet Gynecol* 1988;158:459–470.
14. Jones WE. Traumatic intrauterine adhesions: a report of 8 cases with emphasis on therapy. *Am J Obstet Gynecol* 1964;89:304.
15. Sirbu P, Comen AL, Vexler E. Considerations cliniques sur 20 cas de synechies utereus. *Gynécol Obstet* 1957;56:521–526.
16. Novak F, Andolsek L. The Ljubljana Abortion Study 1971–1973: Comparison of the medical effects of induced abortion by two methods, curettage and vacuum aspiration. NIH Publ. No. 02-039-1.
17. Bergman P. Traumatic intra-uterine lesions. *Acta Obstet Gynecol Scand* (Suppl 4) 1961;40:4.

Endoscopic Management of Gynecologic Disease,
edited by G.D. Adamson and D.C. Martin.
Lippincott-Raven Publishers, Philadelphia © 1996.

CHAPTER 30

Polypectomy and Myomectomy

Philip G. Brooks

PREVALENCE

It is extremely difficult to state with precision the frequency with which endometrial polyps and submucous myomas occur. Because they are most often benign and asymptomatic, their presence usually goes undetected. In a study of women in whom infertility was the indication for hysteroscopy, polyps were discovered in 6–36% of 1034 patients and submucous myomas in 2–22% of 892 patients (1–6). In patients who were asymptomatic but who underwent hysteroscopy for the purpose of inserting intratubal silicone plugs for contraception, Cooper found incidental polyps in four and myomas in five of 323 patients (7). Finally, Townsend, et al. (8) found polyps in 38% and submucous myomas in 48% of menopausal women with uterine bleeding.

CLINICAL FEATURES AND DIAGNOSIS

Endometrial polyps and submucous myomata may be implicated as possible causes of infertility or they may be totally asymptomatic. When they become symptomatic, they most commonly cause abnormal uterine bleeding and usually menorrhagia or menometrorrhagia. Other symptoms can be watery and annoying vaginal discharge and pelvic pain and pressure, the latter depending on the size and location of the tumors. Although the precise mechanism by which intrauterine polyps or myomata cause infertility is unclear, their removal has been reported to reduce reproductive wastage and to increase fertility (9).

Diagnosis of these intrauterine filling defects is suggested by various imaging techniques, such as hysterosalpingography (HSG), ultrasonography, or magnetic resonance (MR). All of these techniques have significant inaccuracy rates and limitations in outlining the three-dimensional characteristics of these lesions. In numerous studies, HSG has been shown to have very high false-positive and false-negative rates (10,11). Both MR and ultrasound can accurately image uterine masses and filling defects, but are unable to differentiate between intracavitary myomas and endometrial polyps (12). In addition, MR and ultrasound cannot define clearly the extent to which the myoma extends into the intrauterine cavity. This is important because a myoma can only be removed hysteroscopically if more than half of it extends into the intrauterine cavity. If less than half of the lesion extends into the intrauterine cavity, laporotomy for myomectomy must be performed. Goldstein reports that the ultrasonographic intracavitary image can be enhanced by instilling a small amount of sterile saline into the endometrial cavity via a 1.8-mm catheter during vaginal sonography (13).

Diagnostic hysteroscopy is the most precise method for diagnosing intrauterine polyps and submucous myomata, and at the same time for assessing the plan for surgical removal hysteroscopically (Figs. 1 and 2). Even dilatation and curettage (D&C), long a standard procedure in the management of abnormal uterine bleeding, is significantly less accurate in detecting polyps and submucous myomata. Gimpelson, in a study comparing the accuracy of diagnostic D&C to that of hysteroscopic biopsy (14), found that the D&C was less revealing in 18% of 342 patients. Brooks found 19 submucous myomata and 4 endometrial polyps in 29 patients undergoing hysteroscopy for persistent bleeding after recent D&C; all were missed during the prior procedure (15).

INDICATIONS AND CONTRAINDICATIONS

As they are almost always entirely benign, endometrial polyps and submucous myomas are usually of no sig-

P. G. Brooks: Department of Obstetrics and Gynecology, UCLA School of Medicine, Cedars-Sinai Medical Center, Los Angeles, California 90048.

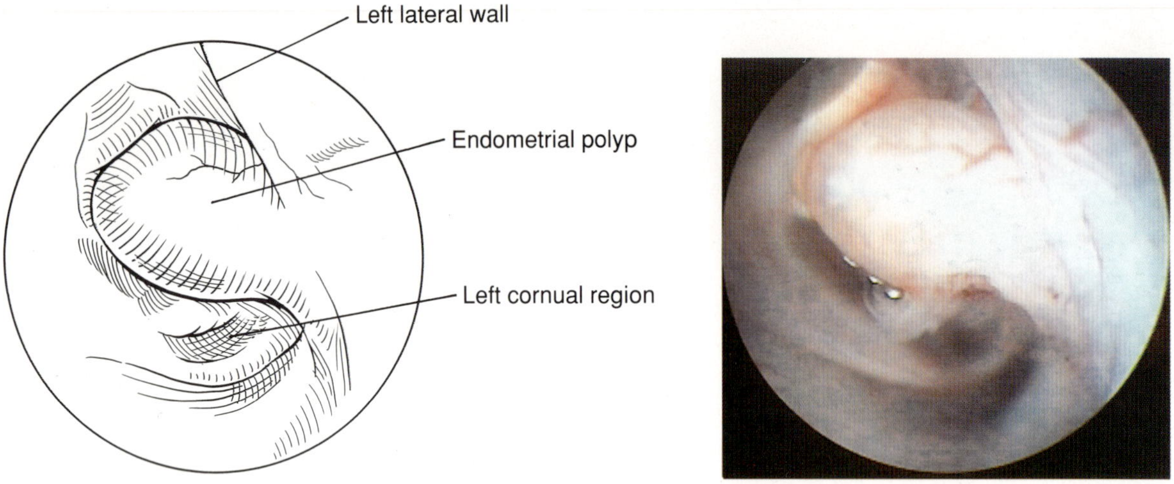

FIG. 1. Endometrial polyp arising from the left lateral wall of the uterus, near the left cornu.

nificant consequence unless they become symptomatic. The major symptom is abnormal uterine bleeding and usually an increase in the intensity and duration of menstrual flow, although intermittent menstrual bleeding often is also present, especially with polyps. Rarely, an increased, watery vaginal discharge that is uncorrectable by the usual vaginal remedies may occur in the presence of intrauterine defects such as these. These symptoms, with or without infertility or repeated pregnancy wastage, bring the patient to her gynecologist and prompt the investigation that results in the diagnosis of polyps or myomas.

When conservation of the uterus is desired, hysteroscopic surgery is the procedure of choice for the treatment of these benign tumors. Contraindications to hysteroscopic management include acute infection, the presence of overt cervical malignancy, medical conditions that contraindicate the use of anesthesias, and a size or configuration of the intrauterine pathology that prevent adequate access transcervically. Although polyps rarely attain sufficient size to make hysteroscopic polypectomy difficult, submucous myomas can become large enough to make the surgery long, tedious, and far more hazardous. In addition, although excessive bleeding often is reduced substantially by partial resection of a sessile myoma, the later regrowth of the myoma or increased extrusion of the residual portion further into the cavity results in a recurrence of symptoms. It is our practice to consider a hysteroscopic approach for removal of sessile submucous myomas only if more than 50% of the tumor protrudes into the endometrial cavity and if it is less than 6 cm in diameter. One should consider an abdominal approach for removal of those lesions not appropriate for hysteroscopic resection.

One way of roughly determining the percentage of the tumor protruding into the cavity is by assessing hysteroscopically the angle between the tumor and the uterine wall. For example, if the angle is greater than 90°, it

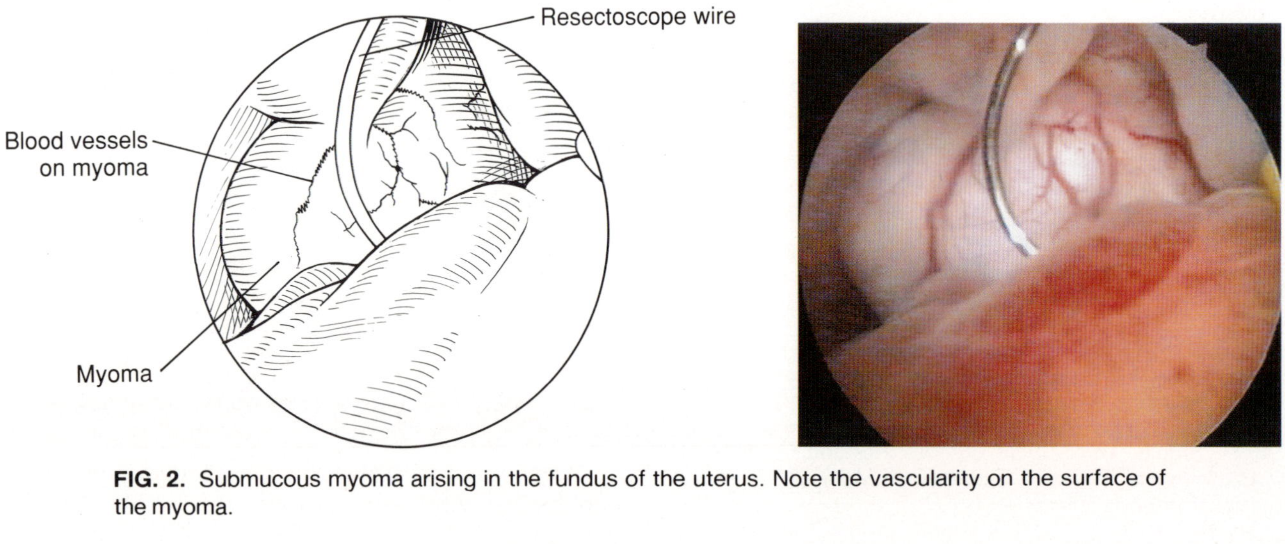

FIG. 2. Submucous myoma arising in the fundus of the uterus. Note the vascularity on the surface of the myoma.

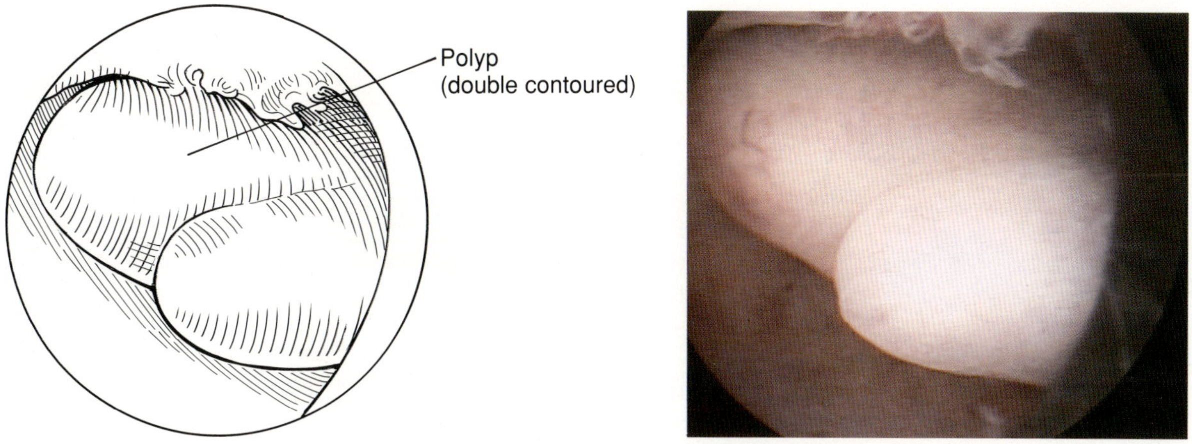

FIG. 3. Double-contoured endometrial polyp.

is likely that the tumor is more intramural than intracavitary.

When the tumor is larger than 5 cm in diameter, it is usually difficult to get the hysteroscope around it and to have adequate room to resect it safely. In such a case, our preference is to attempt to shrink the myoma with the use of a gonadotropin-releasing hormone (GnRH) analog for 3 months prior to resection. Our treatment of choice is leuprolide acetate, depot, 3.75 mg monthly for the 3 months, although nafarelin acetate and buserelin acetate also can be used.

ALTERNATIVE TREATMENT

Alternative treatment of intracavitary myomas and endometrial polyps are hormonal suppression, transabdominal myomectomy, and hysterectomy. Since myomas and, often, endometrial polyps are estrogen-dependent, it is not advisable to use oral contraceptives or estrogen-progesterone regimens for long periods of time to control the bleeding abnormalities caused by these lesions. Hormonal suppression with GnRH analogs generally works well to control bleeding problems, especially for a short time. However, short-term side effects, such as hot flashes, and long-term side effects, such as bone loss, preclude their long-term use. The optimal use of additional medications to avoid these side effects is not yet known.

Transabdominal myomectomy, as stated above, should be considered when more of the myoma is intramural than intracavitary and when the size of the uterus is such that hysteroscopic surgery would be insufficient to correct the uterine condition. In addition, alternative treatment by transabdominal myomectomy should be considered when multiple myomas are present along

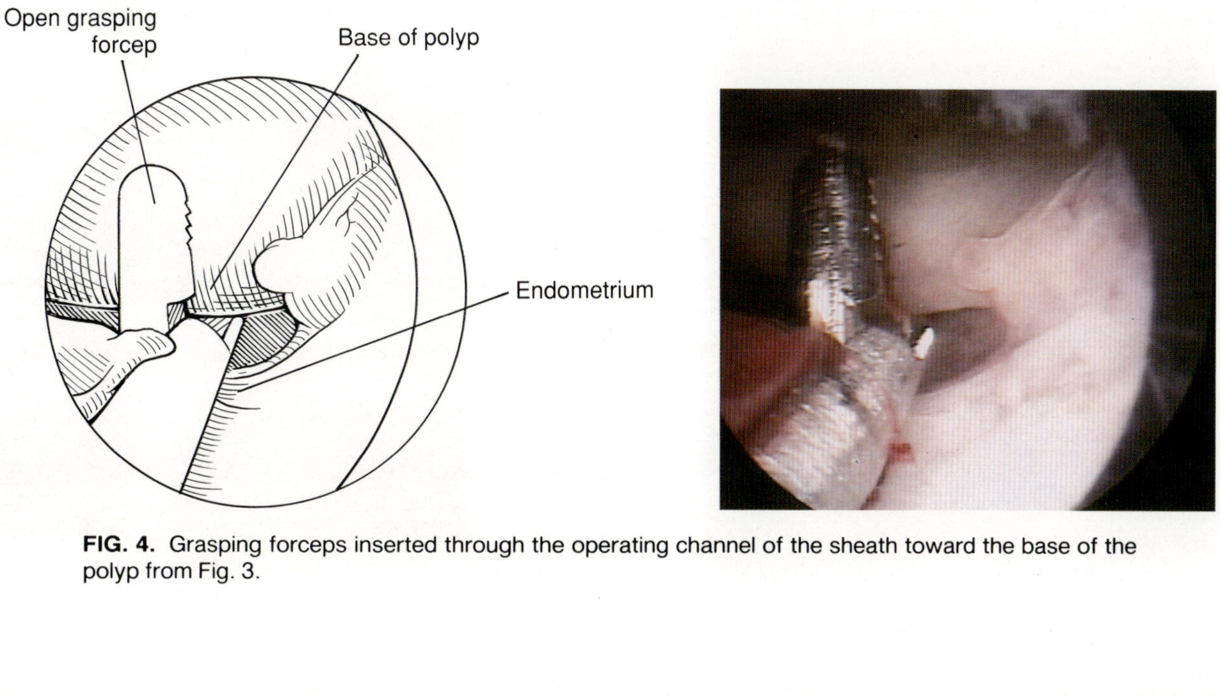

FIG. 4. Grasping forceps inserted through the operating channel of the sheath toward the base of the polyp from Fig. 3.

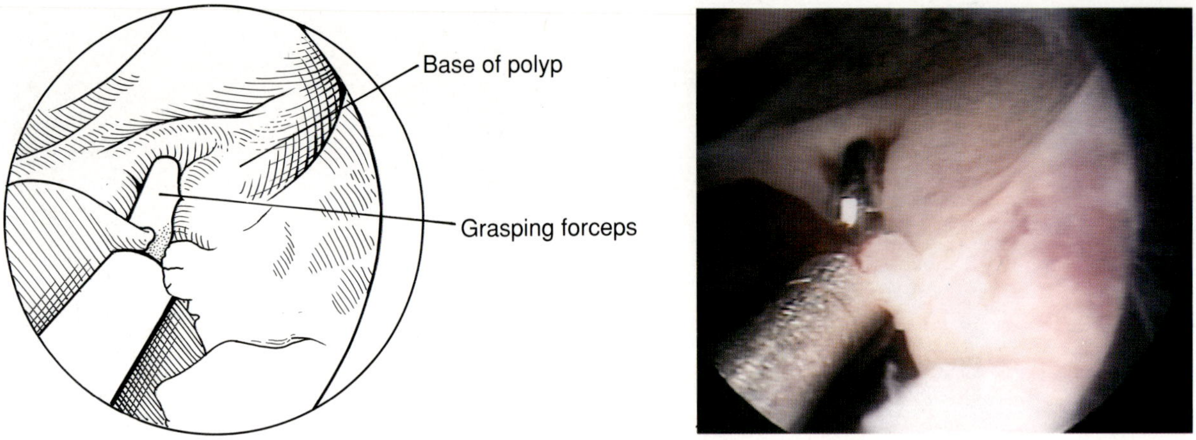

FIG. 5. Grasping forceps is used to bite through the soft and broad base of the polyp from Fig. 3.

with other clinical problems, such as increasing size, pelvic pressure, and pain, such that removal of the intrauterine lesions alone would be insufficient to treat the uterine condition adequately.

SURGICAL TECHNIQUES

In June 1982, the American College of Obstetricians and Gynecologists issued a state-of-the-art commentary on hysteroscopy that contained the following statement: "Clinically applicable therapeutic indications for hysteroscopy include excision of polyps or submucous myomas" (16). No statement of how this could be accomplished with large lesions was included, and since the use of the resectoscope and/or the laser had not yet been reported for these indications, one had to wonder how substantial lesions could be managed. For polyps or small myomas on narrow stalks (Fig. 3), a grasping forceps is inserted through the instrument channel of the operating hysteroscope, or it is passed alongside the sheath if there is no operating channel in the diagnostic hysteroscope that is used. The stalk of the lesion is grasped (Figs. 4 and 5), and the polyp, forceps, and the hysteroscope are removed together through the cervical canal (Figs. 6 and 7). If the cervical canal can be dilated widely enough, grasping instruments or curettes can be inserted blindly into the endometrial cavity to avulse the polyp or myoma. Goldrath (17) reported the use of two or three laminaria initially, then replacement of those with up to six laminaria 6 hr later. This method allowed sufficient dilation of the cervix to grasp pedunculated myomas of up to 5 cm and to twist them off.

Baggish (18), in a small series, reported the use of the neodymium: yttrium-aluminum-garnet (Nd:YAG) laser to vaporize, morcellate, or sever the stalk of intracavitary myomas and leaving the myomas behind to dissolve or be expelled later. Unfortunately, for myomas of substantial size, this technique is slow and tedious and requires experience in the use of laser, which has the economic drawback of being expensive equipment.

Since 1976, as reported by Neuwirth (19), the resecto-

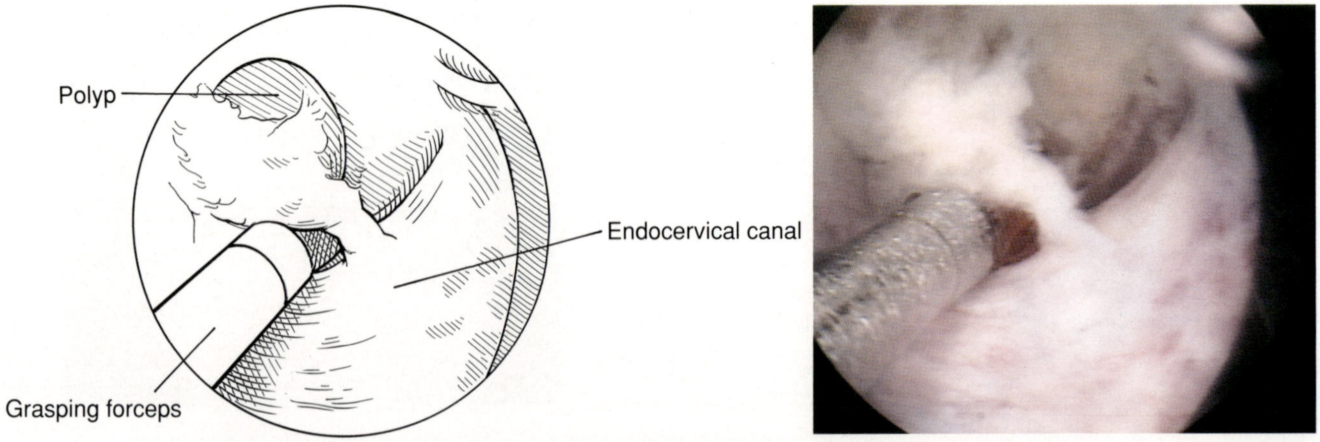

FIG. 6. Grasping forceps and polyp from Fig. 3 are withdrawn through the endocervical canal.

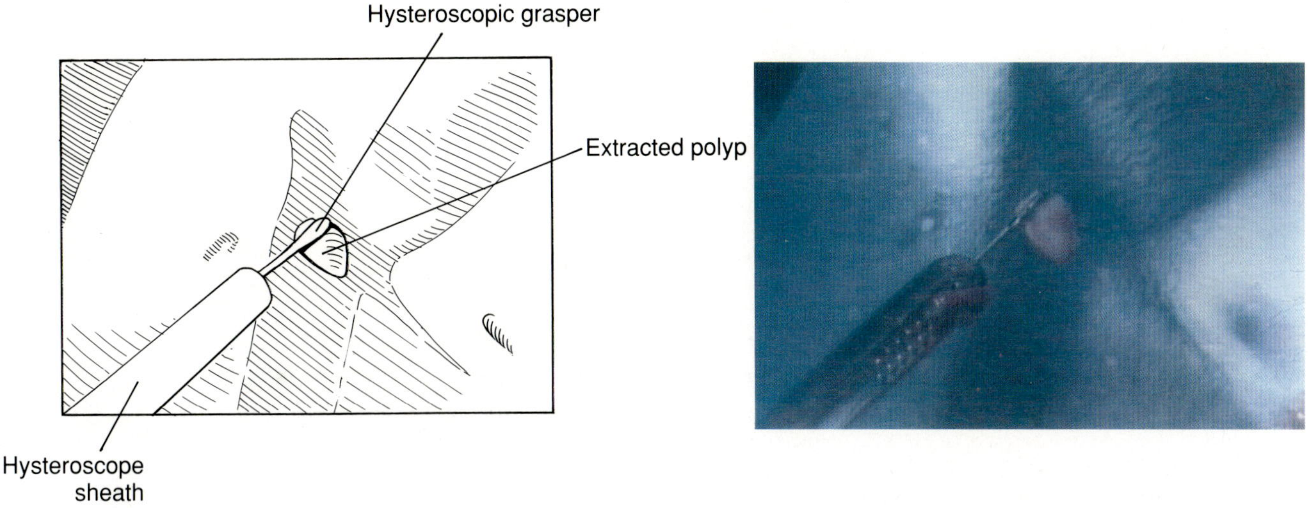

FIG. 7. Extracted polyp still attached to grasping forceps after the entire hysteroscope and operating sheath have been removed from the cervical canal.

scope and electrosurgery have been very successful in morcellating large intracavitary tumors. The standard technique involves the following steps:

1. The patient is placed under light anesthetic, usually a general anesthetic administered by mask. After standard vaginal and cervical preparation, the anterior exocervix is grasped with a tenaculum.
2. For all operative hysteroscopies, and when not contraindicated by medical conditions a small amount (3–4 U total) of vasopressin, diluted 10 U in 20 ml of saline, is injected directly into the cervical stroma in two or three locations. Corson (20), in a prospective, randomized, placebo-controlled study, reported that both blood loss and intravasation of distending media were significantly reduced when vasopressin was used at the beginning of the procedure.
3. The cervix is dilated with Pratt or Hank's dilators up to approximately a 28-French diameter.
4. The resectoscope, usually a 27- or 28-French-diameter instrument, is inserted into the endometrial cavity and the distending medium is instilled. It is essential that, if electrical energy is the power source used to cut through these tumors, the distending media must contain no electrolytes. This ensures that the electricity is concentrated at the tip of the electrode and is not disseminated throughout the medium. The usual distending media include high molecular weight dextran 70 (Hyskon) or low-viscosity fluids, such as sorbitol, glycine, or mannitol.
5. Usually, a pure cutting waveform is used, with the

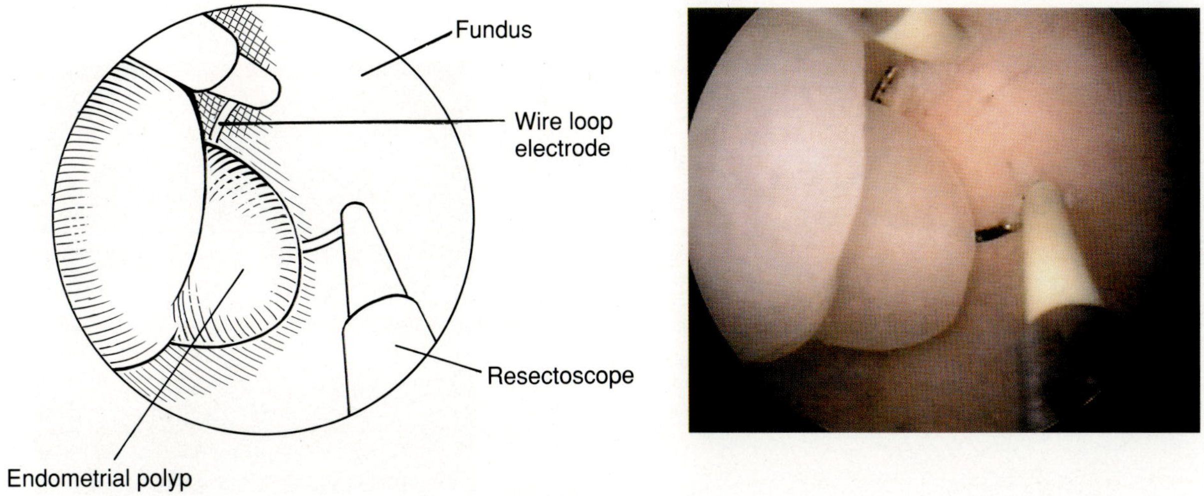

FIG. 8. Endometrial polyp attached to right lateral uterine wall. The resectoscopic wire loop electrode is advanced above the polyp about to be resected.

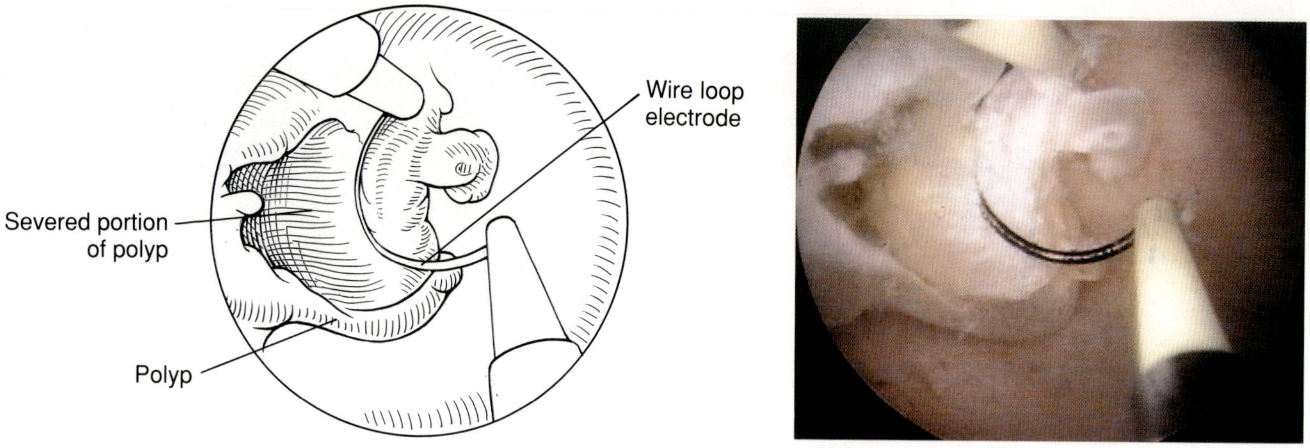

FIG. 9. Appearance of polyp from Fig. 8 after the electrode has shaved through the polyp. Severed portion of polyp is pushed away with the loop.

power setting placed at 90–110 W depending on the size of the electrode and the cutting effect obtained, which can be determined visually.

6. The electrode, usually a 90° wire loop, is extended outward and its tip is placed over the top of the tumor (Fig. 8). For greatest safety, it is mandatory that the current is activated only after the operator starts the movement of the electrode toward himself or herself. The wire loop electrode should glide easily through the tumor, shaving a segment out of the mass (Figs. 9–11).
7. If bleeding points are encountered, they may be fulgurated by placing the electrode tip on or near the bleeding vessel and coagulating the area with a damped (coagulation) current, set at 50–70 W.
8. The remainder of the intracavitary portion of the tumor is shaved with the wire loop electrode until all of the polyp or tumor and its stalk are removed for a pedunculated lesion or down to the concavity of the myometrial surface for a sessile lesion.
9. Either during the procedure, when the pieces of shaved tumor (chips) become so abundant as to interfere with visualization or at the end of the procedure, these chips are removed with a grasping forceps, such as a ring or ovum forceps or a myoma-grasping forceps.
10. The endometrial cavity is reinspected (Fig. 12) for additional tumor that can be resected or for bleeding points to be coagulated, and the instruments are removed.

The resection of pedunculated, submucous myomas and polyps is fairly straightforward: the procedure involves complete removal of the entire lesion and its stalk (Figs. 13–15). However, it is a little more complex when the myoma is partly intramural (Fig. 16). Because of the

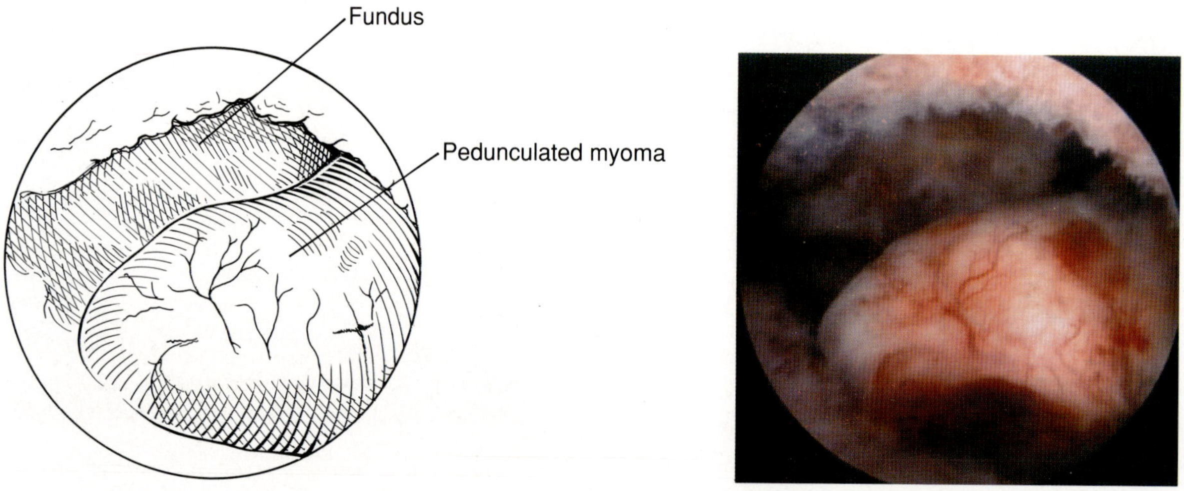

FIG. 10. Pedunculated submucous myoma attached to the left posterior surface of the lower uterine segment.

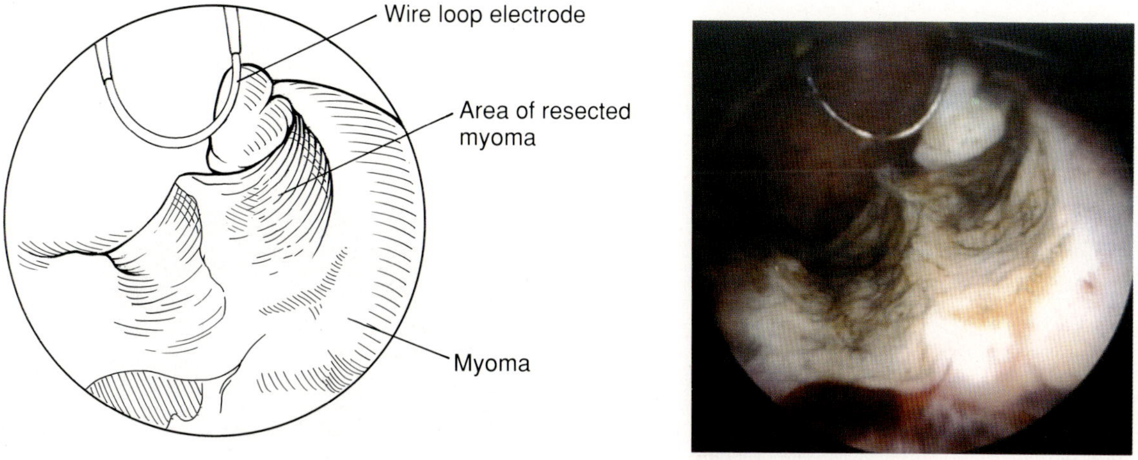

FIG. 11. Myoma from Fig. 10 after several passes of the electrode.

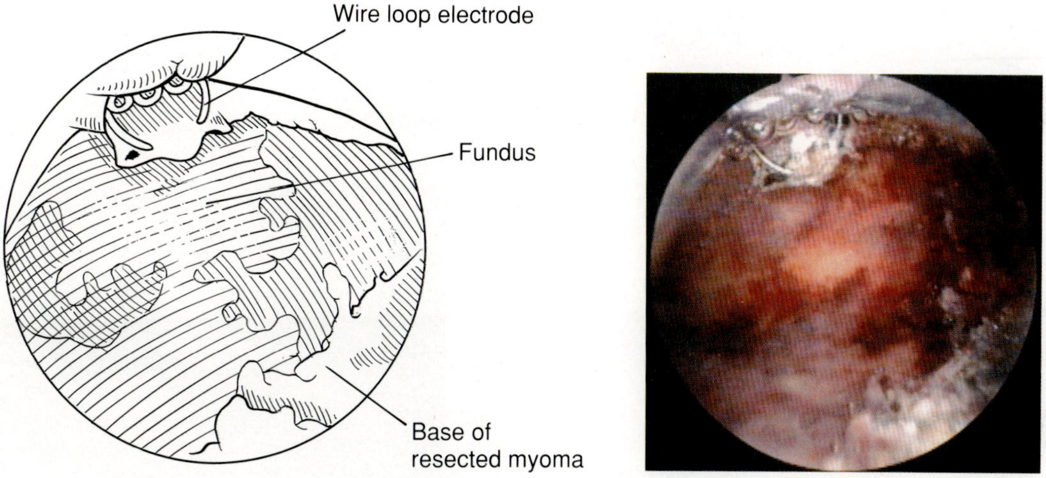

FIG. 12. Endometrial cavity after complete resection of the myoma from Fig. 10.

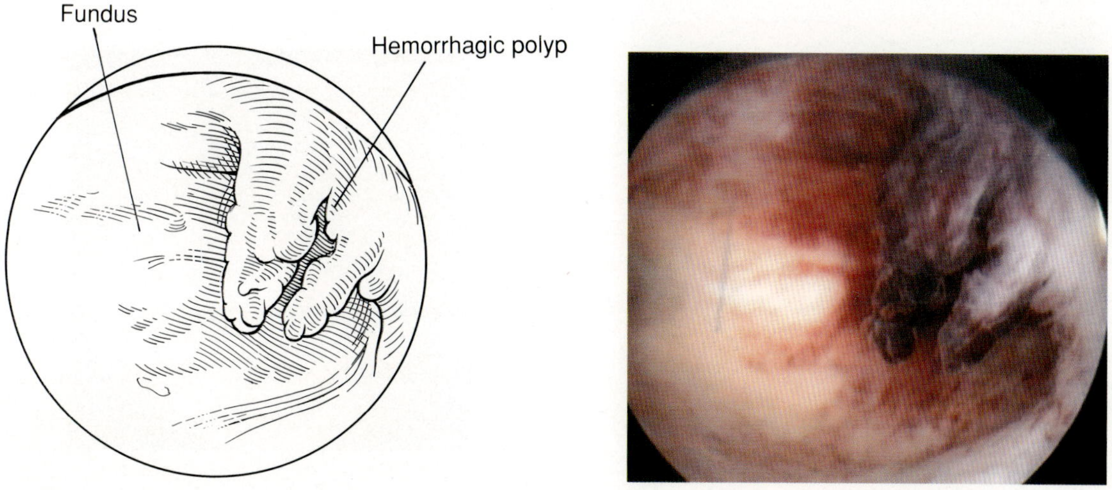

FIG. 13. Hemorrhagic endometrial polyp (histologically benign) arising from the left lateral wall of the uterus.

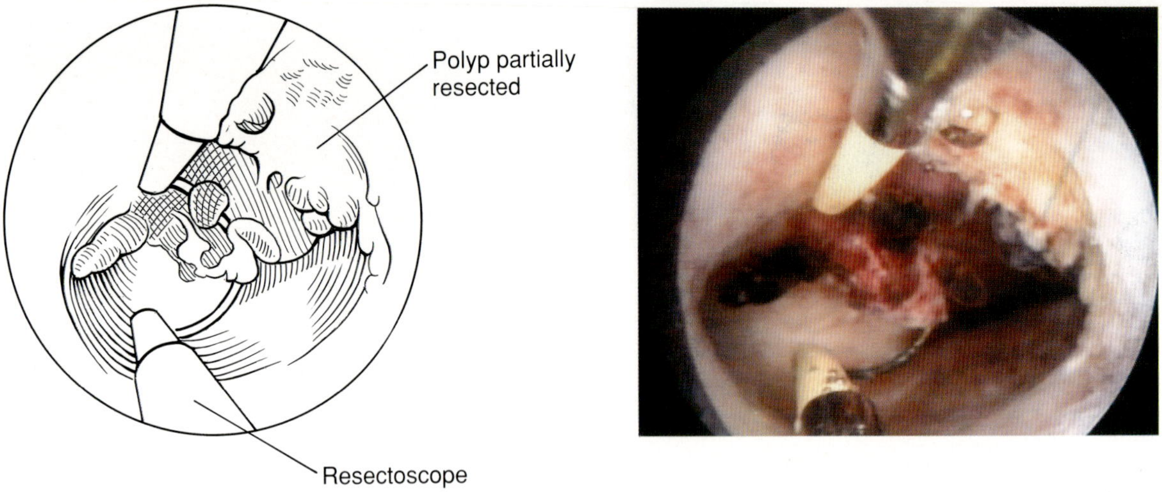

FIG. 14. Resectoscopic resection of part of the polyp from Fig. 13.

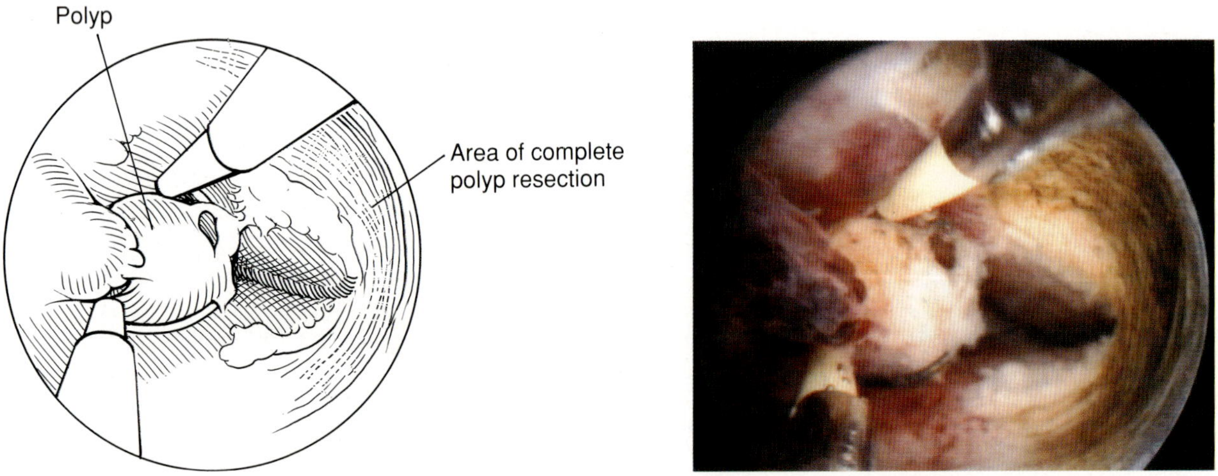

FIG. 15. Appearance of the uterine wall after complete resection of the polyp from Fig. 13.

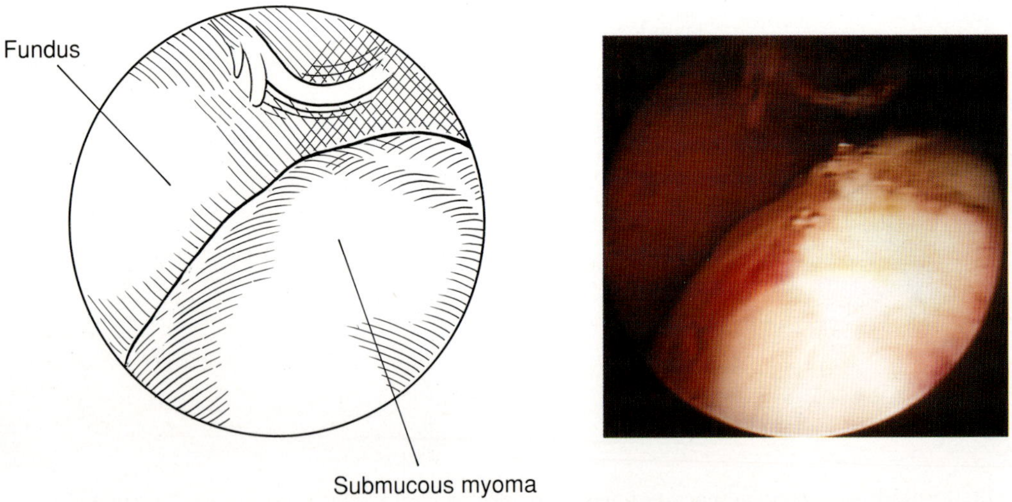

FIG. 16. Submucous myoma approximately 5 cm in diameter and 70% intracavitary.

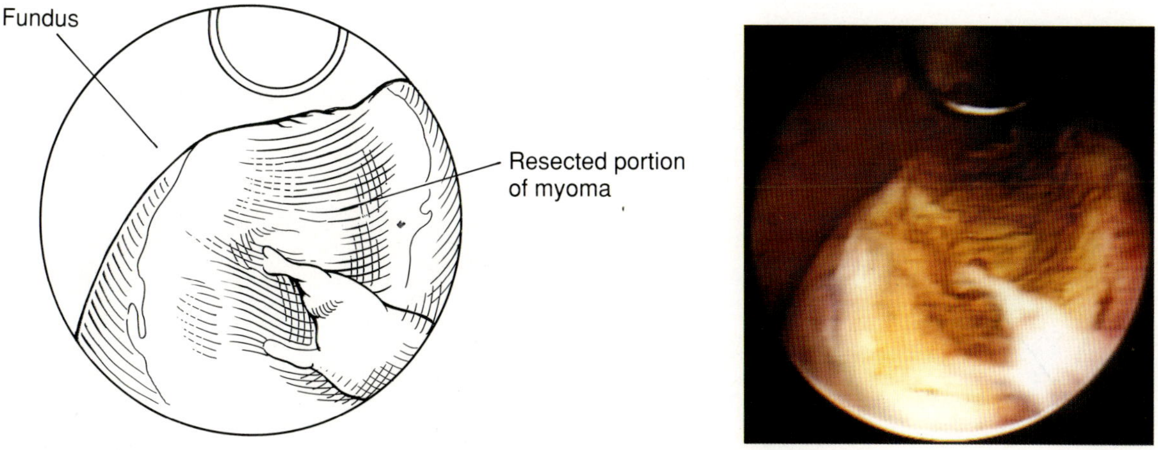

FIG. 17. Myoma from Fig. 16 with portion shaved out.

risk of perforating the uterus and of inducing a thermal injury to adherent or adjacent structures, such as bowel or bladder, it is not recommended that the intramural portion of the lesion be dug out of the wall. Thus, the surgeon should stop the shaving when the myoma surface is flush with the contour of the myometrial surface (Figs. 17 and 18). However, after the resectoscope is removed, the uterine distension is reversed, and the chips of myoma are extracted from the cavity, reinspection of the cavity often shows that more of the myoma extrudes into the cavity and can be shaved a little further without gouging deep into the myometrial wall. It appears that once the resistance of the myoma pushing against the opposite uterine wall is lessened by the partial shaving, the myometrium surrounding the myoma contracts and squeezes more of the tumor into the cavity, allowing more of it to be safely resected.

When the tumor is of a size that allows easy maneuvering of the resectoscope inside the uterus, the tendency is to start on the top or anterior surface (in cases where the myoma is attached posteriorly or superiorly) or on the posterior surface (where the tumor is attached anteriorly) and shave it progressively top to bottom, level by level. However, when the tumor fills the cavity and there is insufficient room to maneuver (Fig. 19), we have found that starting anteriorly or posteriorly in the middle of the tumor (Fig. 20) and shaving repeatedly in the same central furrow allows partial bisection of the lesion (Fig. 21). The two lateral wings of the tumor then collapse on each other, providing much more room within which to work. Often, the thin lateral wings can be grasped with a forceps and avulsed the rest of the way. A view of the endometrial cavity after removal of the myoma is provided in Fig. 22.

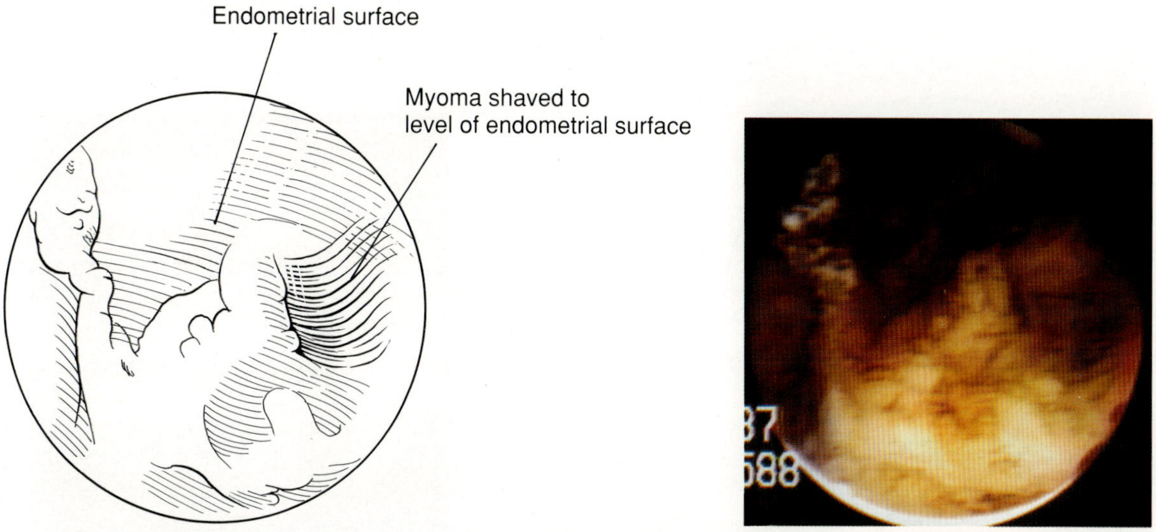

FIG. 18. Appearance of myoma from Fig. 16 after it has been shaved almost to the level of the myometrial surface. Approximately 30% of the myoma is left intramurally.

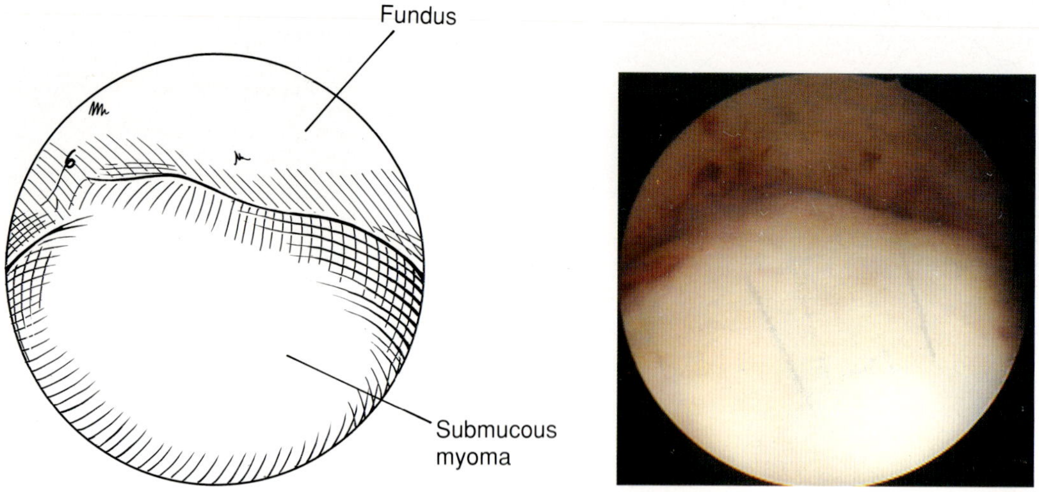

FIG. 19. Large submucous myoma fills the endometrial cavity.

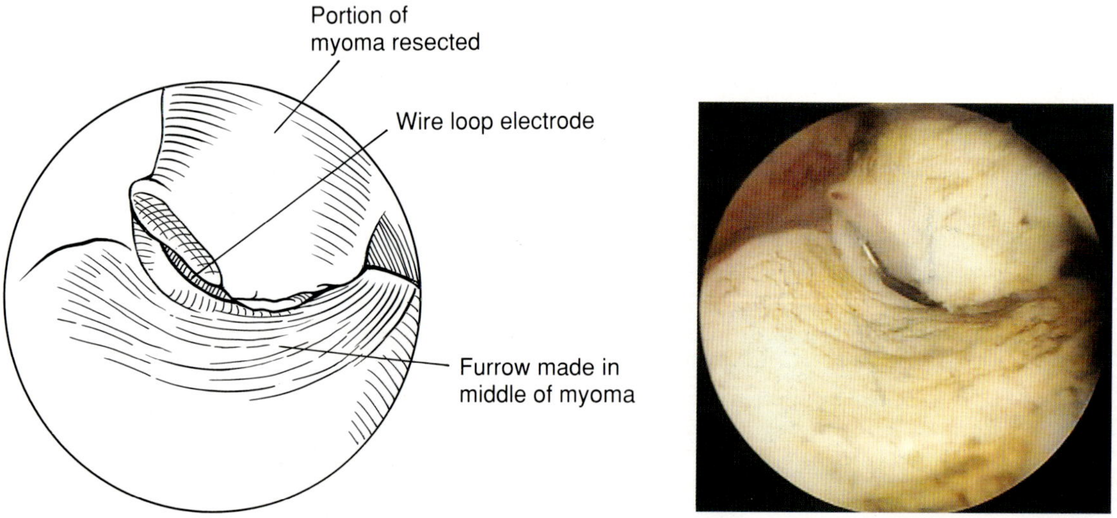

FIG. 20. Beginning of resection of the myoma from Fig. 16. Furrow is begun in middle of the myoma.

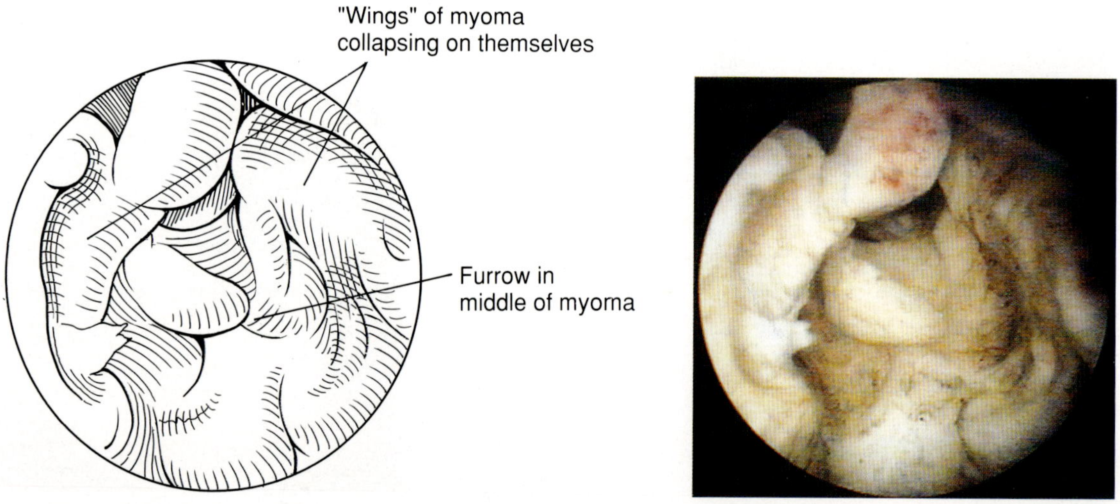

FIG. 21. Furrow is continued down the middle of the myoma from Fig. 16, forming lateral ''wings'' of the myoma, collapsing on themselves.

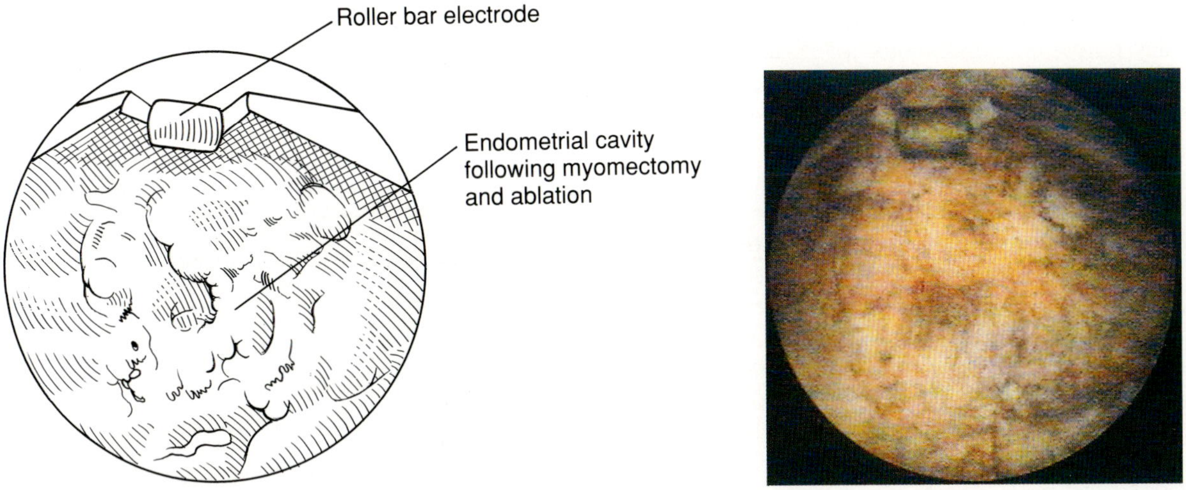

FIG. 22. Inspection of the endometrial cavity after the myoma from Fig. 16 is removed (and after endometrial ablation was performed).

OUTCOME

For all of the three major symptoms that result in the diagnosis of intrauterine polyps or submucous myomata, namely, abnormal uterine bleeding, infertility, and pregnancy wastage, hysteroscopic removal of these lesions results in significant improvement of the complaint. Baggish, in the series of 23 patients with symptomatic submucous myomata and complaints of menorrhagia or infertility and who were treated hysteroscopically with Nd:YAG laser, reported the correction of abnormal bleeding in 22 of the 23 patients; also, 3 of 5 patients desiring fertility conceived (18). Valle reported the results of hysteroscopic removal of submucous myomas in 59 women with abnormal uterine bleeding, dysmenorrhea, and/or infertility. He used only hysteroscopic scissors to sever the stalk of the pedunculated myomas or morcellated ones without pedicles (21). The results were improvement of the bleeding pattern in all patients, and 10 of 16 patients with associated infertility conceived following the hysteroscopic treatment.

In a combined series covering 90 patients with uncontrollable uterine bleeding, Brooks et al. reported improvement in bleeding pattern in 46 of 57 patients with submucous myomas (81%) and in 7 of 9 patients with endometrial polyps (78%) (22). Fifteen patients had complained of infertility and, after hysteroscopic surgery and a very short (3–20 months) follow-up period, five conceived. In a subsequent report of a larger series with a longer (6–36 months) follow-up period, Serden and Brooks reported a 92% improvement in bleeding pattern in 90 patients with submucous myomata (23).

Corson reported on resectoscopic excision of submucous myomas in 92 patients complaining of menorrhagia, dysmenorrhea, pregnancy wastage, and/or infertility, with a mean follow-up period of 17 months (9). Ten of 13 patients (77%) who had been infertile prior to the operation became pregnant. Four of five patients (80%) with prior recurrent midtrimester pregnancy wastage achieved full-term pregnancy and delivery. There was improvement in bleeding pattern in 65 of 80 patients (81%) complaining of menorrhagia and correction of dysmenorrhea in 24 of 28 patients (86%).

Our current series totals 240 patients with resectoscopic removal of submucous myomas and with the complaint of menorrhagia. Of these, five have required repeat resectoscopic surgery: two with regrowth of the same sessile myoma in which only a partial resection had been possible and three with new myomas causing recurrent bleeding. Eight patients (3%) have undergone hysterectomies: three for persistent menorrhagia, one for pelvic pain, one for recurrent menorrhagia 18 months later and due to a new myoma, one for acute pelvic inflammatory disease occurring a year after resection of the myoma, and two because the submucous myomas removed at hysteroscopy were found to be leiomyosarcomas on pathologic examination. Incidentally, at hysterectomy for the latter two patients, both uteri were free of malignancy. Thus, 227 of 240 patients with submucous myomas and menorrhagia (94.6%) were successfully treated with the primary resectoscopic procedure and 232 were improved after either one or two procedures (96.7%).

COMPLICATIONS

Complications of diagnostic and operative hysteroscopy are uncommon and are discussed thoroughly elsewhere in this book. They are an inevitable part of all surgical procedures, but serious complications are particularly infrequent in the hands of experienced surgeons. In our series there have been no serious complications, such as perforation of the uterus, mechanical or electrical bowel injury, or laparotomy for any reason as a result of resectoscopic or mechanical removal of endometrial polyps or submucous myomas. There has been only one case of fluid overload, which occurred during a resectoscopic removal of myomas. The amount was 2500 cm^3 and the overload resulted from a partial perforation (false passage) into the myometrium during the cervical dilation phase of the procedure. This complication did not require hospitalization. Two patients developed endometritis within a week of the procedure and were treated with oral antibiotics as outpatients. Six patients had sufficient bleeding at the termination of the procedure to require placement of an intrauterine balloon for tamponage for several hours, but the bleeding did not require transfusion or admission to the hospital.

HIGHLIGHTS

The removal of submucous myomas and endometrial polyps is very easily and safely accomplished hysteroscopically by mechanical methods (scissors, grasping forceps) or by laser or electric energy. Virtually all patients can be managed as outpatients and, usually, without concomitant laparoscopy. The techniques are fairly simple and vary according to the size of the tumor and the degree of its extension into the endometrial cavity. When these tumors are symptomatic, the presenting complaints are usually abnormal uterine bleeding, dysmenorrhea, infertility, and/or pregnancy wastage. A review of many of the series in the literature shows a significant improvement or cure of all of these presenting complaints. In our series of 240 patients, success rates for improving bleeding problems exceed 95% and few complications have occurred, each of those being relatively minor.

REFERENCES

1. Cohen MR, Dmowski WP. Modern hysteroscopy. Diagnostic and therapeutic potential. *Fertil Steril* 1973;24:905.
2. Mohr J, Lindemann HJ. Hysteroscopy in the infertile patient. *J Reprod Med* 1977;19:161.
3. Salat-Baroux J, Hamou JE, Maillard G, et al. Complications from micro-hysteroscopy. In: Siegler A, Lindemann HJ, eds. *Hysteroscopy: principles and practices.* Philadelphia: JB Lippincott; 1984: 112.
4. Valle RF. Hysteroscopy in the evaluation of female infertility. *Am J Obstet Gynecol* 1980;137:425.
5. Taylor PJ, Leader A, George RE. Combined laparoscopy and hysteroscopy in the investigation of infertility. In: Siegler A, Lindemann HJ, eds. *Hysteroscopy: principles and practices.* Philadelphia: JB Lippincott; 1984:207.
6. Corson SL, Brooks PG. Experience with the Hamou colpomicrohysteroscope. *J Reprod Med* 1983;28:654.
7. Cooper J. Incidence of hysteroscopic abnormalities in "asymptomatic women." *J Reprod Med* 1983;28:659.
8. Townsend DE, Fields G, McCausland A, Kauffman K. Diagnostic and operative hysteroscopy in the management of persistent postmenopausal bleeding. *Obstet Gynecol* 1993;82:419.
9. Corson SL, Brooks PG. Resectoscopic myomectomy. *Fertil Steril* 1991;55:1041.
10. Taylor PJ. Correlations in infertility: symptomatology, hysterosalpingography, laparoscopy and hysteroscopy. *J Reprod Med* 1977;18:339.
11. Lindemann HJ, Mohr J. CO_2 hysteroscopy—diagnosis and treatment. *Am J Obstet Gynecol* 1973;41:685.
12. Fedele L, Bianchi S, Dorta M, Brioschi D, Zanotti F, Vercellini P. Transvaginal ultrasonography versus hysteroscopy in the diagnosis of uterine submucous myomas. *Obstet Gynecol* 1991;77:745.
13. Goldstein SR. Fluid enhanced endometrial assessment by vaginal ultrasound in perimenopausal patients. *Am J Obstet Gynecol* 1994;70(2):565–570.
14. Gimpelson RJ, Rappold HO. A comparative study between panoramic hysteroscopy with directed biopsies and dilatation and curettage. *Am J Obstet Gynecol* 1988;158:489.
15. Brooks PG, Serden SP. Hysteroscopic findings after unsuccessful D&C for abnormal uterine bleeding. *Am J Obstet Gynecol* 1988;158:1354.
16. Hysteroscopy: state-of-the-art commentary. Committee on Gynecologic Practice. American College of Obstetricians and Gynecologists, June 1982.
17. Goldrath MH. Vaginal removal of the pedunculated submucous myoma: the use of laminaria. *Obstet Gynecol* 1987;70:670.
18. Baggish MS, et al. Hysteroscopic treatment of submucous myomata with the Nd:YAG laser. *J Gynecol Surg* 1989;5:27.
19. Neuwirth RS, Amin HK. Excision of submucous fibroids with hysteroscopic control. *Am J Obstet Gynecol* 1976;126:95.
20. Corson SL, Brooks PG, Serden SP, Batzer FR, Gocial B. The effects of vasopressin administration during hysteroscopic surgery. *J Reprod* Med; in press.
21. Valle RF: Hysteroscopic removal of submucous leiomyomas. *J Gynecol Surg* 1990;6:89.
22. Brooks PG, Loffer FD, Serden SP. Resectoscopic removal of symptomatic intrauterine lesions. *J Reprod Med* 1989;34:435.
23. Serden SP, Brooks PG. Treatment of abnormal uterine bleeding with the gynecologic resectoscope. *J Reprod Med* 1991;36:697.

Endoscopic Management of Gynecologic Disease,
edited by G.D. Adamson and D.C. Martin.
Lippincott-Raven Publishers, Philadelphia © 1996.

CHAPTER 31

The Septate Uterus

Stephen L. Corson

A septate uterus is a two-chambered uterus resulting from the failure of absorption of the median system of each hemiuterus during the process of fusion during embryogenic life. The clinical presentation may be totally silent as a congenital anomaly if it does not manifest itself in repetitive abortion.

One of the first therapeutic or operative hysteroscopic procedures to gain popularity was that of uterine septum incision or division (**not resection**). In this section diagnosis, techniques, results, and complications of therapy will be presented.

INCIDENCE

Since the lesion is congenital, incidence is a more appropriate term than prevalence. Older guesstimates were just that and were based on biased populations of women with reproductive wastage or women requiring cesarean section delivery for premature or obstructed labor. Data predicated on radiographic criteria of cavity separation in an attempt to differentiate between bicornate and septate uteri are unreliable, since the separation of the cavity caused by broad septae are easily confused with the bicornate variety. The correct diagnosis is mandatory for operative correction, since attempts to perform surgery hysteroscopically on a bicornate uterus invariably lead to uterine perforation.

Figure 1 schematically illustrates the embryologic differences between bicornate and septate uteri. Normally fusion of the laterally placed anlagen or hemiuteri is well underway by the tenth week and continued fusion takes place from caudad to cephalad. The bicornate uterus is a result of incomplete fusion and is a lesser failure than uterus didelphus or complete duplication of uteri and cervices. A septate uterus, conversely, represents failure of absorption of the medial fused walls of the two hemiuteri. Extension of the septum into the vagina is more commonly seen with complete uterine duplication but may occur with septate uteri. Since associated urologic anomalies emanating from disturbance of urogenital ridge development may occur, an intravenous pyleogram to assess absence, duplication, or malposition of the kidneys and ureters is necessary as a corollary study, although absence is more common with unicollate uterus, and malposition with bicornate uterus. Ultrasonography, which is used diagnostically for uterine identification, can also give information on renal anatomy.

The best prospective study on incidence of the two-chambered uterus was a byproduct of an investigation by Ashton et al. (1) on an office-based method of transcervical sterilization by injection of methylcyanoacrylate to cause proximal tubal obstruction. In 840 postprocedural hysterosalpingograms, 16 anatomic defects were diagnosed (1.9%) with 15 of those being two-chambered uteri with the defect extending down at least halfway from the fundus to the internal cervical os so as to eliminate from consideration the arcuate configuration. Since these were all parous women seeking sterilization, the findings are more applicable to general population demographics than those gleaned from earlier biased groups.

Although the bicornate–septate differential could not be resolved by this study, in our experience the septate uterus is approximately eight times more frequently encountered as the bicornate variety. This is confirmed by a study of Portuondo et al. (2) who found one bicornate uterus in a series of 65 patients with recurrent abortion vs. 11 with septate deformity, although it should be noted that the diagnosis was based on radiographic criteria.

S. L. Corson: Department of Obstetrics and Gynecology, University of Pennsylvania School of Medicine, Pennsylvania Hospital, Philadelphia, Pennsylvania 19107.

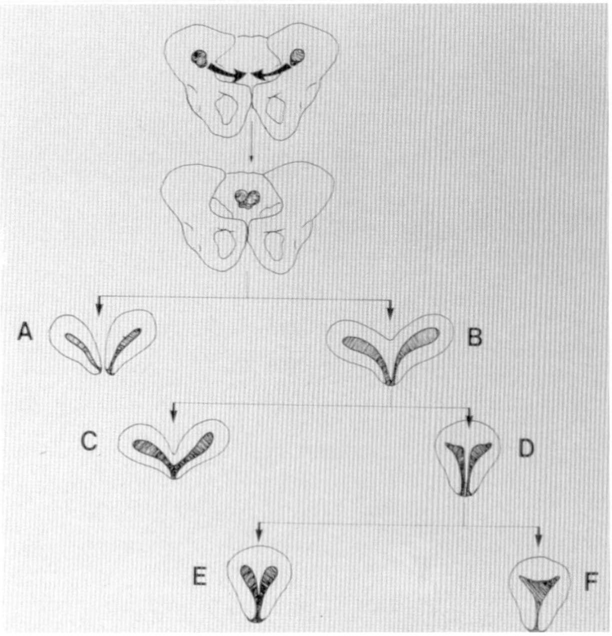

FIG. 1. Schematic diagram of uterine development. A, initial caudal fusion; B, continued fusion cephalad; C, bicornate uterus as fusion failure; D, fusion complete; E, septate uterus as a result of failure of medial wall resorption; F, normal uterine cavity.

DIAGNOSIS

Differential diagnosis is primarily between septate and bicornate deformity. Another anomaly causing confusion is the unicollate uterus. If the tip of the cannula is inserted deeply into one of the cavities of a septate uterus, the radiographic appearance may well be that of a unicollate uterus. Even hysteroscopy can give the same false result. Passing the hysteroscope through the cervical canal under directed vision lessens the chance of this error occurring. The hysteroscopist must assiduously search for another cavity, which sometimes has a rather angulated lateral opening between the septum and the lateral wall of the uterus. Even the most skilled and experienced hysteroscopist has been fooled on occasion. Identification of the tubal recesses and proximal opening into the uterine cavity is sometimes difficult but serves to diagnose correctly the true anatomic condition. A thick midline adhesion may mimic a septum both by radiographic and hysteroscopic examination.

In some cases there is residual hypertrophy of one chamber caused by pregnancy. This is shown in Fig. 2A and 2B, in which hysteroscopy confirms the radiographic appearance. Not infrequently, blind surgical evacuation of the uterus after an unsuccessful pregnancy leaves behind products of conception, which cause filling defects on x-ray (Fig. 3A). However, when viewed by hysteroscopy (Fig. 3B), they are clearly seen to be necrotic or even calcified tissue.

Ultrasonography can usually be used to make the diagnosis of a septate uterus, especially if it is performed vaginally. Figure 4 illustrates a sonogram of a uterus with two cavities separated by myometrium without fundal notching, which is seen with a bicornate uterus. Ultrasonic diagnosis during pregnancy is less reliable because of changes in anatomy. Valdes et al. (3) reported on a series of patients with müllerian anomalies diagnosed ultrasonographically compared with x-ray and/or surgical findings. In the nonpregnant group of 15, sonography was diagnostic in 47%, confirmatory in 40%, and incorrect in 13%.

Magnetic resonance imaging (MRI) is an excellent diagnostic tool, as shown in Fig. 5. However this technique adds great cost to the diagnostic process and does not obviate, in my opinion, the need for laparoscopy during hysteroscopic repair.

Laparoscopy remains the gold standard of diagnosis and is usually performed during the repair procedure with the patient prepared for the alternative operation of laparotomy unification of a bicornate uterus. Figure 6 shows a uterus with a midline whitish area often seen with a septate uterus. Figure 7 shows a uterus with a hallmark feature of a broad fundus filling the laparoscopic panoramic field of view. We repeatedly see patients who have had diagnostic laparoscopy in whom the diagnosis of septate uterus should have at least been entertained because of this feature, but the operators seem to have been oblivious to this possibility.

Although unsupported by the literature, there may be an association between the diethylstilbestrol (DES) malformation and persistent uterine septum. Figure 8 shows a two-chambered small uterus with the typical cornal-tubal deformity of the DES patient; this was later proven to be a septate uterus. Figure 9 illustrates a small, "T"-shaped uterus with a faint, thin, linear, filling defect, which also proved to be a septum. Hysteroscopic surgery in these small uteri is sometimes quite difficult.

OPERATIVE INDICATION

Reproductive wastage is the sole operative indication, unless one cavity becomes obstructed leading to hematometra. Infertility is not caused by septate uteri. Most patients present with a history of two or more first-trimester early losses or early second-trimester loss. This is in contradistinction to patients with bicornate uteri, which usually cause difficulty later in pregnancy and which are more commonly associated with cervical incompetence. Occasionally patients may have a successful term pregnancy in addition to multiple abortions.

A

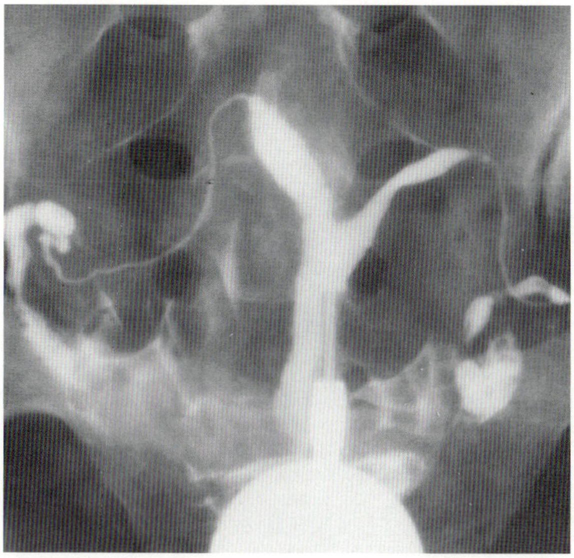

FIG. 2. **A:** Hysterosalpingogram showing residual hypertrophy following pregnancy in a septate uterus. **B:** Hysteroscopic confirmation.

B

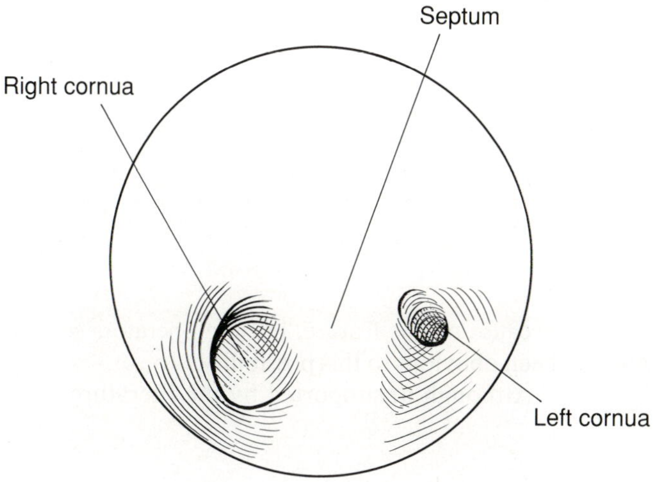

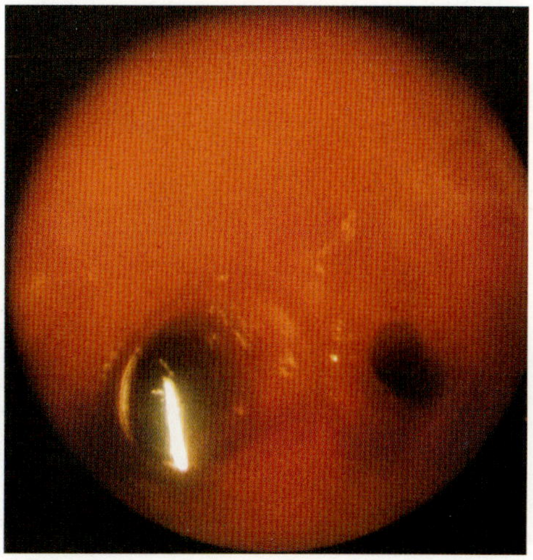

This raises the question of the mechanism of action. Implantation on the poorly vascularized septum has been the traditional answer to explain poor reproductive performance, but this seems an inadequate or incomplete answer. The vascular system supplying a great deal of the endometrium may be altered. Certainly this is a rich area for future research.

Patients who have recurrent abortion and who have two-chambered uteri should still have the remainder of the workup for reproductive wastage, including chromosomal evaluation in selected cases. Chromosomal testing of abortus tissue is increasingly performed, and normal findings decrease the need to screen the parents. Attention should be paid to cardiolipin and lupus-related antibodies, HLA-DR (human lymphocyte antigens) locus antigens, and luteal phase factors. Thyroid disease is an infrequent cause for recurrent abortion. As reported in Ashton et al.'s (1) study, a two-chambered uterus was found in almost 2% of parous women seeking sterilization. We do not find that 2% of the population with recurrent abortion have two-chambered uteri. Therefore, the presence of such a defect does not necessarily indicate future reproductive difficulty. Moreover, the x-ray appearance of a uterus with reference to the apparent length or width of the septum has no reproductive prognostic significance.

Occasionally women with infertility problems have a hysterosalpingographic finding of a two-chambered uterus. Our practice has been not to intervene at that point. If, however, during a later diagnostic laparoscopy for infertility a septate uterus is found, we favor hysteroscopic division of the septum at that time, since the expected morbidity of the procedure is low and the patient is already under general anesthesia. Again, it is empha-

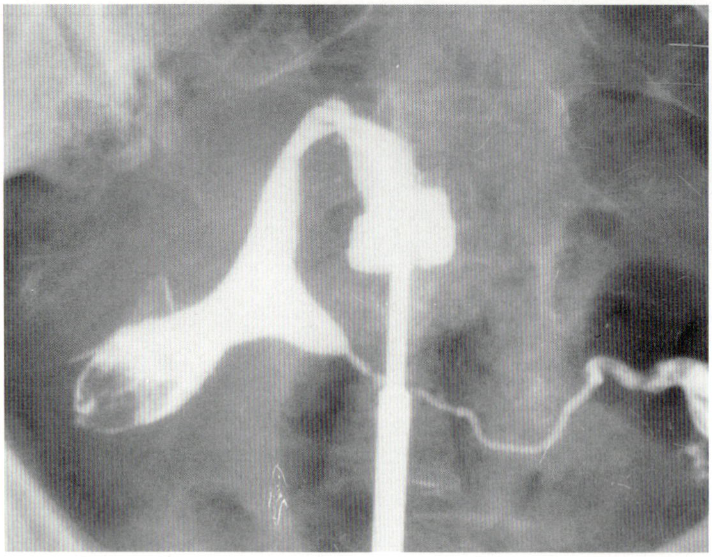

A

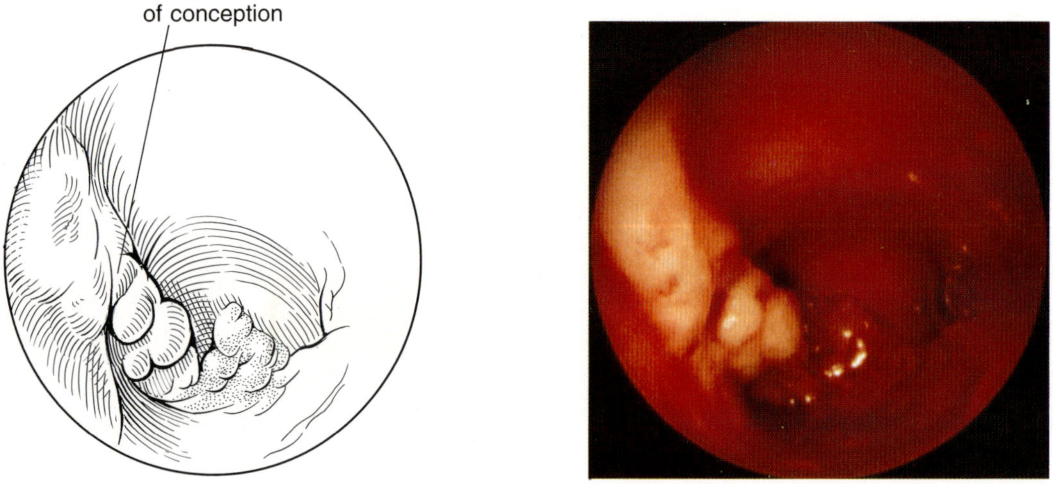

B

FIG. 3. A: Hysterosalpingogram showing two-chambered uterus and products of conception. **B:** Hysteroscopic confirmation of x-ray findings.

sized that septal division is not expected to be a fertility-promoting procedure.

SURGICAL TECHNIQUES

In 1986 Corson and Batzer (4) published a small series of septal incisions performed with optical fixed scissors using either high molecular weight dextran or carbon dioxide for uterine distention in conjunction with an operating hysteroscope. DeCherney's group (5) favored use of the resectoscopic loop to shave the septum electrosurgically.

March and Israel have reported on 91 patients with septate uteri (6). They advocate use of flexible scissors through the operating sheath of a hysteroscope.

Daly (7) also has published his considerable experience with septate uterus and generally uses flexible 6-mm scissors. He describes a special technique to deal with a septum extending down into the cervix (8). The cervical septum can simply be cut with a pair of Metzenbaum scissors high enough to allow entry of the hysteroscope into the cervical canal so that distention can be achieved.

Use of the yttrium-aluminum-garnet (YAG) laser for this indication has been limited to description of a few cases here and there, but a large series has not been described in the literature.

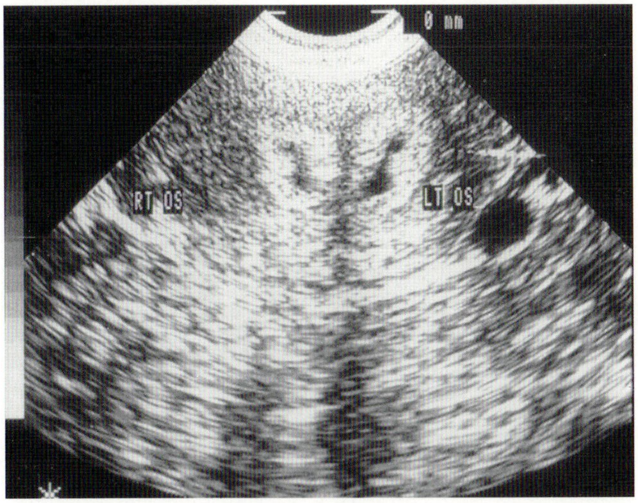

FIG. 4. Ultrasonic appearance of septate uterus.

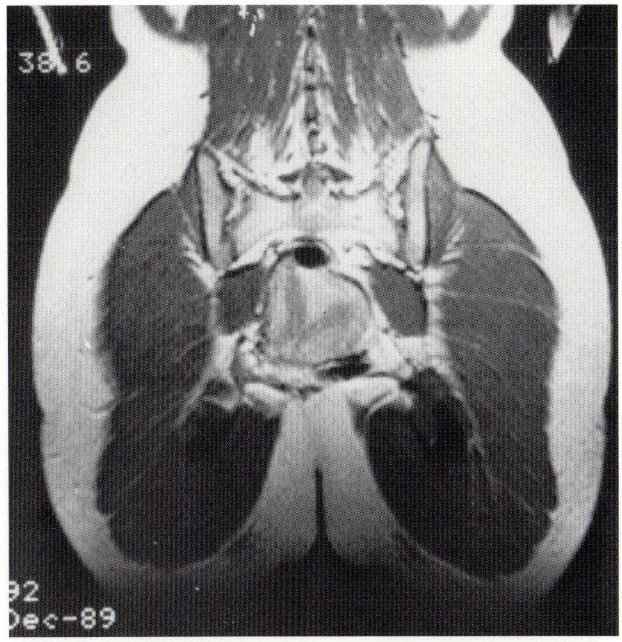

FIG. 5. MR image of septate uterus.

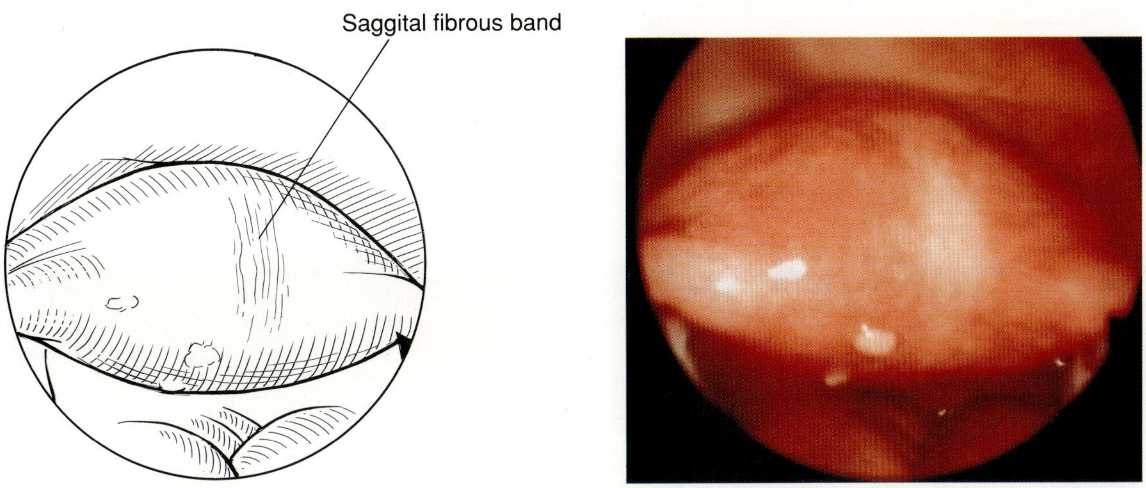

FIG. 6. Laparoscopic appearance of septate uterus with saggital, fibrous band.

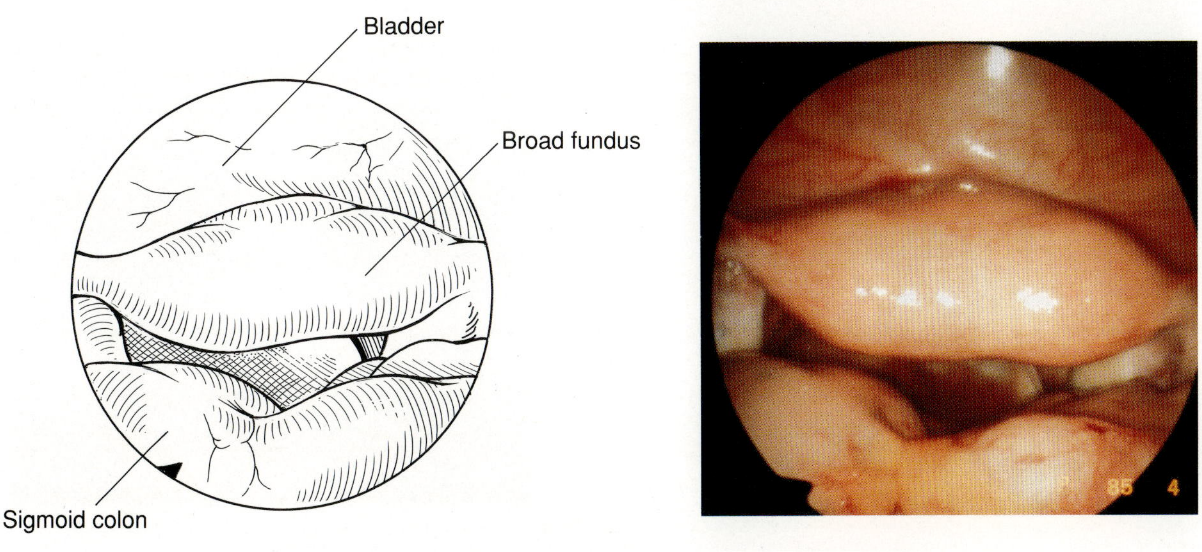

FIG. 7. Broad fundus of a septate uterus seen laparoscopically.

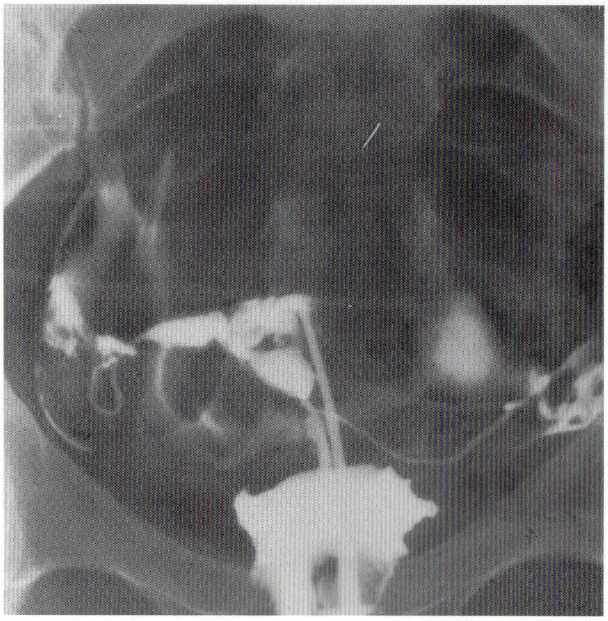

FIG. 8. Diethylstibestrol (DES) and septate uterus.

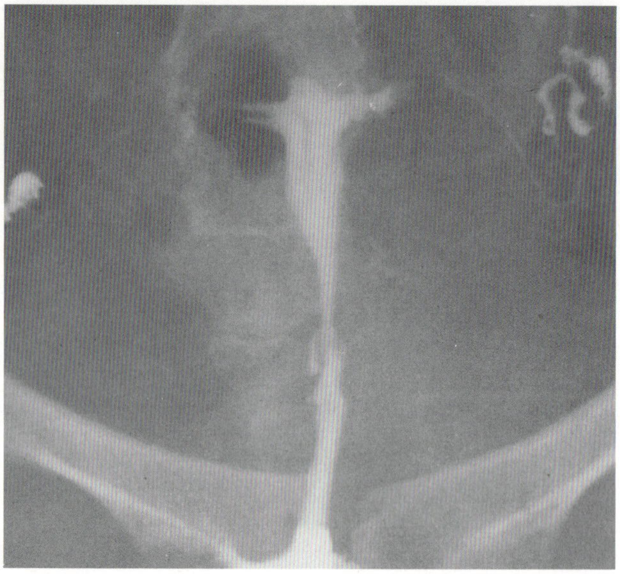

FIG. 9. DES "T"-shaped uterus with thin septum.

General Technique

Hormonal preparation of the endometrium as for endometrial ablation is unnecessary, but surgery is best performed early in the proliferative phase. Laparoscopy is performed under general anesthesia to confirm the diagnosis. The operative hysteroscope is inserted after the cervical canal has been dilated to sufficient diameter. The distending medium is that of operator preference. The septum is a midline fibromuscular structure with poor vascular supply, and bleeding is rarely a problem during or after surgery. In cases involving a broad septum, use of dilute vasopressin (20 U in 50 ml saline) is helpful as a hemostatic agent; it is injected as 4 ml on each side of the cervix at the level of the fornix. If a thin septum such as that seen in Fig. 10 is encountered, use of optical scissors or flexible scissors to incise the septum by encompassing it entirely between the blades is a straightforward technique. Optical scissors offer an advantage of strength to deal with tough fibromuscular tissue but cannot be manipulated independent of the optic. Flexible scissors are more flimsy but are an excellent choice for lateral portions of a wide septum. The incision is made in a line equidistant from the anterior and posterior walls after the entire uterine cavity has been scanned and the tubal recesses and orifices identified. Knowing when to

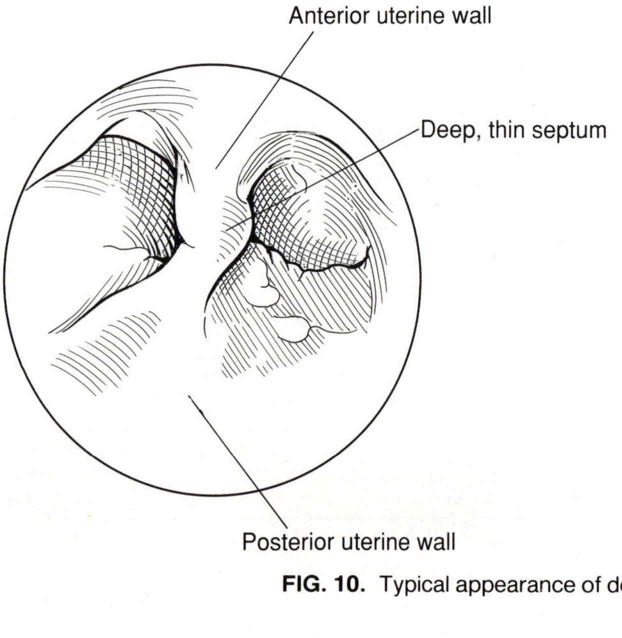

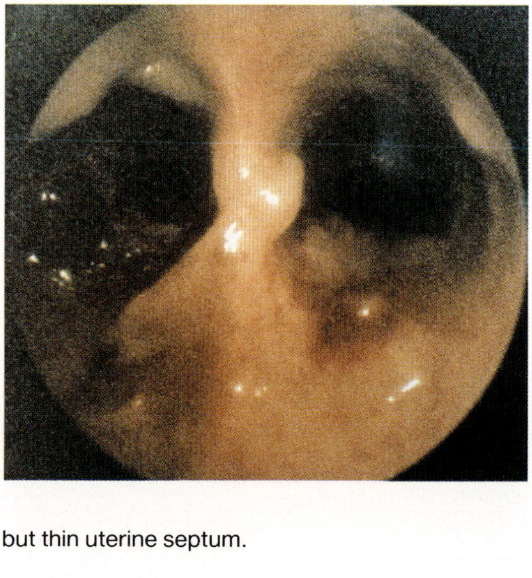

FIG. 10. Typical appearance of deep but thin uterine septum.

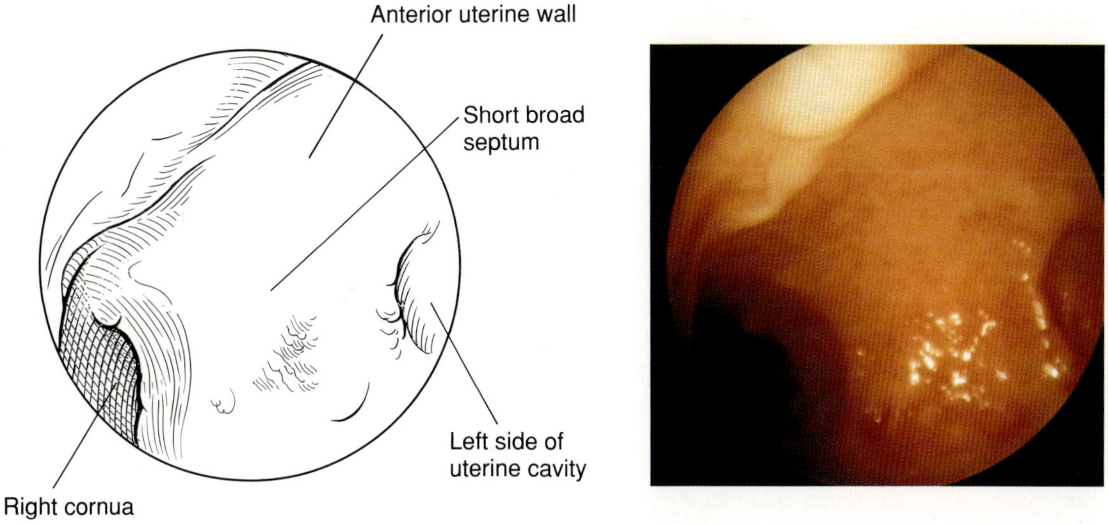

FIG. 11. Short but broad septum.

stop may be difficult because the myometrium in the fundus appears similar to that of the septal fibers. It is helpful to have the laparoscopist dim the light, after which the operator runs the hysteroscope across the fundus from cornu to cornu. The laparoscopist should see an unbroken train of transillumination through the fundus. If the dissection becomes angulated, anterior or posterior perforation may occur. The laparoscopist must observe serosal surfaces of the uterus to check for distortion caused by the scissors biting into the myometrium just below the serosal surface, so perforation can be avoided.

A short, broad septum is shown in Fig. 11. This is more difficult to operate on because the lateral margins must be attacked and the width decreased gradually in a serial fashion. Sometimes a deflecting bridge is necessary in conjunction with the use of flexible scissors. This is one indication for use of an electrosurgical or laser technique as an easier approach. Some authors have expressed fear of scar tissue formation caused by the use of electrosurgical or laser energy within the uterus with possible devascularization of the endometrium and synechiae formation. This fear may be more theoretical than real.

In most cases, hormonal stimulation with exogenous estrogens postoperatively is unnecessary. Office hysteroscopy demonstrates complete endometrial overgrowth of the raw area within 2 months. An exception might be made for broad septae and/or when electrosurgery has been used. In such a case, an equivalent of 6 mg of estrace daily for 30 days with medroxyprogesterone added in the last 10 days should stimulate satisfactory endometrial regeneration. No intrauterine devices are introduced, and no routine antibiotic coverage is employed. Patients may begin efforts to conceive within a month. With experience, follow-up hysterosalpingography or hysteroscopy is confined to cases with suspicion of incomplete division

TABLE 1. *Hysteroscopic division of uterine septum*

		OB Hx preseptal repair						OB Hx postseptal repair						
Author	Patient	Total pregnancies	Abortion	Premature	Term	Ectopic	Live	Patients pregnant	Total pregnancies	Abortion	Premature	Term	Ectopic	Ongoing
Corson and Batzer 1986 (4)	17	43	35	4	0	3	1	13	17	2	1	13	1	0
DeCherney et al. 1986 (5)	72	NR[b]	>144	NR	NR	NR	NR	67	73	10	1	58	0	4
March and Israel 1987 (6)[a]	79	252	212	21	7	0	12	57	63	8	4	44	0	7
Daly 1989 (7)	55	160	130	13	7	0	10	47	79	15	5	55	0	4

[a] Data on 66 women attempting pregnancy postoperatively.
[b] NR, not recorded.

or to insure against adhesion formation after a difficult dissection.

OUTCOME AND COMPLICATIONS

Savings of operating time, hospital bed utilization, and avoidance of a mandatory cesarean section delivery are all obvious advantages of hysteroscopic division of the septum compared with laparotomy metroplasty. However, reproductive results must be at least comparable in order for the procedure to be carried out. Rock and Jones (9) reported 77% salvage, and Capparo (10) reported an 80% success rate after abdominal uterine metroplasty. Table 1 contains data from published series in which pre- and postoperative reproductive data were presented. It is clear that the results via hysteroscopy are at least as good as those following laparotomy. Absence of suture in the endometrium would be expected to diminish significant uterine scar tissue formation, but direct comparisons have not been made. Uterine perforation during division has been reported.

ADDENDUM

Rupture of the uterus following hysteroscopic metroplasty has been reported with use of the resectoscope (11) and after use of scissors (12). An unusual case was reported by Lobaugh et al. (13) in which a KTP laser was used for septal division. The first pregnancy which followed was uncomplicated with a vaginal delivery, but in the next pregnancy the patient presented with a uterine defect noted on ultrasonic scan which proved to be a separation of the uterus with a 3.5 cm fundal defect through which amniotic membranes and placental tissue were seen to protrude. The authors postulated that this was due to an inherent weakness in the wall of the uterus associated with use of the laser. In any event, if perforation occurs during a procedure, regardless of the method employed to divide the septum, the defect should be sutured, preferably via laparoscopy, or even a small mini laparotomy, in an attempt to prevent this late complication.

HIGHLIGHTS

Laparoscopic-guided hysteroscopic incision of the uterine septum offers an excellent chance of reproductive success for patients whose recurrent abortions are causally linked to that diagnosis. This is an outpatient procedure having minimal morbidity and one that allows for future vaginal delivery.

REFERENCES

1. Ashton D, Amin HK, Richart RM, Neuwirth RS. The incidence of asymptomatic uterine anomalies in women undergoing transcervical tubal sterilization. *Obstet Gynecol* 1988;72:28.
2. Portuondo JA, Camara MM, Echanojauregui AD, Calonge J. Müllerian abnormalities in fertile women and recurrent aborters. *J Reprod Med* 1986;31:616.
3. Valdes C, Malini S, Malinak LR. Ultrasound evaluation of female genital tract anomalies: A review of 64 cases. *Am J Obstet Gynecol* 1984;149:285.
4. Corson SL, Batzer FR. CO_2 Uterine distention for hysteroscopic septal incision. *J Reprod Med* 1986;31:713.
5. DeCherney AH, Russell JB, Graebe RA, Polan ML. Resectoscopic management of müllerian fusion defects. *Fertil Steril* 1986;45:726.
6. March CM, Israel R. Hysteroscopic management of recurrent abortion caused by septate uterus. *Am J Obstet Gynecol* 1987;156:834.
7. Daly DC, Maier D, Soto-Albors C. Hysteroscopic metroplasty: six years' experience. *Obstet Gynecol* 1989;73:201.
8. Daly DC, Tohan N, Walters C, Riddick DH. Hysteroscopic resection of the uterine septum in the presence of a septate cervix. *Fertil Steril* 1983;39:560.
9. Rock JA, Jones HW Jr. The clinical management of the double uterus. *Fertil Steril* 1977;28:798.
10. Capparo VJ, Chuang JT, Randall CL. Improved fetal salvage after metroplasty. *Obstet Gynecol* 1968;31:97.
11. Creinin M, Chen M. Uterine defect in a twin pregnancy with a history of hysteroscopic fundal perforation. *Obstet Gynecol* 1992;79:879–880.
12. Howe R. Third-trimester uterine rupture following hysteroscopic uterine perforation. *Obstet Gynecol* 1993;81:827–829.
13. Lobaugh ML, Bammel BM, Duke D, Webster BW. Uterine rupture during pregnancy in a patient with a history of hysteroscopic metroplasty. *Obstet Gynecol* 1994;83:838–840.

Endoscopic Management of Gynecologic Disease,
edited by G.D. Adamson and D.C. Martin.
Lippincott-Raven Publishers, Philadelphia © 1996.

CHAPTER 32

Endometrial Ablation

Franklin D. Loffer

DEFINITION

Destruction of the endometrium or endometrial ablation to control menorrhagia has been tried by a variety of methods. Although, as reported by Vancaillie, an electrical method was described in 1937 and successful clinical results were reported in the German medical literature in 1948 (1), it was not until 1981 that the procedure was popularized with the publication of a successful technique using the neodymium:yttrium-aluminum-garnet (Nd:YAG) laser (2). Since that time, the procedure has gained increasing popularity (3). Endometrial ablation allows women with menorrhagia or menometrorrhagia to avoid a hysterectomy. It is used in women who have normal endometrium and where hormonal manipulation has not been successful or cannot be utilized.

PREVALENCE

There are not yet any statistics indicating the number of patients who have been treated by endometrial ablation. It has been estimated that more than 150,000 hysterectomies have been performed in the United States each year for menorrhagia and menometrorrhagia (4). Many could be avoided if endometrial ablation were offered.

ANATOMY

The anatomy of the endometrium consists of a basal and a functional layer. The latter varies with the menstrual cycle from 1–2 mm to as much as 7–8 mm in height. In normal situations, the functional layer sheds uniformly upon the withdrawal of estrogen and progesterone stimulation, leaving only the basal layer intact to regenerate into the functional layer during the next cycle. The basal layer of the endometrium does not lie uniformly over the myometrium but normally can extend into it. When the extension of the endometrium into the myometrium is greater than normal, adenomyosis exists (5). Adenomyosis is frequently associated with heavy menses and may be a common indication for endometrial ablation. Endometrial polyps and submucous fibroids may also contribute to excessive menstrual flow and endometrial ablation is frequently done at the time of their removal.

CLINICAL PRESENTATION

The presenting complaint of patients who undergo endometrial ablation should be excessive or prolonged menstrual flow not necessarily resulting in anemia. However, this condition should be significant enough that the patient is considering a hysterectomy as a method of management. Although endometrial ablation was originally designed for patients with menorrhagia, those presenting with prolonged and even intermenstrual bleeding can usually be helped. Many patients undergoing endometrial ablation have adenomyosis. However, patients with severe dysmenorrhea should not be considered. Although bleeding may be relieved, pain may continue to be a problem. Patients with bleeding diathesis also are frequent candidates. Although the possible benefit to patients with premenstrual syndrome has been described (6), patients should look on relief from this condition as a possible bonus rather than as the reason for undergoing the procedure.

DIAGNOSIS

Candidates for endometrial ablation should be carefully screened. Not all patients with abnormal uterine

F. D. Loffer: Division of Gynecologic Endoscopy, Maricopa Medical Center, Phoenix, Arizona 85008.

bleeding should be considered. Diagnostic workup should be designed to assure that only appropriate patients are chosen. When a patient presents with a complaint of abnormal uterine bleeding, the severity should be determined to ensure that her expectation of the surgical result will be met. The frequency of menses as well as the length and number of days to be considered excessive should be determined. Included in the history are the number and types of protective pads used, the frequency with which they are changed, the problem of soiling clothing and bedding, and whether there is passage of clots. Endometrial sampling should also be done to ensure that a premalignant or malignant condition does not exist. If there is any question that the problem might be related to anovulation, basal body temperatures, serum progesterone, or endometrial biopsies should be done to determine whether hormonal therapy might be a more appropriate method of management.

INDICATIONS

Endometrial ablation requires a uterine cavity that is or can be made relatively normal in size and contour. It is difficult to identify and destroy all of the endometrium in cavities that are irregular or very large. Cavities are frequently enlarged because they are distorted by intramural or submucous fibroids. If fibroids are submucous, they frequently can be removed at the time of ablation.

Hysteroscopy is the best method for assessing the uterine cavity in women with heavy menses (7). However, it is not always necessary before endometrial ablation if it is determined by palpation that the uterus is normal in size and shape and probes to a normal depth. A submucous myoma found in such a uterus at the time of ablation should be small enough to be removed at the same time. Other methods of assessing the cavity are hystosalpingography and ultrasound.

The author does not believe that anemia is a mandatory prerequisite for endometrial ablation to be considered. Many women have adequate iron stores or dietary iron intake to maintain normal hemoglobin levels despite debilitating and socially embarrassing menstrual flow. It is the author's opinion that endometrial ablation is justified when the menstrual flow creates either a medical or a social problem that requires the patient to consider hysterectomy. It is true that women may consider undergoing endometrial ablation sooner and for less symptomatology than they would consider a hysterectomy. This raises the argument that if this procedure is made available to patients for convenience it will become "cosmetic" surgery for women who simply do not wish to have menses. It has been the author's experience that, since amenorrhea cannot be guaranteed, those women who are looking for the convenience of no menses do not choose to undergo endometrial ablation.

CONTRAINDICATIONS

Contraindications to endometrial ablation are listed in Table 1. No exact uterine dimensions have been established as contraindications to endometrial ablation, but most authors believe that a uterine cavity length of 10 cm or less is appropriate for the Nd:YAG laser ablation and one as large as 14 cm is suitable for a resectoscope ablation. A distorted cavity that cannot be made normal by the removal of an endometrial polyp or fibroid does not allow easy approach to all areas of endometrium and gives poor results because areas of endometrium would be missed.

Patients undergoing this procedure cannot expect to retain their fertility, since the endometrium is completely or almost completely destroyed. Although fertility is certainly compromised, this procedure cannot be described as a sterilization procedure because efficacy rates have not been established. Generally a patient with endometrial changes that predispose her to a high risk of carcinoma of the endometrium should not be considered for this procedure. Those patients at an increased risk for carcinoma of the endometrium, such as very obese patients, should be done only when the benefit of avoiding a hysterectomy outweighs the potential risk of later development of an endometrial cancer.

Hyperplasia per se is not a contraindication to this procedure, unless there are elements of atypia associated with it. Patients not infrequently will have had simple hyperplasia diagnosed at biopsy or dilatation and curettage (D & C). Endometrial ablation still can be considered if the hyperplasia is an incidental finding showing no atypia and relates to exogenous hormonal therapy used in an effort to control bleeding or in an anovulatory patient for whom progesterone alone is not controlling the bleeding. Some patients are predisposed to a high level of endogenous estrogen production or anovulation. These patients should be cycled with a progestational agent following the ablation.

A patient who has significant dysmenorrhea or other concomitant gynecologic problems is better served by hysterectomy and should not be considered for this procedure unless she understands that the other problems might eventually force her to have a hysterectomy. The presence of uterine fibroids alone does not necessarily indicate a hysterectomy or contraindicate this procedure.

TABLE 1. *Contraindications to endometrial ablation*

1. Patient has excessively large or distorted uterine cavity
2. Patient wishes to maintain her fertility
3. Patient has premalignant or malignant endometrial changes
4. Patient has other major gynecologic problems that would require a hysterectomy for management

ALTERNATIVE TREATMENT

Hysterectomy may be a better alternative for some patients, such as those who prefer total amenorrhea or those who do not wish to run the slight risk of continued or recurrent menstrual problems. Although dysmenorrhea is frequently improved, those patients who have a significant problem with it should consider hysterectomy as a better alternative.

Other nonhysteroscopic techniques for endometrial ablation are being investigated. In one such technique, a probe is introduced blindly into the endometrial cavity and thermally destroys the endometrium by radiofrequency, electromagnetic energy (8). Another method destroys the endometrium by heating a water-filled intrauterine balloon (9,10). D&C is not an alternative, since there is no evidence to suggest that it has a therapeutic effect in controlling abnormal bleeding.

SURGICAL TECHNIQUES

Current, clinically available surgical techniques for endometrial ablation involve either the Nd:YAG laser or the gynecologic resectoscope. Two similar techniques exist for each method. One technique destroys endometrium without cutting through it. The second technique physically disrupts the endometrial surface and superficial myometrium.

The technique that does not cut into the superficial myometrium is called—when the Nd:YAG laser is used—a nontouch or blanching technique (11). In this method, the bare fiber is brought in a perpendicular direction as close to the endometrial surface as possible without actually making contact (Fig. 1). In this technique, the laser energy penetrates through the endometrium resulting in the upper portion of the myometrium also being destroyed. However, the surface of the endometrium is not broken. A similar technique with the resectoscope is the roller bar or ball (12,13). In this technique, the electrode rolls over the intact endometrial surface causing it to "melt" away and expose the underlying myometrium (Fig. 2). Although the energy used in this technique removes the endometrium, the rollers do not cut into the myometrial tissue. The speed with which the electrode crosses the surface is critical. If drawn too quickly, adequate myometrial penetration is not achieved. It is important that the electrode be moved slowly enough that the electrical effect on tissue is seen to precede it (Fig. 3). The basal layer of the endometrium and any adenomyosis lying within the myometrium are destroyed by thermocoagulation in both techniques.

The second technique, which does cut through the endometrium and into the myometrium, is called—when the Nd:YAG laser is used—a touch or dragging technique. It results when a bare Nd:YAG laser fiber is dragged through and cuts into the endometrium and myometrium (2). The initial dragging forms furrows (Fig. 4A), which are connected by lateral movement of the fiber (Fig. 4B). The laser energy both cuts and vaporizes tissue. A comparable technique with the resectoscope involves the loop electrode to resect endometrium and the superficial myometrium (14) (Fig. 5).

Combination techniques exist with both techniques. With the Nd:YAG laser, the fundal portion is blanched and the lower uterine segment is treated by dragging. When the resectoscope is used in a combination technique, the endometrium first is resected and then the surface is rolled for further destruction.

At the end of the procedure regardless of the tech-

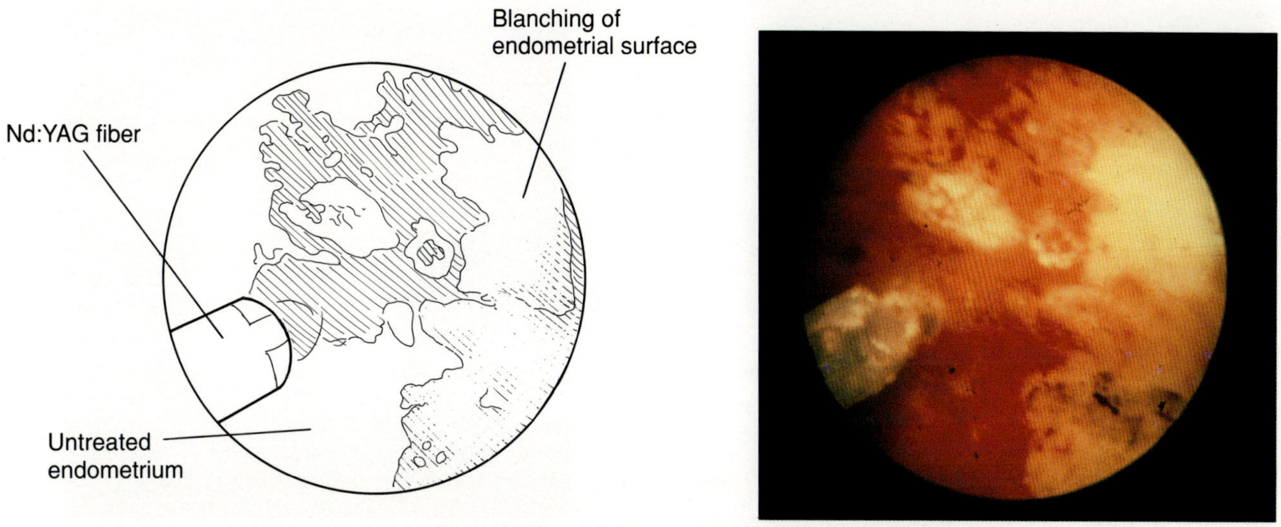

FIG. 1. The Nd:YAG nontouch or blanching technique. The fiber is seen coming from the lower left-hand corner of the picture. It is brought perpendicular and as close to the endometrial surface as possible. It is swept slowly across the surface creating blanched areas seen here primarily on the right.

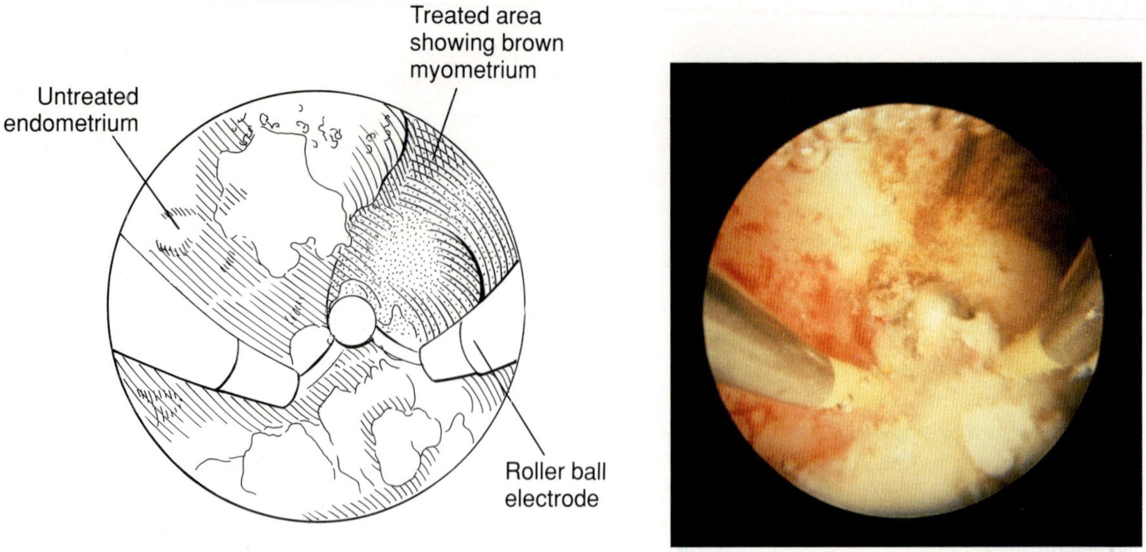

FIG. 2. The roller ball or bar electrode technique. The rolling electrode (shown here using a ball) "melts" the spongy endometrium and reveals a harder, brown surface, which is the myometrium. Further rolling may provide further in-depth electrical destruction to the myometrium but will not cause the electrode to sink further into it. Untreated endometrium is seen on the left.

nique, the uterine cavity has a brownish-yellow, rough tissue surface (Fig. 6) with the configuration of a normal uterine cavity. The endometrium has disappeared and the myometrium is exposed. The success of the procedure depends in large part on the destruction of the blood vessels supplying the superficial myometrium.

Most authors use some form of endometrial suppression to thin the endometrial surface prior to ablation. This is done to allow easier penetration through the basal layer. Danazol and depot leuprolide acetate are the most commonly used drugs but nafarelin acetate is another option. Equal results can be obtained by simply scheduling the patient in the immediate postmenstrual phase and mechanically removing the endometrium prior to the procedure (15). This latter technique is probably more satisfactory with the electrical techniques than with Nd:YAG laser since the laser energy is absorbed in dark colors. The blood created by the endometrial curettage may limit penetration by the Nd:YAG laser energy into the deeper endometrial basal layer.

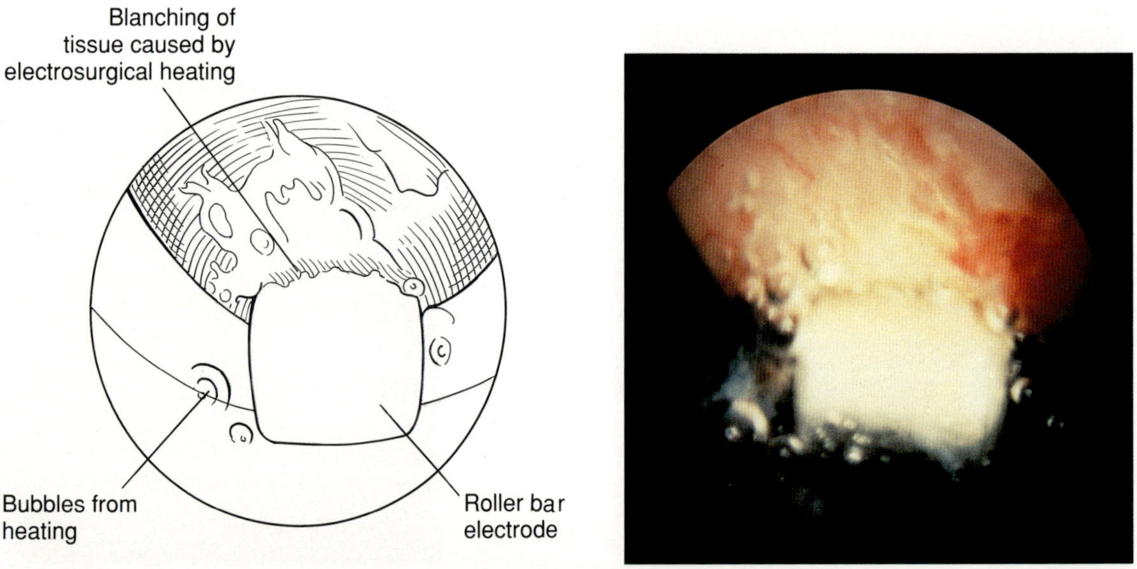

FIG. 3. Electrical effect on the myometrium. The roller electrode (shown here as a bar) should cover the surface of the endometrium slowly enough that electrical activity should be seen to precede the electrode. This activity appears as "lightening bolts" darting ahead of the roller.

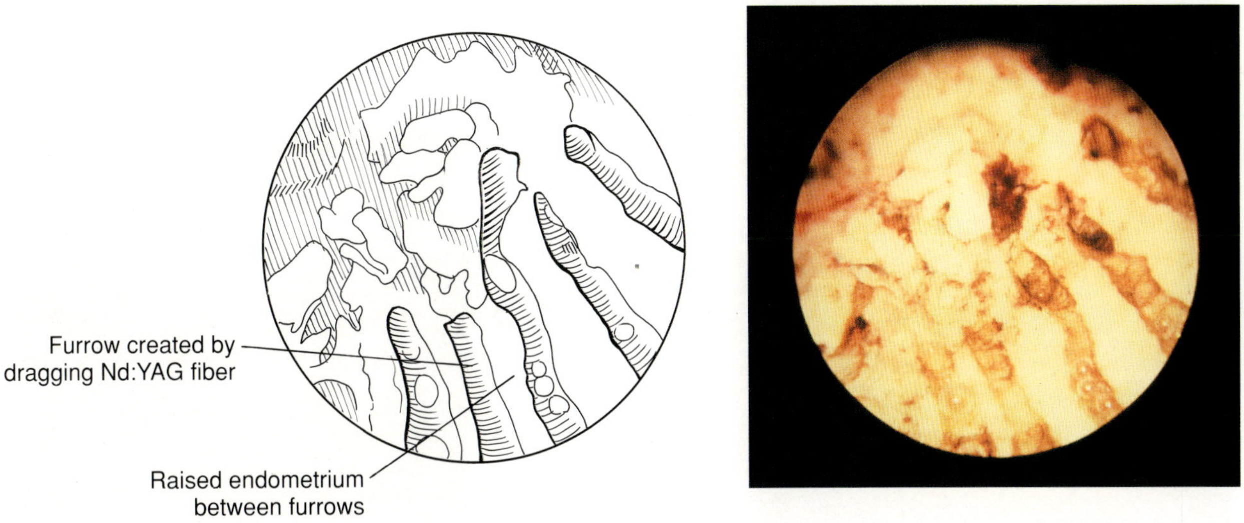

A

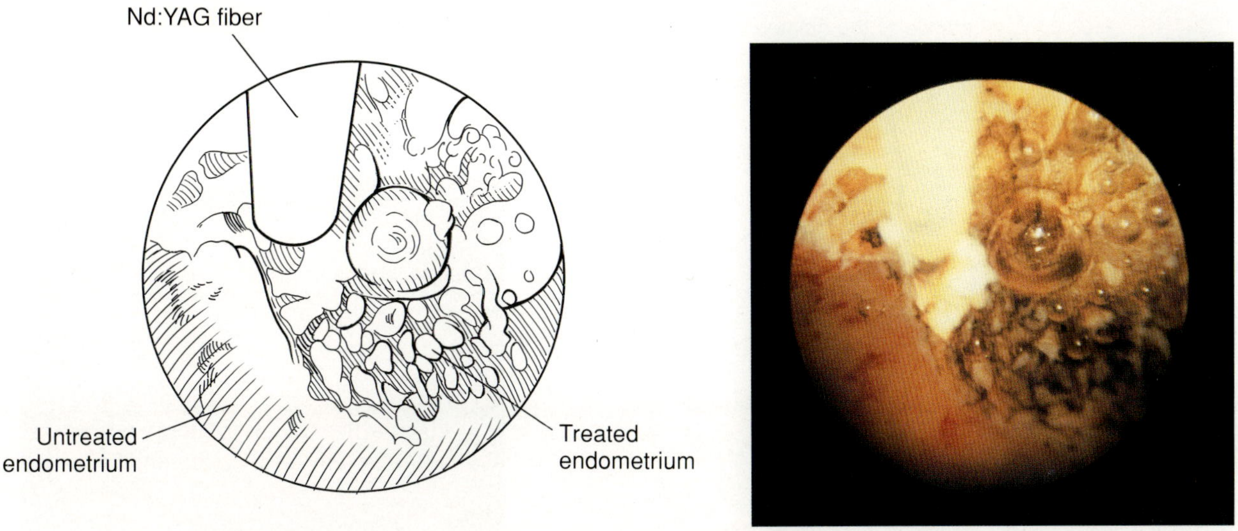

B

FIG. 4. The Nd:YAG laser touch or dragging technique. **A:** the initial dragging of the fiber creates furrows into the myometrium leaving a raised area of endometrium. **B:** Moving the fiber back and forth across the rows destroys the intervening endometrium. Normal, untreated endometrium appears in the lower left-hand portion of this picture.

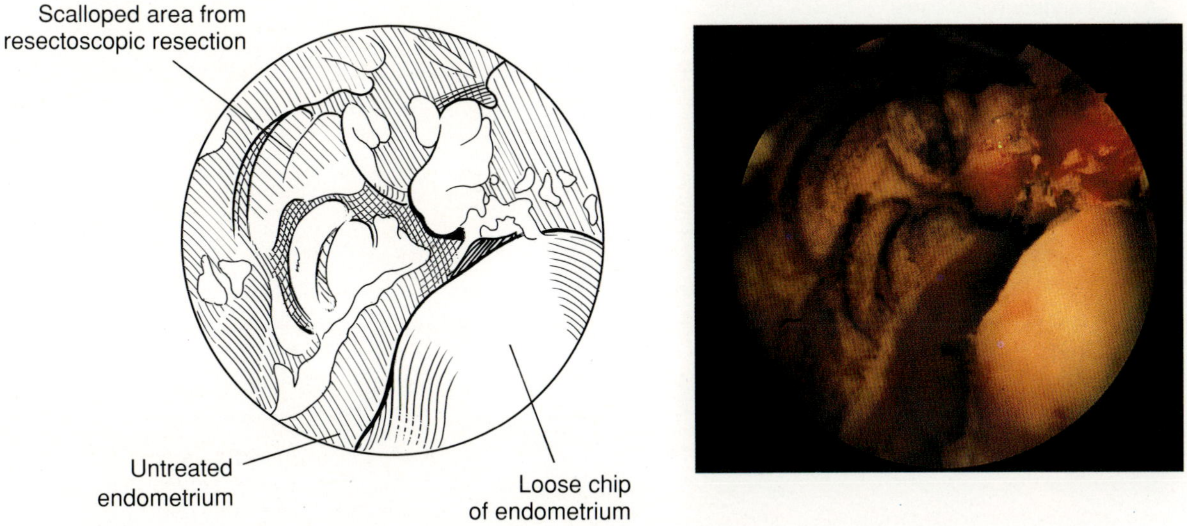

FIG. 5. The resection technique of endometrial ablation. The resected areas of endometrium give a scalloping effect of the exposed myometrium. Loose chips are seen in the lower portion of the picture and a small area of untreated endometrium in the 9 o'clock position.

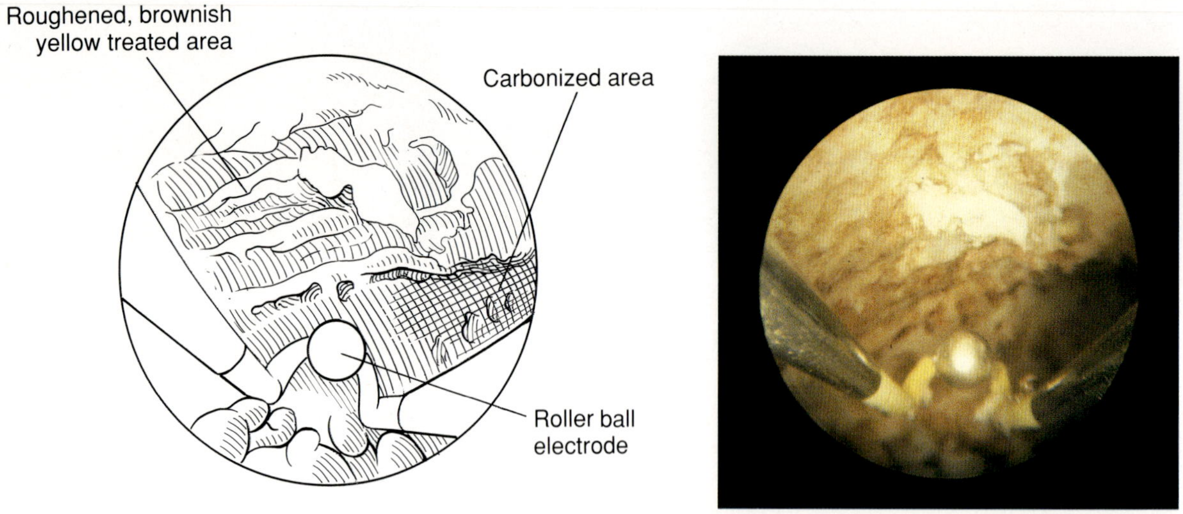

FIG. 6. Appearance of the ablated endometrial cavity. Although there are subtle differences between techniques, the endometrial cavity retains its shape. It is irregular, roughened, and has a brownish-yellow appearance. Black areas representing carbonization may also be seen.

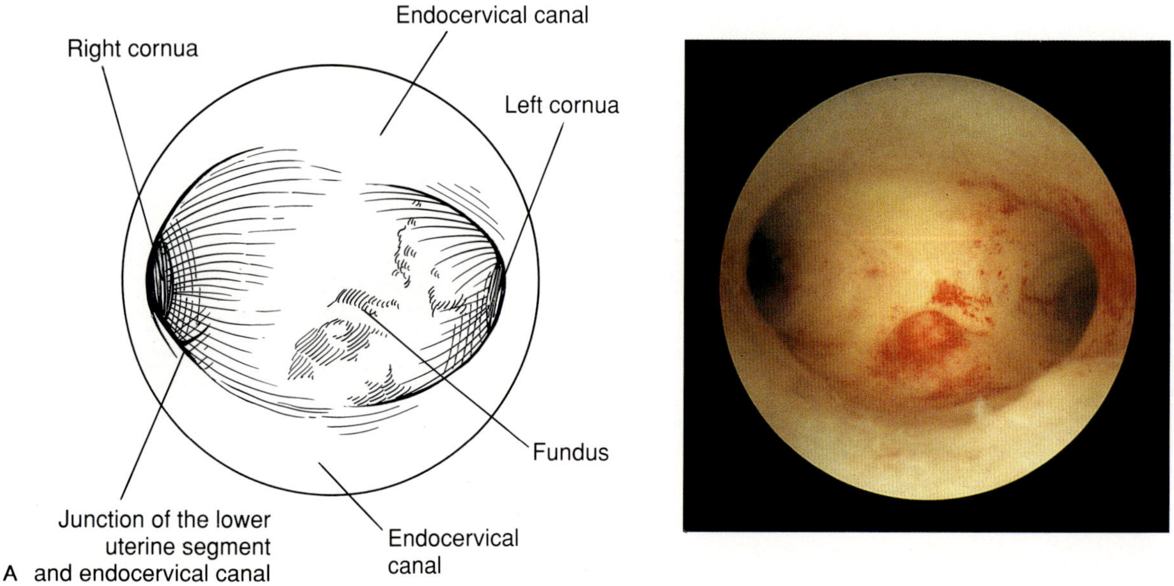

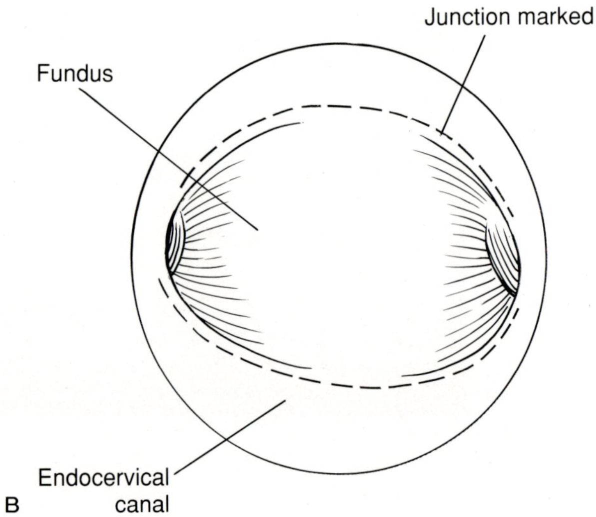

FIG. 7. A: Identification and marking of the junction of the lower uterine segment and endocervical canal is necessary prior to endometrial ablation. **B:** Junction to be marked before initiating ablation.

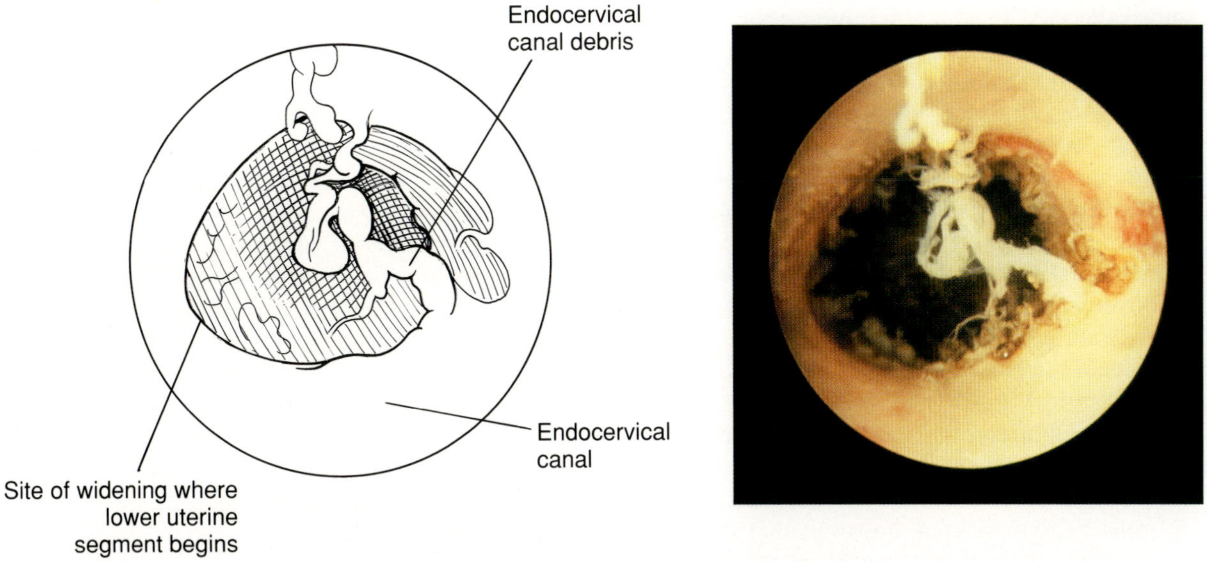

FIG. 8. The lower uterine segment subtley narrows into the canal and it frequently is difficult to determine this junction as the scope is withdrawn. It is more clearly delineated by withdrawing the hysteroscope into the canal and slowly advancing it until the canal starts to widen into the lower uterine segment.

When submucous fibroids coexist, they can be removed by a variety of techniques (16). Usually the same instrumentation is used for their removal as for endometrial ablation. Endometrial ablation usually is done prior to removal of the fibroid, except in those cases where a loop resectoscope electrode resection technique is used. The reason for this sequence is that visualization decreases as pieces of the fibroid are resected and fill the uterine cavity.

Power settings for endometrial ablation with the Nd:YAG laser in the dragging technique are usually 55 W and up to 70 W in the blanching technique. Resection of endometrium with the resectoscope loop is usually accomplished with 100–110 W of pure continuous (cut) current. The best wattage for roller ball or roller bar ablation has not been determined. The author finds that 75 W of a modulated (coagulation) current slowly rolled over the surface provides satisfactory results. Others prefer a continuous (cutting) current. There is no evidence that there is a difference in results with the two types of current.

Cleansing of the uterine cavity during ablation is required because of the debris, bubbles, and bleeding that occurs. This is accomplished with the resectoscope using a continuous flow system and with the Nd:YAG by providing an outflow catheter through a double-channeled instrument (17).

A systematic approach must be undertaken in the destruction of the endometrial cavity to avoid missing or incompletely treating areas. Except in the case of endometrial resection, the anterior wall is usually first treated followed by the lateral and posterior walls. In endometrial resection, the posterior wall is first treated since the resected chips that are produced cover the posterior wall and soon obscure visualization. Generally the ablation procedure is started in the cornual areas, and the fiber or electrode is brought out of the cornual area along the surface. Since the cornual area is the thinnest area of the uterus, care must be taken not to destroy too great a depth in this area.

The optics and mechanics of hysteroscopy do not easily allow the operator to sweep from the cornual area down through the lower uterine segment in a continuous stroke. Generally the upper third or fourth of the cavity is done followed by similar segmental areas until the lower uterine segment is treated. The junction of the lower uterine segment and endocervical canal is not always clear. It is best to mark this junction after studying its location by destroying a small area (Fig. 7A,B). Then ablation can be carried down to this mark. It is not necessary or desirable to destroy into the endocervical canal. To determine the start of the endometrial canal as well as assess if all areas of the cavity have been ablated, the hysteroscopist needs to withdraw the hysteroscope into the very upper portion of the endocervical canal to get a full overview of the cavity (17) (Fig. 8). Then the scope can be reintroduced into the cavity to view the area more closely when further ablation is necessary.

OUTCOME

Postoperatively patients have minimal discomfort and are generally sent home with only mild analgesics. They should be instructed that they will have a serosanguineous discharge for at least 3 weeks and possibly heavy bleeding at the time of the first menses. This bleeding does not predict the ultimate outcome. It has been suggested that continued postoperative suppression may have some value (18). In addition, some authors perform a postoperative curettage. Patients must understand that endometrial ablation cannot guarantee amenorrhea. It is a procedure designed to help women avoid a hysterectomy for heavy menses, and therefore satisfactory results should be defined as the avoidance of a hysterectomy or other subsequent uterine surgical procedures, including repeat ablation. However, the greatest degree of decreased menstrual flow possible is desired not only for patient convenience but to decrease the risk of endometrial regrowth and long-term failure.

The results of the Nd:YAG laser ablation and the resectoscope electrical ablation have been reviewed and are similar (19). Failure, defined as continued menorrhagia, hysterectomy, or repeat ablation, occurred in 8% of the Nd:YAG laser cases and in 10% of the resectoscope cases. It must be remembered, however, that these figures are from reports published by authors who have developed the technique and reflect not only their learning curve in performing the procedure but also in their selection of appropriate patients. They also are not reported as a life table analysis. Excellent results, as defined as amenorrhea or hypomenorrhea, were found in 86% of the Nd:YAG cases and in 84% of the resectoscope ablation cases. Normal menses occurred in 6% of the Nd: YAG patients and in 7% of the resectoscope patients. There does not appear to be a great deal of difference in results whether or not the ablation technique disrupts the endometrial surface.

COMPLICATIONS

Complications related to the procedure should be few (3) but are greatly increased by inexperience (20). The most commonly reported problem is fluid overload. This problem is more common when the endometrial surface is disrupted, thus opening the myometrial vascular channels. The role of uterine distending pressure is critical. Pressures above 75–100 mm Hg are not necessary and are dangerous (21). The risk of postoperative bleeding is also increased with those techniques that open vascular channels. Physical perforation of the uterine wall and damage to intraabdominal contents by transmission of energy without actual perforation have been reported (22,23). These risks should be minimal if appropriate power settings are used and the laser fiber or electrode are always kept in sight and drawn back toward the telescope rather than being advanced.

Most authors do not use prophylactic antibiotics. However, there may be an advantage in patients with a history of pelvic inflammatory disease (24).

Long-term complications have not been identified. The risk of pregnancy in women not protected would appear to be about 1% (3). Detractors of this procedure raise the question that if carcinoma of the endometrium were to develop in the future it would be hidden from early detection. It would appear that most cavities contract down rather than scar from wall to wall. Therefore, bleeding from carcinoma should be seen as frequently in women who have had an endometrial ablation as in those who have not (25,26). It is possible that the reduction in the volume of endometrium remaining after ablation may reduce the risk of the development of an endometrial cancer. The development of pelvic pain and dysmenorrhea occurs in some patients. This may be related to localized areas of hematometrium/hematosalpinx in patients who are sterilized by tubal closure (27). There is no evidence that the procedure creates adenomyosis, although patients who preoperatively have significant dysmenorrhea are not good candidates. Although many experience pain relief, those with extensive adenomyosis usually continue to have problems. This is not from the creation of adenomyosis but rather from its persistence.

HIGHLIGHTS

Hysteroscopic endometrial ablation has become an established method for managing menorrhagia in women who do not desire further pregnancies and who wish to avoid a hysterectomy. It is an efficacious, safe, outpatient procedure, which should be considered, if appropriate, as an alternative to all women with heavy menses.

REFERENCES

1. Vancaillie TC. Endometrial electro ablation. In: Sutton C, Diamond M, eds. *Endoscopic surgery for gynaecologists.* London: WB Saunders; 1993:307–316.
2. Goldrath MH, Fuller TA, Segal S. Laser photovaporization of endometrium for the treatment of menorrhagia. *Am J Obstet Gynecol* 1981;140:14–19.
3. Loffer FD. Endometrial ablation—where do we stand? *Gynecol Endosc* 1992;1:175–179.
4. Carlson KJ, Nicholas DH, Schiff I. Indications for hysterectomy. *N Engl J Med* 1993;328:856–860.
5. Vercellini P, Ragni G, Trespidi L, Oldani SA, Panazza S, Crosignani PG. Adenomyosis: a déjà vu? *Obstet Gynecol Surv* 1993;48: 789–794.
6. Lefler HT, Lefler CF. Ablation of the endometrium: three-year follow up for premenstrual symptoms. *J Reprod Med* 1992;37:147–150.
7. Loffer FD. Hysteroscopy with selective endometrial sampling compared with D&C for abnormal uterine bleeding: the value of a negative hysteroscopic view. *Obstet Gynecol* 1989;73:16–20.
8. Phipps JH, Lewis BV, Prior MV, Roberts T. Experimental and clinical studies with radio frequency induced thermal endometrial ablation for functional menorrhagia. *Obstet Gynecol* 1990;76: 876–881.
9. Neuwirth RS, Duran AA, Singer A, Bolduc LR. The endometrial ablator: a new instrument. *Obstet Gynecol* 1994;83:792–796.
10. Singer A, Almanza R, Gutierrez A, Haber G, Bolduc LR. Preliminary clinical experience with a thermal balloon endometrial ablation method to treat menorrhagia. *Obstet Gynecol* 1994;83:732–734.
11. Loffer FD. Hysteroscopic endometrial ablation with the Nd:Yag laser using a non-touch technique. *Obstet Gynecol* 1987;69:679–682.

12. Lin BL, Miyamoto N, Tomomatu M, et al. The development of a new hysteroscopic resectoscope and its clinical application on transcervical resection (TCR) and endometrial ablation (EA). *Jpn J Obstet Gynecol* 1988;4:56–61.
13. Vancaillie TG. Electrocoagulation of the endometrium with the ball and resectoscope. *Obstet Gynecol* 1989;74:425–427.
14. DeCherney AH, Diamond MP, Lavy G, Polan ML. Endometrial ablation for intractable uterine bleeding: hysteroscopic resection. *Obstet Gynecol* 1987;70:668–669.
15. Lefler HT, Sullivan GH, Hulka JF. Modified endometrial ablation: electrocoagulation with vasopression and suction curettage preparation. *Obstet Gynecol* 1991;77:949–953.
16. Loffer FD. Removal of large symptomatic intrauterine growths by the hysteroscopic resectoscope. *Obstet Gynecol* 1990;76:836–840.
17. Loffer FD. Hysteroscopy. In: Stangel JJ, ed. *Infertility surgery; a multi-method approach to female reproductive surgery.* Norwalk, CT: Appleton and Lange; 1990:72–85.
18. Goldrath MH. Use of danazol in hysteroscopic surgery for menorrhagia. *J Reprod Med* 1990;35:91–96.
19. Loffer FD. Endometrial ablation—a comparison of hysteroscopic techniques. In: Lewis BV, Magos AL, eds. *Endometrial ablation.* Edinburgh: Churchill Livingstone; 1992:143–155.
20. Macdonald R, Phipps J, Singer A. Endometrial ablation: a safe procedure. *Gynecol Endosc* 1992;1:7–9.
21. Loffer FD. Complications from uterine distension during hysteroscopy. In: Corfman RS, Diamond MP, DeCherney A, eds. *Complications of laparoscopy and hysteroscopy.* Boston: Blackwell Scientific; 1993;177:86.
22. Perry PC, Daniell JF, Gimpelson RJ. Bowel injury from Nd:Yag endometrial ablation. *Gynecol Surg* 1990;6:199–203.
23. Sullivan B, Kenney P, Seibel M. Hysteroscopic resection of fibroid with thermal injury to sigmoid. *Obstet Gynecol* 1992;80:546–547.
24. McCausland VM, Fields GA, McCausland AM, Townsend DE. Tuboovarian abscesses after operative hysteroscopy. *J Reprod Med* 1993;38:198–200.
25. Copperman AB, DeCherney AH, Olive DL. A case of endometrial cancer following endometrial ablation for dysfunctional uterine bleeding. *Obstet Gynecol* 1993;82:640–642.
26. Istre O, Skajaa K, Holm-Neilsen P, Forman A. The second-look appearance of the uterine cavity after resection of the endometrium. *Gynecol Endosc* 1993;2:159–163.
27. Townsend DE, McCausland V, McCausland A, Fields G, Kauffman K. Post-ablation-tubal sterilization syndrome. *Obstet Gynecol* 1993;82:422–424.

Endoscopic Management of Gynecologic Disease,
edited by G.D. Adamson and D.C. Martin.
Lippincott-Raven Publishers, Philadelphia © 1996.

CHAPTER 33

Salpingoscopy and Falloposcopy

Eric S. Surrey, Mark W. Surrey, and John F. Kerin

Significant technical advances have allowed reproductive surgeons to visualize the entire length of the fallopian tube lumen from the fimbriated end to the uterotubal ostium. Two microendoscopic techniques that aid in achieving this end shall be presented in this chapter: salpingoscopy and falloposcopy. Salpingoscopy allows for visualization of the ampulla, infundibullum, and fimbria through a transfimbrial approach performed at laparoscopy. Falloposcopy affords visualization of the entire length of the fallopian tube by a nonincisional transcervical approach.

ANATOMY AND PHYSIOLOGY

The average length of the human fallopian tube is 8–13 cm (1). The intramural portion of the tube extends 1.5–2.0 cm from the uterotubal ostium. It is the narrowest segment measuring between 0.4 and 0.5 cm in diameter and has three distinct muscle layers: outer spiral, inner longitudinal, and intermediary circular. The mucosa contains a high degree of secretory elements with a greater proportion of ciliated cells than in the isthmus. The isthmic region extends from the cornua to the ampulla and measures 2–3 cm in length and 1–2 cm in diameter. The longitudinal muscle layer becomes more attenuated as it approaches the ampulla. On cross-section, the isthmus takes on a cruciate appearance. There is a relative dearth of ciliated cells. The normal ampulla represents the distal two thirds of the fallopian tube extending from the ampullary-isthmic junction to the infundibulum. The diameter widens dramatically to approximately 1 cm. The muscular layers become significantly attenuated with virtual loss of the longitudinal layers and extensive thinning of the middle circular layer. Secretory and ciliated cells are abundant in this region.

The fallopian tube represents a complex neuroendocrine organ. The lush folds within the ampulla, infundibulum, and fimbria serve as the sites for ovum capture, fertilization, and early embryo development. The time course of ovum transport in the human fallopian tube is approximately 80 hr, of which 72 are spent in the ampulla after rapidly traversing the distance from the fimbria (2). Ampullary embryo transport appears intimately related to the presence of an adequate number of cilia located on the mucosal ridges, although other factors play a role. The functioning muscularis and secretory activity of glands within the folds create a turbulent system. Secreted cytokines and growth factors may also be a factor in enhancing early embryo development and uterine receptivity. More proximally, the isthmus and intramural regions with a more distinctive muscularis and relative dearth of ciliated cells are characterized by rapid embryo transport, which may reflect the function of enhanced muscular contractility in this region.

PATHOPHYSIOLOGY

Distal tubal occlusion and hydrosalpinx formation primarily results from ascending or descending infection or a noninfectious inflammatory response (e.g., endometriosis, surgical adhesions). The pathophysiology of this disorder has been extensively reviewed elsewhere in this book. It had previously been assumed that the etiologies of proximal and distal tubal occlusion are identical. Re-

E. S. Surrey and M. W. Surrey: Center for Reproductive Medicine and Surgery, Beverly Hills, California 90210.

J. F. Kerin: Department of Obstetrics and Gynecology, Flinders University, Bedford Park, South Australia 5042.

cent studies have raised questions regarding this concept. Intraluminal adhesions, fibrosis, debris, polyps, mucous plugs, and endometriosis have been described as causes of proximal obstruction (3–6). Sulak and co-workers reported pathologic findings in 18 patients who underwent resection and reconstruction of proximal tubal segments thought to be obstructed based on hysterosalpingogram and laparoscopic chromotubation (5). No occlusion was noted in 11 patients, whereas in 6 patients an amorphous material compatible with a mucous plug was noted.

Salpingitis isthmica nodosa (SIN), a disorder uniquely limited to the isthmic region, is characterized by nodular thickening, which may contain glandular elements. Multiple diverticulae lined by tubal epithelium, which penetrate the muscularis and are in communication with the tubal lumen, are pathognomonic of SIN. Inflammatory cells are rarely present, which calls into question the likelihood of an infectious etiology. This disorder appears to be progressive and is associated with proximal occlusion and an increased incidence of tubal pregnancy (7,8).

Hysterosalpingography, laparoscopy, and hysteroscopy have been the traditional means for assessing the fallopian tube. Correlation between findings achieved with these modalities has been variable (9–11). The diagnosis of proximal tubal occlusion can also be confused by tubal spasm, which may provide a false-positive finding. Others would suggest that this finding may be associated with intrinsic tubal abnormalities and lower pregnancy rates (12). Needless to say, these techniques primarily afford information regarding tubal patency, degree of dilation, and peritubal disease. Direct visualization of the tubal lumen and endothelial lining cannot be achieved.

SALPINGOSCOPY

Technique

Salpingoscopy affords visualization of the oviductal lumen from the ampullary–isthmic junction to the fimbria. The salpingoscope is introduced transfimbrially at the time of laparoscopy or laparotomy. Both flexible (Olympus Corp., Lake Success, NY) and rigid (Karl Stortz, Culver City, CA) salpingoscopes with outer diameters (OD) of 1.5–2.8 mm have been employed (13–16) (Fig. 1). The size of these instruments prevents direct access to the isthmic and intramural segments. Flexible salpingoscopes are less traumatic and can more closely approach the ampullary-isthmic junction, whereas rigid endoscopes afford greater image quality.

The salpingoscope is introduced into the peritoneal cavity through a 3-mm reducer placed through an accessory trocar during laparoscopy. The fimbriated end of the tube is stabilized with atraumatic grasping forceps (Fig. 2A). The salpingoscope is advanced gently until resistance is reached. In the absence of obstruction, this should be at the point of the ampullary–isthmic junction. Heparinized Ringer's lactate solution is gently infused by a hand-held syringe through extension tubing connected to the irrigating channel of the salpingoscope (Fig. 2B). The use of carbon dioxide as a distention medium may hamper adequate visualization by flattening ampullary folds. The endothelial lining and tubal lumen are visualized in a retrograde fashion as the salpingoscope is slowly withdrawn. A separate standard camera chip, light source, and video monitor are employed. The procedure is performed after prophylactic antibiotics have been administered.

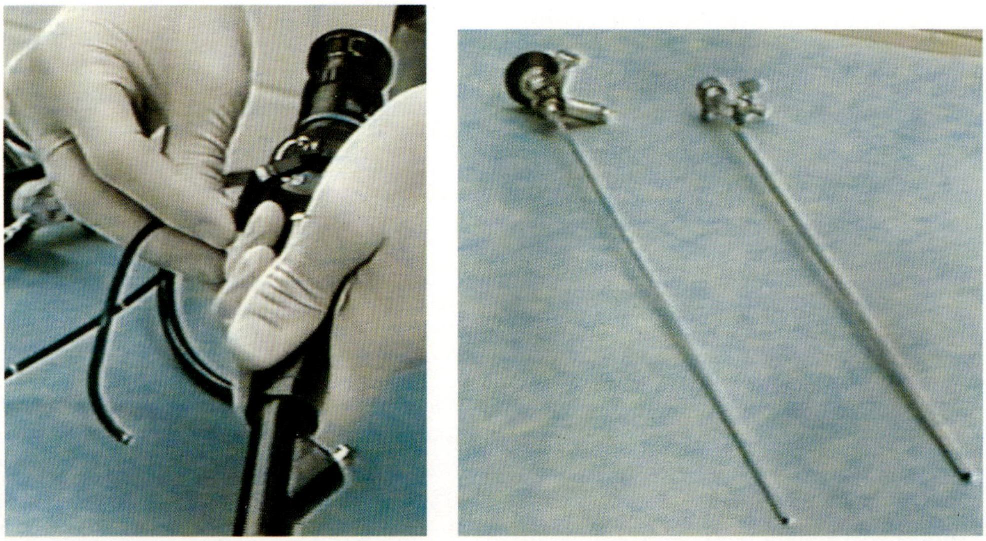

A B

FIG. 1. A: Flexible salpingoscope (Olympus Corp., Lake Success, NY). **B:** Rigid salpingoscope (*left*) and sheath (*right*) (Karl Storz, Culver City, CA).

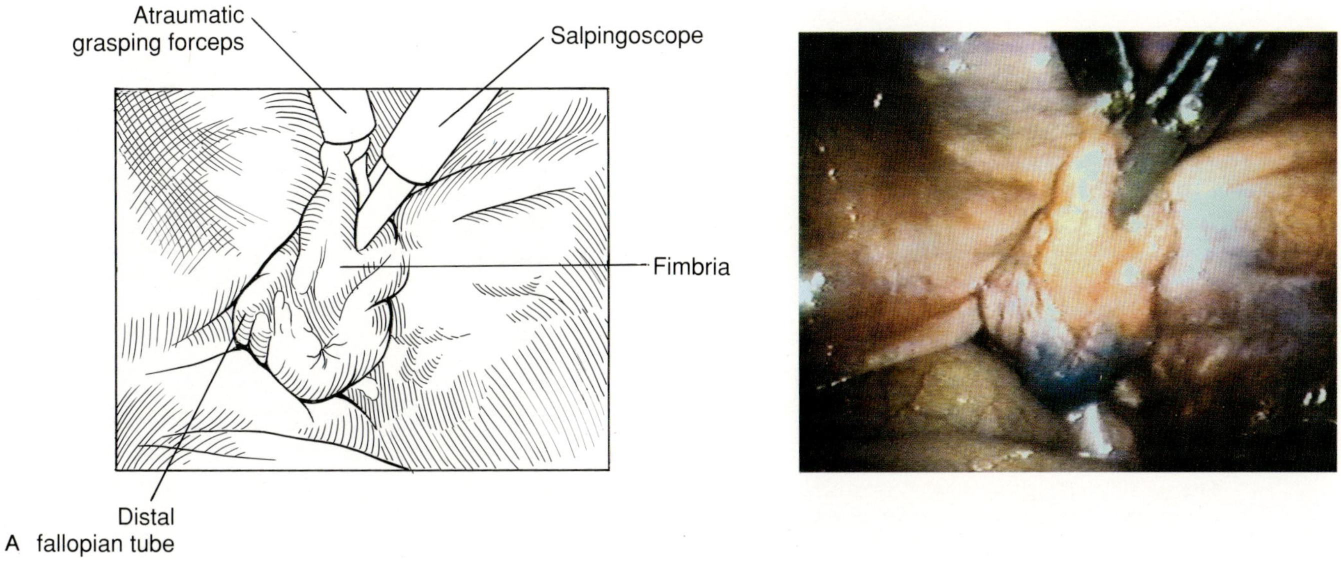

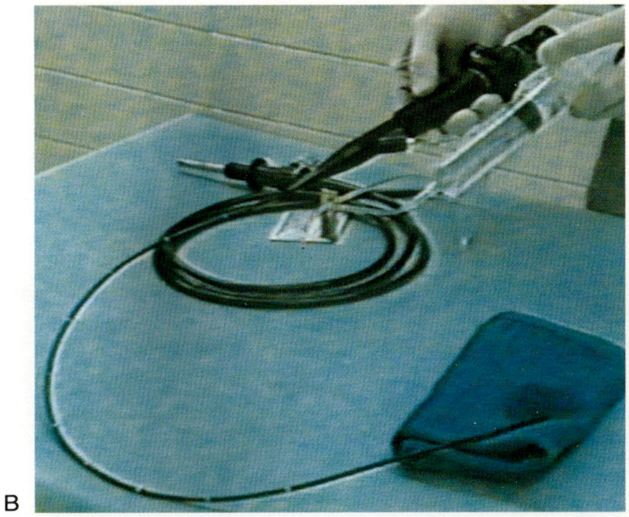

FIG. 2. **A:** Flexible salpingoscope introduced into fimbriated end of fallopian tube. The serosal surface has been grasped just proximal to the fimbria with atraumatic grasping forceps. **B:** Heparinized lactated Ringer's solution is infused through the accessory port of the salpingoscope as a distension medium.

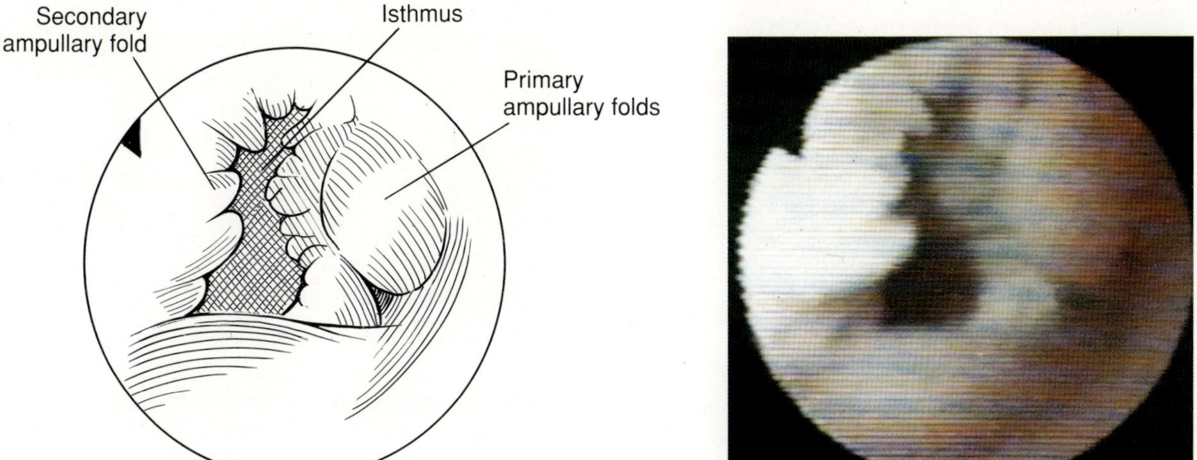

FIG. 3. Salpingoscopic view of the ampullary–isthmic junction. Note initiation of primary radial folds with rare secondary folds.

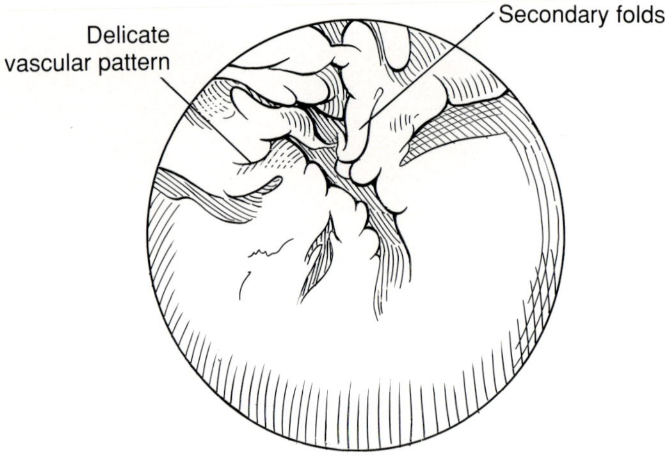

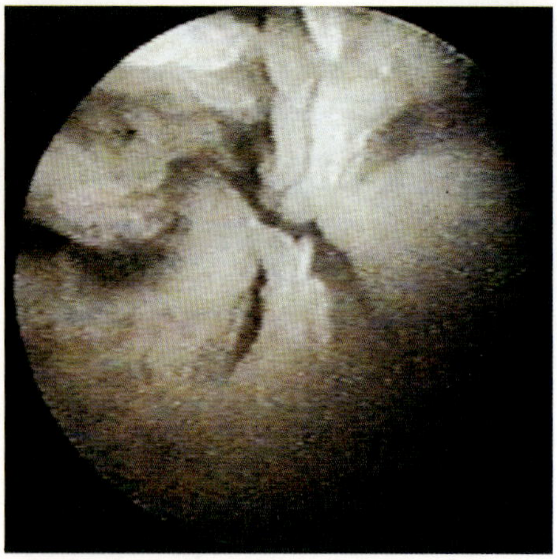

FIG. 4. Salpingoscopic view of distal ampulla-infundibulum. Note delicate vascular pattern and presence of extensive network of secondary folds.

If a hydrosalpinx is encountered, access to the tubal lumen is obtained by creating a small terminal neosalpingostomy, which is made only large enough to accommodate the salpingoscope, using standard endoscopic techniques. This opening can serve as an initiating point for a more complete reconstructive procedure should the quality of the endothelial lining be acceptable. If this is not the case, the opening can easily be closed with coagulation or laser techniques or the tube can be removed entirely as appropriate.

Normal Anatomy and Pathologic Findings

As the surgeon progresses from the ampullary–isthmic junction into the ampulla, a series of radially arranged primary folds approximately 4 mm in height can be viewed (Fig. 3). Secondary folds with delicate vascular patterns approximately 1 mm in height become more pronounced in the distal aspect of the tube. The number of folds increases toward the fimbriated end (Fig. 4).

A variety of abnormal findings have been reported. These include intraluminal synechiae (Fig. 5), stenoses (15), ampullary diverticulae (Fig. 6), inflammatory vascular patterns (Fig. 7), mucosal atrophy and loss of endothelial folds (Fig. 8). Several authors have attempted to classify the severity of luminal abnormalities detected at salpingoscopy (14,17).

The prognostic value of salpingoscopic findings in the management of distal tubal disease or unexplained infertility has been investigated. Henry-Suchet et al. reported that of 136 women who underwent a tuboplasty, intrauterine pregnancies were achieved only in those with at least one tube which was normal at salpingoscopy (18). Cornier described intraluminal adhesions in 37% of tubes visualized in patients with prior diagnosis of unexplained infertility with normal findings at laparoscopy and hysterosalpingogram (15). We recently reported that a relation between salpingoscopic findings and those noted at laparoscopy was high in patients with moderate to severe disease but poor in patients with laparoscopically staged mild disease (19).

Complications are extremely rare after salpingoscopy. A single case of postsalpingoscopy infection has been reported (13). Minimal bleeding at the point of the anti-

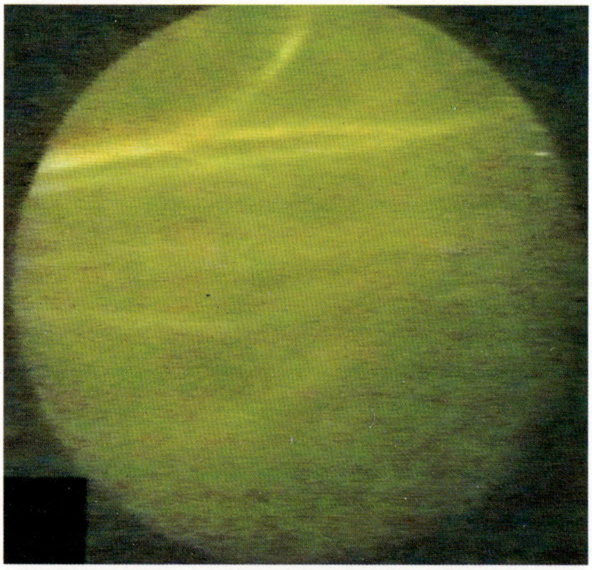

FIG. 5. Close-up view through salpingoscope of intraluminal adhesions in the midampullary region of the oviduct. This patient had a history of primary infertility and pelvic inflammatory disease. Hysterosalpingogram was normal and laparoscopy revealed minimal peritubal adhesions with normal-appearing fimbria.

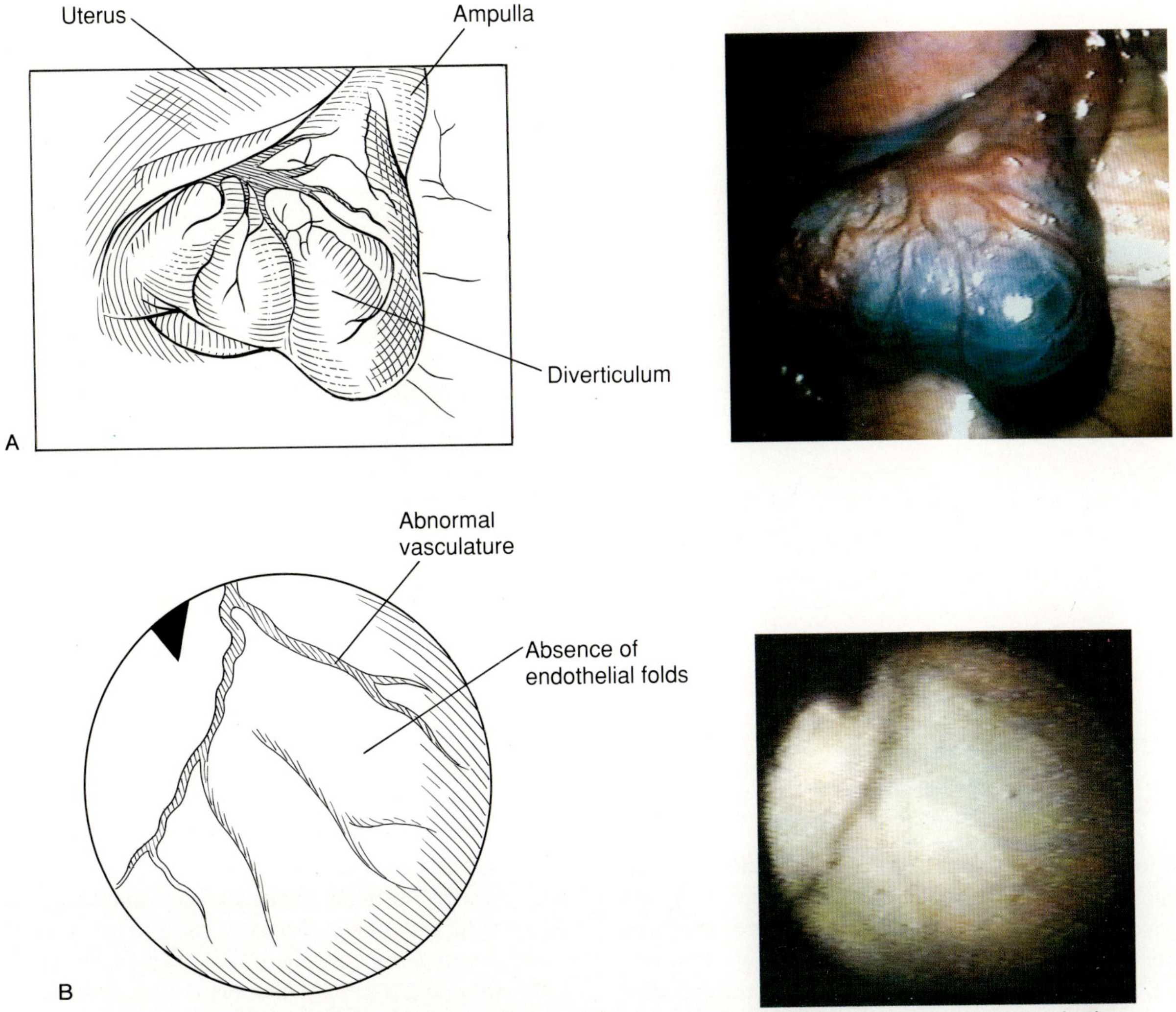

FIG. 6. A: Apparent diverticulum in distal ampullary region noted after distention during chromotubation in patient with unexplained infertility. Hysterosalpingogram and tubal appearance prior to chromotubation were normal. **B:** Salpingoscopic view of diverticulum described in Fig. 6A. Note complete absence of primary or secondary ampullary endothelial folds and abnormal vascular pattern.

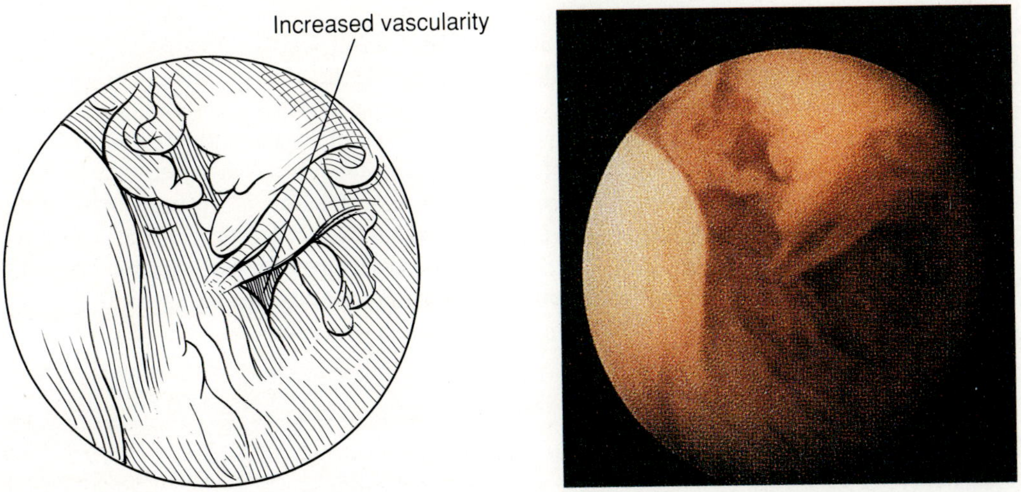

FIG. 7. Increased vascularity in patient with moderate tubal disease as viewed through the salpingoscope. (From ref. 14, with permission.)

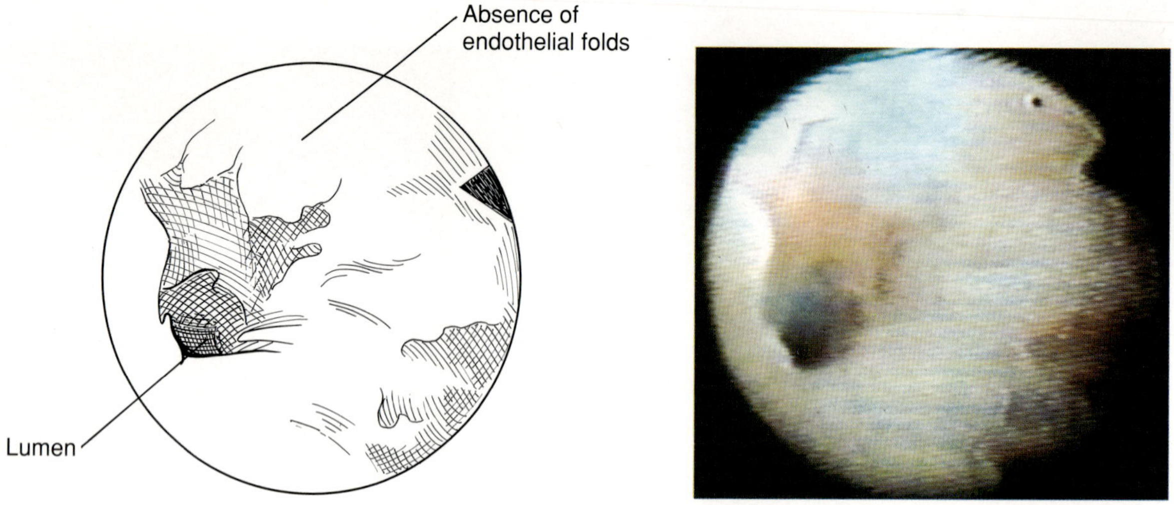

FIG. 8. Loss of endothelial folds and absence of normal vascular pattern in patient with hydrosalpinx as viewed through a flexible salpingoscope.

mesenteric border at which the tube is grasped can occur. This should resolve spontaneously.

FALLOPOSCOPY

Technique

Falloposcopy involves a transvaginal, transcervical approach to visualization of the tubal lumen. This can be performed with either a coaxial or a linear everting catheter delivery system. Kerin and colleagues first described the successful visualization of the entire length of the fallopian tube lumen by a coaxial technique in 1990 (20,21). This procedure is ideally performed during the midfollicular phase of the menstrual cycle after cessation of menses. Antibiotic prophylaxis should be administered.

A flexible hysteroscope with 1.5–3.5 mm OD (Olympus Corp., Lake Success, NY; Intramed Laboratories, San Diego, CA; Mitsubishi Cable Industries, Atami, Japan) is introduced into the uterine cavity under video monitoring. The uterine cavity is sounded but the cervix is not dilated. The hysteroscope is directed to within 1–2 mm of the uterotubal ostium. A Tuohy-Borst Y connector (Cook Ob-Gyn, Spencer, IN) is attached to the accessory port of the hysteroscope. Ringer's lactate is infused as a distension medium through one arm of the Y connector. A platinum-tipped, floppy guidewire coated with Teflon or stainless steel and with an OD of 0.3–0.8 mm (Conceptus, Inc., San Carlos, CA; Target Therapeutics, San Jose, CA; Cook Ob-Gyn; Guidewire Medi-Tech, Watertown, NH) is then introduced through the other arm of the Y connector. It is advanced through the ostium under direct visualization for a distance of 15 cm or until resistance is met. To avoid perforation, the operator should not advance the wire past a point of resistance. Gentle torque may be required to advance the wire through the acute angles of the intramural portion of the fallopian tube. A flexible Teflon catheter with OD 1.2–1.3 mm (Conceptus Inc; Target Therapeutics; Cook Ob-Gyn) and a second Y connector attached to its proximal end is introduced over the wire for a similar length. Care should be taken to avoid manipulation of the uterotubal ostia during spasm to avoid bleeding and traumatic entry into the tube (Fig. 9). The guidewire is then withdrawn. A falloposcope is then introduced through the straight arm of the Y connector. These devices vary from 1.0 to 1.5 cm in length and from 0.35 to 0.5 mm OD (Mitsubishi Cable; Olympus Corp.; Intramed Laboratories; Medical Dynamics, Englewood, CO). The surrounding catheter provides protection for the highly flexible and fragile falloposcope (Fig. 10). A high-resolution camera chip is attached to a second video monitor. Ringer's lactate is infused with minimal pressure through the angled arm of the Y connector. Visualization is performed in a retrograde fashion while maintaining the falloposcope just within the catheter lumen to avoid a white-out.

FIG. 9. View 1(A): Hysteroscopic view of the uteroutubal ostium in the relaxed state. View 2(B): Same ostium several seconds later during contraction. Note typical four-segment puckered appearance. View 3(C): Ideal distance and end-on view of ostium prior to guidewire insertion. View 4(D): Introduction of the guidewire along the intramural tubal lumen visualized hysteroscopically.

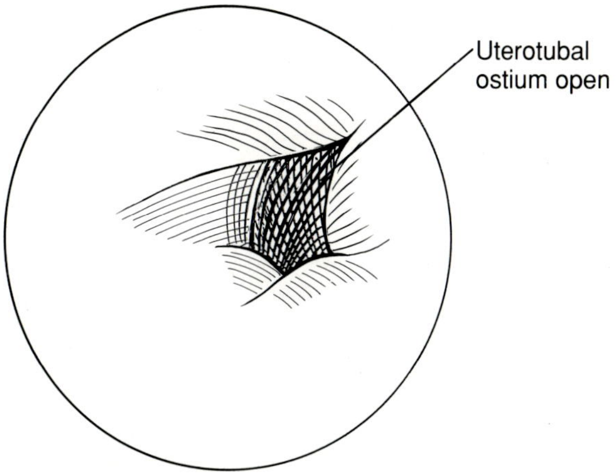
Uterotubal
ostium open

A

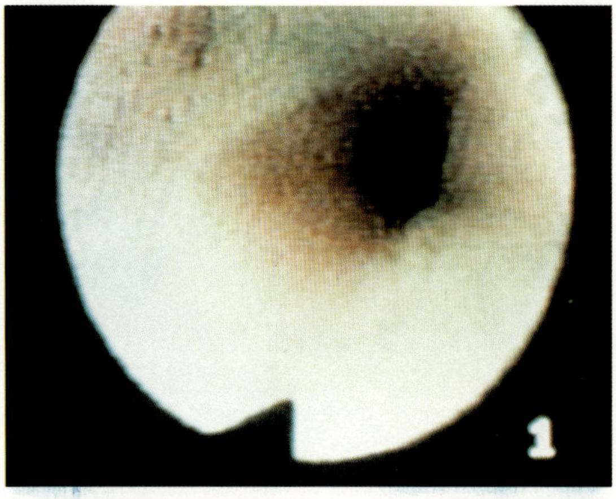
1

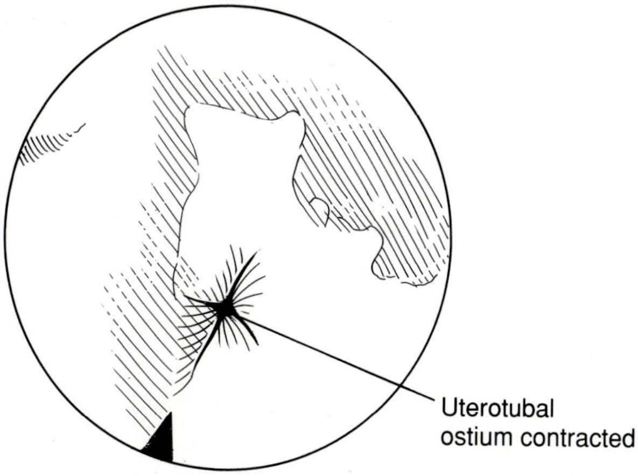
Uterotubal
ostium contracted

B

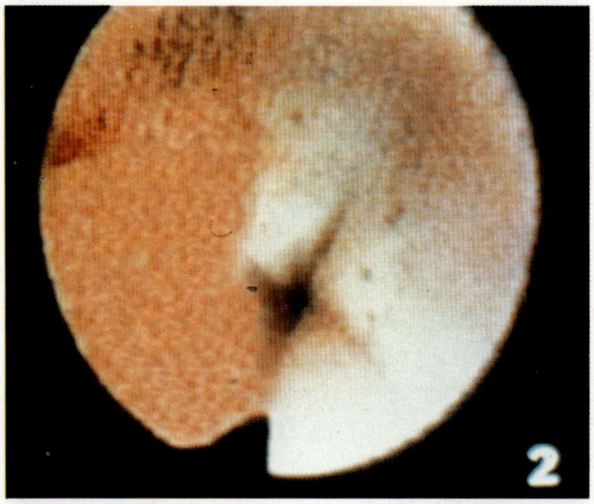
2

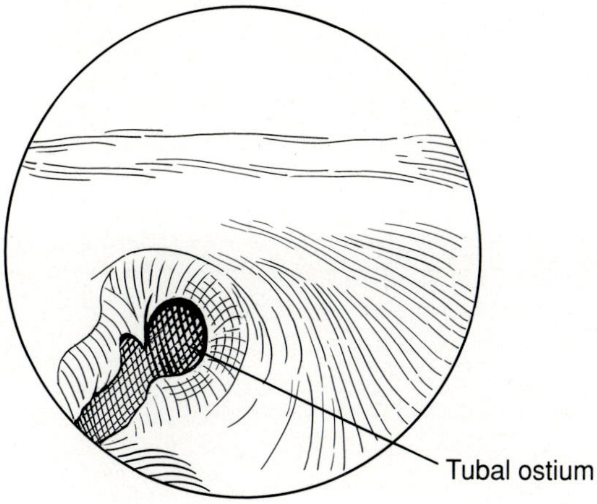
Tubal ostium

C

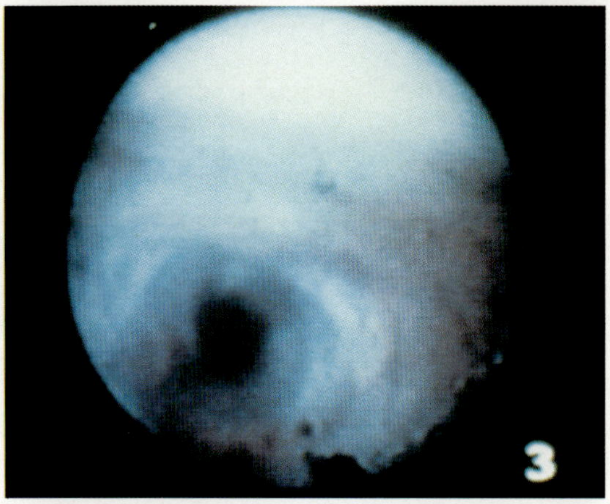
3

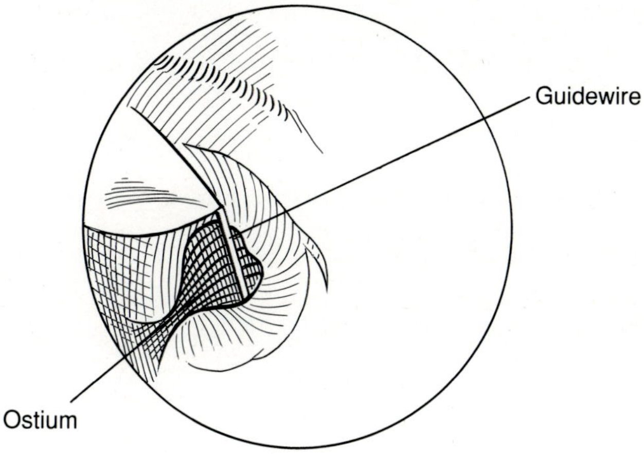
Guidewire
Ostium

D

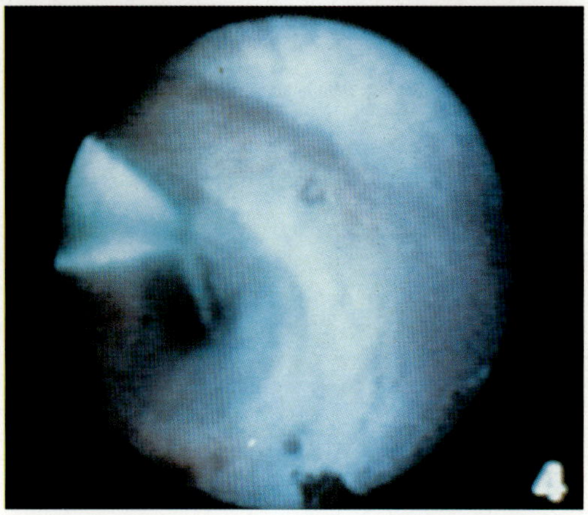
4

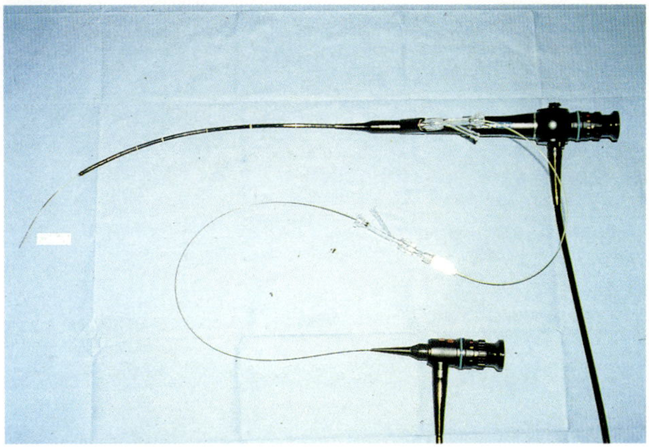

FIG. 10. Falloposcope introduced through Y connector attached to over-the-wire Teflon catheter. Entire system has been previously thread through the operating channel of flexible hysteroscope.

The linear everting catheter (LEC) represents an alternative means of transcervically accessing the proximal portion of the fallopian tube for falloposcopy (22). This system (Imagyn, Laguna Niguel, CA) is composed of outer and inner catheter bodies joined by a distal balloon, which everts as the inner body is advanced (Fig. 11). The balloon is pressurized, resulting in a slow eversion of the catheter tip (Fig. 12). This process allows the balloon to conform to the tortuous course of the tube and results in a reduction of lateral shear forces. The falloposcope is introduced through the catheter lumen. Imaging is performed in a retrograde fashion as well.

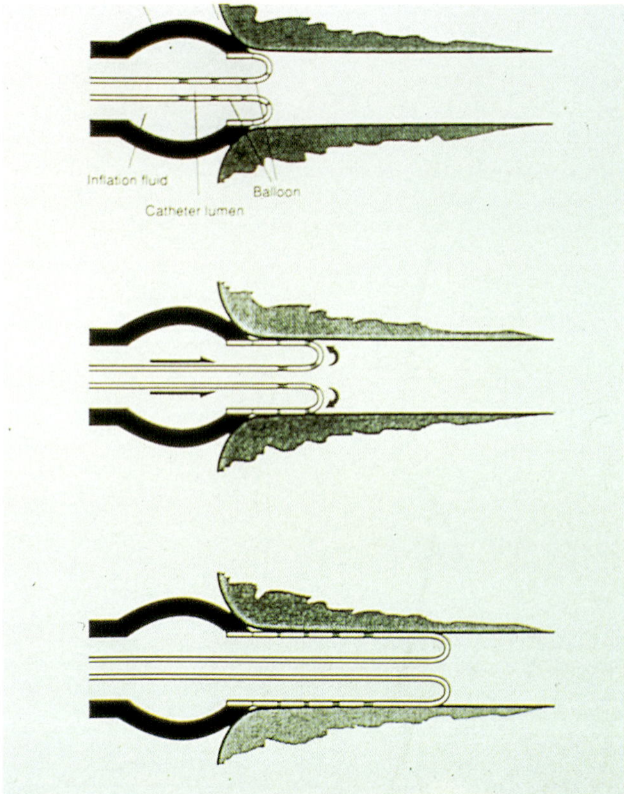

FIG. 12. Mechanism of eversion with LEC falloposcopy system. (From ref. 22, with permission.)

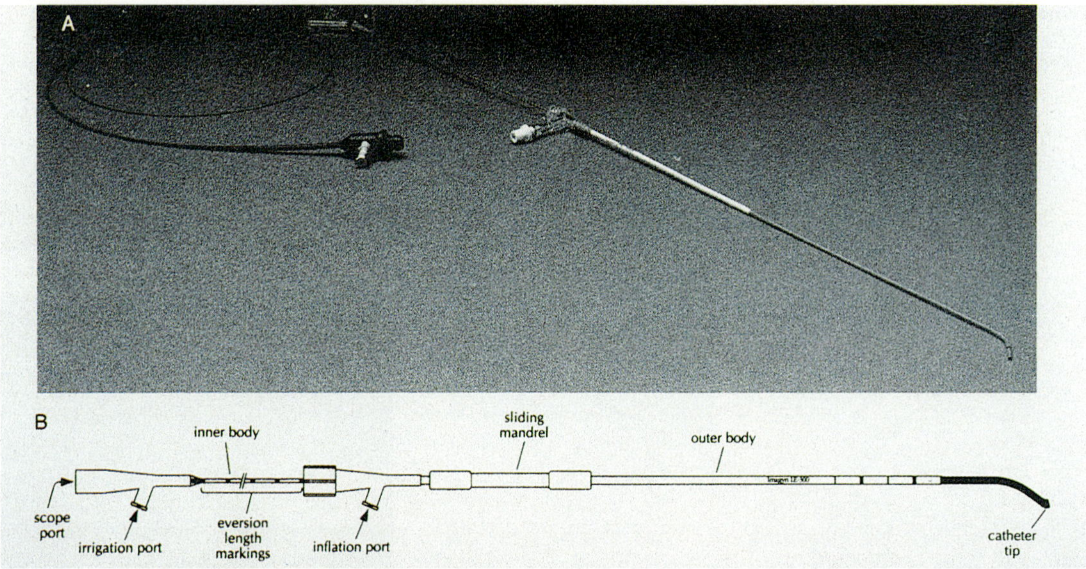

FIG. 11. Linear everting catheter. **A:** Actual photograph. **B:** Labeled diagram. (From ref. 22, with permission.)

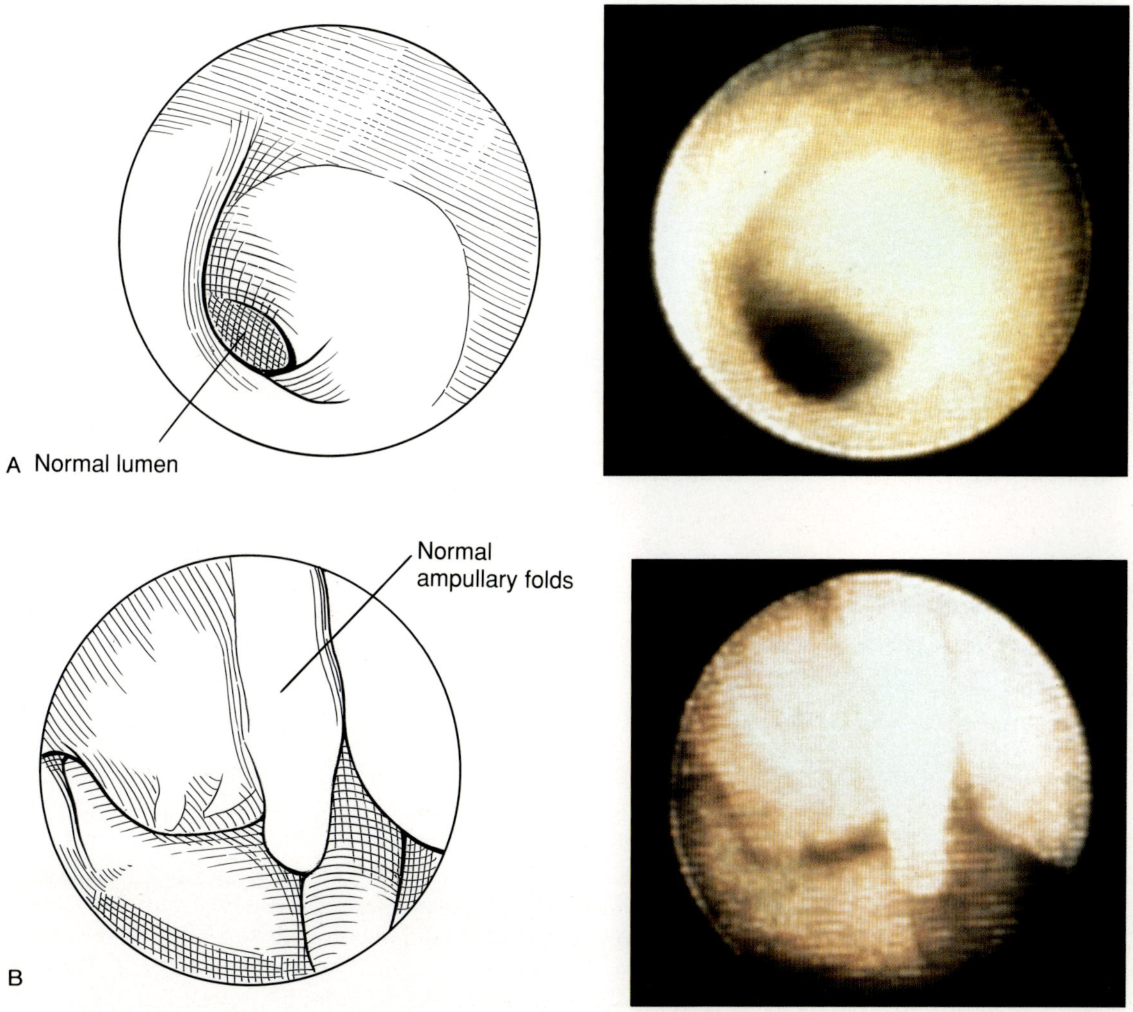

FIG. 13. A: Image of normal isthmus obtained with LEC falloposcopy system. **B:** Image of normal ampulla obtained with LEC falloposcopy system. (From ref. 22, with permission.)

Technical failure, defined by the inability to advance the falloposcope or to visualize the tubal lumen in the absence of detectable lesions, has been reported in only 8.5% of coaxial- and 13.4% of LEC-directed procedures (22,23).

Normal Anatomy and Pathologic Findings

The intramural portion of the oviduct is generally fairly straight in its course, but it may form an acute angle with the endometrial cavity. Its lining has several flattened folds. It is important to note that once emerging from the uterine wall the tube may bend in as much as a 60° angle. The normal isthmus is pink with four to six longitudinal folds. A falloposcopic view of this region is shown in Fig. 13A. The endotubal appearance of the more distal aspects of the fallopian tube have been described above. An image of the normal ampulla obtained at falloposcopy with the LEC is shown in Fig. 13B. Although the wider salpingoscopes currently provide enhanced image resolution of this region, falloposcopy has the potential of being performed as an office procedure for circumstances in which laparoscopy would otherwise be unnecessary (24).

Endotubal lesions recognized at falloposcopy were initially described by Kerin and co-workers (25). Intraluminal adhesions and mucous plugs are often best detected after performance of selective chromotubation with dilute methylene blue dye (Fig. 14). Polyps protruding into the tubal lumen may present as incidental findings or represent an etiology of partial tubal occlusion (Fig. 15). Progressive stenosis leading to complete fibrotic obstruction has also been characterized (Fig. 16). Intraluminal diverticulae have been recognized in patients with classical findings of salpingitis isthmica nodosa at laparascopy

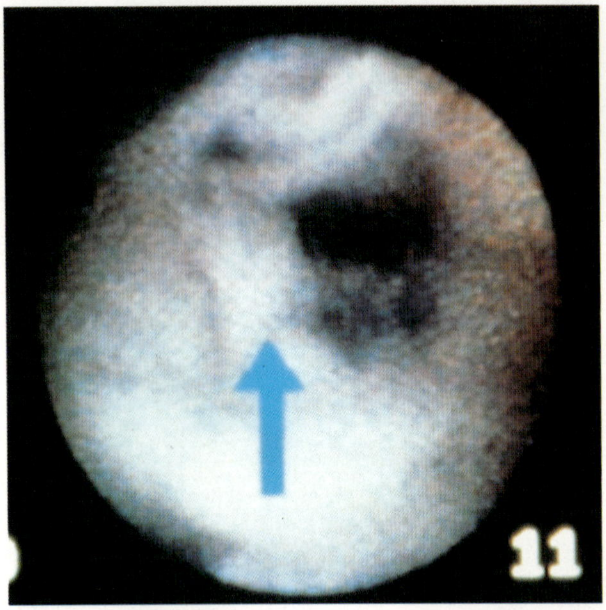

FIG. 14. Stringy intralumenal isthmic adhesions. These are nonobstructive but are coupled with devascularized atrophic epithelium. Hysterosalpinogram and laparoscopy were normal in patient with otherwise unexplained infertility. (From ref. 3, with permission.)

and hysterosalpingography (Fig. 17). A classification system based on such falloposcopic findings as epithelial pallor, vascularity, luminal narrowing, and adhesions has been presented (3). In one series in which 112 tubes were adequately visualized in patients with suspected tubal disease, no disease was noted in 46% (23). Severe obstruction was noted in 25% of patients, none of whom had conceived within a year of surgery. Of 72 patients with mild-to-moderate disease, only 2 had conceived spontaneously a year postoperatively.

OPERATIVE FALLOPOSCOPY

Several minimally invasive approaches to proximal tubal occlusion with wire probes or balloons have been described. Investigators have achieved access to the fallopian tube employing tactile, sonographic, and fluoroscopic techniques (26–29). Unfortunately, these modalities do not allow for direct visualization of the cause of the occlusion. With the use of concomitant falloposcopy, the appropriate means for approaching proximal tubal obstruction may be selected based on identification of etiology. Intraluminal debris, mucous plugs, and filmy adhesions may be effectively managed by either aquadissection or gentle advancement of the flexible guidewire (Fig. 18). In our reported experience, aquadissection and/or guidewire cannulation was successfully used to lyse nonobstructive intraluminal adhesions in 60% (9 of 15) cases (20,25). Thicker adhesions, moderate stenoses, and intraluminal polyps may be effectively treated by gently advancing flexible dilation wires with up to 0.8 mm OD (Target Therapeutics; Cook Ob/Gyn). Thicker adhesions and narrower stenoses may also respond to the use of small balloon catheters (1.0 cm deflated, 2.5 cm inflated) (Target Therapeutics) (20,25). These balloons are passed to the point of obstruction, inflated, deflated,

A

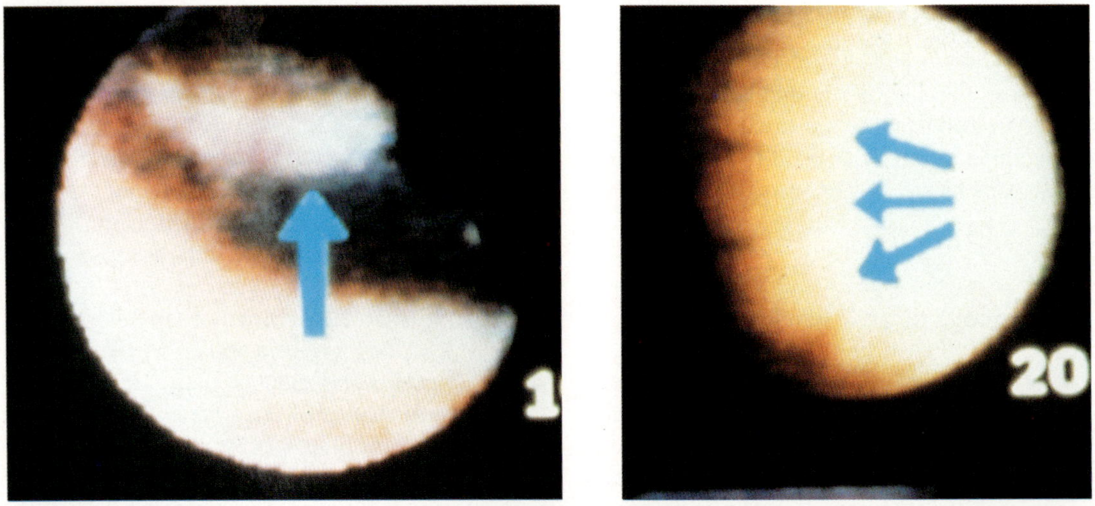

B

FIG. 15. **A:** Intralumenal polyp appreciated at the ampullary-isthmic junction noted during falloposcopy. This 1 × 0.3-mm simple polyp was an incidental finding in an otherwise normal tube. **B:** A broad-based papillary isthmic polyp noted at falloposcopy in a patient with primary infertility and normal hysterosalpingogram. (From ref. 3, with permission.)

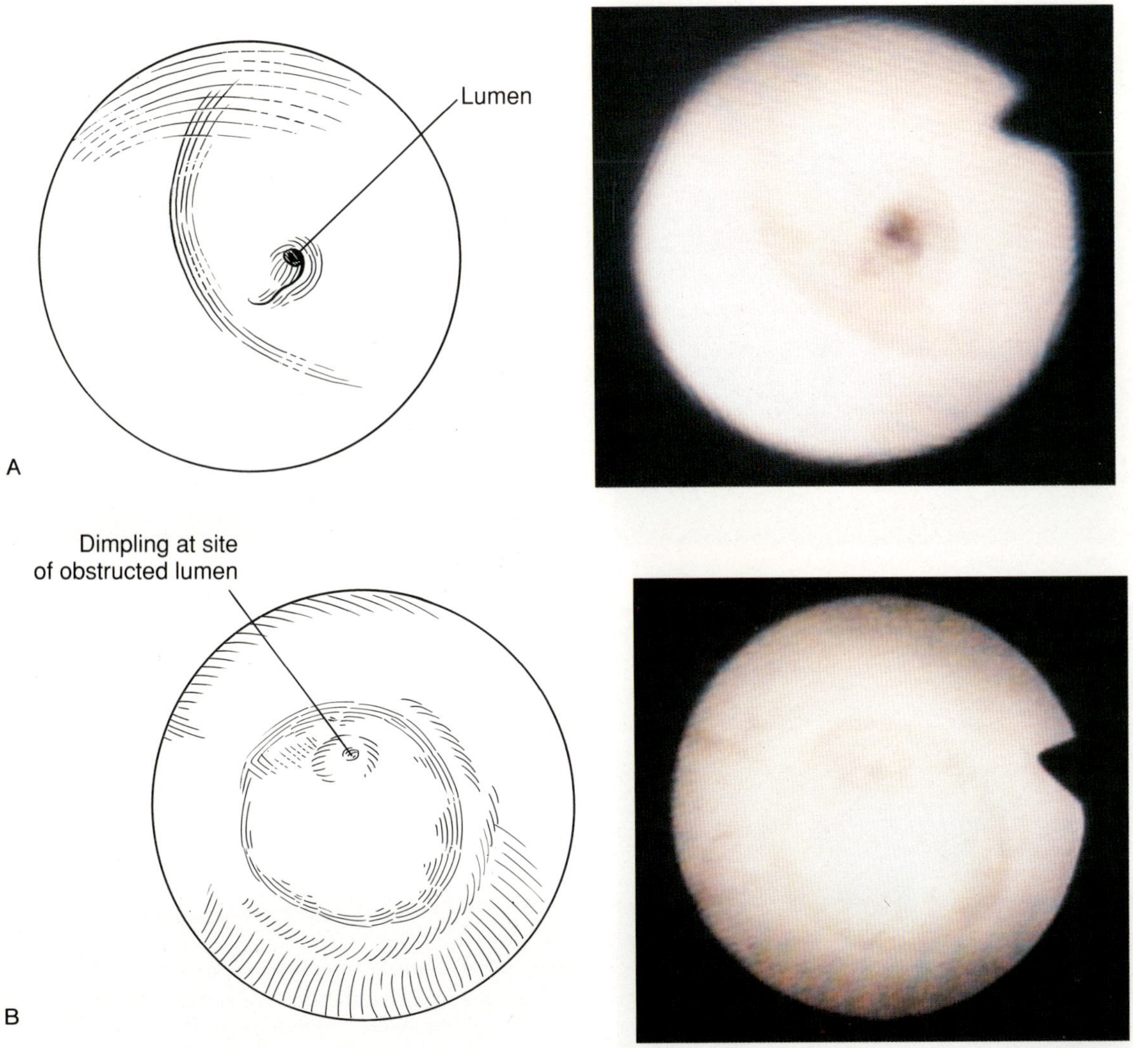

FIG. 16. A: Falloposcopic view of severe isthmic stenosis. **B:** View of complete fibrotic isthmic obstruction noted during coaxial falloposcopy. Note dimpling at site of obliterated lumen.

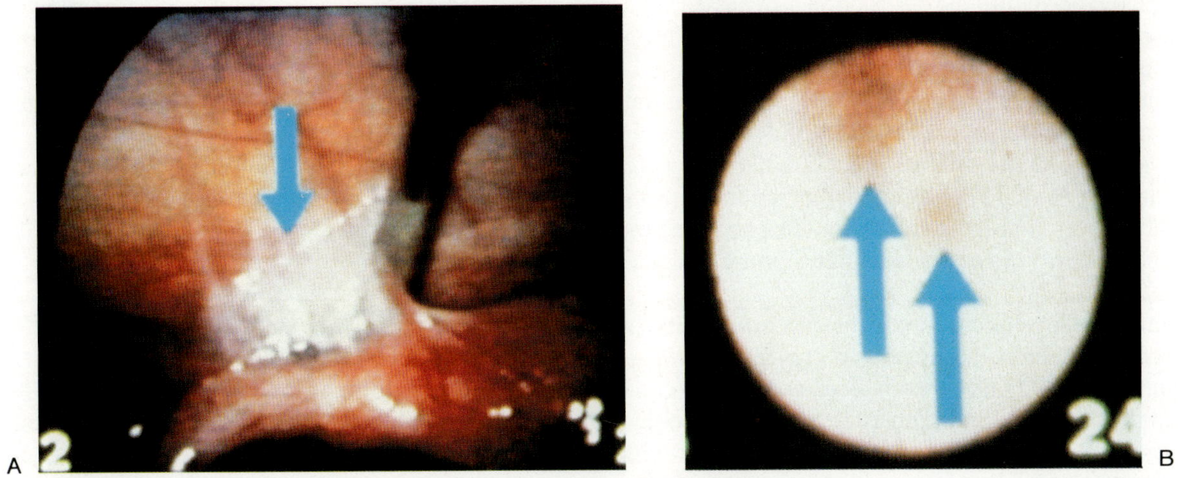

FIG. 17. A: Peritubal adhesions between fibrotic left isthmus and bladder peritoneum in patient with hysterosalpingogram findings compatible with salpingitis isthmica nodosa. **B:** View through falloposcope of lumen of the same tube demonstrating stenosis, fibrosis, and two diverticular openings from lumen (*arrows*) extending into muscularis. (From ref. 3, with permission.)

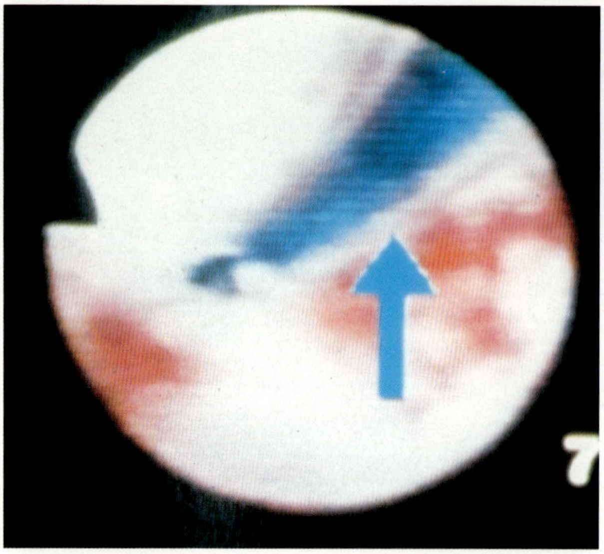

A

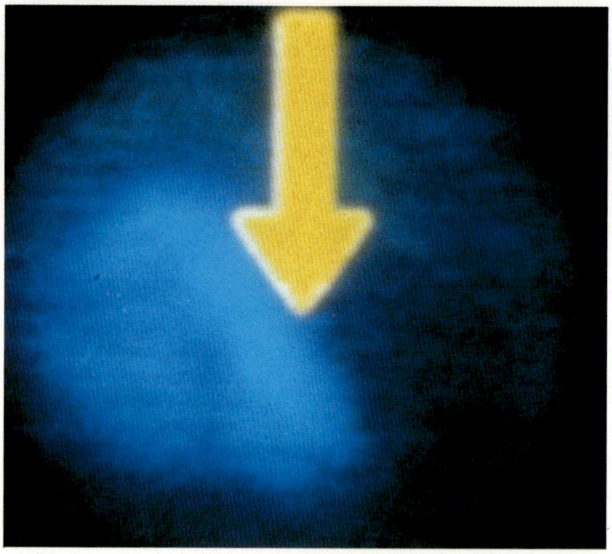

B

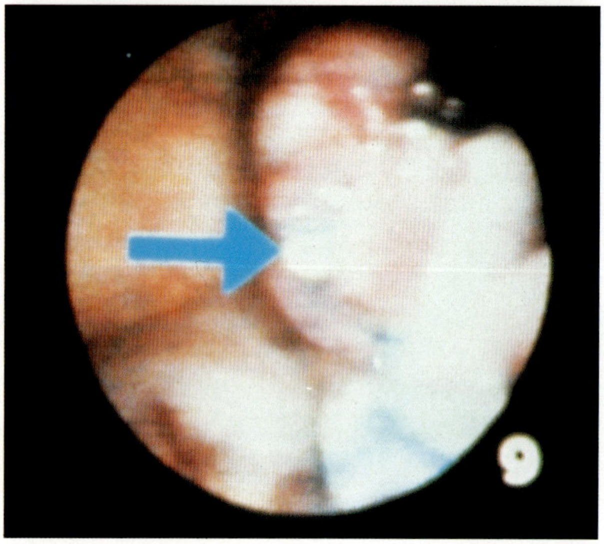

C

FIG. 18. Aquadissection through Teflon catheter employing dilute methylene blue dye (**A**) to mobilize intraluminal mucous plug (**B**). Subsequently, plug was noted at laparoscopy to extend through fimbriated end of tube (**C**). Pathologic analysis confirmed the presence of an amorphous cast. (From ref. 3, with permission.)

and then advanced until the obstruction is bypassed. The falloposcope is removed prior to passage of the balloon or wire and subsequently replaced both to confirm patency and to rule out intraluminal damage. In our initial report, moderate stenoses were successfully dilated in 39% (5 of 13) of cases, whereas moderate stenoses were dilated in 33% (4 of 12) of cases employing these techniques. However, no tubal patency could be achieved by these techniques in 11 cases of complete fibrotic obstruction (20,25).

Operative falloposcopy should be performed under laparoscopic guidance in an effort to prevent tubal perforation. Diagnostic falloposcopy does not require concomitant laparoscopy unless otherwise indicated. No significant complications have been reported in over 120 cases of diagnostic falloposcopy. Six perforations without sequelae have been described; all occurred in patients with severe fibrotic occlusion in over 60 operative procedures (30). The most frequent sites for tubal perforation are diagrammed in Fig. 19. Peritubal adhesions, which kink the tube, intraluminal adhesions, and stenoses all predispose to perforation.

HIGHLIGHTS

Falloposcopy and salpingoscopy represent complementary, minimally invasive means of visualizing one of the last frontiers of the female reproductive system: the fallopian tube lumen. Falloposcopy has great promise for use as an office-based procedure. Both techniques allow reproductive surgeons to diagnose and create management strategies more appropriately for patients with suspected tubal disease and unexplained infertility.

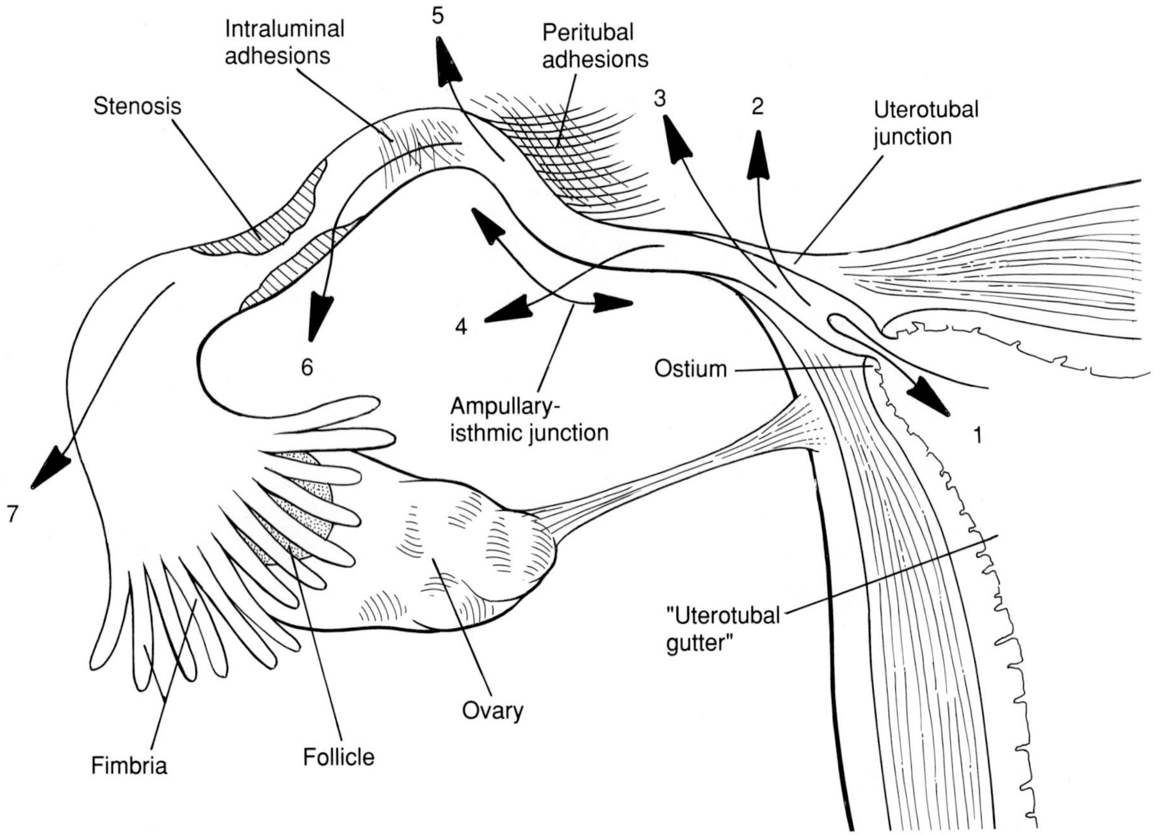

FIG. 19. Most vulnerable sites for perforation during tubal cannulation prior to falloposcopy. (From ref. 30, with permission.)

REFERENCES

1. Hoffman JJ. Anatomy and physiology of the fallopian tube. In: Hunt RB, ed. *Atlas of female infertility surgery.* Chicago: Year Book Medical; 1986:3–10.
2. Croxatto HB, Ortiz ME, Diaz S, Hess R, Balmaceda J, Croxatto HD. Studies on the duration of egg transport by the human oviduct. II. Ovum location at various intervals follow luteinizing hormone peak. *Am J Obstet Gynecol* 1978;132:629–634.
3. Kerin JF, Williams DB, San Roman GA, Pearlstone AG, Grundfest WS, Surrey ES. Falloposcopic classification and treatment of fallopian tube lumen disease. *Fertil Steril* 1992;57:731–741.
4. Letterie GS, Sakas EL. Histology of proximal tubal obstruction in cases of unsuccessful tubal canalization. *Fertil Steril* 1991;56:831–835.
5. Sulak PJ, Letteire GS, Coddington CC, Hayslip CC, Woodward JE, Klein TA. Histology of proximal tubal obstruction. *Fertil Steril* 1987;48:437–441.
6. Siegler AM. Evaluation of tubal factors in infertility and management of tubal obstruction. *Clin Obstet Gynecol* 1978;22:81.
7. McComb PF, Rowe TC. Salpingitis isthmica nodosa: evidence it is a progressive disease. *Fertil Steril* 1989;51:542–545.
8. Majmudar B, Henderson PH, Semple E. Salpingitis isthmica nodosa: a high risk factor for tubal pregnancy. *Obstet Gynecol* 1983;62:73–78.
9. World Health Organization. Comparative trial of tubal insufflation, hysterosalpingography, and laparoscopy with dye hydrotubation for assessment of tubal patency. *Fertil Steril* 1986;46:1101–1107.
10. Snowden EU, Jarrett JC II, Dawood MY. Comparison of diagnostic accuracy of laparoscopy, hysteroscopy, and hysterosalpingogram in evaluation of female fertility. *Fertil Steril* 1984;41:709–713.
11. Gabos P. A comparison of hysterosalpingography and endoscopy in evaluation of tubal function in infertile women. *Fertil Steril* 1976;27:238–243.
12. Gleicher N, Pratt D. Transvaginal procedures for infertility. In: Behrman SJ, Patton GW Jr, Holtz G, eds. *Progress in infertility.* Boston: Little Brown; 1994:225–248.
13. Henry-Suchet J, Tesquier L, Pez JP, Loffredo U. Prognostic value of tuboscopy vs. hysterosalpingography before tuboplasty. *J Reprod Med* 1984;29:609–612.
14. Herschlag A, Seifer DB, Carcangiu ML, Patton DL, Diamond MP, DeCherney AH. Salpingoscopy: light microscopic and electron microscopic correlations. *Obstet Gynecol* 1991;77:399–405.
15. Cornier E. Ampullosalpingoscopy. In: Siegler AM, ed. *The fallopian tube: basic studies and clinical contributions.* White Plains, NY: Futura; 1986;383–390.
16. Shapiro BS, Diamond MP, De Cherney AH. Salpingoscopy: an adjunctive technique for evaluation of the fallopian tube. *Fertil Steril* 1988;49:1076–1079.
17. Puttemans P, Brosens I, Delattin P, Vasquez G, Boeckx W. Salpingoscopy versus hysterosalpingography in hydrosalpinges. *Hum Reprod* 1987;2:535–540.
18. Henry-Suchet J, Loffredo V, Tesquier L, Pez JP. Endoscopy of the tube (tuboscopy): its prognostic value for tuboplasty. *Acta Eur Fertil* 1985;16:139–145.
19. Surrey ES, Surrey MW. The role of transfimbrial salpingoscopy in the management of distal tubal disease: correlation with traditional criterion. Program of the 42nd Annual Meeting of the Pacific Coast Fertility Society; April 20–24, 1994, (Abstract P-1).

20. Kerin J, Daykhovsky L, Grundfest W, Surrey E. Falloposcopy: a microendoscopic transvaginal technique for diagnosing and treating endotubal disease incorporating guide wire cannulation and direct balloon tuboplasty. *J Reprod Med* 1990;35:606–612.
21. Kerin J, Daykhovsky L, Segalowitz J, Surrey E, et al. Falloposcopy: a microendoscopic technique for visual exploration of the human fallopian tube from the uterotubal ostium to the fimbria using a transvaginal approach. *Fertil Steril* 1990;54:390–400.
22. Pearlstone AC, Surrey ES, Kerin JF. The linear everting catheter: a nonhysteroscopic, transvaginal technique for access and microendoscopy of the fallopian tube. *Fertil Steril* 1992;58:854–857.
23. Kerin JF, Surrey ES. Tubal surgery from the inside out: falloposcopy and balloon tuboplasty. *Clin Obstet Gynecol* 1992;35:299–312.
24. Scudamore IW, Dunphy BC, Cooke ID. Outpatient falloposcopy: intra-luminal imaging of the fallopian tube by trans-uterine fiberoptic endoscopy as an outpatient procedure. *Br J Obstet Gynecol* 1992;99:829–835.
25. Kerin JF, Surrey E, Daykhovsky L, Grundfest WS. Development and application of a falloposcope for transvaginal endoscopy of the fallopian tube. *J Laparosc Surg* 1990;1:47–56.
26. Thurmond AS. Selective salpingography and fallopian tube recanalization. *AJR* 1991;156:33–38.
27. Confino EC, Tur-Kaspa I, DeCherney A, et al. Transcervical balloon tuboplasty: a multicenter study. *JAMA* 1990;264:2079–2082.
28. Maroulis GB, Yeko TR. Treatment of cornual obstruction by transvaginal cannulation without hysteroscopy or fluoroscopy. *Fertil Steril* 1992;52:1136–1138.
29. Lisse K, Sydow P. Fallopian tube catheterization and recanalization under ultrasonic observation: a simplified technique to evaluate tubal patency and open proximally obstructed tubes. *Fertil Steril* 1991;56:198–201.
30. Kerin JF, Pearlstone A, Surrey ES. Cannulation of the fallopian tube and falloposcopy: difficulties and complications. In: Corfman RS, Diamond MP, DeCherney A, eds. *Complications of laparoscopy and hysteroscopy.* Boston: Blackwell Scientific; 1993:223–232.

PART VI

Intraoperative and Postoperative Management

Endoscopic Management of Gynecologic Disease,
edited by G.D. Adamson and D.C. Martin.
Lippincott-Raven Publishers, Philadelphia © 1996.

CHAPTER 34

Complications of Operative Laparoscopy

Wayne S. Maxson, David I. Hoffman, Farr Nezhat, and G. David Adamson

The applications of the laparoscope have extended rapidly from the simple diagnosis of pelvic pathology to tubal sterilization, and—over the past two decades—to the treatment of multiple intraabdominal diseases previously performed by laparotomy. The avalanche of new laparoscopic techniques and instruments has been triggered primarily by uncontrolled demonstrations of feasibility rather than by controlled prospective evaluations of utility and safety.

The complications of operative endoscopy arise from poor technique, poor judgment, inadequate instrumentation, or unavoidable misadventure. The precipitous assimilation of untested novel procedures into routine surgical practice challenges the novice and potentially increases the operative risks.

This chapter outlines some of the more common or most dreaded complications of operative laparoscopy and offers clues for their avoidance and treatment. The photographs in this chapter are from the collections of the authors and of Dr. Dan C. Martin. Fortunately, these complications are from cases from many sources and are not just our own. The quality of the photographs is inevitably influenced by the recording methods available and the composure (or blissful unawareness) of the surgeon.

PREOPERATIVE PLANNING

Proper preoperative planning is essential to minimize intraoperative problems that otherwise could have been anticipated, and adequate counseling before surgery can make the expectations of patient and families more realistic (see the Chapter by Sgarlata, "Preoperative Patient Preparation"). Preparation for the patient considering operative endoscopy must include a review of previous medical records, a discussion of the differential diagnosis and therapeutic alternatives, an accurate assessment of the costs and outcomes, a review of the risks of each alternative, the potential necessity for laparotomy, and an analysis of the anesthetic alternatives. Whenever possible, these discussions should involve both the patient and the partner or parent. Preoperative consultation should include a consideration of special circumstances, such as autologous blood donation, bowel preparation, and antibiotic prophylaxis for mitral valve prolapse. A preoperative vaginal ultrasound scan is recommended for all patients about to undergo pelvic laparoscopy to detect an unsuspected ovarian cyst or uterine tumor that could alter the operative approach.

OVERVIEW OF LAPAROSCOPIC COMPLICATIONS

Since many surgical complications go unreported, it is difficult to accurately estimate the prevalence of a given adverse outcome. The American Association of Gynecologic Laparoscopists (AAGL) has conducted regular evaluations of complications by reviewing and tabulating responses to questionnaires mailed to all members. Results from three of those questionnaires are provided in Table 1.

The Carbon Dioxide Laser Laparoscopy Study Group reviewed 821 operative laparoscopies performed for multiple indications (4). Complications occurred in 14 women (17.1 per 1000) and all were treated laparoscopically. A single, unplanned laparotomy was performed for suspected small bowel injury, but none was noted in this patient. No deaths were reported in this series.

W. S. Maxson and D. I. Hoffman: Northwest Center for Infertility, Margate, Florida 33063.
F. Nezhat: Department of Obstetrics and Gynecology, Stanford University, Palo Alto, California 94304.
G. D. Adamson: Fertility Physicians of Northern California, Palo Alto, California 94301.

TABLE 1. *Evaluation of complications conducted by the American Association of Gynecologic Laparoscopists (AAGL)*

Date	Response rate (%)	Number of procedures	Total major complications[a]	Complication rate per thousand	Complications leading to death	Deaths per 100,000 procedures	Ref.
1973	NA	12,182	82	6.8	3	25.0	1
1988	24	36,928	568	15.4	2	5.4	2
1991	17	56,536	573	10.1	1	1.8	3

[a] These numbers perhaps reflect increasingly aggressive gynecologic endoscopy.

Lehmann-Willenbrock et al. summarized the German experience with pelviscopy from 1949 through 1988 (5). Questionnaires were sent to 800 clinics and 215 consultants (private practitioners) in two mailings with a response rate of 44.9% from the former and 66% from the latter. Operative laparoscopies were performed in 98.9% of the clinics and 90.9% of the private practices of those responding. Serious complications occurred in 3.56 per 1000 cases in the summary of procedures from 1949 to 1977, decreasing to 2.36 per thousand in 1986–1988. Deaths from laparoscopy were 24 (90 per 100,000) in 1949–1977, compared to 6 (24 per 100,000) in 1983–1985, and 2 (8 per 100,000) in 1986–1988. In this last series, one patient died from intestinal perforation after leakage from a repaired trocar injury and one from agranulocytosis after bipolar, high-frequency adhesiolysis.

Compared to Laparotomy

No well-controlled studies have directly compared laparoscopy and laparotomy complication rates. The most serious common laparoscopic injuries are injuries to the internal organs (especially the bowel), hemorrhage, and anesthetic complications. The earlier postoperative ambulation following operative laparoscopy should reduce the rate of pneumonia and thrombophlebitis (6). Laparoscopic surgery may be safer than laparotomy for the surgeon because of a lower risk of percutaneous injury from scalpels or other sharp instruments (7).

Although complications associated with operative laparoscopy may be lower than those associated with laparotomy, certain complications are unique to laparoscopy (8). Anesthesia complications, such as respiratory embarrassment because of increased intraabdominal CO_2 gas pressure and/or deep Trendelenburg position, can occur. Subcutaneous emphysema, pneumothorax, and pneumomediastinum are more common. Cervical laceration and/or uterine perforation can occur with placement of manipulating instruments. Inadvertent intravascular Veress needle placement and CO_2 embolism can result in cardiovascular collapse, as can laceration of a major blood vessel. Injury to organs from blind placement of instruments occurs more often than at laparotomy. Unipolar electrosurgical injury poses a greater risk at laparoscopy than at laparotomy. These injuries may also be less recognizable at laparoscopy than at laparotomy. Hemorrhage may be more difficult to control because of reduced ability to apply pressure. In addition, some operations, such as myomectomy, may take longer at laparoscopy. It is important for all surgeons to be aware of these differences in the nature and potential complications between laparotomy and laparoscopy.

EQUIPMENT AND ANESTHESIA COMPLICATIONS

Equipment

Major complications can occur at laparoscopy because of inadequate visualization. It is imperative that the surgeon use an adequate laparoscope with matching light cable and an adequate light source. The surgeon requires a high-flow insufflator as well as a sharp Veress needle to maintain the pneumoperitoneum. Gas recirculators may be helpful during laparoscopy when a CO_2 laser is used. Also required are adequate trocars with matching sleeves, so as to avoid electrosurgical capacitance, and matching gaskets. Electrosurgical equipment, both unipolar and bipolar, and matching cords must be available. A laser and a staff knowledgeable in all aspects of its function are necessary when this equipment is a primary modality of energy. Different types of graspers, scissors, and sutures must be available. There must be adequate backup for all of the described instrumentation or else the surgeon may find it impossible to complete the laparoscopic procedure. In addition, working with suboptimal equipment can markedly increase the risk of complications.

Anesthesia

The 1973 AAGL survey documented an anesthesia complication rate of 0.7 per 1000 cases. No such adverse reactions were reported in the 1991 summary.

Anesthetic morbidity can follow hypoventilation (esophageal or endobronchial), aspiration of gastric contents, arrhythmias (rapid insufflation of carbon dioxide at pneumoperitoneum), vascular gas embolism, and gastric distention. These complications can be minimized by the routine use of a nasogastric tube, a short and cuffed endotracheal tube, slow induction of pneumoperitoneum with CO_2, maintenance of adequate relaxation, automatic control of maximum intraabdominal pressure, pulse oximetry, and measurement of expired CO_2 levels (see the Chapter by Collins and Jackson, "Anesthesia in Hysteroscopic and Laparoscopic Infertility Procedures.")

INTRAOPERATIVE SURGICAL COMPLICATIONS

Needle and Trocar Injuries

Most complications from laparoscopy have been reported to occur at the time of Veress needle or trocar insertion (9). Superficial introduction of the needle can lead to extraperitoneal insufflation and emphysema, which can dissect the peritoneum from the posterior rectus sheath and limit entry into the peritoneal cavity. Alternative approaches to the establishment of a pneumoperitoneum in these cases include open laparoscopy, passage of the needle vaginally through the posterior cul-de-sac or the uterine fundus, introduction of the needle in the left upper quadrant, or suprapubic needle insertion under visualization by the extraperitoneally placed laparoscope (10).

Responses (50.9% response rate) to a questionnaire mailed to the Society of Obstetricians and Gynecologists of Canada indicated that 26.7% of 407 gynecologists had encountered at least one Veress needle injury (11). The majority of these injuries involved the bowel (30.3%) and significant blood vessels (28.4%).

Techniques to minimize or identify a needle-induced injury include umbilical introduction with the patient supine and the abdominal wall elevated, minimal advancement of the needle after feeling two levels of resistance, and use of a needle placement test, such as the hissing sound, the aspiration test, the hanging drop test, or identification of low intraabdominal pressure (12).

Even after apparent successful induction of pneumoperitoneum, intraabdominal injuries can follow the insertion of the primary umbilical trocar. In the Canadian review, the majority of respondents indicated that they established a large pneumoperitoneum first. Nevertheless, in this summary, 25.6% of physicians had encountered a vascular or organ injury attributed to the primary trocar (11).

Direct insertion of the umbilical trocar without prior pneumoperitoneum reduces the number of blind insertion steps and avoids the risks of extraperitoneal insufflation, gas embolism, and pneumointestine (13). Further, the Veress needle has been implicated in more major vascular injuries than has the trocar (14).

Copeland et al. (15) used the direct trocar insertion technique in more than 2000 unselected patients with only three major complications. In a high-volume training center at Tripler Army Medical Center, 937 laparoscopies involving direct trocar insertion were reviewed (16). No major complications were reported and minor adverse effects decreased with departmental experience from 5.3% to 1.3% over 3 years. Interestingly, in this series the skill level of the surgeon did not affect the complication rate. Two thirds of the minor complications encountered occurred in obese patients.

Nezhat et al. compared the Veress needle method to the direct trocar technique in 200 patients, none of whom had had previous laparotomy (13). No major complications were associated with either approach. Minor adverse effects (emphysema of the retroperitoneum or omentum) occurred in 22% of the Veress group, whereas only 3% of the trocar group experienced complications (omental perforation and subcutaneous emphysema). All three of the direct trocar problems were seen in the 50 patients receiving the conventional reusable instrument. No complications occurred in the 50 women who received the disposable trocar, but 20% (10 patients) in each direct trocar group required two insertion attempts; 8% of those with the reusable and 4% of those with the disposable resulted in failed insertions.

Vascular Injuries

Whereas some gastrointestinal perforations at laparoscopy may be inevitable, the majority of injuries to the great vessels of the abdomen and pelvis should be avoidable. Indeed, most vascular trauma affects the smaller blood vessels of the omentum, mesentery, pelvic viscera, and abdominal wall.

Although vascular injuries account for 30–50% of surgical trauma at laparoscopy (11), the frequency of perforation of the aorta, iliac vessels, or vena cava is probably less than 1 per 1000. A survey of the Royal College of Obstetricians and Gynaecologists in 1978 reported injury to the great vessels in 0.9 per 1000 laparoscopies (17). A contemporaneous review of 100,000 laparoscopies in France identified 31 major vascular injuries (0.3 per 1000 cases) (18). The Veress needle accounted for 36% of vascular perforations, whereas the primary and secondary trocars each caused about 32%.

The usual site of trauma to the large vessels is the terminal aorta near its bifurcation and the common iliac arteries. Only 1 woman out of 15 with major vascular injuries reviewed by Baadsgaard et al. had an injury to the external iliac vessels (14). The vena cava and the iliac veins may also be lacerated and may be more difficult to repair.

The anatomy of the abdomen and the alterations in organ relationships consequent to the Trendelenberg position help to explain these serious injuries. In nonobese women, the distance from the umbilicus to the aortic bifurcation averages 6 cm (19), and the umbilicus is directly over or cephalad to the bifurcation in 53% (20). In obese women, the umbilicus lies directly over the aorta in only 30% of cases. The Veress needle and the trocar should be inserted with the patient flat and not in the Trendelenberg position, since this displaces the umbilicus upwards, brings the common iliac vessels closer to the horizontal plane, and decreases the distance between the umbilicus and the aortic bifurcation (12).

Vascular perforation, like bowel injuries, can be minimized by careful attention to anatomy and by smooth needle and trocar introduction. Adequate skin incisions, sharp instruments, and controlled insertion are all necessary. For the auxilliary trocars, introduction under direct visualization is mandatory, following identification of the inferior epigastric and external iliac vessels.

Deep Epigastric Vessels

Injury to the deep epigastric vessels is the most common vascular injury at operative laparoscopy. The deep epigastric artery and its veins come off the external iliac artery near its transition to the femoral artery and lie in the medial peritoneal fold of the internal inguinal ring. The round ligament curls around these vessels on entrance into the inguinal canal. Deep epigastric vessels are adjacent to the obliterated umbilical ligaments and beneath the lateral margin of the rectus muscle (Figs. 1 and 2) (21). The deep epigastric vessels can be seen through the laparoscope intraabdominally. Placement of trocars lateral to this region will minimize injury. The lower quadrant secondary puncture trocars should be placed under direct vision. Transillumination aids primarily in visualization of the superficial epigastric vessels. Should bleeding occur from the deep epigastric vessels, the first approach to diagnosis and management includes rotation of the trocar through 360° to determine where the bleeding site is, followed by immediate control of the bleeding (Fig. 3A). The Kleppinger bipolar electrosurgical forceps can then be used to desiccate the deep epigastric vessels above and below the site of injury (Fig. 3B). Should this not be successful, pressure can be placed in the region by passing a Foley catheter through the 5-mm sheath, insufflating the balloon and pulling it snugly up against the abdominal wall, and maintaining pressure by placement of a Kelly or similar clamp over a 4 $\times$ 4 gauze wedged against the skin. The Foley catheter can be released approximately 10 min later to facilitate evaluation of bleeding and/or to attempt to maintain hemostasis with the Kleppinger bipolar electrosurgical forceps, since bleeding may well be reduced. Copious irrigation of the area helps to identify the bleeding site. Should this approach be unsuccessful, a figure-of-eight suture with either a straight or a curved needle can be placed through-and-through the anterior abdominal wall; alternatively, a figure-of-eight suture can be placed laparoscopically, although this is more technically difficult (Fig. 3C). In the unlikely event that these approaches are unsuccessful, the lower quadrant should be explored from the skin

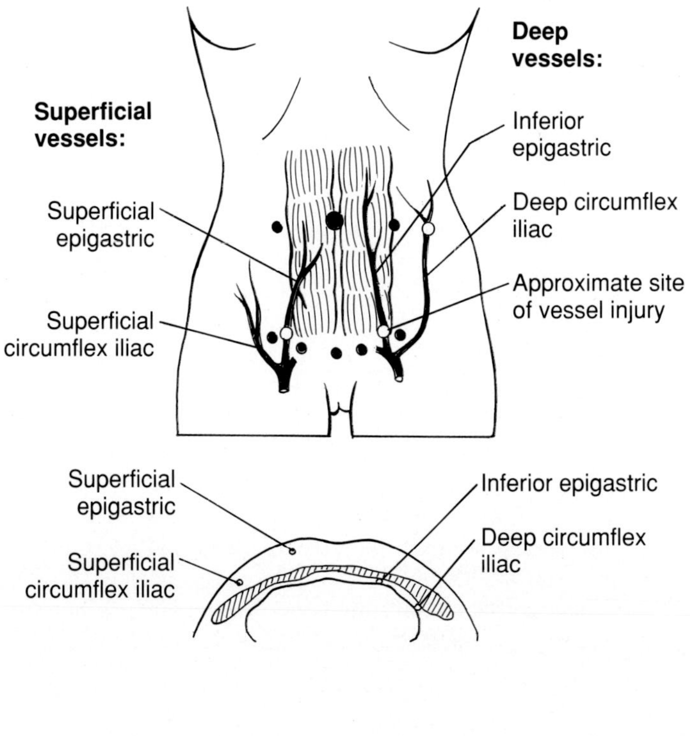

FIG. 1. Approximate location of the superficial and deep vessels of the anterior abdominal wall, frontal and axial views. In the frontal view, dashed lines indicate the relative location of the lateral margin of the rectus abdominis muscle, and solid circles indicate ideal laparoscopic trocar placement sites. The open circles indicate the approximate sites of vessel injuries in three reported cases (21). In the axial view, taken at a level 1 cm below the umbilicus, soft tissue layers are indicated in gray and bone in white.

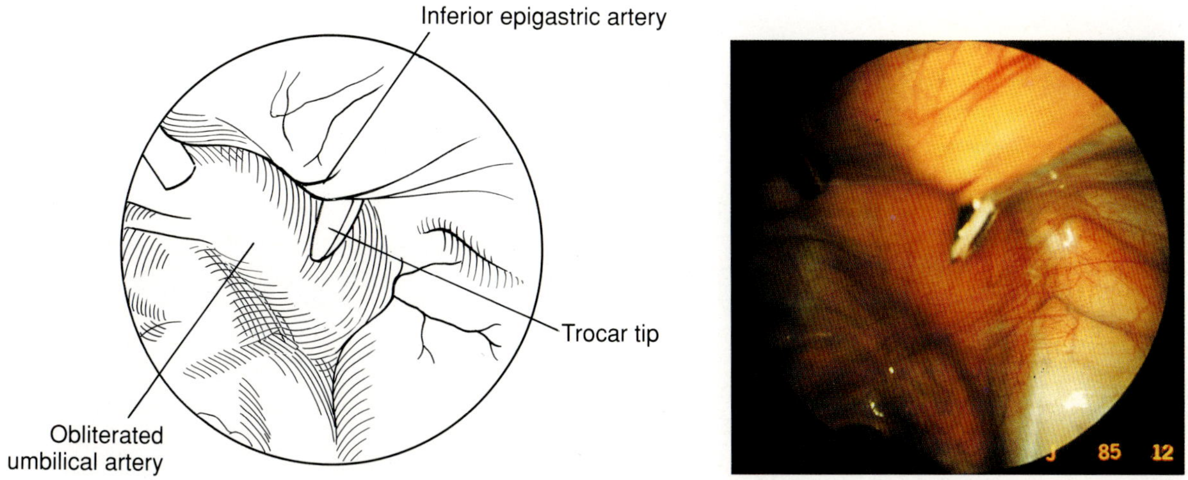

FIG. 2. Identification of the inferior epigastric vessels. The inferior epigastric vessels lie retroperitoneal and lateral to the easily identified obliterated umbilical arteries. Here the inferior epigastric artery is stretched across the sharp tip of the trocar. Bipolar coagulation was used for hemostasis through a separate puncture site.

and ligature of the vessels carried out. After hemostasis is obtained, copious irrigation and aspiration should be performed to evacuate any hematoma. Small hematomas will resolve spontaneously (Fig. 4).

Anterior Abdominal Wall

Bleeding from the anterior abdominal wall can also occur from the superficial epigastric vessels, the rectus muscle, or from small vessels in the skin and subcutaneous tissue. In general, this bleeding can be controlled with external pressure. Should this not be successful, ligature or an electrosurgical approach is necessary. It is imperative that the abdominal puncture sites be observed carefully with and without the pneumoperitoneum upon removal of trocars at the completion of the operation to ensure that vascular injury that was unrecognized because of pressure of the transabdominal instruments is now identified. Intrarectal sheath bleeding, in particular, can be difficult to diagnose.

Large Vessels

Large-vessel injury to the aorta, inferior vena cava, or common iliac artery or vein can be life threatening. Frequency of perforation is approximately 1 per 1000 cases or less (17,18). The usual site of injury is the terminal aorta near its bifurcation and the common iliac arteries (14). Such injuries are usually caused by the Veress needle or the trocar (Fig. 5A). Risk of injury can be reduced by the supine position, elevation of the abdominal wall, advancement of the needle through two layers of resistance in a Z fashion, placement of cervical traction to move the fundus inferiorly, and use of tests of needle placement such as the hissing sound, the aspiration test, the hanging drop test, and identification of a low intraabdominal pressure (12). Careful attention to anatomy, adequate skin incisions, and sharp instruments is also important. In one series, 2 of 15 patients with major vascular injuries died (14). These injuries may result in immediately obvious, copious intraabdominal hemorrhage, in which case immediate laparotomy and management by a vascular surgeon is indicated (Fig. 5B). However, such injury may not appear immediately because of increased intraabdominal pressure (10–15 mm Hg) caused by insufflation of CO_2 gas, decreased venous pressure from Trendelenburg position, and retroperitoneal hematoma, which may tamponade the large vessels. However, postoperatively, when pressure returns to normal, bleeding may occur. Therefore, it is essential that the large intraabdominal vessels be examined at the beginning and end of the operative procedure to evaluate their integrity. The Veress needle tends to produce a round hole in a vessel and may be observed postoperatively with the patient in the intensive care unit if there appears to be no active bleeding. However, a triangular hole is created by a trocar and merits immediate laparotomy and exploration with a vascular surgeon. Retroperitoneal hematomas can be exceedingly difficult to identify, and merit very careful examination and exploration to prevent major morbidity and mortality. Retroperitoneal injury occurs more commonly in thin patients.

Intrapelvic Vessels

Intrapelvic vessels, including the ovarian and uterine vessels, can bleed profusely if injured during surgery (Fig.

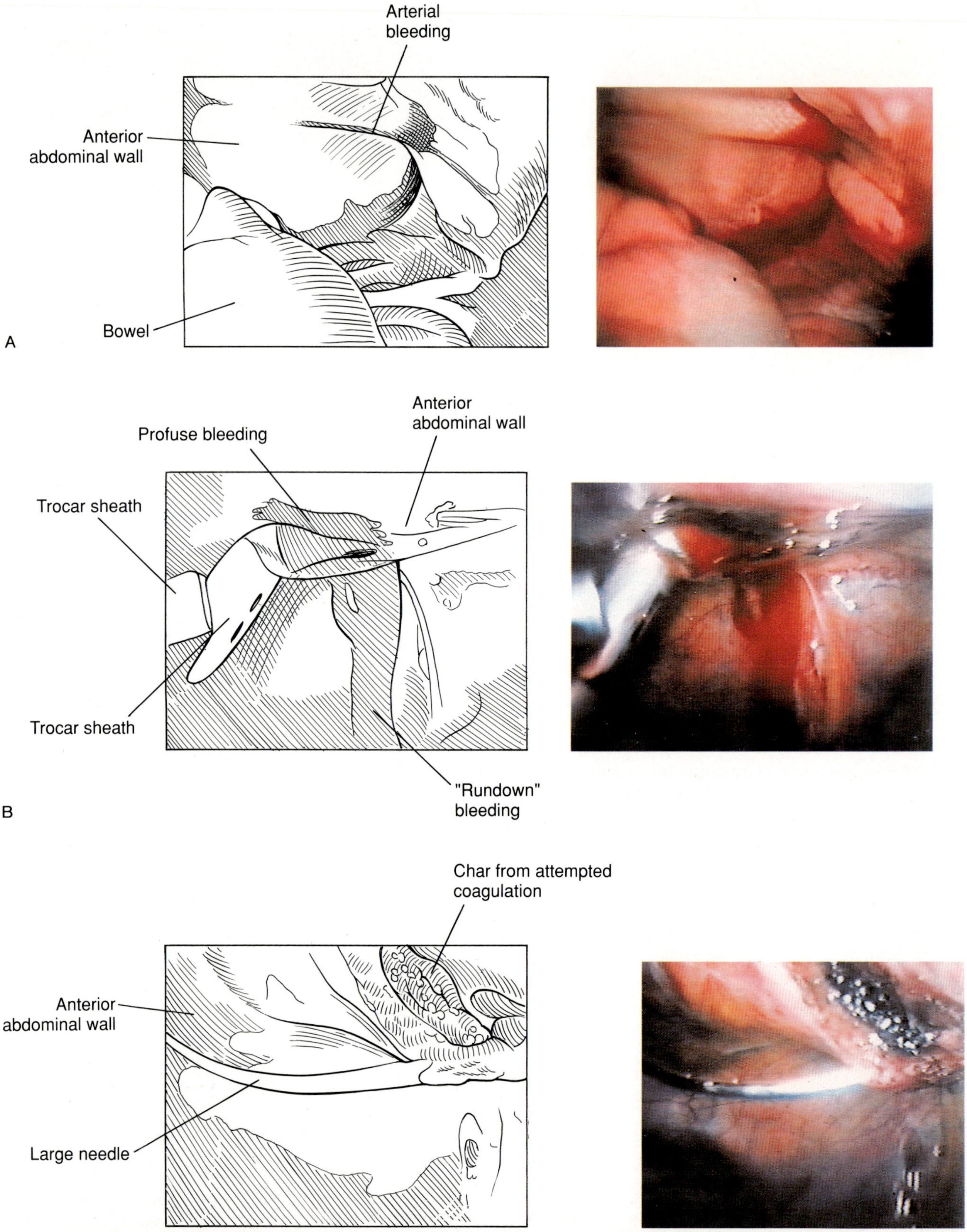

FIG. 3. A: Arterial bleeding from the inferior epigastric vessels cut with the secondary trocar. Attempts at tamponade are unsuccessful. **B:** Bleeding continues. Bipolar cauterization of the trocar track may be beneficial, but the inferior epigastric vessels often retract and require suturing. **C:** In this case, a large needle is passed and tied on the anterior abdominal wall for hemostasis.

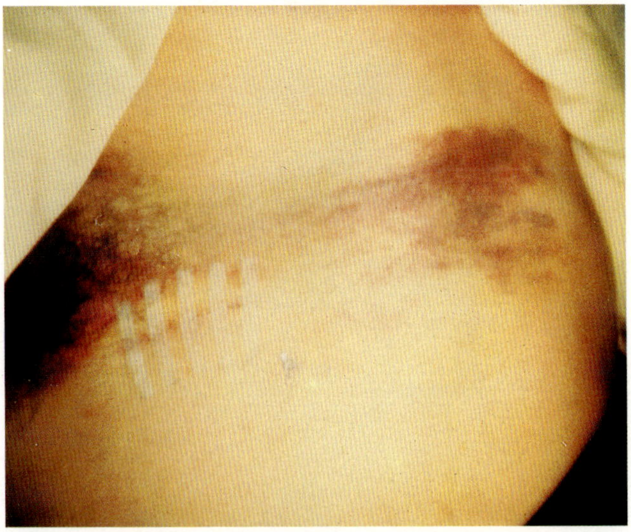

FIG. 4. Subcutaneous hematoma after ligation of the inferior epigastric vessels. This small hematoma with impressive ecchymosis resolved spontaneously.

6A,B). The initial approach is to obtain hemostasis through application of a blunt clamp to the vessel to enable adequate visualization of the vessel and surrounding structures, such as the ureter. Hemostasis can then be obtained by use of bipolar electrosurgery, clips, or occasionally loop ligature (Fig. 6C). Injury to these vessels can be avoided by careful identification of the anatomy, use of backstops when laser is used, hydrodissection to identify tissue planes and structures, and placement of fluid in the cul-de-sac to produce a backstop for CO_2 laser energy (Fig. 7). Power density needs to be appropriate for the nature of the disease, anatomic location, and surgeon's skill. Finally, pulsing of the pedal when using the laser, and/or the use of small strokes with the electrosurgical needle, and/or small bites with the endoscopic scissors will reduce the risk of injury. Adequate hemostatic control also can be enhanced throughout the operation by the surgeon's ensuring that bleeders are identified and controlled immediately rather than allowing multiple bleeders to develop within the pelvis.

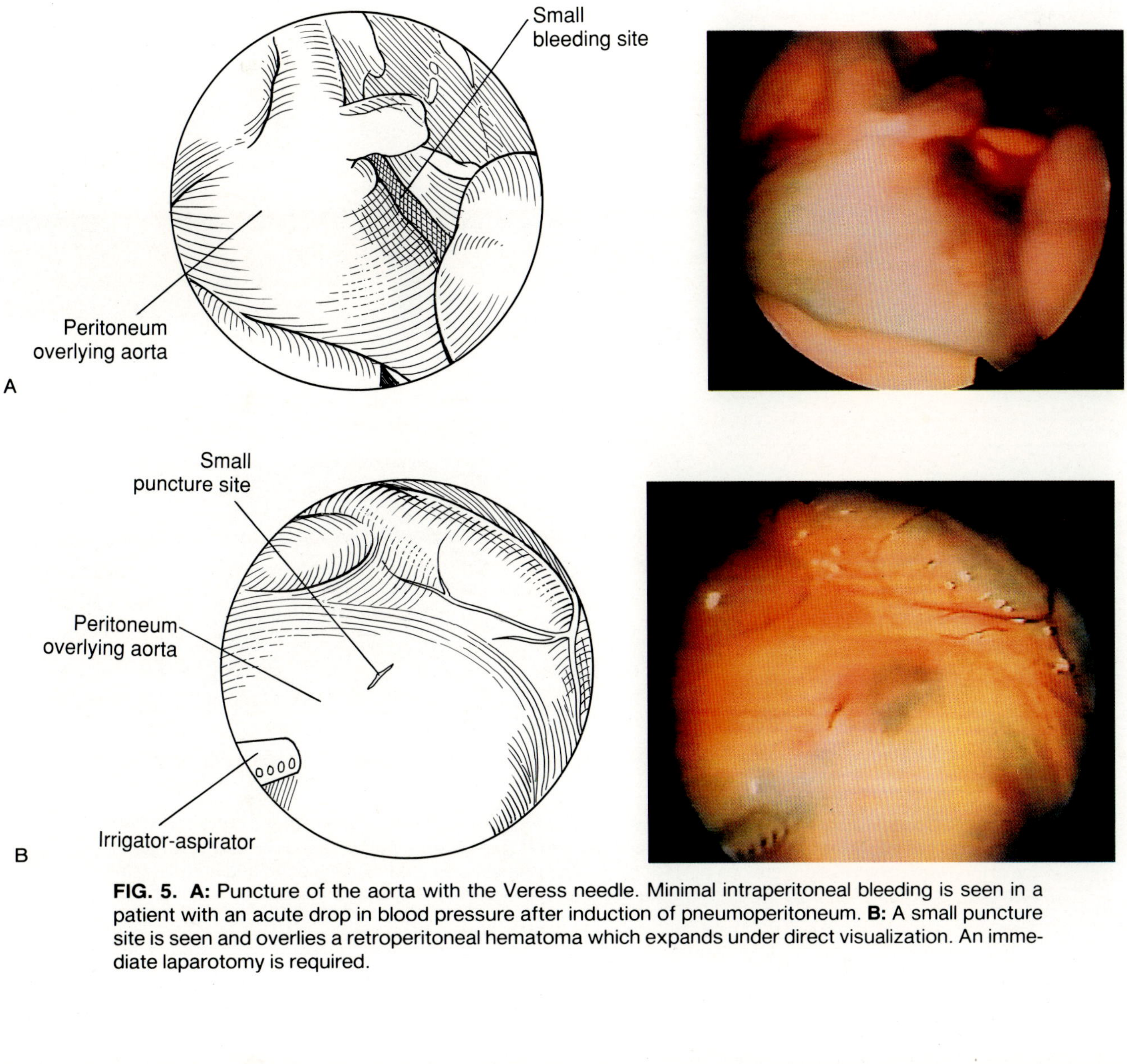

FIG. 5. A: Puncture of the aorta with the Veress needle. Minimal intraperitoneal bleeding is seen in a patient with an acute drop in blood pressure after induction of pneumoperitoneum. **B:** A small puncture site is seen and overlies a retroperitoneal hematoma which expands under direct visualization. An immediate laparotomy is required.

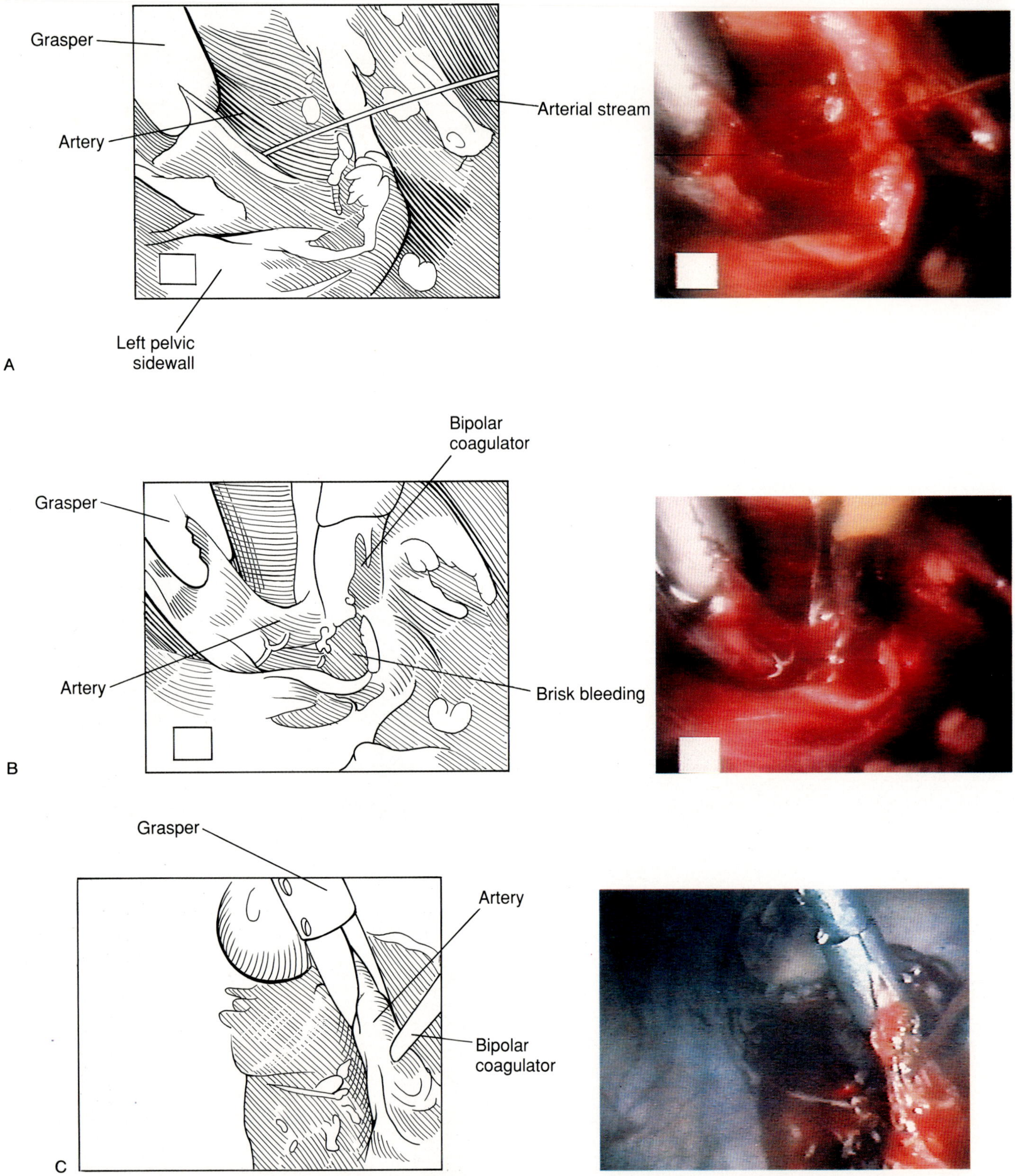

FIG. 6. A: Coagulation of a lacerated pelvic artery. Dissection of adhesions to the lateral pelvic side wall cut a small but persistent artery. **B:** Bipolar coagulation is hampered by brisk bleeding. **C:** Elevation of the artery with compression reduces the blood flow and permits successful coagulation and hemostasis. Alternatively, clips or sutures could be used as long as the location of the ureter is known.

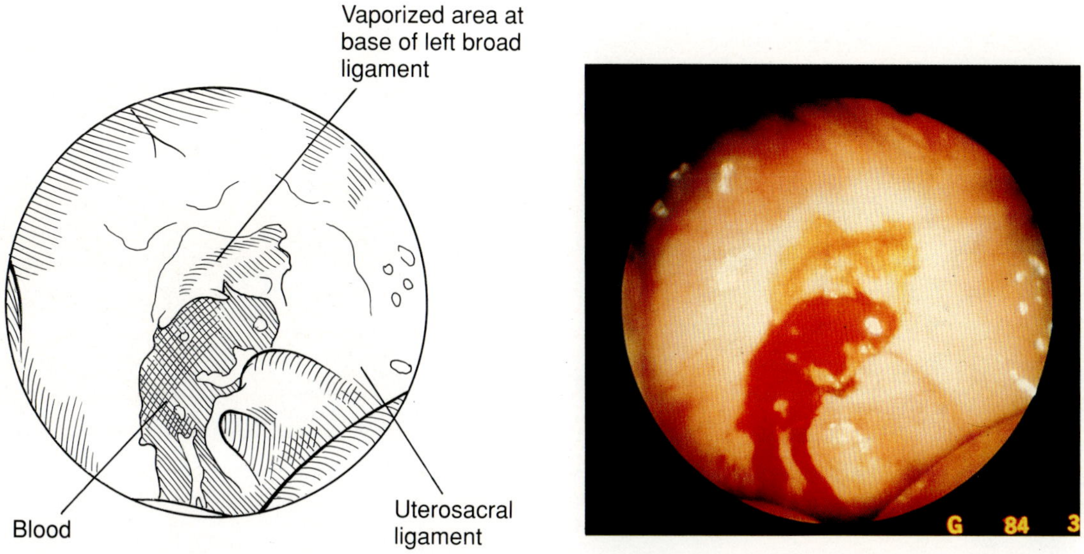

FIG. 7. Arterial bleeding lateral to the uterosacral ligament. Resection or vaporization of the uterosacral ligaments risks perforation of the branch of the vaginal arteries, which courses just lateral to and sometimes beneath the ligament. Bipolar cauterization is usually effective, but care must be taken to avoid the ureter, which can lie immediately lateral to the uterosacral ligament.

Peritoneum

Bleeding from the peritoneum can be prevented by careful attention to the anatomy and appropriate use of titanium backstops for laser as well as by placing fluid in the pelvis to act as a backstop for CO_2 laser. Small bleeders can be observed, as these may stop on their own. The CO_2 laser beam coagulates small vessels adequately. Electrosurgical bipolar and unipolar units can be utilized for hemostasis. In addition, pressure with instruments or clamps, use of the argon beam coagulator in selected circumstances, and warm Ringer's solution may assist in obtaining hemostasis on peritoneal surfaces. It is imperative that the pneumoperitoneum be decompressed for at least 3 min "by the clock" at the end of surgery to allow small bleeders tamponaded by the pneumoperitoneum to be identified through direct visualization and the finding of trailers in a fluid bath placed in the pelvis. The patient should also be placed in reverse Trendelenburg position near the end of the procedure to allow intraabdominal fluid and blood, which may have accumulated in the upper abdomen, to flow into the pelvis and be aspirated. Bleeding may also occur from mesosalpingeal tears as a result of inappropriate traction on the fallopian tube. These vessels must be coagulated carefully to avoid devascularization of the fallopian tube. Vascular adhesions may also bleed; these should be coagulated prior to division. These procedures will help ensure that intraoperative and postoperative bleeding will be minimized and not result in postoperative hematomas (Fig. 8).

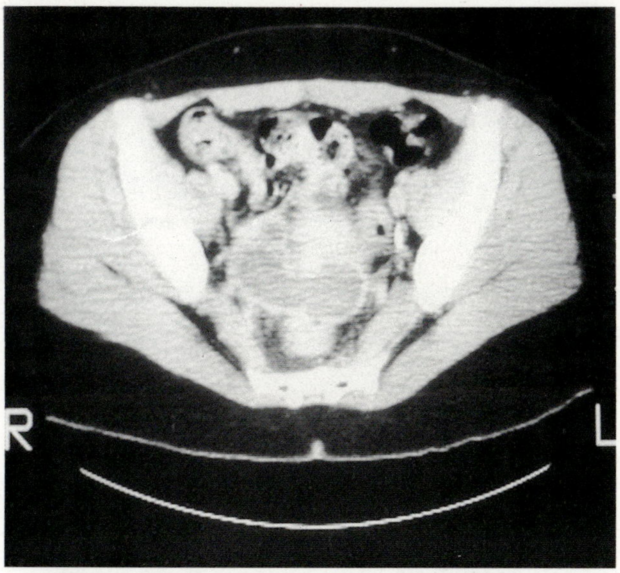

FIG. 8. CT scan of a hematoma in the posterior cul-de-sac. Eighteen days prior, the patient had a laparoscopy with lysis of dense right ovarian and bowel adhesions and resection of severe recurrent pelvic endometriosis. Postoperatively, the patient was transfused two units of packed cells and discharged. Despite absence of infection and evidence of gradual resolution of the hematoma by serial untrasound scans, a laparotomy was performed with evacuation of the hematoma 42 days after initial surgery because of persistent pelvic pain.

Cervix and Uterus

Cervical laceration following placement of the cervical clamp for uterine manipulation is usually minor but in selected instances merits repair with an interrupted su-

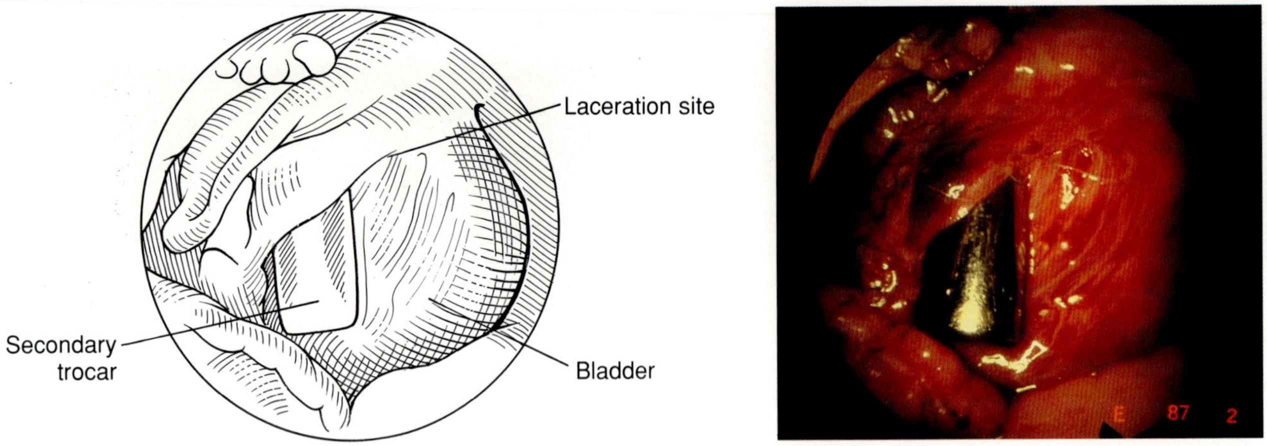

FIG. 9. Laceration of bladder muscularis with the secondary trocar. Four hundred ml of saline and methylene blue were instilled into the bladder and no leakage was seen. The patient was treated with 10 days of an indwelling Foley catheter without complication.

ture. Uterine perforation can also occur with the uterine manipulator or through injury from the primary or secondary abdominal puncture sites. Hemostasis should be obtained with the electrosurgical bipolar unit. Further repair of the uterus is generally unnecessary.

Abdominal Wall

Abdominal wall vessel injury occasionally results in a hematocele. This should be treated with drainage and copious irrigation and appropriate hemostasis with electrosurgery or suture.

Omental Vessels and Bowel Mesentery

Bleeding from omental vessels or bowel mesentery can occur from injury associated with placement of the Veress needle or trocar. Such bleeding is often self-limited but can be controlled with bipolar electrosurgical desiccation.

Urinary Tract Injuries

Bladder

Bladder perforation can result from placement of the Veress needle or the primary or secondary trocars in the lower abdomen (11) (Fig. 9). Since the routine use of a transurethral catheter to drain the bladder, needle or trocar perforations of the bladder have been rare. A survey of Canadian gynecologists indicated that the occurrence of Veress needle injuries equaled those caused by trocars and that the trocar perforations were evenly distributed between the primary and accessory instruments (11).

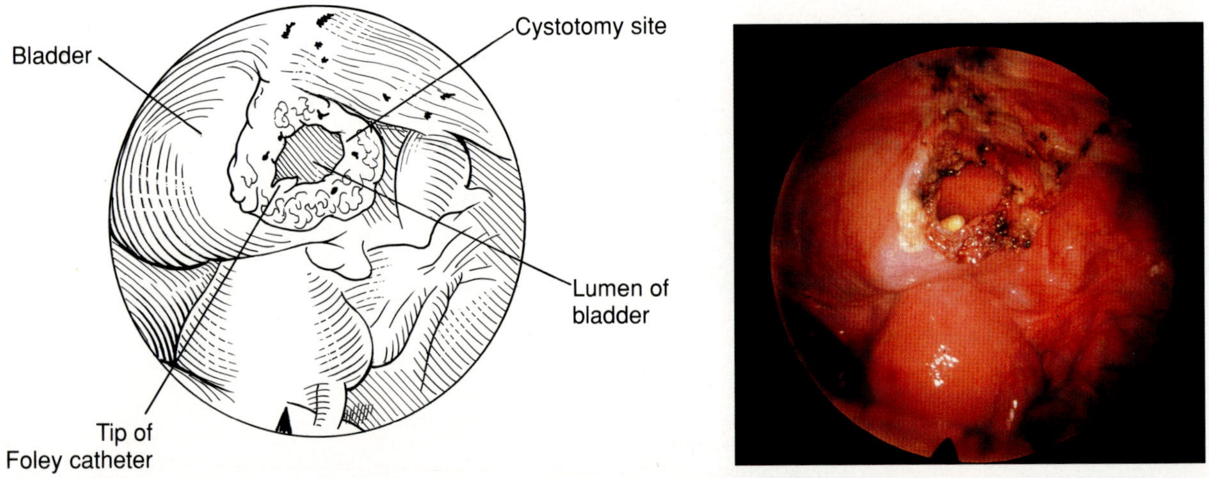

FIG. 10. Cystotomy during adhesiolysis. A bladder laceration during lysis of extensive adhesions was repaired by minilaparotomy and a two-layer closure. A Foley catheter was left in place for 10 days and the patient recovered uneventfully.

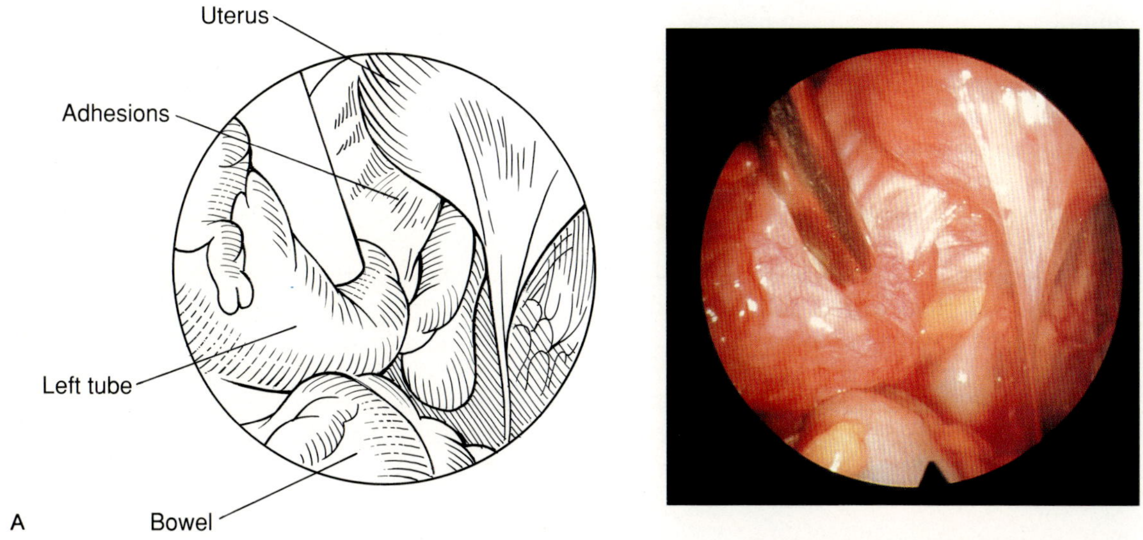

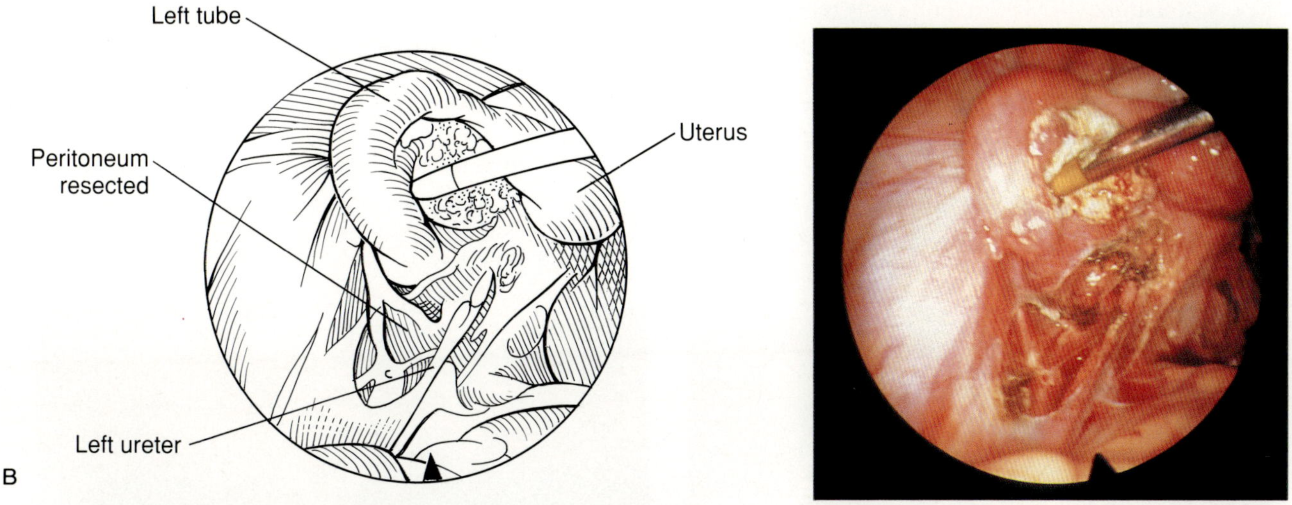

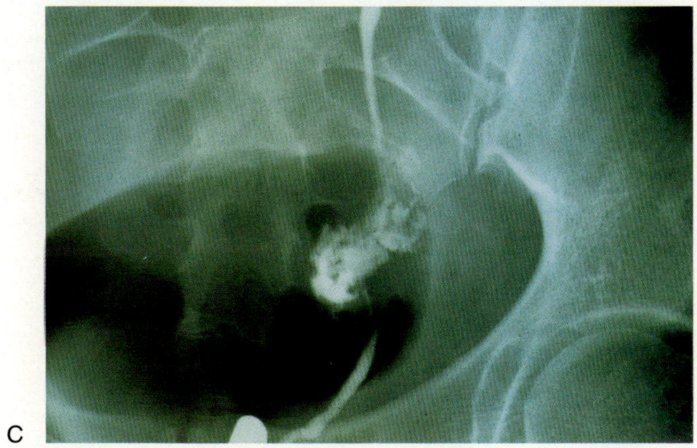

FIG. 11. A: Left tube and ovary adherent to the broad ligament. Severe left adnexal adhesions are seen with nonvisualization of the left ovary and distal tube. **B:** The adhesions have been lysed and the broad ligament endometriosis resected. The left ureter is visualized after superficial coagulation to stop bleeding from an ureteral vessel. **C:** A ureteral fistula is diagnosed 4 days postoperatively and treated with a stent for 4 weeks. Replacement of the stent was required because of persistence of the fistula, which healed after another 4 weeks.

Bladder injuries are more common in patients with severe anterior cul-de-sac endometriosis, previous bladder surgery, and prior cesarean sections, although the most common cause remains bladder distention (12) (Fig. 10). Recently, the laparoscopically assisted vaginal hysterectomy in the hands of the neophyte has also increased the frequency of bladder laceration. Bladder injuries usually can be avoided by placement of a Foley catheter preoperatively and by placement of the secondary puncture site under direct vision. Injury has also been documented from transvaginal placement of the Rubin's cannula into the bladder, and an urachal sinus perforation has also been reported (22,23).

The diagnosis of bladder perforation can be made by the finding of gas in the Foley bag, and it can be confirmed by cystography, retrograde instillation of indigo carmine or methylene blue solution, or cystoscopy. Treatment includes a double-layer, watertight closure with polydioxanone (PDS) (24). Following repair, indigo carmine should be injected in a retrograde fashion to confirm the watertight closure. An indwelling catheter is then left for 7–10 days and the patient is treated with prophylactic antibiotics for a similar period of time. Urologic consultation should be obtained if there is any question regarding the adequacy of management and repair.

Ureters

Ureteral injury is not common (25). It is usually caused by unipolar or bipolar electrosurgery and most commonly occurs near the uterosacral ligaments (Fig. 11A–C). Injury by trocar has also been reported. Injury generally results in ureteral narrowing and hydroureter. This damage can be significant since in one study 3 of 13 patients suffering injury lost renal function and 2 required nephrectomy (25). The diagnosis of ureteral injury is suggested by the presence of flank, pelvic, low back, or abdominal pain as well as fever, leukocytosis, and peritonitis in the early postoperative period (48–72 hr). However, diagnosis may be delayed for up to 3 weeks (12). Increased blood urea nitrogen (BUN) may also occur by urinary contact with the peritoneum. Suspicion of injury should be immediately confirmed by intravenous pyelogram (Fig. 12A, 12B). Treatment with a retrograde or percutaneous stent left in situ for approximately 2 months may be effective, but surgery for resection and reanastomosis of the injured segment of ureter frequently is needed. Urologic consultation is obviously indicated.

Prevention of ureteral injury is most easily accomplished by careful identification of the course of the ure-

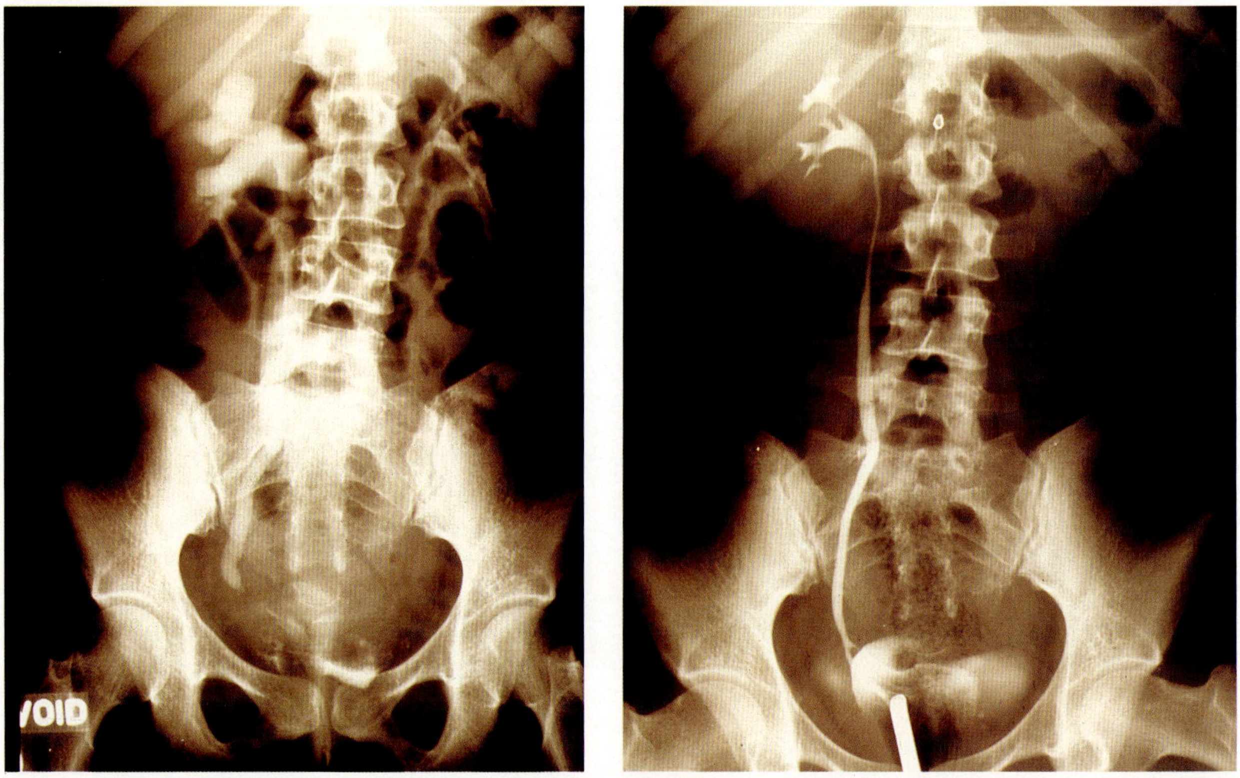

A B

FIG. 12. A: Intravenous pyelogram showing a hydroureter and hydronephrosis due to a fistula and stenosis of the right ureter. This followed extensive lysis of right adnexal adhesions and was manifested by fever and abdominal pain. **B:** A retrograde study in the same patient with ureteral injury.

ter (Fig. 13A–C). This should be done at the initiation of the operative laparoscopy when peristalsis is still active and the peritoneum has not lost its translucency, as occurs in prolonged operative laparoscopy procedures. Special care should be taken to identify the location of the ureter at the pelvic brim and its relation to the infundibulopelvic ligaments, as well as its location with respect to the uterine vessels in the cardinal ligament region. Continued evaluation of the course and location of the ureter throughout the procedure should be performed. Extraperitoneal dissection of placement of catheters may be of assistance. Should any concern be present regarding potential injury, 5 cm^3 of indigo carmine can be injected intravenously by the anesthesiologist. This should appear in the Foley catheter bag within approximately 10 min. Underwater exploration of the ureter for trailers suggesting ureteral injury can then be performed. If suspicion of injury is present, a cystoscopy with placement of an ureteral stent can be performed and/or appropriate intraoperative repair effected. Postoperative diagnosis can be assisted by intravenous pyelography.

Gastrointestinal Injuries

The reported prevalence of gastrointestinal injury is estimated to be 1–3 per 1000 laparoscopies (12,26)—a rate higher than the 6.2 per 10,000 incidence of bowel penetration extracted from the literature in 1975 by Loffer and Pent (27). The actual occurrence of bowel perforation is unknown and may be somewhat higher, since such injuries may go unnoticed or unreported. Soderstrom personally reviewed 66 cases brought to litigation for bowel perforation after laparoscopy (28).

Of the 20 case reports prior to 1975, 9 represented injuries to the stomach (4 needle-induced and 5 trocar-induced), 5 to the small bowel (3 needle and 2 trocar), and 6 to the colon (4 needle and 2 trocar) (27).

The majority of intestinal injuries are secondary to mechanical trauma. Electrosurgical or laser perforations are relatively rare. Utilizing careful histologic analysis, only 6 of 66 laparoscopic bowel perforations were caused by direct electric dessication, 2 were the result of defective equipment, 3 were due to operator error, and 1 was a "calculated risk" of extensive adhesiolysis (28).

Small Bowel

The open technique of laparoscopy may reduce but does not eliminate the risk of bowel injury (28). Small bowel laceration generally occurs with extensive enterolysis for small bowel adhesions (Fig. 14A–C). Injury has been reported in up to 25% of patients undergoing complex operations for small bowel adhesions. Another very common cause of small bowel injury occurs with placement of secondary lower quadrant puncture sites when this is not done under direct vision. Often such injury goes unrecognized. Repair should be carried out with 3-0 or 4-0 silk or PDS on a tapered SH needle (Fig. 14D). At the completion of the repair, sterile milk can be instilled to detect occult perforations. A nasogastric tube is also indicated, and a general surgical consultation should be obtained.

Large Bowel

Large bowel injury is frequently caused by the Veress needle and probably is often undiagnosed. Diagnosis is made by the presence of foul-smelling gas. Injury to the large bowel from a small hole made by the Veress needle can usually be managed expectantly. Other Veress needle placement sites that can be utilized to avoid bowel injury include the left costal margin in the midclavicular line, lateral to the umbilicus in the midclavicular line, or transvaginally through the posterior cul-de-sac and suprapubically in the midline.

Injury to the large bowel by a trocar may occur when there is complete transfixation of large bowel to the anterior abdominal wall (Fig. 15). This complication is often undiagnosed, and it can only be determined through careful observation through the laparoscope as the laparoscope is entirely removed from the abdominopelvic cavity back through the abdominal wall. Should an injury be diagnosed in this area, the trocar should be left in situ to identify the site of injury while a laparotomy is performed, and double-layer closure with 3-0 or 4-0 PDS or silk performed, or bowel resection and reanastomosis carried out if the extent of injury so merits.

The most common site of large bowel injury is the rectosigmoid. This occurs most frequently as a result of treatment of endometriosis or dense adhesions in the pelvis or from injury with the Veress needle or trocar. Superficial injury may be managed simply by observation (Fig. 16). Deep injury requires surgical repair, preferably in two layers, with 3-0 or 4-0 PDS or silk suture (Fig. 17A,B).

The majority of intestinal injuries are secondary to mechanical trauma (28). However, injury to the large bowel is not uncommon. Superficial thermal injury may be treated by a pursestring suture placed beyond the thermally damaged tissue. However, deep thermal injury requires resection and repair of the damaged tissue in two layers, with 3-0 or 4-0 silk or PDS. The bowel should be checked following repair by placement of a 30-cm^3 Foley catheter in the rectum with clamping of the bowel above the site of repair, followed by injection of a dilute solution of 50% betadine. Underwater exploration documents trailers of iodine antiseptic solution. A 100-cm^3 syringe can also be utilized to inject air into the bowel to look for bubbles and ensure that complete closure has been effected.

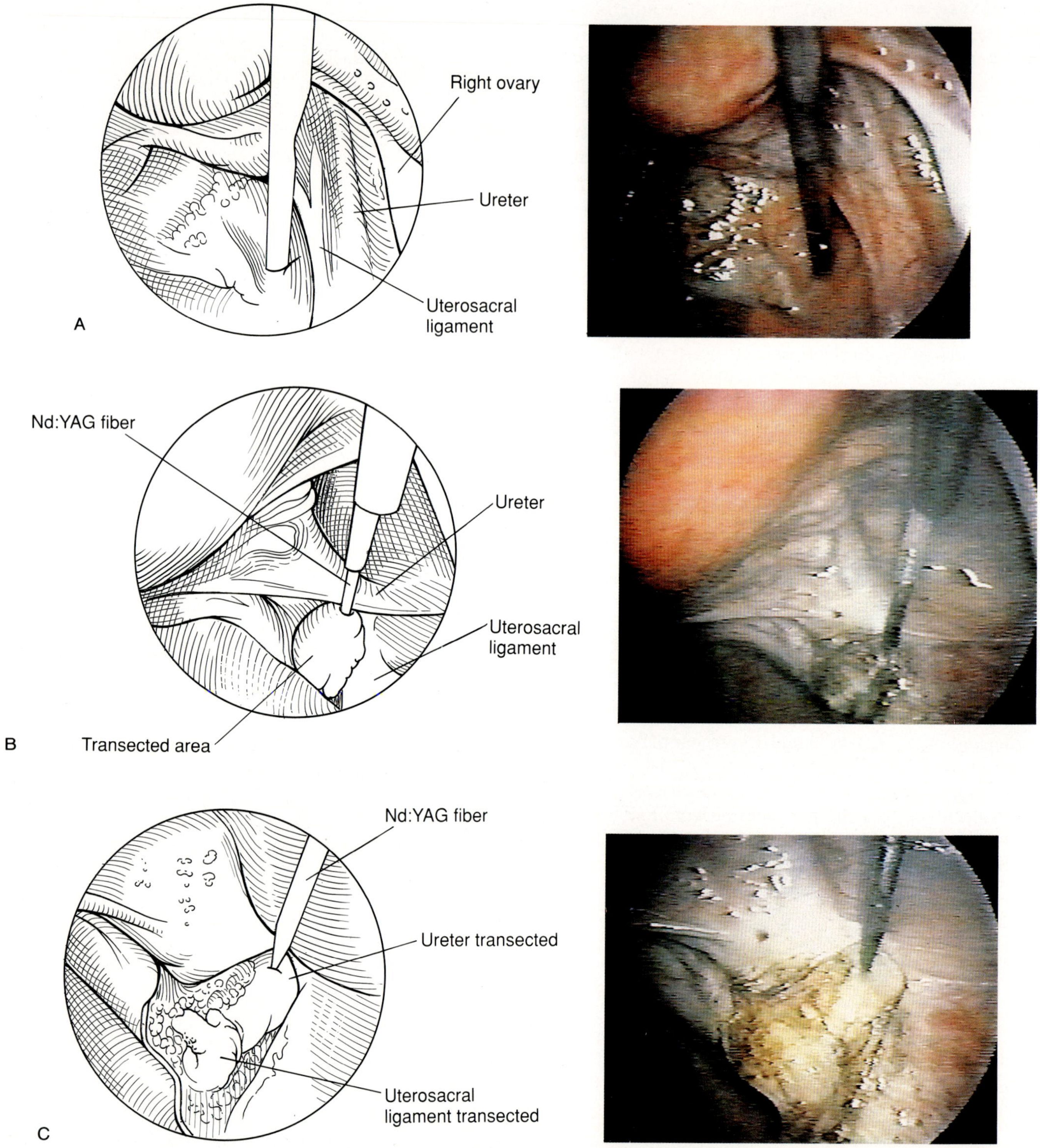

FIG. 13. **A:** Close approximation of the ureter to the uterosacral ligament prior to a laser uterosacral nerve ablation (LUNA). **B:** Transection of the uterosacral ligament and the ureter with the neodymium: yttruim-aluminum-garnet (Nd:YAG) laser fiber. **C:** Further dissection through the ligament and ureter. The ureter is apparently not noticed by the operator, and the ablation of the uterosacral ligament is carried too far laterally. The patient was subsequently anuric and required ureteral implantation.

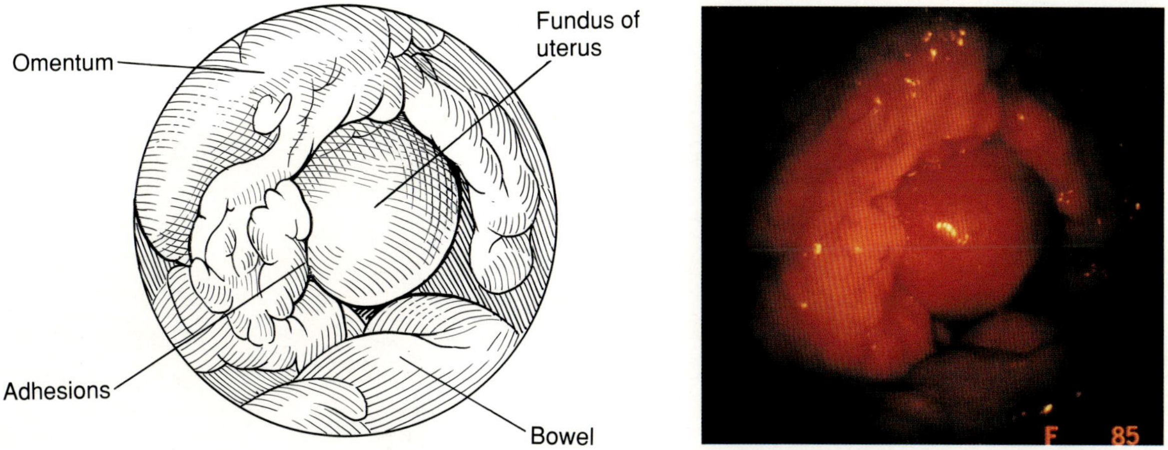

A

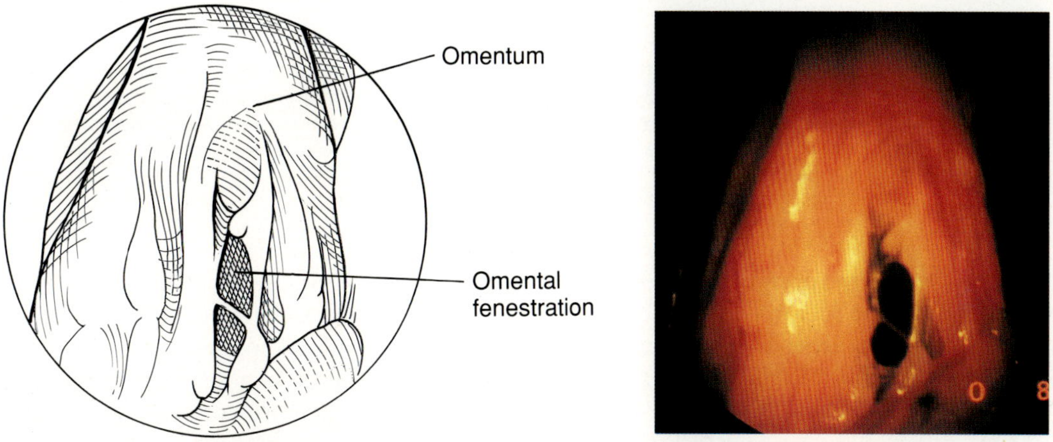

B

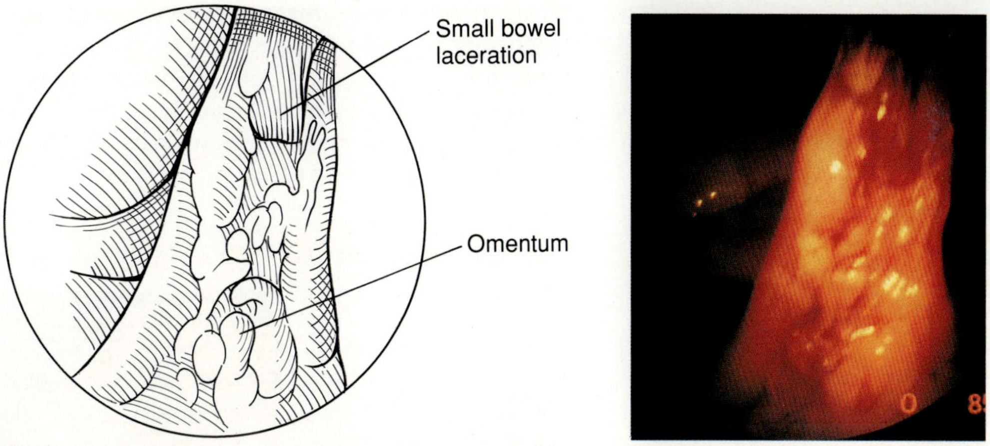

C

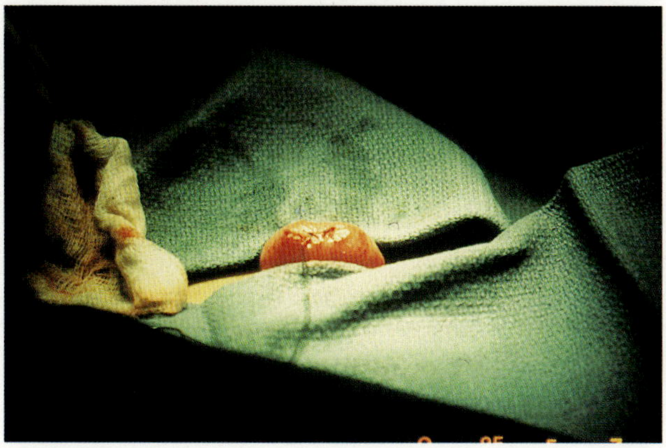

D

FIG. 14. A: Omental adhesions with small bowel laceration. In this case, the omentum was adherent to the uterine fundus and pelvis following a previous laparotomy. Because the omentum obscured the pelvic viscera, the risk of injury to bowel or vasculature was increased when the primary or secondary trocars are introduced. **B:** The omentum was fenestrated with rather blunt scissors without adequate visualization of structures lying behind. **C:** The small bowel, adherent to the omentum, has been cut. **D:** A minilaparotomy was performed and the small bowel was oversewn. The patient was observed in the hospital for 2 days and then discharged.

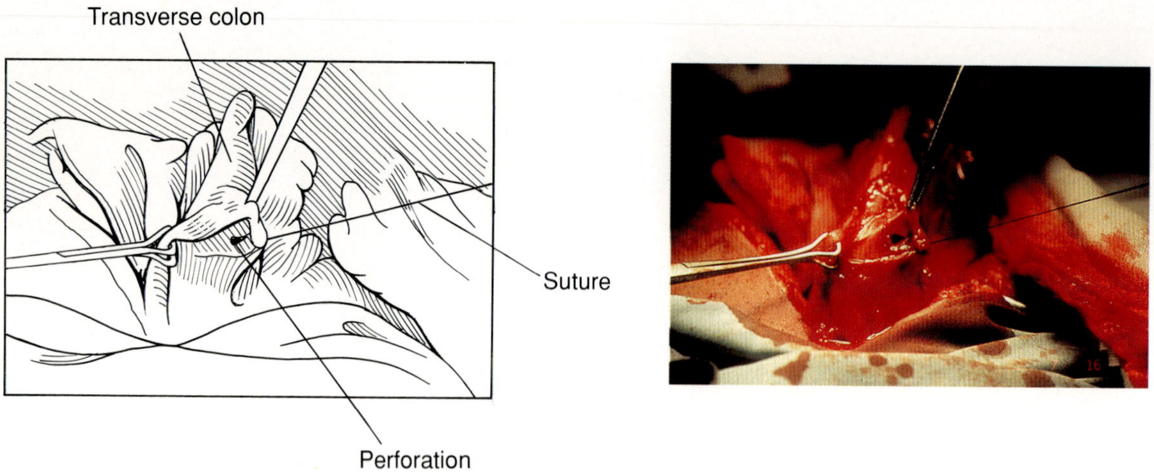

FIG. 15. Trocar perforation of the transverse colon. This patient had a history of an automobile accident and a consequent laparotomy with splenectomy. The colon was adherent to the anterior abdominal wall. Subsequent laparotomy showed essentially no anterior parietal peritoneum and dense adhesions to the entire upper abdominal wall extending 6 cm below the umbilicus. The bowel was oversewn and the patient was discharged in 6 days.

Many patients undergo operative laparoscopy with an unprepared bowel. The decision on the method of bowel repair in this situation depends on the amount of fecal spillage. A large amount of spillage merits laparotomy, whereas a small amount of spillage may be treated by laparoscopic suture and copious irrigation. It may not be necessary to perform a colostomy with bowel injuries associated with laparoscopy. Nevertheless, much greater safety for the patient and comfort for the surgeon can be effected by ensuring that a full-bowel preparation is performed on patients who are undergoing extensive operative laparoscopy, especially those with suspected disease around the bowel (Fig. 18A–D).

It is common for injury to large bowel to go unrecognized intraoperatively. Traumatic injury generally presents with symptoms within 24–48 hr, but electrosurgical injury may not cause symptoms for 4–10 days. The patient then presents with abdominal pain, fever, leukocytosis, and often nausea and vomiting. Delayed symptoms of bowel injury can also occur after perforation of bowel that has been devascularized mechanically or by hemorrhagic ischemic necrosis, although such situations are rare. Treatment of bowel injury after delayed diagnosis requires bowel resection of all necrotic tissue with end-to-end anastomosis, copious lavage, use of antibiotics, and minidose heparin therapy. General surgical and

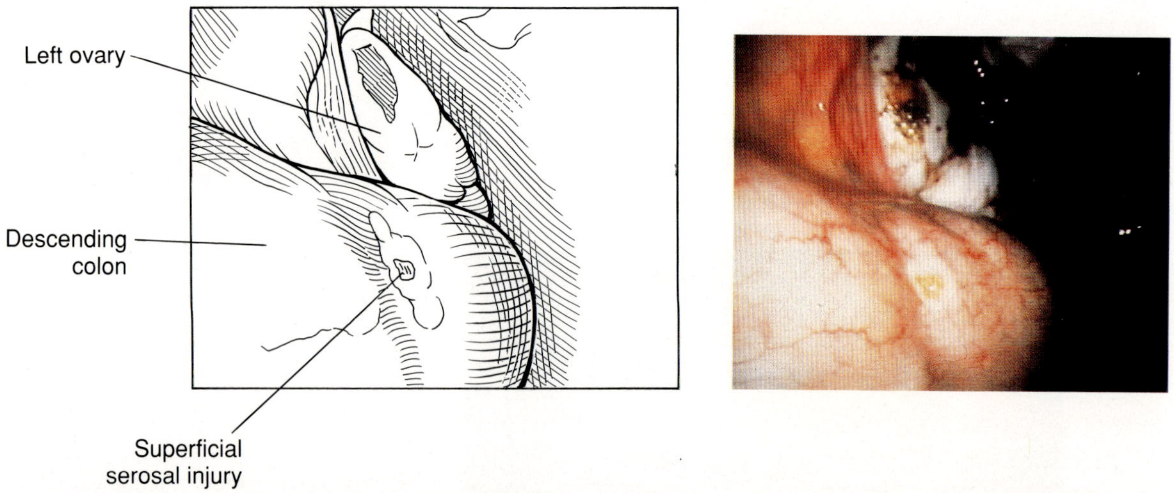

FIG. 16. Serosal burn of the descending colon with the CO_2 laser. The serosa of the colon is grazed with the laser beam during vaporization of endometriosis of the left ovary. No perforation is seen and the patient recovered without event. These patients should be cautioned about signs of peritonitis which can be delayed for as long as 2 weeks after surgery.

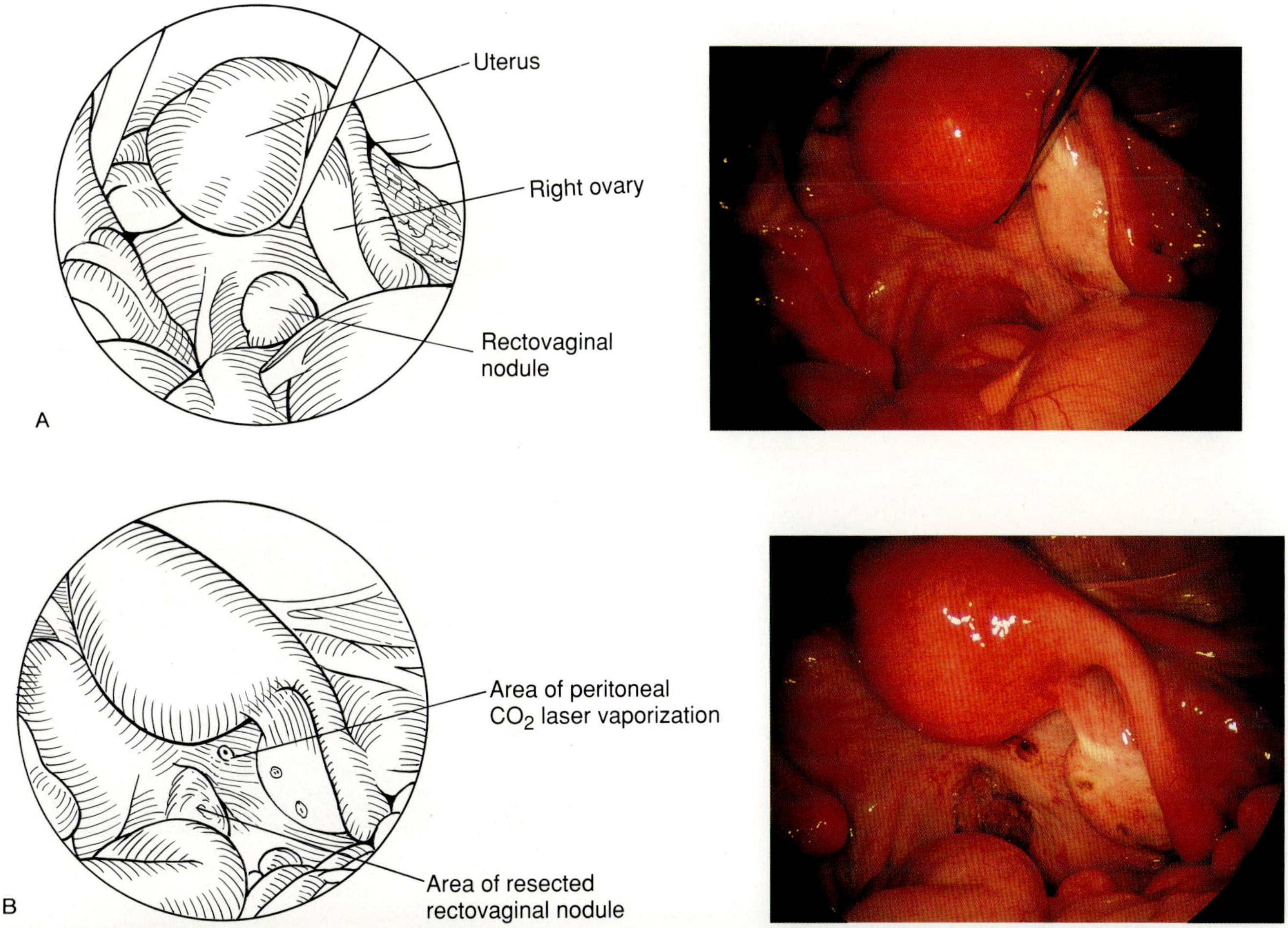

FIG. 17. A: Delayed peritonitis following CO_2 laser resection of a rectovaginal nodule of endometriosis. Prior to resection, a painful, 2-cm nodule of endometriosis is seen medial to the right uterosacral ligament. **B:** The pelvis is inspected after the nodule has been resected utilizing a sponge stick in the rectum to delineate the rectal margins. Recovery was uneventful until 11 days after surgery, when the patient presented with an acute abdomen. No perforation was seen and peritoneal cultures were negative, but a temporary diverting colostomy was performed. An intraoperative indigo carmine or gastrografin enema may have avoided the colostomy.

other appropriate consultation should be obtained (Fig. 19).

Stomach

Stomach injury is usually caused by the Veress needle or laparoscopic trocar. It is especially common following difficult intubations and resultant gastric distention. It can be prevented by use of an orogastric tube. When a stomach injury is recognized through direct visualization of the stomach mucosa, treatment can be effected by leaving the trocar in place and incising over it to produce a minilaparotomy, thereby assisting the identification of the injury site. The stomach can be repaired with a pursestring suture or figure-of-eight suture in a two-layer closure of 2-0 or 3-0 PDS. A nasogastric tube should be left in place for 2 days and appropriate general surgery consultation obtained.

Subcutaneous and Subfascial Emphysema and Edema

Emphysema is a common minor complication of operative laparoscopy. Emphysema can occur in the omentum, anterior abdominal wall, space of Retzius, retroperitoneum, or bowel mesentery as a result of inappropriate placement of the Veress needle and/or passage of CO_2 gas through defects created by the instrumentation or surgical procedure (Fig. 20). Such emphysema is rarely of much significance, although it can be of concern to the patient. It generally subsides within a few hours but can be present for a couple of days. It can be recognized in the anterior abdominal wall and even in the thoracic wall through the finding of crepitus. Emphysema involving the face is usually of limited clinical significance because it resolves spontaneously, but patient reassurance is necessary.

Edema, the presence of fluid in the tissues, occurs in the same location as subcutaneous emphysema, but usu-

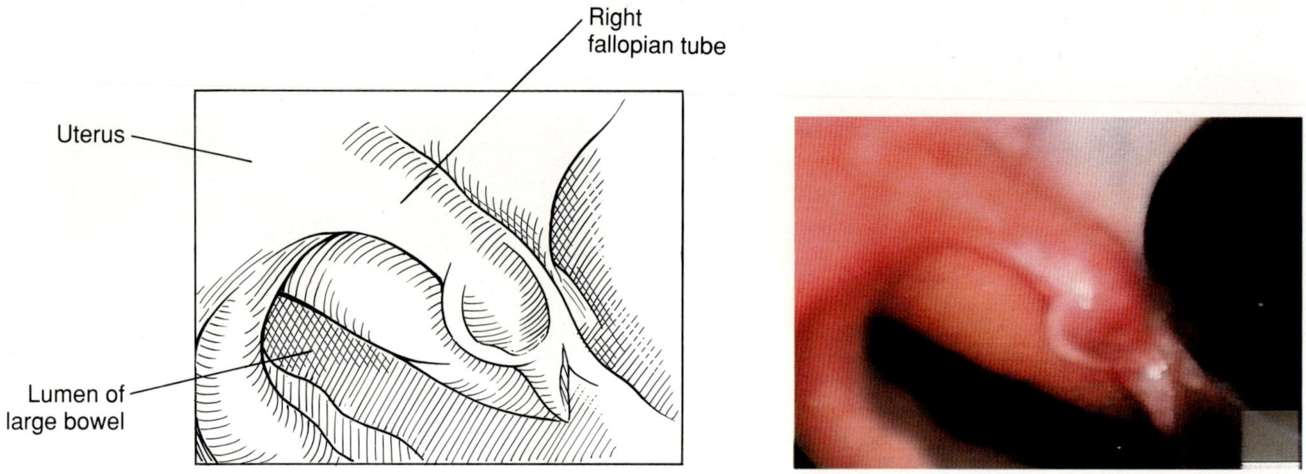
Right
fallopian tube
Uterus
Lumen of
large bowel
A

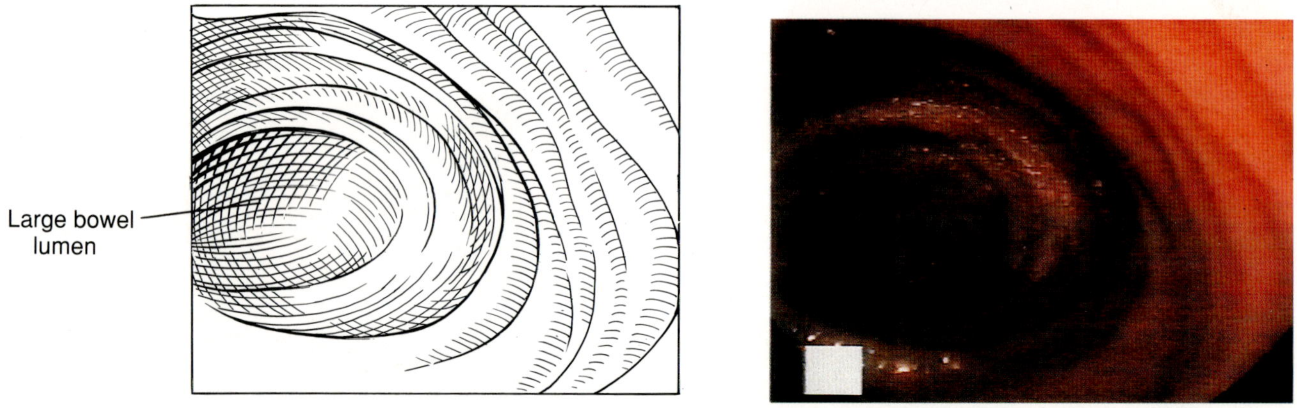
Large bowel
lumen
B

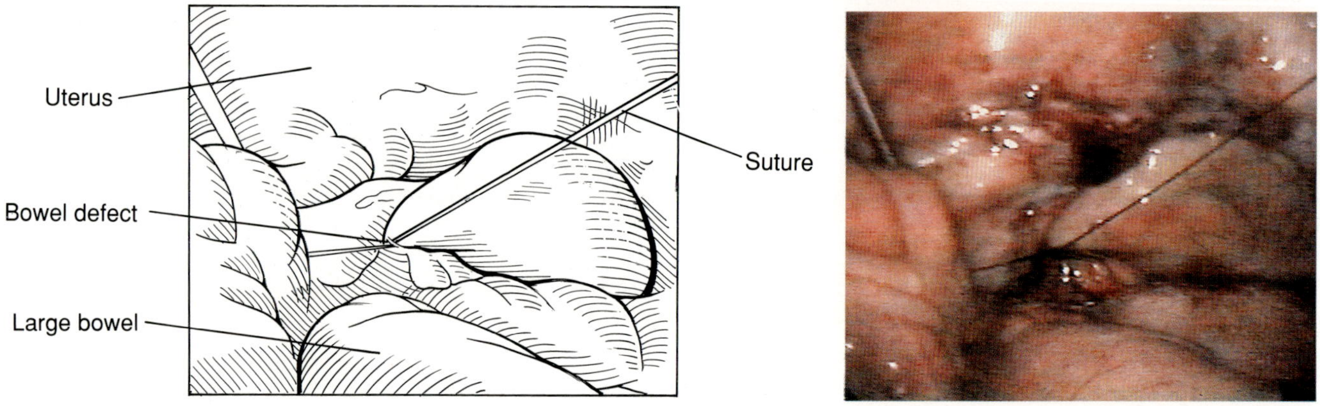
Uterus
Suture
Bowel defect
Large bowel
C

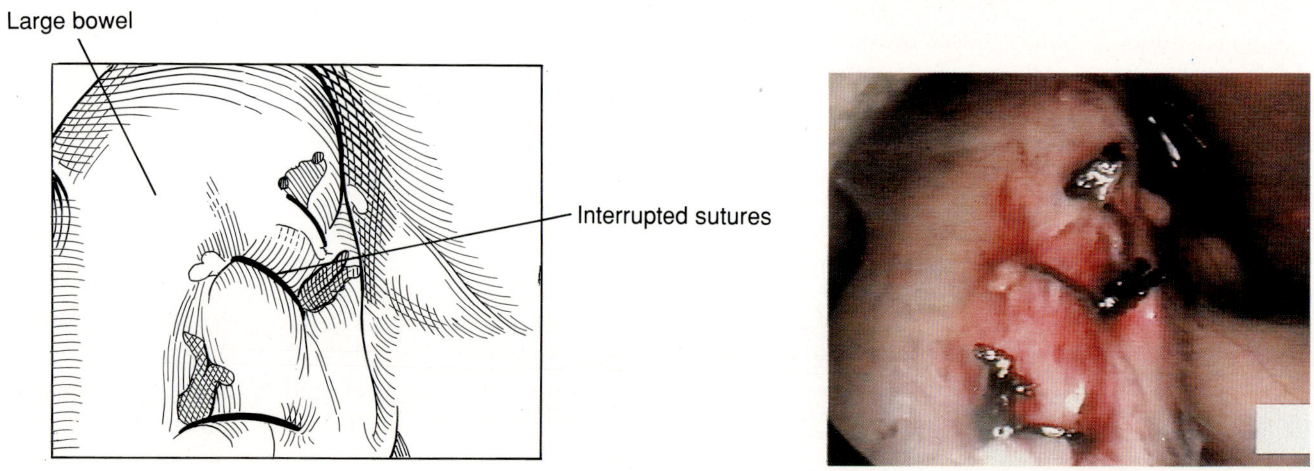
Large bowel
Interrupted sutures
D

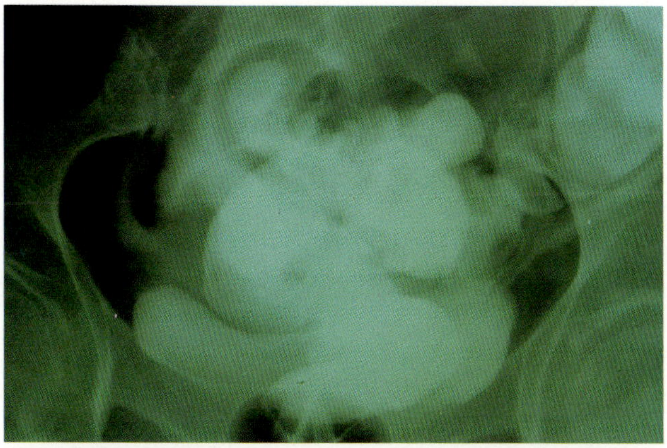

FIG. 19. Gastrografin enema demonstrating bowel perforation. Five days after extensive cul-de-sac dissection the patient developed right chest pain. Pelvic tenderness was minimal, a white cell count was normal, and free air was seen under the diaphragm on upright x-ray. A computed tomography (CT) scan of the pelvis showed an abnormality in the region of the rectum but no obvious perforation.

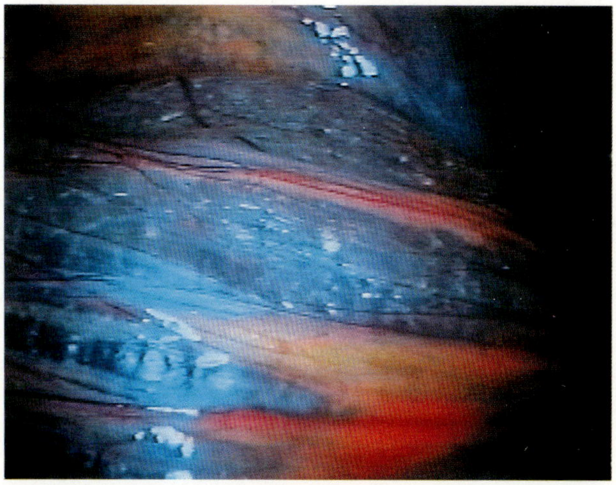

FIG. 20. Omental insufflation. The omentum has been pierced by the Veress needle and is distended with CO_2. The bowel is inspected and appears normal, and no omental or mesenteric vessels have been severed.

ally in more dependent areas, especially the flanks and vulva. Subcutaneous edema may occur concurrently with subcutaneous emphysema. Severe vulvar edema may rarely require the placement of a Foley catheter. Fascial edema is proportional to the length of the procedure and the degree of Trendelenburg position, usually resolving within hours after surgery.

Vasopressin Complications

Vasopressin is a potent vasoconstrictor that can cause hypertension and severe coronary vasoconstriction. It may be used during ectopic salpingostomy and laparoscopic myomectomy. Prevention of complications is facilitated by the use of dilute solutions and by careful injection with aspiration to avoid intravascular injection. The minimum amount necessary should be utilized, and the anesthesiologist should be informed prior to its injection.

Carbon Dioxide Laser Complications

A recent study found that only 1.2% of laparoscopic injuries were directly attributable to CO_2 laser use (4). Prevention of CO_2 laser complications includes adequate training and experience for the surgeon, use of a backstop to prevent the laser beam striking distant tissues, placement of fluid in the cul-de-sac, hydrodissection, and careful observation of the bowel at all times. Care should be taken never to fire the laser unless the HeNe aiming beam can be visualized. Recognition that a blind region occurs out of the field of view of the laparoscope, close to the end of the laparoscope, is mandatory. Carbon particles should be washed off tissue and removed from the pelvis. Currently, there are no known clinically significant sequelae of these carbon particles, but it seems prudent to remove as much carbon as possible (Fig. 21A–D).

Impairment of Normal Function

Care should be taken to avoid aspiration of the fimbria into the aspiration cannula, grasping of the fimbria, or creation of other thermal or mechanical injury near the fimbria. In the treatment of ectopic pregnancy, intraluminal damage should be minimized. Adhesiolysis should be performed with a view to maintaining the serosa of the fallopian tube as much as possible.

Ovarian adhesiolysis can easily result in injury to the ovarian surface, which tends to form adhesions postoperatively very easily. Ovarian cystectomy should be

FIG. 18. A: During lysis of dense posterior cul-de-sac adhesions, the large bowel is entered. **B:** An inadvertent laparoscopic colonoscopy is performed, showing excellent results from the patient's preoperative bowel preparation. **C:** The defect is repaired with interrupted sutures laparoscopically. **D:** A watertight seal is created. Less bold endoscopists may choose to repair this type of defect with a minilaparotomy and with the assistance of a general surgeon. The use of a bowel preparation obviated the need for a temporary diverting colostomy.

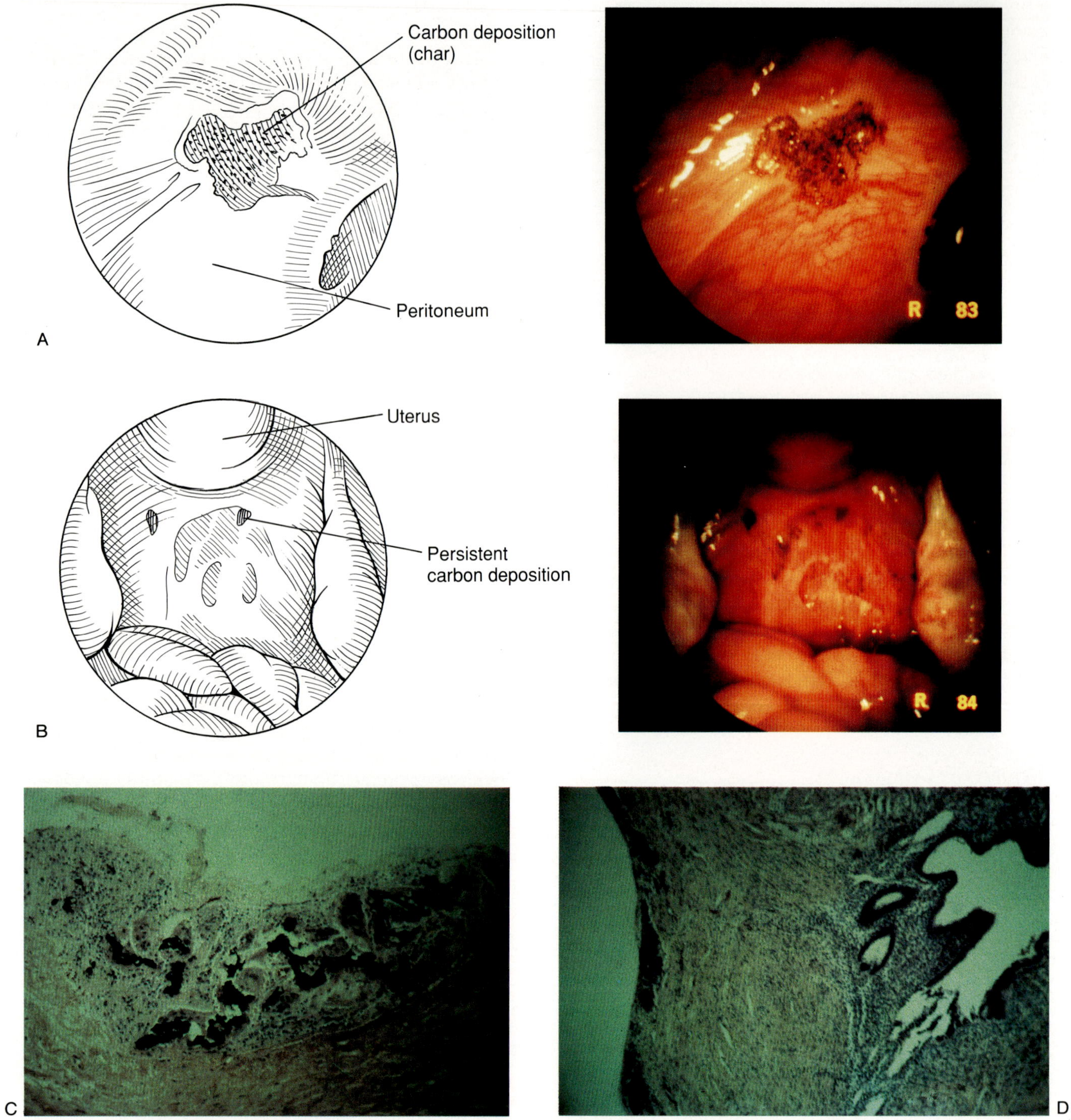

FIG. 21. A: Extensive carbon deposition after CO_2 laser vaporization of endometriosis using low-power densities. **B:** Second-look laparoscopy on the same patient shows persistent carbon. These spots can mimic recurrent endometriosis but may be differentiated by their irregular margins on close inspection under magnification. **C:** Residual carbon produces a foreign body giant cell reaction. **D:** Endometriosis may be hidden behind the carbon and foreign body reaction.

effected with a view to maintaining the maximum amount of normal ovarian tissue. Failure to remove all of the ovarian cyst, and especially an endometrioma, can result in persistence of disease associated with the cysts. Oophorotomy by electrosurgery or laser for treatment of polycystic ovarian disease can potentially lead to ovarian adhesions and should only be performed in highly selected patients. Excessive resection of ovarian tissue, cortical damage, or vascular compromise can potentially result in premature ovarian failure. As a general rule, an ovary should always be conserved unless oophorectomy is absolutely mandatory.

The uterus can be injured at the time of myomectomy. It is important to leave as much uterine tissue as possible when removing leimyomata. In addition, the uterine cavity should be left intact if possible. Suturing of the myoma site is necessary when large myomas are removed, although adhesion formation will likely be greater.

Failure to Complete Procedure

Failure to complete the operative laparoscopy procedure can result in inadequate treatment for the patient. The patient should always be counseled preoperatively regarding the potential necessity of laparotomy. Laparotomy should be performed to complete the operation when necessary to obtain the optimum result for the patient. Different surgeons have different skill levels and different thresholds for performing a laparotomy. Performance of a laparotomy by itself does not constitute a complication, but the surgeon and the patient need to understand preoperatively that such an outcome may be necessary to obtain the optimal surgical result. Patients with extensive pelvic adhesions or endometriosis and who have infertility as their only symptom are often best treated with in vitro fertilization (IVF), therefore avoiding the risks of complex pelvic surgery.

EARLY POSTOPERATIVE COMPLICATIONS

Abdominal Pain

Early postoperative complications include abdominal pain. This can be minimized by using the smallest possible abdominal incisions, ensuring careful closure with hemostasis of the abdominal wounds, placing 0.25–0.5% bupivacaine into the wound margins at the completion of the surgery, and avoiding abdominal overdistention. Abdominal pain as a result of postoperative ileus can be reduced through the use of preoperative bowel preparation. Postoperative analgesics are appropriate to help manage pain.

Shoulder Pain

Shoulder pain, in particular on the right side, may be the result of diaphragmatic stimulation of C4 as a result of gas or air left intraabdominally. The CO_2 gas should be expelled at the termination of the procedure through pressure placed on the abdominal wall. Shoulder pain, when it occurs, can be quite severe and last for several days. Assumption of the knee–chest or Trendelenberg positions can "float" the bubble of gas away from the diaphragms and afford immediate relief.

Neurologic Injury

Neurologic injury can occur postoperatively from injury to the peroneal nerve as a result of pressure on the lateral aspect of the knee and lower leg. This results in foot drop and paresthesias. This condition is generally self-limiting over a period of several days. It can be avoided by proper positioning of the patient, use of well-designed stirrups, and avoidance of pressure on the lateral aspect of the lower limbs. In addition, the legs can be exercised by the operating room staff approximately every 2 hr during the operation.

Sciatic nerve injury can occur from inappropriate placement of the patient on the operating room table. Brachial nerve injury can occur from the use of shoulder braces and can be a very significant complication. This can be avoided by not using these braces but using pads underneath the patient and/or a Trendelenburg position that is not quite as steep. Femoral nerve injury can occur as a result of extreme flexion, abduction, and lateral rotation of the hip joint. This can also be prevented by careful patient positioning (29).

Urinary Retention

Postoperative urinary retention can occur in cases lasting longer than 2 hr, especially when large volumes of intravenous fluids have been administered. Prevention of this problem can include the delay of Foley catheter removal until the patient is awake and aware of the catheter, which occurs approximately 1–2 hr after completion of the operation. In selected situations, the patient may receive bethanechol chloride (Urecholine) 25 mg. If the patient has not voided by 4 hr postoperatively, she can be straight-catheterized and treated again with bethanechol chloride 25 mg (24) or observation.

Infection

Infection is not a common postoperative complication with operative laparoscopy. Nevertheless cystitis and urinary tract infection can occur and should be diagnosed and treated in a standard fashion. Peritonitis and abscess are extremely uncommon and most often associated with bowel injury. Pelvic infection is similarly very uncommon. Cellulitis and infection in the abdominal wall can result in pain, swelling, and erythema. This should be treated by warm compresses, drainage, and appropriate antibiotics. Pneumonia is rare and should be treated in the usual fashion.

Prevention of infection can be enhanced by the use of appropriate sterile technique, appropriate sterilization of instruments, and prophylactic antibiotics. One regimen utilizes doxycycline 100 mg by mouth the night prior to surgery and 100 mg intravenously at the initiation of surgery. It should be noted that contamination of the peritoneal cavity occurs 90% of the time with hydrotubation (30). Nevertheless, infection is uncommon in the abdominal cavity. Copious lavage at laparoscopy also reduces the risk of infection. It is also important not to perform an unnecessary appendectomy, especially in young patients desiring future fertility, since such procedures occasionally result in pelvic infection and reduction in fertility.

Other

Other early postoperative complications include fluid overload and pulmonary edema, as well as urinary retention, incisional hematoma, and vulvar edema. Drug allergies can occur in any patient and should be treated in a standard fashion.

LATE POSTOPERATIVE COMPLICATIONS

Late postoperative complications include bowel injury and pelvic abscess. Uterine rupture may occur at the time of subsequent pregnancy if large defects have been left in the uterine wall. Ectopic pregnancy also is a potential complication of reconstructive tubal surgery. Intrauterine or ectopic pregnancy is a complication of tubal ligation. Dissemination of cancer may result from inappropriate management of adnexal masses; guidelines for management of adnexal masses should be followed carefully to prevent this problem. Psychological complications may occur rarely in selected patients who have not been appropriately selected for surgery.

Incisional hernias can occur following operative laparoscopy. Omental herniation is possible (31), and herniated tissue may become incarcerated (32, 33). Hernias usually occur more than 7 days postoperatively, although they have been reported earlier. Prevention includes the use of a Z track with placement of large instruments, the use of smaller trocars whenever possible, shaking of the abdominal wall or passage of a probe at the end of surgery to drop bowel or omentum out of incisions, and the placement of fascial sutures with the aid of skin hooks through skin incisions greater than 7 mm.

HIGHLIGHTS

It is clear that operative laparoscopy has brought many benefits to our patients. Nevertheless these operations are associated with complications that may cause significant morbidity or even mortality. It is imperative that we as surgeons become well trained before attempting operative laparoscopy. Most complications occur in a surgeon's first 50 cases. There are fewer complications after 200 cases. Experience can only be gained slowly, and it is incumbent on each surgeon to attempt only procedures for which he or she is technically competent.

The most important decision for surgeons to make to reduce complications is whether or not to operate. The decision to perform surgical procedures should not be influenced by personal, psychological, financial, or other professional needs, or be unduly influenced by the referring physician or patient. In addition, surgeons should not be unduly influenced by literature results or other surgeons' anecdotal experiences. Each surgeon must understand his or her own unique set of skills and weaknesses and develop enough rapport with each patient to understand and respect the uniqueness of the clinical situation.

By doing this, surgeons will be able to exercise good judgment and not violate basic surgical principles, while modifying each surgical decision to optimize the benefit for the patient and to minimize the risk of complication. Avoidance of complications is possibly the most critical factor in creating benefit for our patients once the decision to operate has been made. Awareness of potential complications is necessary to avoid them, diagnose them early when they occur, and manage them appropriately to minimize their sequelae.

REFERENCES

1. Hulka JF, Soderstrom RM, Corson SL, et al. Complications Committee of the American Association of Gynecologic Laparoscopists: first annual report. *J Reprod Med* 1975;10:301–306.
2. Peterson HB, Hulka JF, Phillips JM: American Association of Gynecologic Laparoscopists 1988 membership survey on operative laparoscopy. *J Reprod Med* 1990;35:587–589.
3. Hulka JF, Peterson HB, Phillips JM, Surrey MW. Operative laparoscopy. American Association of Gynecologic Laparoscopists 1991 membership survey. *J Reprod Med* 1993;38:569–571.
4. Diamond MP, Daniell JF, Feste J, et al. Initial report of the carbon dioxide laser laparoscopy study group: complications. *J Gynecol Surg* 1989;5:269–272.
5. Lehmann-Willenbrock E, Riedel H-H, Mecke H, Semm K. Pelviscopy/laparoscopy and its complications in Germany, 1949–1988. *J Reprod Med* 1992;37:671–677.
6. Method MW, Keith CG. Economic impact of gynecologic endoscopy. In: Sanfilippo JS, Levine RL eds. *Operative gynecologic endoscopy.* New York: Springer-Verlag; 1989.
7. Tokars JI, Bell DM, Culver DH, et al. Percutaneous injuries during surgical procedures. *JAMA* 1992;267(21):899–904.

8. Murphy AA. Operative laparoscopy. *Fertil Steril* 1987;47(1):1–18.
9. Ohlgisser M, Sorokin Y, Heifetz M. Gynecologic laparoscopy: a review article. *Obstet Gynecol Surv* 1985;40:385–396.
10. Kabukoba JJ, Skillern LH. Coping with extraperitoneal insufflation during laparoscopy: a new technique. *Obstet Gynecol* 1992;80:144–145.
11. Yuzpe AA. Pneumoperitoneum needle and trocar injuries in laparoscopy. A survey on possible contributing factors and prevention. *J Reprod Med* 1990;35:485–490.
12. Smith S. Complications of laparoscopic and hysteroscopic surgery. In: Azziz R, Murphy AA, eds. *Practical manual of operative laparoscopy and hysteroscopy.* New York: Springer-Verlag; 1992:199–215.
13. Nezhat FR, Silfen SL, Evans D, Nezhat C. Comparison of direct insertion of disposable and standard reusable laparoscopic trocars and previous pneumoperitoneum with Veress needle. *Obstet Gynecol* 1991;78:148–150.
14. Baadsgaard SE, Bille S, Egeblad K. Major vascular injury during gynecologic laparoscopy. Report of a case and review of published cases. *Acta Obstet Gynecol Scand* 1989;68:283–285.
15. Copeland C, Wing R, Hulka JF. Direct trocar insertion at laparoscopy: an evaluation. *Obstet Gynecol* 1983;62:655–659.
16. Byron JW, Fujiyoshi CA, Miyazawa K. Evaluation of the direct trocar insertion technique at laparoscopy. *Obstet Gynecol* 1989;74:423–425.
17. Chamberlain G, Brown JC, eds. Gynaecological laparoscopy: the report of the Confidential Inquiry into Gynaecological Laparoscopy. London: Royal College of Obstetricians and Gynaecologists; 1978:114.
18. Mintz M. Risks and prophylaxis in laparoscopy: a survey of 100,000 cases. *J Reprod Med* 1977;18:269–272.
19. Hurd WW, Bude RO, DeLancey JO, Gauvin JM, Aisen AM. Abdominal wall characterization by MRI and CT imaging: the effect of obesity on laparoscopic approach. *J Reprod Med* 1991;36:473–476.
20. Hurd WW, Bude RO, DeLancey JO, Pearl ML. The relationship of the umbilicus to the aortic bifurcation: implications for laparoscopic technique. *Obstet Gynecol* 1992;80:48–51.
21. Hurd WW, Pearl ML, DeLancey JO, Quint EH, et al. Laparoscopic injury of abdominal wall blood vessels: a report of three cases. *Obstet Gynecol* 1993;82(4):673–676.
22. McLucas B, March C. Urachal sinus perforation during laparoscopy: a case report. *J Reprod Med* 1990;35(5):573–574.
23. Sherer DM. Inadvertent transvaginal cystotomy during laparoscopy. *Int J Gynecol Obstet* 1990;32:77–79.
24. Reich H, McGlynn F. Laparoscopic repair of bladder injury. *Obstet Gynecol* 1990;76:909–910.
25. Grainger DA, Soderstrom RM, Schiff SF, Glickman MG, DeCherney AH, Diamond MP. Ureteral injuries at laparoscopy: insights into diagnosis, management, and prevention. *Obstet Gynecol* 1990;75:839–843.
26. Bayer SR: Trocar injuries to the large intestine. In: Corfman RS, Diamond MP, DeCherney AH, eds. *Complications of laparoscopy and hysteroscopy.* Boston, Blackwell Scientific; 1993:46–49.
27. Loffer FD, Pent D. Indications, contraindications, and complications of laparoscopy. *Obstet Gynecol Surv* 1975;30:407–426.
28. Soderstrom RM. Bowel injury litigation after laparoscopy. *J Am Assoc Gynecol Laparoscop* 1993;1:74–77.
29. Hershlag A, Loy R, Lavy G, DeCherney AH. Femoral neuropathy after laparoscopy: a case report. *J Reprod Med* 1990;35(5):575–576.
30. Pyper RJ, Ahmet Z, Houang ET. Bacteriological contamination during laparoscopy with dye injection. *Br J Obstet Gynecol* 1988;95:367–371.
31. Rajapaksa DS. Asymptomatic omental herniation following laparoscopic sterilisation. *Ceylon Med J* 1983;28:35.
32. Kiiholma P, Makinen J. Incarcerated Richter's hernia after laparoscopy: a case report. *Eur J Obstet Gynecol Reprod Biol* 1988;28:75–77.
33. Thomas AG, McLymont F, Moshipur J. Incarcerated hernia after laparoscopic sterilization: a case report. *J Reprod Med* 1990;35(6):639–640.

Endoscopic Management of Gynecologic Disease,
edited by G.D. Adamson and D.C. Martin.
Lippincott-Raven Publishers, Philadelphia © 1996.

CHAPTER 35

Anesthesia in Hysteroscopic and Laparoscopic Infertility Procedures

Mary Jane Carroll Collins and Stephen H. Jackson

The infertility patient brings to the anesthesiologist a unique set of challenges. Often presenting as the culmination of several years of unsuccessful attempts at achieving pregnancy, the infertility patient harbors highly charged emotional and intellectual issues. The infertility workup is demanding and invades the most private aspects of her life. Both medications and infertility techniques may lead to extreme demands on the sexual behavior and interpersonal relationships of the patient and her mate. Her anxiety may be far reaching and self-esteem low, as concerns with her fertility encompass her entire future. Small wonder, then, that these patients frequently are found by the anesthesiologist to be extremely anxious and questioning.

In the preoperative setting, anesthesiologists have the unique opportunity to interact with these women in a refreshingly positive and humanistic fashion. It is the development of this relationship that enables the anesthesiologist to allay the patient's anxieties regarding both the anesthesia and the surgery. Indeed, the anesthesiologist should empathetically acknowledge that the infertility patient brings with her not only a reproductive pathophysiology but also the full complement of her intellectual, spiritual, and psychological being. Of all the procedures done in the outpatient arena, the prolonged infertility laser laparoscopy is among the most physiologically rigorous. Furthermore, the patient often has significant postoperative abdominal discomfort, shoulder pain, and nausea and vomiting. In addition, if the procedure has been replete with extensive peritoneal ablation, the patient may experience severe malaise in the recovery phase. In our surgery center, we have performed over 1000 general anesthetics for hysteroscopy and laser laparoscopy, and this clinical experience serves as the springboard for the ensuing chapter.

M. J. Carroll Collins: Sereno Surgery Center, Los Gatos, California 95032.

S. H. Jackson: Department of Anesthesiology, Good Samaritan Hospital of Santa Clara Valley, San Jose, California 95124.

PREOPERATIVE MANAGEMENT

Perhaps the single most important technique that has been helpful in allaying anxiety preoperatively is the preoperative phone call by the anesthesiologist. In this humanistically-oriented interview, the anesthesiologist and patient develop a dialogue during which the patient's anxieties are addressed, medical problems are chronicled, and the patient is informed about her anticipated perioperative experience in detail (1). During the phone interaction, the patient is informed about the admitting routine, induction of anesthesia, emergence from anesthesia, and the nature of the postoperative course. We believe that the patient who understands that she may experience postoperative abdominal discomfort, shoulder pain, and nausea and vomiting does significantly better than the patient who is unaware of these potential side effects of surgery and anesthesia. A meaningful doctor–patient relationship developed in this manner can generate within the patient a strong sense of caring and trust, which can have powerful therapeutic and healing potential.

When possible, we arrange for the patient to take a long-acting histamine-2 blocking drug, either famotidine (40 mg) or rizantidine (150 mg), at bedtime. These drugs reduce acid secretion during the fasting phase and well into the day of surgery (2,3). Omeprazole (20 mg) at bedtime is an effective supplemental drug, as it is a gastric ATPase pump inhibitor that further reduces acid secretion (4). Metoclopramide (10 mg) with a sip of water 1 hr before the patient is expected to arrive at the surgery center will promote emptying of the stomach and simultaneously tone the gastroesophageal junction. The recent literature is replete with studies that have challenged the classical wisdom of 6–8 hr of preoperative fasting. There now is ample data to support shortening the period of preoperative fasting and to permit water and even clear liquid intake closer to the operative time (5). However, our practice remains that of adhering to the more traditional approach of "prolonged" fasting.

On admission to the surgery center, the patient is asked to read an information form, which reiterates many of the points made by the anesthesiologist in the preoperative telephone interview. The admitting nurse again prepares the patient as to how she is likely to feel postoperatively. Stress-reducing activities at this time include earphone music of the patient's choice, or meditation or self-hypnosis tapes, as well as a wide selection of reading materials.

The anesthesiologist then reviews any appropriate laboratory information and personally performs a limited physical examination on the patient while further enhancing the doctor–patient interaction. We have made the clinical observation that an increased incidence of temporomandibular joint (TMJ) dysfunction exists among infertility patients. This may be a physical reflection of the chronic stress associated with their infertility. These patients may be unable to open their mouths widely (4,6). This limited ability to open the mouth also may interfere with a more extensive inspection of the oropharynx for visualization of the soft palate, uvula, and tonsillar (faucial) pillars, an examination that helps predict the potential degree of difficulty of endotracheal intubation (4,7). However physical examination may help in determining the intraanesthetic reversible component, if any, of this functional limitation. Patients with TMJ dysfunction are more prone to experience postanesthetic TMJ pain following airway manipulation.

For those patients with a history of significant nausea and vomiting following a previous anesthetic experience, transdermal scopolamine patches have been successfully employed prophylactically when applied sufficiently in advance of scheduled surgery (8). In fact, when applied at bedtime, transdermal scopolamine can provide preoperative sedation and drying of oral secretions (anticholinergic effects), as well as assuring antiemetic serum levels. In our experience, these patches are particularly helpful for patients who give strong histories of motion sickness, and this is consistent with the fact that much postoperative nausea and vomiting is related to motion such as sitting up, moving out of bed, and ambulation (2). Because the risk for nausea and vomiting may be significantly greater during the 3 days preceding menstruation and the first 8 days of the cycle, it seems beneficial to schedule infertility surgery so as to avoid this period of time (9).

INTRAOPERATIVE MANAGEMENT

In many facilities, it is possible to arrange for the patient, who should be wearing comfortable facility clothing, to walk from the preoperative area into the operating room in the company of the circulating nurse. This increases the atmosphere of wellness surrounding the patient's surgical experience. The patient should be covered with warm blankets as she assumes the supine position on the operating table. If there is a history of back problems, the patient is placed in modified lithotomy stirrups prior to the induction of anesthesia. Monitors should include electrocardiograph, pulse oximeter, blood pressure cuff, precordial stethoscope, and end-tidal carbon dioxide and inhalational anesthetic concentration analyzer. Intravenous cannulation should be accomplished with a 20-gauge or larger catheter. However, in some situations, a 22-gauge catheter inserted into an antecubital vein can be used for induction and can be replaced at a later time under anesthesia with a larger catheter in a more distal vein.

Planning for every anesthetic regimen should include consideration of the parenteral administration of antiemetic drugs, such as droperidol, phenothiazines, metoclopramide, and even scopolamine if it has not been applied transdermally.

Following induction of anesthesia with propofol (which may be associated with a lower incidence of postoperative nausea and vomiting than the barbiturates) or barbiturate the patient is intubated, preferably with a nondepolarizing muscle relaxant, and a urinary drainage catheter is inserted. The patient's legs are placed in modified lithotomy stirrups fitted with additional gel-type padding. Peripheral nerve injuries are the most common of the serious complications following anesthesia. Ulnar nerve injury, brachial plexopathy, and lower extremity motor neuropathy may occur without an obvious mechanism but they are often attributed to presumed errors in intraoperative care (improper positioning and/or padding) or in judgment (excessively prolonged use of lithotomy position). Lower motor nerve neuropathies are most likely to be associated with the lithotomy position and may occur at a rate as high as 1 per 3600 (10). The risk factors for lower extremity motor neuropathy include being in the lithotomy position for four hours or longer, a body mass of less than 2 kg/m^2 (thin women), and a history of cigarette smoking within a month of the surgery. Diabetes mellitus with its predisposition to neuropathy and/or peripheral vascular disease may be another factor leading to the increased likelihood of peripheral nerve injury. Therefore, it is extremely important that the patient's legs be positioned carefully in the stirrups especially because common peroneal nerve injuries are a known sequela of prolonged procedures conducted in the lithotomy position. Similarly, proper positioning and padding of the upper extremities is essential for preventing nerve injuries at the level of the neck, shoulder, and elbow (11). Following intubation, the anesthesiologist should insert an orogastric sump tube to reduce the likelihood of the complication of gastric perforation by the surgeon, as well as to empty the stomach of any fluid and gas accumulated by the end of the anesthetic.

Immediately postintubation, it is advisable to note the peak inspiratory pressure and tidal volume so as to estimate pulmonary compliance. In this manner, acceptable ventilatory parameters can be established for when the patient is placed in Trendelenburg position while intraperitoneal carbon dioxide is being insufflated.

Hysteroscopy

Both high- and low-viscosity fluids may be employed for uterine distention and surgical visualization for operative hysteroscopy. Each medium possesses unique physiologic and biochemical properties and, in turn, carries its own potential for morbidity and even mortality (12). All of these fluids can be absorbed into the systemic circulation. The most important factors affecting the extent of absorption are the intrauterine distention pressures, the extent of resection and transection of vascular beds, and the duration of distention and surgical resection (13).

Dextran-70 (32%) in 10% glucose (Hyskon) is a high-viscosity fluid composed of dextrans (average molecular weight 70,000) that are slowly metabolized by the reticuloendothelial system and have an intravascular half-life measured in days. Its intravascular absorption increases intravascular volume most significantly by increasing plasma oncotic pressure. Dextran-70 (32%) expands blood volume by ten times its directly absorbed volume (14). Therefore, seemingly minor absorption effects a marked hypervolemia and the potential for circulatory overload. In fact, more than 500 ml of intrauterine instillation, a volume considered to predispose to pulmonary edema (14,15), is not uncommon with the resection of intrauterine synechiae and submucous leiomyomata. Such procedures mandate both meticulous measurement of the volume instilled and a preoperative agreement between surgeon and anesthesiologist as to the maximal acceptable absorbed volume before ceasing the hysteroscopy. Clearly, judicious restriction of intravenous fluids is an appropriate adjuvant to circulatory management.

These precautions notwithstanding, anticipatory vigilance for the signs of pulmonary edema—and its precursor, intravascular overload—must be maintained and include (a) inspiratory rales and rhonchi, especially in the dependent lung fields; (b) decreasing arterial oxygen saturation with an unchanged inspiratory concentration of oxygen; (c) decreasing lung compliance; (d) increasing end-tidal carbon dioxide tension (late occurrence); (e) frothy sputum. Treatment of this hyperoncotic-hypervolemic pulmonary edema includes (a) 100% inspired concentration of oxygen; (b) positive pressure ventilation or adding positive end-expiratory pressure to preexisting positive pressure ventilation; (c) discontinuation of dextran-70 (32%) instillation and its evacuation from the uterine cavity; (d) fluid restriction; (e) elimination of the Trendelenburg and lithotomy positions and even providing a reverse Trendelenburg posture; (f) administration of diuretics, such as furosemide or ethacrynic acid, or, in more extreme or poorly responsive situations, bumetidine or chlorothiazide; (g) administration of vasodilator drugs, such as hydralazine, nitroprusside, or nitroglycerine; (h) judicious use of inotropes with vasodilator properties, such as dopamine or dobutamine. Pulmonary edema may manifest itself upon emergence from anesthesia when positive pressure ventilation is terminated, vasodilatory effects of anesthetic drugs and techniques are dissipated, and vasoconstriction is induced by pain, anxiety, and the hypothermia developed during anesthesia.

Thirty-two percent dextran-70 also has been associated with the development of coagulopathies, anaphylactic shock, noncardiogenic pulmonary edema, hyperglycemia, and oliguria.

The low-viscosity fluids most commonly used for operative hysteroscopy are either 1.5% glycine (a rapidly metabolized amino acid) or a premixture of 2.7% sorbitol–0.54% mannitol (the former is rapidly biodegraded to fructose and glucose, the latter being a largely inert osmotic diuretic that is rapidly excreted unchanged). Both solutions are nonelectrolytic; glycine is slightly hypoosmolar (200 Mosml/L) and inexpensive while the alditol isomer mixture is more hypoosmolar (178 Mosml/L), and more costly. A vast literature exists for the use of both fluids for transurethral prostate resection (TURP). During or immediately after this procedure a small percentage of patients exhibit overt signs of increased circulatory volume and dilution of serum electrolytes (16). What is pertinent is that the pathophysiologic sequelae of the intravascular absorption of instillates also are occasionally encountered during and after hysteroscopic surgery: hypervolemia, hypoosmolemia, and hyponatremia (17). This pathophysiologic state can be worsened by the use of vasopressin to control surgical bleeding. This variant of water intoxication can result in pulmonary edema, the diagnosis and treatment of which are discussed above for high-viscosity fluids. However, menstruant women have been shown to be at high risk for death or brain damage (seizures, cerebral edema, and cerebral herniation) from even modest hyponatremia and, perhaps even more importantly, hypoosmolemia (18). Five percent mannitol is an alternate low-viscosity instillate that may have a wider margin of safety because it is isoosmolar (278 Mosml/L) (19). In fact, mannitol is commonly administered intravenously during neuroanesthesia, often in volumes and concentrations greater

TABLE 1. *Early and later signs and symptoms of hyponatremic syndrome*

Early
Bradycardia
Systolic and diastolic hypertension
Later
Hypotension
Cyanosis/dyspnea
Cardiac dysrhythmia
Restlessness
Mental confusion
Agitation
Lethargy
Nausea and vomiting
Headache
Visual disturbances
Skeletal muscle twitching or tremors
Seizure
Coma

than those encountered in operative hysteroscopy, and without pathophysiologic sequelae. Excessive intravascular absorption of instilled 5% mannitol causes hyponatremia, but serum osmolarity does not change. Furthermore, mannitol initiates a diuresis that self-corrects volume overload.

The earliest signs of this potentially lethal, operative hysteroscopy intravascular absorption (OHIA) syndrome (20) are bradycardia with systolic and diastolic hypertension (Table 1). Following a variable latency period, these are succeeded by hypotension, cyanosis, cardiac dysrhythmias, seizures, and coma. Because the patient receiving general anesthesia does not readily or reliably manifest signs of cerebral edema and dysfunction, it might be advantageous—as with TURP—to employ regional anesthesia, when not contraindicated or refused, for extensive operative hysteroscopy without laparoscopy. A regionally anesthetized, awake or lightly sedated patient may show *precursor* symptoms and signs, such as restlessness, mental confusion, agitation, lethargy, nausea, vomiting, headache, visual disturbances (especially with glycine), skeletal muscle twitching or tremors, and dyspnea. These portend impending cardiac dysrhythmias, cardiovascular collapse, seizures, or other advanced clinical manifestations of cerebral dysfunction and injury. Detection of precursor symptoms or signs should prompt cessation of surgery and evacuation of instillate until clinical and laboratory evaluation determines the extent, if any, of pathophysiologic alterations related to the low-viscosity fluids.

Hyponatremia must be cautiously and judiciously corrected (21). Patients under regional anesthesia with serum sodium concentrations below 125 meq/L who are not symptomatic (that is, there are no precursor clinical manifestations) usually do well clinically when treated with water restriction and/or intravenous administration of normal saline while diuresis occurs spontaneously. However, a loop diuretic will hasten the mobilization of free water. The regionally-anesthetized patient with a sodium level below 120 meq/L who is symptomatic certainly should be treated with hypertonic saline and a pharmacologically-induced diuresis. Electrocardiographic changes—widened QRS complexes as well as ST segment alterations—usually follow when the serum concentration of sodium falls to 115 meq/L. Visual symptoms may appear in the 102–115 meq/L range although visual changes independently may be caused by hyperglycinemia. Seizures, coma, and cardiac arrest are inevitable when serum sodium falls below 102 meq/L.

Because hysteroscopic surgery is most commonly performed under general anesthesia, the majority of warning signals for hyponatremia seen with regional anesthesia are not available to the anesthesiologist. Indeed, the diagnosis of morbid hyponatremia may be subsequent to a catastrophic intraanesthetic or early postanesthetic event, or it may arise in the differential diagnosis of an unexplained failure to emerge from general anesthesia or prolonged effect of neuromuscular blocking drugs. To mitigate against this increased risk for delayed recognition of the hyponatremic syndrome in patients under general anesthesia, an ongoing tabulation of the input and output of low-viscosity instillates and a predetermined time schedule for blood sampling for rapid determination of serum sodium concentration should be established in selected cases. Hyponatremia indicates fluid absorption but does not necessarily correlate with the volume absorbed. Ethanol 1% added to instillates as a biological marker has been used to estimate fluid absorption by measuring the ethanol content of end-tidal breath during TURP procedures (22), this technique has been successfully extended to operative hysteroscopy. When a patient under general anesthesia is found to have a serum sodium level less than 125 meq/L, termination of surgery and withdrawal of instillate should be immediate, and therapy should be started with intravenous saline while initiating a diuresis with furosemide or ethacrynic acid.

One must guard against a false sense of security engendered by the sympathetic blockade of a regional anesthesia and its vasodilatation with enhanced venous capacitance: as the block wears off, borderline hypervolemia may progress to circulatory overload. The same precaution applies to the termination of a general anesthetic's vasodilatation. The onset of postoperative pain and the inevitable hypothermia upon emergence from any form of anesthesia also provide the stimulus for vasoconstrictor activity.

It has been controversially stated—and inadequately documented—that too rapid correction of hyponatremia may cause the syndrome of central pontine myelinosis (a cerebral demyelinating process), the neurologic sequelae of which may involve severe morbidity or even mortality (21). In light of this controversy, the therapy for clinically significant hyponatremia should be cautious use of hypertonic saline at a rate of infusion which should not exceed 100 ml/hr and should not cause the serum sodium concentration to increase at a rate exceeding 2 meq/L/hr until the level is greater than 125 meq/L. However, the therapeutic goal should not exceed 135 meq/L. Acute hypokalemia may be a concomitant finding and may itself require judicious correction.

Glycine itself, when metabolized, may result in a hyperammonemia, which in turn may cause an encephalopathy. Glycine also is metabolized to oxalate, and acute renal crystal and stone formation can occur.

Ringer's lactate, its variants containing gluconate and acetate in place of lactate, and isotonic saline are alternative low-viscosity fluids used for diagnostic hysteroscopy. Their systemic absorption is the equivalent of an intravenous infusion and can progress to pulmonary edema.

Laparoscopy

For laparoscopy the patient is placed in Trendelenberg position and carbon dioxide is insufflated into the peritoneal cavity. Systemic absorption of carbon dioxide from the peritoneal surface leads to hypercarbia relative to preinsufflation levels if ventilation is not adjusted. The capnogram reflects any progressive hypercarbia and serves as a guide to altering the ventilatory parameters so as to maintain normocarbia. Capnography also rapidly detects any significant entry of carbon dioxide into the systemic circulation through surgically induced vascular rents (23). The increased intraabdominal pressure from the insufflate effects a reduction of the functional residual capacity, which leads to atelectasis and potential hypoxemia, both of which are countered by positive pressure ventilation and an appropriate inspired concentration of oxygen. The pulse oximeter monitors the outcome of these opposing physiologic forces. Positive inspiratory pressure should be measured and recorded prior to the establishment of the Trendelenburg position, and it remains an important parameter to monitor throughout the case. The respiratory frequency is adjusted so as to keep the positive inspiratory pressure within an acceptable range—preferrably less than 20–25 torr—while maintaining adequate respiratory gas exchange. The use of laryngeal mask airway is contraindicated because of the risk for regurgitation and aspiration during laparoscopic procedures.

Subcutaneous emphysema, pneumomediastinum, pneumopericardium and pneumothorax are complications that may stem from the barotrauma of positive pressure ventilation, particularly in the Trendelenberg position. However, these complications also can be surgically induced either through surgical technique or through equipment mismanagement (23–28).

Subcutaneous emphysema and pneumomediastinum are the more commonly encountered of these complications, and usually run a benign clinical course with conservative therapy. Subcutaneous emphysema is nonetheless quite disconcerting to the patient and family as well as to the physician despite its relatively rapid resolution. Moreover, it is mandatory to rule out any accompanying pneumothorax or pneumopericardium, and this is accomplished by both physical examination and radiographic evaluation. In over 1000 cases we have observed several subcutaneous emphysemas, but the only pneumothorax occurred in a patient with recurrent pneumothoraces secondary to pleural endometriosis.

Tension pneumothorax, a not uncommon complication of laparoscopy, is potentially life threatening. Its diagnosis in the anesthetized patient is prompted by decreased blood pressure, increased positive inspiratory pressure with decreased lung compliance, decreased oxygen saturation, decreased breath sounds over the affected lung (or lungs), and evidence for diminished carbon dioxide elimination. It can progress very rapidly to cardiovascular collapse. Diagnostic confirmation may be obtained by needle aspiration of the anterior pleural space. Treatment involves (a) pleural cavity decompression by needle, catheter, or chest tube as is clinically indicated; (b) discontinuance of nitrous oxide; (c) administration of 100% inspired oxygen concentration by positive pressure ventilation; and (d) cessation of surgery and evacuation of the insufflate from the peritoneal cavity. Not all pneumothoraces are immediately life threatening, and clinical judgment must be exercised in determining the urgency and extent of aggressive treatment. X-ray confirmation of the diagnosis and/or effectiveness of therapy is obtained at the appropriate time during the care of the patient.

Fortunately, pneumopericardium is a very rarely encountered complication of laparoscopy, but it leads to cardiovascular collapse by causing cardiac tamponade. The treatment of this entity is beyond the scope of this chapter.

It has been suggested that careful management of ventilatory parameters might reduce the incidence of complications related to barotrauma during anesthesia. As mentioned previously, one should consider employing smaller tidal volumes and faster respiratory rates in an attempt to minimize inspiratory pressures. The utilization of nondepolarizing muscle relaxants to reduce peak positive inspiratory pressures should be an integral part of any anesthetic technique mitigating against barotrauma. These ventilatory objectives are more difficult to accomplish in obese patients and in those with restrictive or obstructive pulmonary impairment. Frequent variations in the intraabdominal pressure secondary to suctioning of the plume by the surgeon or alterations of insufflation settings necessitate continuous vigilance directed to all ventilatory parameters.

Use of a peripheral nerve stimulator to monitor neuromuscular blockade is helpful in determining appropriate doses of muscle relaxants. Adequate abdominal muscle relaxation also facilitates the surgeon's ability to keep the abdominal viscera out of the pelvis during the surgery. Increases in the degree of Trendelenburg position also may be necessary to keep the bowel out of the pelvis and away from the potentially harmful beam of the laser.

Numerous anesthetic drug combinations and techniques have been successfully utilized for maintenance of patients undergoing laser laparoscopy. The technique must be individualized for each patient and remains under the discretion of the anesthesiologist. One should be cognizant of the fact that the concentration of nitrous oxide in the peritoneal cavity can reach a level that can support combustion of bowel gases (methane and hydrogen) should there be an unintentional bowel perforation (28).

Because there is a high incidence of nausea following laparoscopic procedures, it is advisable to hydrate these patients so that they have a fluid and electrolyte reserve in the event they are unable to drink in the early postoperative period. The second liter of fluid probably should contain dextrose as prophylaxis against any tendency toward hypoglycemia (29). The Foley catheter collection can provide a useful monitor of hydration.

The data correlating prolonged duration in the lithotomy position with the development of lower extremity motor neuropathy (10) supports our policy that two hours after the patient's legs have been placed in padded stirrups, the circulating nurse should remove each lower extremity from its stirrup and massage it before replacing it in the stirrup. These maneuvers are repeated at 1-hr intervals during the remainder of the surgical procedure. Since we instituted this regimen, we have detected no incidents of common peroneal nerve injury. Prior to the institution of this policy, we had experienced two cases in which transient peroneal nerve palsies followed prolonged procedures. These manipulations also could have beneficial effects in terms of deep vein thrombosis prophylaxis. Others have advocated the use of elastic stockings, sequential compression stockings, and even low-dose heparin prophylaxis for patients at risk for deep vein thrombosis.

As discussed earlier, attempted maintenance of euthermia is another important goal. A heating pad under the patient is used during surgery, and exposed skin is covered to prevent heat loss. All surgical irrigating fluids and intravenous fluids should be warmed to body temperature. Furthermore, inspiratory gases should be inexpensively humidified with passive heat and moisture exchangers so as to minimize the loss of heat via the respiratory tract. Only 10% of the total loss of body heat is through ventilation (30).

At the end of surgery, the surgeon should evacuate as much CO_2 as possible from the abdominal cavity. This maneuver might minimize the incidence or duration of postoperative, referred shoulder pain.

POSTOPERATIVE PERIOD

In the postanesthesia recovery unit, the patients are covered with inexpensive passive insulators such as warm blankets (31); supplemental oxygen is administered; and as soon as the patient is conscious, she is encouraged to resume the upright position gradually. After she tolerates the sitting position she is transferred to a reclining chair, which in turn is gradually brought to the upright position. Most patients who experience nausea do so when they are moved: with elevation of the head of the bed, with transfer from bed to chair, or when voiding or dressing themselves (2). Delay of alimentation prevents some nausea and vomiting. Administration of intravenous fluids can preclude the perceived necessity for early alimentation. Certainly, in the well-hydrated patient there is no reason to demand alimentation as a criterion for discharge from the facility.

There are, of course, numerous antiemetic regimens available for treatment of postoperative nausea. It may be that specific drug combinations are more effective for certain patients, but the individualization of this pharmacology remains more of an art than a science. We have found that a combination of 10 mg metoclopramide and 5–10 mg ephedrine IV frequently is effective and does not make patients sleepier, a point of particular concern in the outpatient setting. Droperidol has a penchant for increasing drowsiness and causing an occasional dysphoric reaction, so it is avoided in the recovery room. Promethazine also will induce drowsiness, but it can be a valuable drug when dispensed in the rectal suppository form, which in appropriate doses can serve as an effective agent for managing postdischarge (home) nausea and vomiting.

Ondansetron, a 5-hydroxytryptamine antagonist, may possess some distinct advantages—greater antiemetic efficacy and absence of sedative and dysphoric reactions—over the current armamentarium of antiemetic drugs (32). However, ondansetron may be most useful when developed prior to induction of anesthesia in a prophylactic manner in order to prevent or significantly reduce postoperative nausea and vomiting (33,34). In doses of 4-8 mg IV ondansetron may be effective in this respect. Because of its comparatively high cost, ondansetron might most be indicated in patients with a strong positive history for postoperativeness nausea and emesis and/or motion sickness. However, when one considers its being a prophylactic as well as therapeutic agent devoid of sedative action, it may be cost effective in an expanded context as it potentially shortens recovery room (discharge) time. Granisetron is a newer 5-hydroxytryptamine agonist that has yet to be studied as extensively as ondansetron.

Postoperative analgesia must be addressed, and a wide variety of narcotic drugs are available as are an increasing array of nonsteroidal antiinflammatory drugs (NSAIDs) (35). Ketorolac is one such intramuscular nonopioid with analgesic effects equivalent to those of morphine and meperidine (36). We anticipate that its success will stimulate the use of other NSAIDs postoperatively. The addition of intramuscular ketorolac as a supplemental analgesic to therapeutic doses of narcotics can result in unmasking the respiratory depressant effect of the narcotics. Moreover, ketorolac possesses a mild sedative effect.

Ketorolac shares the risks of the other NSAIDs. Gastropathy, postoperative hemorrhage, and renal toxicity have been reported even following brief courses of postoperative ketorolac therapy. Ketorolac is contraindicated in any patient with active peptic ulcer disease, recent gastrointestinal bleeding or performation, and with a history of peptic ulcer disease or gastrointestinal hemorrhage. The incidence and severity of gastrointestinal complications increases in a dose- and time-dependent manner. The concurrent administration of misoprostol, a prostaglandin E_1 analog, to protect against the development of NSAID-induced gastropathy, may find increasing acceptance (37,38). Histamine-2 blockers and omeprazole have been effective for duodenal ulcer prophylaxis.

Ketorolac's predisposition to bleeding related to platelet dysfunction should be a precaution against its use postoperatively when hemostasis of the surgical site remains a concern.

Ketorolac contraindicated for use in patients with advanced renal dysfunction and in those at risk for renal failure due to volume depletion, as in the chronically diuresed, salt-restricted patient. Ketorolac can precipitate renal failure in patients with minimally impaired—or even normal—renal function. The recommended initial and total daily dose of ketorolac has recently been reduced by the manufacturer, especially for patients greater than 65 years of age, renally impaired, and less than 50 kg body weight.

Discharge instructions must address the issues of postoperative pain, nausea and vomiting, voiding, ambulation, and diet. Follow-up phone interviews with patients are essential elements of quality care for both the patients and the surgical facility.

CONCLUSIONS

We believe that the foregoing text offers a rational approach to the administration of anesthesia for hysteroscopic and laparoscopic infertility procedures. Patients can do very well if the anesthesiologist and operating team are attentive to details. Constant vigilance is mandatory. As an integral part of the infertility team, the anesthesiologist can derive a genuine sense of accomplishment and fulfillment from having helped the patient through this major life experience.

REFERENCES

1. Jackson S. Humanism and anesthesia safety. *Curr Rev Clin Anesth* 1988;8:194–199.
2. Berry F. Postoperative vomiting—causes and treatment. *Curr Rev Clin Anesth* 1991;11:89–96.
3. Ostheimer G. Pulmonary acid aspiration. II. Prevention of complications. *J Drug Dev* 1989;2(Suppl):18–32.
4. Jackson S, Lampe G, Silcox D. Anesthetic considerations. In: Oloff L, ed. *Musculoskeletal disorders of the lower extremity.* Philadelphia: WB Saunders; 1992.
5. McKinley A, James R, Mims G. NPO after midnight before elective surgery is no longer common practice for the majority of anesthesiologists. *Amer J Anesthesiology* 1995;22:88–92.
6. Block C, Brechner V. Unusual problems in airway management. II. The influence of the temporomandibular joint, the mandible, and associated structures on endotracheal intubation. *Anesth Analg* 1971;50:114–122.
7. Mallampati S, Gatt S, Gugino L, et al. A clinical sign to predict difficult tracheal intubation: a prospective study. *Canad Anesth Soc J* 1985;32:429–434.
8. Jackson SH, Schmitt L, McGuire J, Hall MV. Transdermal scopolamine as a preanesthetic drug and postoperative antinauseant and antiemetic. *Anesthesiology* 1982;57:A330.
9. Beattie W, Lindblad T, Buckley D, et al. Menstruation increases the risk of nausea and vomiting after laparoscopy. A prospective randomized study. *Anesthesiology* 1993;78:272–276.
10. Warner M, Martin J, Schroeder D, et al. Lower-extremity motor neuropathy associated with surgery performed on patients in a lithotomy position. *Anesthesiology* 1994;81:6–12.
11. Stoelting R. Postoperative ulnar nerve palsy—is it a preventable complication? *Anesth Analg* 1993;76:7–9.
12. Witz C, Silverberg K, Burns W, et al. Complications associated with the absorption of hysteroscopic fluid media. *Fertil Steril* 1993;60:745–756.
13. Liu W, Wong K: Anesthesia for genitourinary surgery. In: Barash P, Cullen B, Stoelting R, eds. *Clinical anesthesia.* Philadelphia: JB Lippincott; 1992:1157–1168.
14. Mangar D, Gerson J, Constantine R, et al. Pulmonary edema and coagulopathy due to Hyskon (32% Dextran-70) administration. *Anesth Analg* 1989;68:686–687.
15. Golan A, Seidner M, Bahar M, et al. High output left ventricular failure after dextran use in an operative hysteroscopy. *Fertil Steril* 1990;54:939–941.
16. Mebust W, Holtgrewe H, Crockett A, et al. Transurethral prostatectomy—immediate and postoperative complications: a cooperative study of 13 participating institutions evaluating 3885 patients. *J Urol* 1989;141:243–247.
17. Baggish M, Brill A, Rosensweig B, et al. Fatal acute glycine and sorbitol toxicity during operative hysteroscopy. *J Gynecol Surg* 1993;9:137–143.
18. Arieff A, Ayas J. Endometrial ablation complicated by fatal hyponatremic encephalopathy. *JAMA* 1993;270:1230–1232.
19. Allgen LG, Norlen H, Lolmert T, et al. Absorption and elimination of mannitol solution when used as an isotonic irrigating agent in connection with transurethral resection of the prostrate. *Scand J Urol Nephrol* 1987;21:177–184.
20. Jackson S, Lampe G. Operative hysteroscopy intravascular absorption syndrome. *West J Med* 1994;162:53–54.
21. Jackson S. Hereditary hepatic porphyrias. In: Katz J, Benamof J, Kadis L, eds. *Anesthesia and uncommon disease.* Philadelphia: WB Saunders; 1990:84–99.
22. Hahn RG. Monitoring of TURP with ethanol. *Lancet* 1991;338: 1602.
23. McGrath B, Zimmerman J, Williams J, et al. Carbon dioxide embolism treated with hyperbaric oxygen. *Can J Anaesth* 1989;36: 586–589.
24. Kalhan S, Reaney J, Collins R. Pneumomediastinum and subcutaneous emphysema during laparoscopy. *Cleveland Clin J Med* 1990;57:639–642.
25. Shah P, Ramakantan R: Pneumoperitoneum and pneumomediastinum: unusual complications of laparoscopy. *J Postgrad Med* 1990;36:31–32.
26. Bard P, Chen L. Subcutaneous emphysema associated with laparoscopy. *Anesth Analg* 1990;71:101–102.
27. Whiston P, Eggers K, Morris R, et al. Tension pneumothorax during laparoscopic cholecystectomy. *Br J Surg* 1991;78:1325.

28. Neuman G, Sidebotham G, Negolanu E, et al. Laparoscopy explosion hazards with nitrous oxide. *Anesthesiology* 1993;78:875–879.
29. Jackson S, Brill J. Hypoglycemia. In: Katz J, Benumof J, Kadis L, eds. *Anesthesia and uncommon diseases.* Philadelphia: WB Saunders; 1990:30–43.
30. Bickler P, Sessler D. Airway humidification. *Anesth Analg* 1990;71:415–418.
31. Sessler D, McGuire J, Sessler A. Perioperative thermal insulation. *Anesthesiology* 1991;74:875–879.
32. Scuderi P, Wetchler B, Sung Y-F, et al. Treatment of postoperative nausea and vomiting after outpatient surgery with the 5-HT_3 antagonist ondasetron. *Anesthesiology* 1993;78:15–20.
33. McKenzie R, Kovac A, O'Connor T, et al. Comparison of ondansetron versus placebo to prevent postoperative nausea and vomiting in women undergoing ambulatory gynecologic surgery. *Anesthesiology* 1993;78:21–28.
34. Khalil S, Kataria B, Peearson K, et al. Ondansetron prevents postoperative nausea and vomiting in women outpatients. *Anesth Analg* 1994;79:845–851.
35. Dahl J, Kehlet H. Non-steroidal anti-inflammatory drugs: rationale for use in severe postoperative pain. *Br J Anaesth* 1991;66: 703–712.
36. Oosterlinck W, Philip N, Charig C, et al. A double-blind single dose comparison of intramuscular ketorolac tromethamine and pethidine in the treatment of renal colic. *J Clin Pharmacol* 1990;30:336–341.
37. Roth S, Fries J, Aladi I, et al. Prophylaxis of nonsteroidal antiinflammatory drug gastropathy: a clinical opinion. *J Rheumatol* 1991;18:956–957.
38. Gabriel S. Is misoprostol prophylaxis indicated for NSAID induced adverse gastrointestinal events? An epidemiologic opinion. *J Rheumatol* 1991;18:957–961.

Endoscopic Management of Gynecologic Disease,
edited by G.D. Adamson and D.C. Martin.
Lippincott-Raven Publishers, Philadelphia © 1996.

CHAPTER 36

Visual Documentation in Endoscopy

Joseph S. Sanfilippo and John M. Leventhal

We have indeed come a long way from first recording the "written word." The capability to take digital video camera equipment to the moon represents one such hallmark in the technological advances that have directly impacted operative endoscopic surgical procedures.

New advances in the arena of video documentation include magnetic monomedia, frame grabbing, laser disk technology, archiving and retrieval, and three-dimensional endoscopy. It is the objective of this chapter to explore the technological advances in photographic and electronic imaging as applied to the documentation of pelviscopic surgical procedures. The following should provide an orderly sequence for the clinician to evaluate video equipment and to discern the most appropriate armamentarium for specific endoscopic surgical procedures.

METHODS OF DOCUMENTATION

Methods of documentation are as follows:

Cerebral
Written
Drawings
Diagram(s)
Photography

Perhaps the most obvious is cerebral. The human memory—while not always reliable with the passage of time—literally sets the stage for exquisite imaging and recording of immediate and past events. The written documentation allows for a permanent record and reflects the knowledge and know-how of the operating surgeon. Theoretically, the written documentation is always available and certainly is a cost-effective means of documentation (1).

Drawing material is another means of facilitating communication with respect to documentation. Three-dimensional effects can be suggested and cross-sections can be drawn.

Diagramming is an often used technique with laparoscopic surgical procedures. Although diagrams primarily are two-dimensional, they are an effective means of recording.

High-quality still and cine photographic imaging—in the form of still prints, slides, and videotapes—continues as state-of-the-art documentation for the permanent record (2). An instant hard copy documentation that complements the operative report lends further elucidation of the exact intraoperative findings, the procedure performed, and the potential benefits of the procedure.

VISUAL IMAGING

Ideally, video imaging and documentation is supplemented by audio recording on the same tape. This procedure allows communication of the surgeon's interpretation(s) of what is seen, and it greatly assists the subsequent viewer in understanding the original findings. Among the numerous uses for the recorded video image are:

1. Patient information and education
2. Review by the health care team
3. Communication with referring and other physicians
4. Documentation for the patient record
5. Follow-up review

All imaging requires the recording on light-sensitive medium of an observed image. The medium may be directly sensitive to light, e.g., silver halide film, or it may be influenced secondarily by magnetic fields that, in

J. S. Sanfilippo: Department of Obstetrics and Gynecology, University of Louisville School of Medicine, Louisville, Kentucky 40292.

J. M. Leventhal: Department of Obstetrics and Gynecology, Harvard Medical School, Boston, Massachusetts 02115.

turn, provide dimension by signals, the value of which is determined by light, e.g., digital disks and laser disks. The degree of sensitivity of the medium to light in any documentation system depends greatly on the type of recording equipment used. Usually it is necessary to provide more light for photographic recording than for electronic imaging; thus, even very fast film usually is not as sensitive as the electronic light sensors of a microprocessor chip. Nevertheless, the desired result of every recording is an image reproduced in a manner that renders it recognizable to the eye and that accurately represents the original object of observation. There must be sufficient light available to the documentation system to achieve intelligible imaging.

Surgeons can look forward to the use of miniature electronic cameras, which are expected to be reasonably cost-effective. Indeed, the combination of high-powered light sources and increased sensitivity of chip cameras allows the surgeon adequate resolution of the video image to permit the undertaking of appropriate surgical procedures. Recording of the procedure is an integral part of the video capabilities. A video printer allows a still picture to be obtained instantaneously for the patient's record and complements the documentation (3).

Appropriate light sources are mandatory for proper resolution and illumination of the subject material. The lens system or optical axis through which the light travels is a critical component of the camera laparoscope video system. The optical characteristics of the axis are subject to a host of factors that may directly influence image quality.

Sufficient light for useful documentation depends on four variables: the sensitivity of the recording system, the light transmission efficiency of the lens system used with the recording equipment, the illuminating power (usually expressed in lumens) of the light source, and the size of the exposed image.

Sensitivity of the Recording System

Laparoscopic still photography primarily involves the use of color slide film, which is balanced for electronic flash. Film specified for daylight use, which emphasizes the blue light spectrum and is balanced for color temperatures between 5000 K and 6100 K, should be used (3). As a rule, the film should be stored at $\leq$13°C and should be removed from the refrigerator 1 hr before its use. Ideally, the film should be processed as quickly as possible after completion of the photographic task. Film sensitivity is designated by the ASA (American Standards Association), DIN (German equivalent), or ISO (comparable to ASA) numbers. In general, laparoscopic photography is best accomplished with ASA values of 200 or 400; if the illumination of the subject is low or if the desired area to be imaged is large, then ASA values of 800 or 1600 are preferable.

Light Transmission Efficiency of the Lens System

The quality of the lenses incorporated in the endoscopic lens bundle also are determinants of the amount of light passing through the system. The better the quality and precision of the lens crafting, the more light that is transmitted.

Illuminating Power of the Light Source

Illuminating power is nothing more than brightness (expressed in *lumens*). The greater the number of lumens emitted, the greater the light available.

Size of the Exposed Image

Given the same amount of transmitted illumination, a small exposure area receives a greater quantity of light per surface area than does a larger one. Thus, from a practical standpoint, it takes less light to expose a single 16-mm movie frame correctly than it does to expose a 35-mm slide correctly.

Most camera systems are provided with adapters suitable to any laparoscope eyepiece (Fig. 1). In order to fill the entire film frame when using a 10-mm laparoscope, the operator must employ a lens with a focal length of 100–110 mm.

Separate flash generators or ring light sources also have been used with still photography. The camera should be a single-lens reflex system, preferably with a clear glass

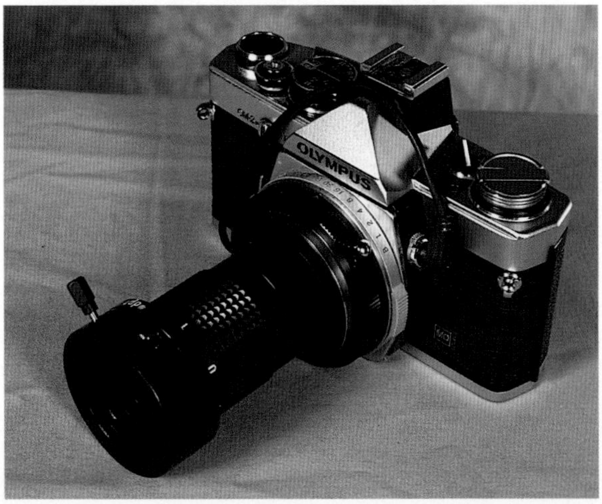

FIG. 1. A 35-mm photographic setup for endoscopy with a 110-mm lens. (Courtesy of Dr. Daniel C. Martin.)

screen (not ground glass focusing). A motor drive winder for film advancement and record data-back for superimposing appropriate information are most helpful.

ELECTRONIC IMAGING

Electronic imaging for the endoscopist involves the use of a video camera and monitor, videotape and video cassette recorder, and possibly other imaging devices such as optical laser recorders and frame grabbers. The use of a video camera as an aid in both performing and recording gynecologic laparoscopic and hysteroscopic procedures is increasingly common. Taking the surgeon's view from the endoscopic eyepiece and to the color video monitor has brought the previously hidden procedure into the immediate visual realm of the entire operating team. This results not only in better understanding by the team but in more efficient utilization of assistants and instruments.

VIDEO SYSTEMS

Half-inch VHS format tapes, with 200 lines of horizontal resolution, are the standard for high-quality video imaging. This soon may be replaced by Super VHS (400 lines) or 8-mm tapes of equal imaging quality. The $\frac{1}{2}$-in. Beta format, originally developed by Sony, is excellent in reproductive quality but is little used in medical imaging systems. If the surgeon's purpose is to produce a very high-quality tape for editing and formal presentation, the $\frac{3}{4}$-in. U-Matic tape probably remains the best for mastering. However super VHS requires smaller equipment than is associated with $\frac{3}{4}$-in. tape imaging and is of even better mastering quality. Its disadvantage, though, lies in its incompatibility with all other standard VHS equipment, including monitors, making it very poorly transportable to other areas for viewing. One-inch and the older two-inch broadcast-quality master videotapes generally are unavailable for operating room use and are not necessary. With duplication of tapes it should always be remembered that no generation of tape beyond the master, regardless of the size of the tape, will ever be of higher quality than the master tape itself. Each duplication has some loss in image quality.

VIDEO RECORDING

Formats

In recent years the ideal electronic format for video recording equipment has been the subject of numerous international meetings. Unfortunately a universal format has not yet emerged. In North America, parts of South America, Japan, and parts of Asia, the National Television Standards Committee (NTSC) format is in general use. In most of Europe and Australia, the Phase Alternation Line (PAL) format is the usual standard; the standard in France generally is Sequence de Coulers avec Memoire (SECAM). NTSC format provides 525 horizontal lines of digital information, and PAL and SECAM formats provide 625 horizontal lines. Other standards exist and newer ones are being studied throughout the world. Each format has its advantages and disadvantages with respect to the quality of the image recorded, and it is likely that no universal format will emerge for a number of years. From the practical standpoint, the surgeon must keep in mind that, should it be desired to show videotapes in Europe and in some parts of the Caribbean, it is necessary in most cases to have the NTSC tapes converted to PAL before leaving the United States. Facilities for conversion in Europe are scarce in all but the largest metropolitan areas. Until there is universal agreement on a standard, it is best to create tapes in the format in use at the desired place of showing.

Cameras

Although the vacuum tube video camera continues to provide (by the smallest of margins) the highest image resolution, it has been, for all practical purposes, completely replaced by the single, solid-state microprocessor chip camera for medical use, and by the three-chip camera for broadcast and some professional applications. Advances in solid-state camera technology have been rapid, and these cameras provide resolution densities almost indistinguishable from those of the larger, bulkier tube cameras. The solid-state camera has the advantages of being extremely small and light-weight (Figs. 2 and 3), which is ideal for endoscopy. There are two basic types

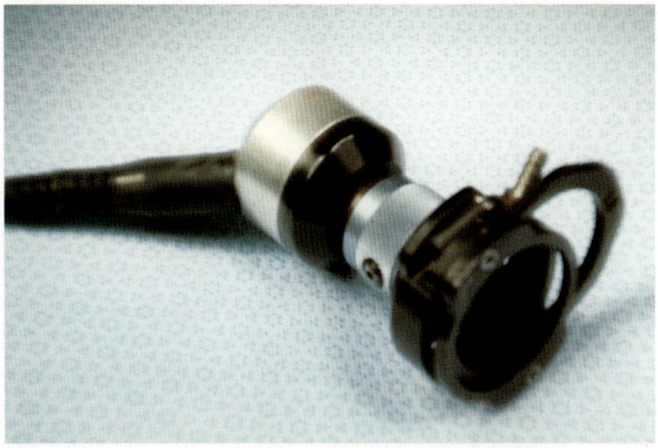

FIG. 2. Endoscopic CCD camera with the endoscopic adaptor. (Courtesy of Dr. Daniel C. Martin.)

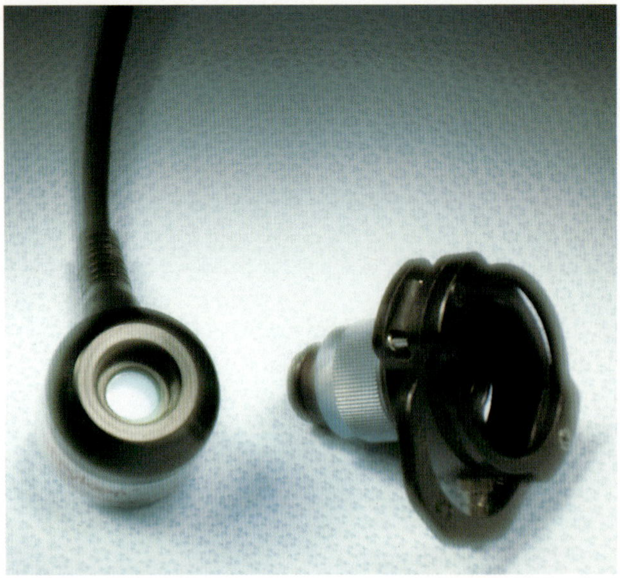

FIG. 3. Disassembled camera and adaptor. The CCD chip is seen within the camera head, which is attached to the camera cable. The endoscopic adaptor is to the right. (Courtesy of Dr. Daniel C. Martin.)

of microprocessors used in video cameras. They are the charge-coupled device (CCD) chip and the metal oxide semiconductor (MOS) diode chip. In general, the CCD chip is more sensitive but is capable of lower resolution than the MOS chip. Improvements aimed at correcting the deficiencies in each type of chip, however, have proceeded quickly. The addition of a negative charge to the MOS chip resulted in the negative MOS (NMOS) diode chip and in a marked increase in light sensitivity for this device. In its present form, the MOS or NMOS diode chip strikes a state-of-the-art compromise between sensitivity, dynamic range, noise, and lag (the effect of light contaminating the image before it can be moved from the diode to the storage register). Even greater advances in CCD technology include the hole accumulator diode (HAD) sensor and the frame interline transfer (FIT) CCD by Sony; the latter is an ingenious combination of the older frame transfer CCD and the interline transfer CCD. This technology provides some outstanding advantages over the conventional CCD or MOS sensor.

Both the CCD and MOS microprocessors are integrated circuit devices that utilize the principle of changes in electrical resistance of a metallic or silicon oxide in response to varying intensities of light striking its surface. The chip is divided into an array of *pic*ture *el*ements, called pixels, which are arranged along horizontal scanning lines. The NTSC format of 525 horizontal lines contains 700 pixels/line, whereas the PAL and SECAM formats of 625 horizontal lines contain 833 pixels/line; these values provide the usual aspect ratio of 4:3. Since one of the major measurements of resolution can be roughly calculated as the number of horizontal lines times the number of pixels per line, it can be seen that the PAL and SECAM formats have inherently better resolution. Light striking the pixel induces changes in resistance which are stored in the *image register.* The electronic circuitry controlling the microprocessor chip allows for a rapid sequential sweeping of the information stored in the image register to temporary storage in the *storage register,* thereby freeing the image elements (pixels) for the next fragment of light stimulation. The rate at which this occurs is the frame rate and is measured in images per second. The frame rate for NTSC is 30 and that for PAL and SECAM is 25.

The solid-state camera used in endoscopy is lightweight (2–6 oz.), can be sterilized by immersion, and has many features that make both monitoring and recording simple and of high quality. For the physician contemplating the purchase of a video system in today's market, desirable features for a modern video camera are as follows:

1. Horizontal resolution of at least 610 lines
2. Automatic light intensity control
3. Simple one-hand focusing at camera head
4. Automatic white balancing
5. Recorder control at the camera head
6. NTSC format (PAL in Europe)

Recording Devices and Storage Media

The standard for video recording media has long been analog magnetic videotape. Videotape remains the most widely used medium, primarily because of its low cost and its compatibility with the vast majority of video equipment. However, technology never stands still, and video recording has moved significantly into the digital age, primarily to accommodate the use of the computer for image enhancement and data incorporation. The microprocessor chip camera produces a digital signal which, in order to be displayed on most commonly used monitors, must be converted to an analog signal. This digital-to-analog (D-A) conversion introduces an additional step in image processing, which results in more electronics and some loss in image quality. Recently, digital monitors that obviate the need for conversion have become available, but they represent significant replacement cost for the analog systems now in use and still do not relieve the user of the disadvantages of magnetic storage media (i.e., videotape).

The inconveniences inherent in magnetic tape are those of storage and the time required for specific image access. The storage of VHS videocassettes after 1 or 2 years of surgery becomes a significant space problem. Spooling back and forth in a videotape to find a specific part of a procedure is an annoyance with which all of us are all too familiar. These drawbacks are obviated with the optical laser disk. The optical disk uses the digital output of the microprocessor chip to control a laser beam, which records by engraving microimpressions on the surface of the disk. The density (capacity for recorded data) of this media is many orders of magnitude greater than that available on magnetic tape. The access time for the recovery of digital data is measured in microseconds. Disks with densities of hundreds of gigabytes are commercially available; they allow for very compact storage and make virtually instant image access a reality. The archiving of video data in digital format allows for the marriage of video imaging to many of the potential applications of the computer, making possible real-time annotation, image manipulation, and virtually instant access. Whole segments of video imaging can be archived on a single disk and, with the application of data compression technology, many videotape equivalents can be archived on a single disk. The optical laser disk is small (up to 13 in. in diameter) and almost indestructible with respect to physical abuse and magnetic influence. At present, its cost is still much more than that of videotape, and most optical disks can be written to only once, although erasable disk technology is already beyond the experimental stage. Unfortunately, the cost of replacement equipment, at a time when hospitals face financial obstacles, serves to slow the widespread introduction of this next generation of video technology into the medical marketplace. However, there is little doubt that the replacement of the 35-mm still image and the magnetic videotape by laser optical disks in the endoscopy operating room is just around the corner.

VIDEO COMMUNICATIONS

Laser energy is applied in a number of frequencies to video imaging. Solid-state lasers are used to encode digital signals and transmit them with virtually no energy loss in fiberoptic cables to distant locations where decoding back to digital information is accomplished. Digitization of 35-mm slides can allow for conventional telephone or satellite transmission to distant sites. It is now possible, for instance, to place 15,000 color slides in digital format on a single optical disk as files similar to those organized on a personal computer magnetic disk. They can be accessed and displayed instantaneously by such simple instruments as a microcomputer or a bar code reader, which identifies and calls up the file. Live video conferencing of laparoscopic procedures via satellite or land line link is a reality and will become far more common in the near future as satellite capacities increase and the uplink and downlink facilities become more numerous.

TECHNOLOGIC IMPROVEMENTS

Imaging

The rapidity with which imaging technology is changing has guaranteed that the future is no farther than tomorrow morning. Never has it been more so than in the field of endoscopy. We are on the verge of witnessing the complete replacement of the optical lens endoscope by the electronic endoscope with the camera chip embedded in the distal portion of the instrument. Very soon it will not even be *possible* for the surgeon to look through the endoscope. Image quality, even now approaching that of color film, will become almost identical to that previously reserved for direct visual observation through a system of lenses.

As three-dimensional imaging has already become a part of the radiologist's armamentarium, its introduction to endoscopy is probably not very far away. There are three systems in commercial use for three-dimensional viewing of imaged objects: holography, stereo pairing, and virtual reality or multiplanar display. Holography, although suitable for three-dimensional printing on two-dimensional surfaces or spatial projection, is extremely cumbersome and expensive and cannot at present accommodate real-time imaging. Virtual reality is a newer concept and provides the viewer with a projected object volume in space allowing for full three-dimensional viewing. Since it requires that the dimen-

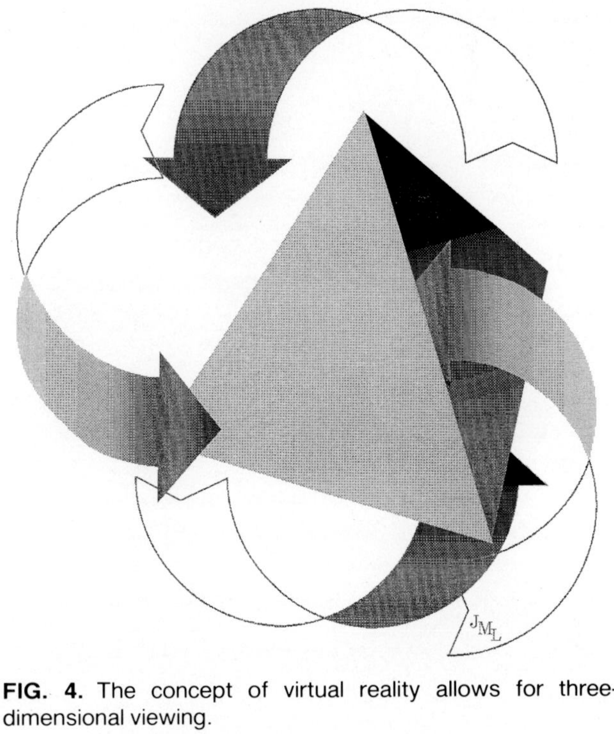

FIG. 4. The concept of virtual reality allows for three-dimensional viewing.

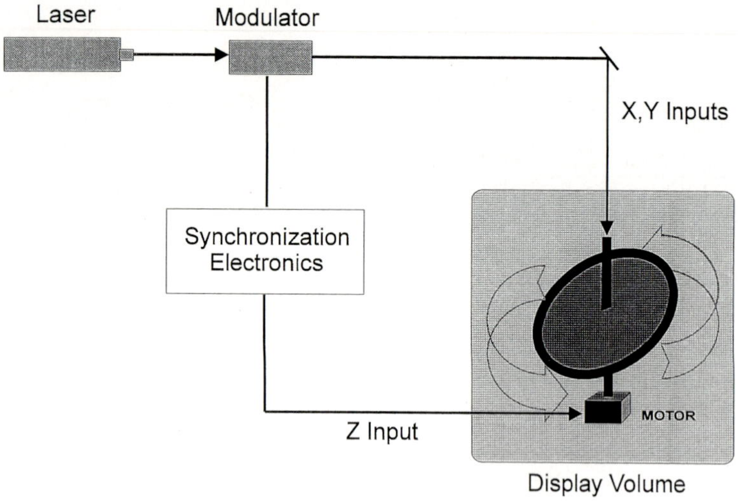

FIG. 5. The multiplanar display, allowing for the input of three dimensions (X, Y, Z), illustrates the principle of operation of a virtual reality system.

sions of an object in all three planes be registered before synchronization and projection into the display volume can be accomplished, it would appear to be impractical for real-time endoscopy but quite applicable for radiologic or magnetic resonance imaging. Figures 4 and 5 illustrate the principles of virtual reality. Stereo pairing requires the use of special glasses for viewing as well as the utilization of two stereoscopically spaced cameras. Such a system is theoretically possible for endoscopy and shows some promise of development. Its implementation, however, must await the evolution of extremely small video cameras that can be fitted to the distal end of the endoscope.

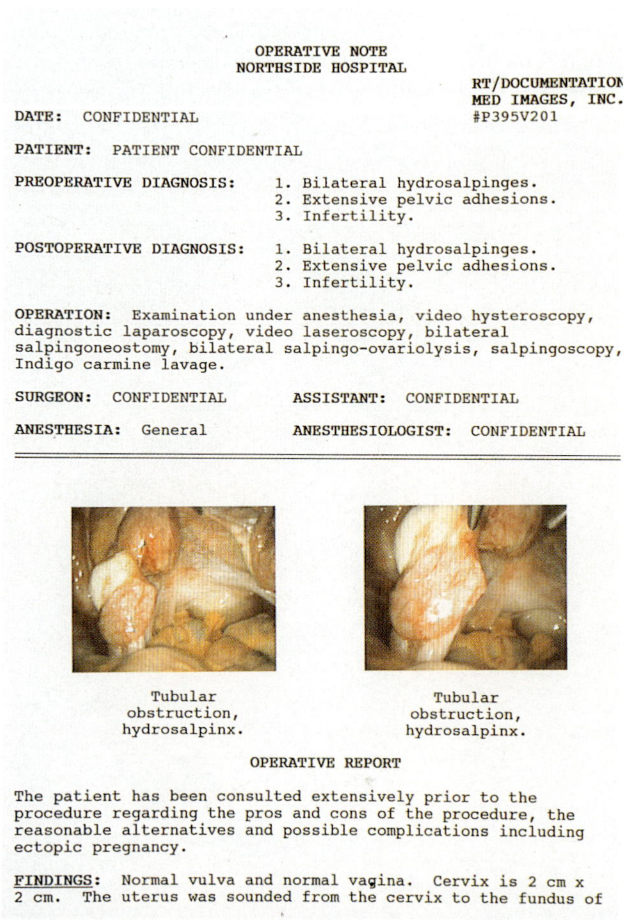

OPERATIVE NOTE
NORTHSIDE HOSPITAL

RT/DOCUMENTATION
MED IMAGES, INC.
#P395V201

DATE: CONFIDENTIAL

PATIENT: PATIENT CONFIDENTIAL

PREOPERATIVE DIAGNOSIS: 1. Bilateral hydrosalpinges. 2. Extensive pelvic adhesions. 3. Infertility.

POSTOPERATIVE DIAGNOSIS: 1. Bilateral hydrosalpinges. 2. Extensive pelvic adhesions. 3. Infertility.

OPERATION: Examination under anesthesia, video hysteroscopy, diagnostic laparoscopy, video laseroscopy, bilateral salpingoneostomy, bilateral salpingo-ovariolysis, salpingoscopy, Indigo carmine lavage.

SURGEON: CONFIDENTIAL ASSISTANT: CONFIDENTIAL

ANESTHESIA: General ANESTHESIOLOGIST: CONFIDENTIAL

Tubular obstruction, hydrosalpinx.

Tubular obstruction, hydrosalpinx.

OPERATIVE REPORT

The patient has been consulted extensively prior to the procedure regarding the pros and cons of the procedure, the reasonable alternatives and possible complications including ectopic pregnancy.

FINDINGS: Normal vulva and normal vagina. Cervix is 2 cm x 2 cm. The uterus was sounded from the cervix to the fundus of

FIG. 6. Typical operative dictation with frame-grabbed images. (Courtesy of Med Images, Inc.)

Record Keeping

Video images can be preserved in records or in hard copy. *Frame grabbing* is a technique whereby a single frame of a videotape or real-time image can be captured in digital form and printed out on material such as paper. A number of color printers are available. This technology has been combined by at least one company into a system for recording multiple, frame-grabbed images obtained by simply pressing a foot pedal at any desired time during the video-imaged procedure. The resultant still images then are combined with the operative dictation, sent by telephone to a central office, and returned as an integrated document containing both the color still images and the typed operative report (Med Images, Inc., Knoxville, TN). Figure 6 illustrates an example of a final operative dictation involving this form of frame grabbing. Because the image is digitized, frame grabbing allows for image notation and enhancement with a personal computer loaded with the appropriate software.

Storing and Archiving

It is certain that in the near future the large storage space required for videotape archiving will be put to better use, and video-imaged procedures will be accessible from optical disks sorted on a short bookshelf. Bar coding of various segments of the imaging with corresponding bar codes placed in the patient record or logbook will allow for virtually instant access to interesting aspects of any procedure. Lecturers eventually will not need to carry pages of slides with them to seminars and meetings; a simple modem connection through the telephone with the home database will allow the presentation of any previously digitized color slide or segment of digitally stored video.

HIGHLIGHTS

Electronic video imaging for endoscopic procedures of every sort will probably replace the 35-mm camera in all but a few institutions within the next few years. Continuing refinements of existing instruments and development of techniques not yet imaged will result in procedures that are more easily accomplished, better understood, and more often successful.

REFERENCES

1. Yuzpe A, Gamel B, Taylor P, Rioux J. Endoscopic documentation. In: *Laparoscopy and hysteroscopy.* Chicago: Yearbook; 1986.
2. Leventhal J. Documentation of laparoscopy with polaroid cinematography. *J Reprod Med* 1981;26:5.
3. Wimsteker K. Documentation in laparoscopic surgery. *Bailliere's Clin Obstet Gynaecol* 1989;3:625.

SUGGESTED READING

1. Leventhal J. In: Sanfilippo J, Levine R, eds. *Visual documentation in operative gynecologic endoscopy.* New York: Springer-Verlag; 1987.
2. Morton R. Image permanence: the video disk—a hope for the future. *J AV Media Med* 1986;9:5.
3. Wigton R. The new knowledge bases: CD/ROM and medicine. *MD Compute* 1987;4:34.
4. Lardennois B, Adnet J, Oismayo C, et al. The storing of medical images on video disc, lasers: presentation of the first instructional video disc with In. *Urol Acta Urol Belg* 1987;55:113.
5. Berci G, Brooks P, Paz-Partlow M. TV laparoscopy: a new dimension in visualization and documentation of pelvic pathology. *J Reprod Med* 1986;1:585.

PART VII

The Present and the Future

Endoscopic Management of Gynecologic Disease,
edited by G.D. Adamson and D.C. Martin.
Lippincott-Raven Publishers, Philadelphia © 1996.

CHAPTER 37

A Scientific Appraisal of Gynecologic Endoscopy

David L. Olive

There are four types of lies: lies, damned lies, IVF statistics, and success rates with endoscopy.
—ANONYMOUS, 1991

Endoscopic surgery has grown, in the span of little more than a decade, from an occasionally utilized technique to the predominant mode of surgical interaction in gynecology. Along with this growth spurt has come a myriad of techniques and equipment previously unimagined by early pioneers in the field. As with any rapidly expanding technology, the ability to perform specific procedures endoscopically has leaped far ahead of our critical evaluation of such procedures. However it is incumbent on the modern gynecologic surgeon, as a physician and scientist, to perform procedures not only because they *can* be done but because they *should* be done.

The appraisal of gynecologic endoscopic techniques has taken many forms in the literature. Some reports are designed simply as glorified case reports: in essence they show that in expert hands a given surgical approach can be performed endoscopically. Manuscripts such as these abound in the gynecologic journals. A second, more complex type of study, involves assessing the value of such "performable" procedures. These investigations require hypotheses to be tested, study designs that actually test the hypotheses, and methods of analyzing the resulting data so that valid conclusions may be drawn. Without this latter type of research, endosurgery would remain on par with charlatanism and hucksterism, a field where wild claims can be neither supported or refuted by available evidence. To appraise gynecologic endoscopy honestly, one must first have the discipline to evaluate it scientifically.

This chapter will endeavor to provide the structure and tools for analyzing endoscopic research. Application of these tools will allow the reader to cut through the haze of conflicting claims and be able to evaluate the literature critically, as it exists, for applicability of these procedures to routine patient care. The chapter will also provide guidelines for those wishing to fill in the gaps of the existing literature and conduct appropriate trials appraising gynecologic endoscopic techniques.

D. L. Olive: Section of Reproductive Endocrinology and Infertility, Department of Obstetrics and Gynecology, Yale University School of Medicine, New Haven, Connecticut 06510.

FORMULATING AN HYPOTHESIS

The first question to be asked of any investigative endeavor is, "What is the hypothesis?" The hypothesis to be tested ultimately will influence subsequent design and analysis, and a clear determination of the outset of the study will often prevent the investigator from becoming bogged down in tangential issues. When reviewing studies already conducted, the discerning reader must likewise ask what hypothesis is being tested; lack of clarity regarding this point often is indicative of a "shotgun" approach by the authors, who are looking for anything significant to help justify use of a procedure.

Once a hypothesis is raised, the next decision involves selection of the appropriate outcome measure. Examples of such measures in endoscopy may include pregnancy rates (for treatment of fertility problems), pain relief (for treatment of pain syndrome), or even operating time or blood loss (when comparing endoscopy to laparotomy). Whatever outcome measure is selected, it must address the original hypothesis. For instance, if it is hypothesized that endoscopic myomectomy will increase subsequent fertility when compared to laparotomy, it is inappropriate to use intraoperative blood loss as a primary outcome measure for this effect.

DESIGNING THE STUDY

Types of Clinical Trials

Research design may be divided into two categories: (a) descriptive, such as delineation of prognostic factors or the clinical course of a disease, and (b) analytic, in which an interventional cause–effect relationship is investigated. The latter category encompasses those studies evaluating the role of endoscopy in the treatment of gynecologic disease. Within the category of analytic research, there are two basic structures: the experimental trial and the observational survey (1). A study design qualifies as an experimental trial when more than one study group is involved and when study subjects are allocated to each of the study groups in a random fashion. If, on the other hand, only a single study group is evaluated or if treatment options are assigned not randomly but for a reason, the research is an observational survey.

Observational surveys can be classified further by when the data were collected in relation to the present time (real-time relationship). Studies with data accumulated in the past, prior to hypothesis development, can be called retrospective, whereas those performed after the study was conceived and designed are termed prospective (2,3).

Another way to classify observational surveys is by their research pursuit direction, i.e., from what point in the diagnosis–treatment–outcome continuum was the patient selected for inclusion in the study (3,4). If the subject was selected based on a diagnosis or treatment modality and was subsequently followed for outcome evaluation, the direction is termed antecedent-to-outcome, or *cohort*. Conversely, if a study enrolls patients because of a given outcome and then follows their records back to see what treatment was administered, the research pursuit direction is outcome-to-antecedent, or *trohoc*.

The primary advantage of a study performed in present time (the randomized trial and the prospective cohort study) is the ability to collect data in a complete and dependable fashion. Thus, the presence or absence of a factor of importance in the study can be determined uniformly and without bias among study participants. Furthermore, since the means of evaluation are determined before initiation of data collection, uniformity of outcome assessment is more likely in this situation. Despite these advantages, there are problems with prospective trials. Experimental studies are expensive, time consuming, and often of insufficient size to address adequately the hypothesis being tested. They also may be so rigid in their inclusion criteria that the results only apply to a very narrow subset of the patient population. Prospective cohort studies suffer from the lack of random assignment of patients, with the resulting bias sure to affect study results. Both study types must make allowances for the failure of some subjects to complete the designated study protocol.

In the retrospective study, data are gleaned from medical records or patient recall; both can be significantly unreliable to the point of severely prejudicing the conclusions. In addition, these studies are limited to those methods of evaluation recorded in the chart, prompting questions about any preexisting conditions that may or may not have been recorded, the degree and intensity of observation, and whether or not there was uniformity of outcome assessment. Although such studies are rapid and inexpensive to perform, the results often are highly suspect due to these shortcomings in design.

When a retrospective analysis of endoscopic surgery is performed, the authors must consider and discuss each of these issues. What qualified the patient for inclusion into the study, and were these criteria uniformly applied? Were all women operated on in the same manner by surgeons of comparable skill and experience? If the outcome was pregnancy, what test was used and was it performed at the same time for all subjects? Inconsistencies in any of these areas will substantially decrease the value of a study, and information extracted from such investigations should be considered preliminary and in need of prospective confirmation.

Control Groups

To determine the value of a therapeutic maneuver, it must be clear as to what would have happened had the therapy not been administered. This concept, the determination of baseline values as a source of comparison, is termed *control* (3). A study may be controlled in a variety of ways or it may remain uncontrolled; the decision as to whether and how to control a trial can impact greatly on the value of a clinical investigation.

In endoscopic treatment trials, the appropriate choice of a control group depends on the hypothesis being tested. If the study is an attempt to study the efficacy of endoscopic treatment, one must consider what is known to occur in the absence of treatment or with alternative treatment. If it is well known that the absence of treatment never leads to a favorable outcome, demonstration of an improvement via endoscopy would require only evidence that successful outcome follows endoscopic intervention, without the need for a comparable control group of untreated patients. For example, if the hypothesis is that women with bilateral distal tubal obstruction will have increased pregnancy rates following laparoscopic cuff salpingostomy, any pregnancies resulting after the procedure can be deemed to have resulted from the procedure itself, as no woman would achieve pregnancy without the surgery.

Conversely, if the study hypothesis is that women with unilateral distal tubal obstruction will have increased pregnancy rates following laparoscopic cuff salpingostomy, the issue is quite different. In this situation, untreated women will achieve pregnancy; the question is whether or not they will do it more often after surgery. To test this hypothesis, a control group of untreated women is essential so that the baseline success rate can be identified, and it can be seen if the treated group performs better.

If, however, a standard treatment exists that is of known efficacy, the hypothesis to be tested may not be whether the intervention is efficacious but rather how it compares to standard therapy. For the above example of bilateral distal tubal obstruction, control group selection might include women undergoing microsurgical cuff salpingostomy or even in vitro fertilization. Pregnancy rate would certainly be one outcome measure; but others might include cost, recovery time, and complication rates. Again, the outcome measure(s) selected depend on the precise hypothesis under consideration.

Aside from the composition of the control group, the method of accumulating controls is an important issue. In a randomized therapeutic trial, patients are arbitrarily allocated to either the experimental or the control group. This method is optimal in that it minimizes effects of confounding variables on the outcome measure (5). However, most studies are not of this design but rather exist as observational surveys. For such trials, patients may be assigned at the same time to either the experimental or the control group, but the assignment is based upon clinical discretion rather than random assignment. This type of control group is referred to as *concurrent* and *nonrandomized.* This method of control has the obvious limitation of the introduction of bias due to the method of allocation (6,7). Clearly, the factors that influence a clinician to place the patient in one group or the other might also affect the rate of successful outcome in the two groups.

Another type of control group is the *historical control.* With this technique, patients treated with the experimental procedure are compared to subjects previously treated with the control approach. Thus, the two groups are not treated during the same time span but rather sequentially. Historical control creates many difficulties, including the fact that the historical data usually are gathered retrospectively—with all the inherent problems of a retrospective study. Furthermore, other substantive factors may have changed over time besides the therapeutic change under study; these factors may contribute to significant alterations in the outcome of the study. For example, consider a study comparing endometrial ablation by resectoscope from 1983 to 1987 vs. ablation by Nd:YAG laser from 1988 to 1991. Aside from a change in technique in 1988, the patients treated in the second group were subjected to surgery by a more experienced hysteroscopist with considerably improved video equipment. If the laser group were shown to have an improved outcome, the cause might be any of these factors and the improvement could not necessarily be attributed solely to the ablative instrument.

Confounding Variables

Patient characteristics known to effect the outcome measure in an endoscopic treatment trial may have substantial impact on study results. For example, if the outcome measure is pregnancy, variables such as age, duration of infertility, gravidity, and additional infertility factors might have considerable effect. The best way to minimize the effect of confounders on a study outcome is the randomized experimental design discussed earlier. Random allocation of subjects should virtually equalize the effects of such confounding variables—whether known to the investigator or not! However, even with randomization, there is the possibility that some critical factor may unduly influence one group over another. To protect against this, the prevalence of all known confounding variables should be assessed for each study group. If the research involves a nonrandomized but comparative trial, specific regression techniques can be utilized to help determine the value of treatment independent of such confounders. A thorough understanding of biases present in the study population will always aid in determining the applicability of results to specific clinical circumstances.

ANALYZING A STUDY

In research involving endoscopic surgery, there are two types of outcome measures. The first type involves measures related to the surgical procedure or the immediate postoperative period. In this situation, there is a one-to-one relationship between the procedure and the outcome measure, and standard statistical techniques are applicable. Examples include such outcomes as time of surgery, amount of blood loss, number of lymph nodes recovered, agreement of surgical and tissue diagnosis, and length of hospital stay.

A second type of outcome measure is much more complex: the time-dependent outcome. With this measure, the result may vary given the length of follow-up after surgery. Thus, the outcome at 1 month postoperatively may differ from that of 6 or 12 months following surgery. Most outcomes related to symptom relief fall into this category. Examples include pregnancy, pain relief, restoration of continence, and reduction/elimination of abnormal uterine bleeding. Statistical methodology applied to these types of trials differ markedly in that follow-up time must be considered; methods that fail to take this factor into consideration prove grossly inadequate in analyzing such data.

Two common types of endoscopic surgery studies, i.e., infertility treatment trials and attempts to produce pain relief, prove to be excellent examples for application of the techniques available given a time-dependent outcome. A review of such methods is provided here.

INFERTILITY TREATMENT TRIALS

Noncomparative Data Reporting

When there is no need for a control group, single treatment group trials are performed and reported. The time-dependent nature of pregnancy creates specific issues in data reporting that may be approached in several ways. Listed are the numerous approaches to noncomparative reporting of pregnancy rates, with the advantages and disadvantages of each.

Simple Pregnancy Rates

The most common calculation in endoscopic treatment trials is the simple (or crude) pregnancy rate fol-

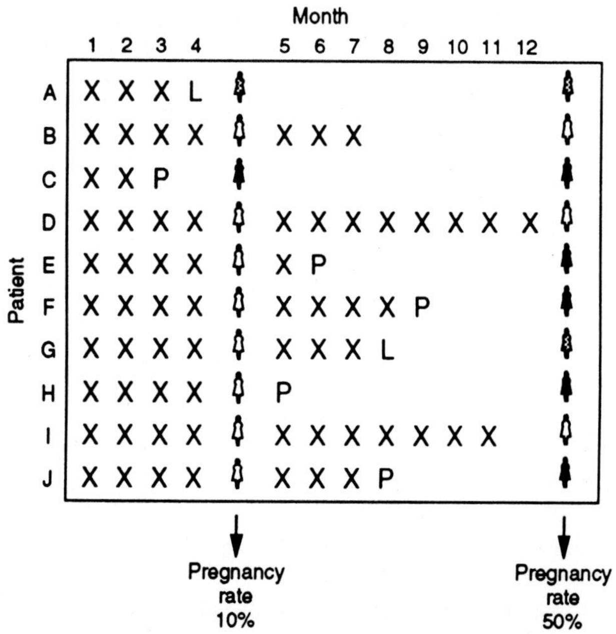

FIG. 1. Variation in pregnancy rate as a function of length of follow-up study. A trial of these ten women ended at 4 months follow-up would have yielded a pregnancy rate of 10%; the same ten women followed up for 12 months provide a 50% pregnancy rate. X, cycle without conceptions; P, cycle with conception; L, lost to follow-up. (From ref. 4.)

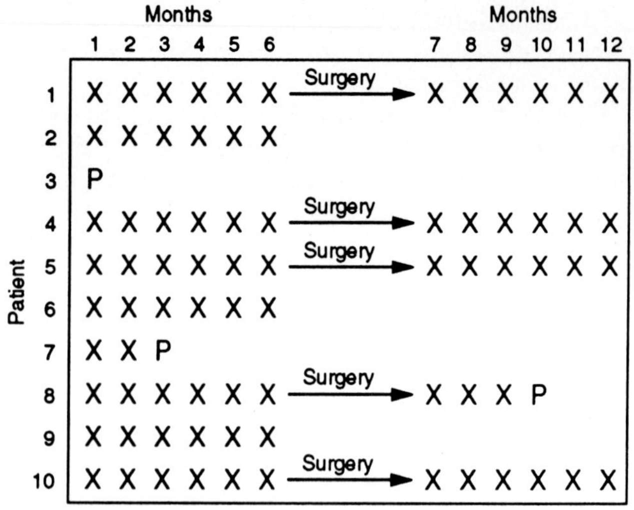

FIG. 2. Overestimation of pregnancy rate because of removal of treatment failures. A trial of laparoscopic surgery in ten women is illustrated, with two achieving pregnancy. X, cycle without conception; P, cycle with conception. (From ref. 4.)

lowing endoscopic surgery. This value is defined as the number of pregnancies divided by the number of patients treated. It is among the easiest of analyses to perform yet there are a number of critical problems associated with this method.

First, the method does not inherently adjust for simple bias, i.e., confounding variables that may affect fertility. Additional adjustments must be applied if this is to be considered.

Second, the simple pregnancy rate varies depending on the length of follow-up after surgery. Clearly, women undergoing endoscopic treatment are less likely to conceive if followed 2 months postoperatively, than if followed for 6 or even 12 months (Fig. 1). The principle is a simple one: women are more likely to conceive the longer they attempt to conceive.

It has been argued that simple pregnancy rates at least provide a minimum rate of conception expected for a therapeutic intervention. However, even this is untrue. Take, for example, a study of ten women undergoing laparoscopic surgery for endometriosis (Fig. 2). At the conclusion of 6 months follow-up, two women are pregnant and eight are not. Of the eight, five now undergo laparotomy for excision of the disease and over the next 6 months one of these women achieves pregnancy. The data might then be reported as a 40% pregnancy rate with laparoscopic treatment (two of five) and a 20% pregnancy rate with combined laparoscopy and laparotomy (one of five). Of course, such figures are greatly misleading and illustrate how inadequate the reporting of simple pregnancy rates can be.

If a study is performed whereby all patients enroll for the entire investigative period and none is lost to follow-up over a set period of time, the simple pregnancy rate can provide a reasonable and rapid means of comparing study groups. However, for analyzing data with censored patients (women not completing the full follow-up period), comparing groups with varying duration of follow-up, or simply understanding the effect of time upon pregnancy, the simple pregnancy rate is an inadequate method.

Corrected Pregnancy Rates

Corrected pregnancy rates are calculated similarly to simple pregnancy rates, except that couples with additional infertility factors are excluded from the statistics. In this way, a more homogeneous patient population is obtained for study. However, the same problems with variable follow-up seen with crude pregnancy rates make this analytic approach of little value to the clinical investigator. Furthermore, there is an additional difficulty: a lack of standardization among researchers as to what defines a confounding factor in the infertile couple. The phrase "corrected for additional infertility factors" can have different meanings with different researchers, making it virtually impossible to draw generalizable conclusions from such studies.

Corrected pregnancy rates also can be manipulated to provide highly misleading information. An example is data reporting 12 of 20 women treated surgically for endometriosis achieving pregnancy (60%). An addendum to this report noted that six of the eight couples failing to conceive suffered from oligospermia; when corrected for this, the pregnancy rate grew to 12 of 14 (86%). What the authors failed to report is that 8 of the 12 couples achieving pregnancy had oligospermia, and the true corrected pregnancy rate is 4 of 6, or 67%. The principle is straightforward: if "correction" for other factors is to be performed, it must be done on all study patients, not simply those failing to conceive.

Cumulative Pregnancy Rate

A method to deal with variable length of follow-up among study subjects is to produce a graphic display of the cumulative rate of pregnancy as length of follow-up increases (Fig. 3). The technique generally used to construct this cumulative curve is commonly referred to as life table methodology, after its original use as a descriptor of patient survival in oncology studies (8–11). This curve has the advantage of identifying the rate of conception at any particular time during postoperative follow-up. In addition, if patients drop out of the study without conceiving, these censored patients can be mathematically corrected for to give an estimate of what would have happened had all patients continued to the completion of the trial period. Details of how to calculate a cumulative pregnancy curve using life table methodology is provided elsewhere (3,12).

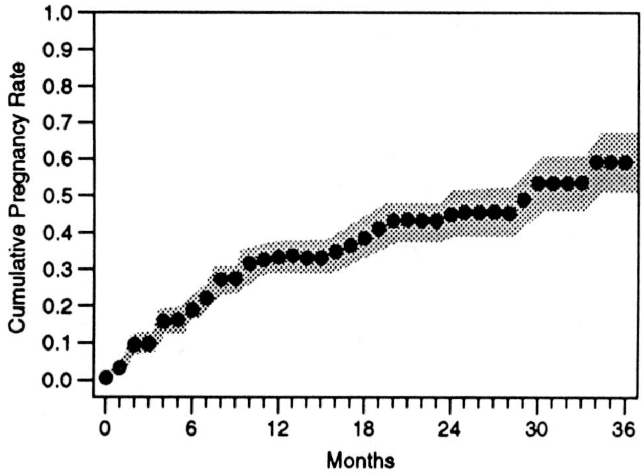

FIG. 3. Graphic representation of a life table based on the conception rate of 88 women undergoing conservative surgery for endometriosis-associated infertility. *Shaded area* indicates variance of each time point. (From ref. 4.)

Although this method represents a tremendous improvement over the simple calculation of pregnancy rates, there is one potentially misleading facet of this technique. In life table calculations, after some patients are censored (lost to follow-up), those remaining in the study are presumed to represent all patients (censored or not) who have failed to conceive. Thus, women who are lost to follow-up are assumed to be identical to those who continue to be followed up. Unfortunately, this premise frequently is untrue; often the woman lost to follow-up has circumstances different from those remaining in the study. Computer simulations of fertility trials have demonstrated that if pregnant patients are more likely to be followed up than those women who remain infertile, the cumulative pregnancy curve will appear substantially more successful than it would had all patients been followed uniformly (Doody M, personal communication, 1991). Fortunately, strategies to deal with this statistical quirk have been suggested for incorporation into study design.

Monthly Fecundity Rates

Although cumulative pregnancy curves are an excellent means of visualizing data over prolonged time intervals, relating a curve from a study to other existing data is both operationally and conceptually difficult. In order to reduce data with variability in follow-up to a single number, the follow-up period can be reduced to a series of universal units that may be additive. For surgical studies, the unit is a month. Calculating the pregnancy rate per month following surgery gives equal weight to each attempt at pregnancy by each study patient. This statistic is called the monthly fecundity rate (MFR). It is calculated by taking the number of pregnancies and dividing by the total number of months of follow-up for all study patients. Advantages include ease of calculation as well as easily defined confidence limits. Methods for statistical comparisons with other MFRs are well elucidated (13). Furthermore, it suggests what the expected chance of conception is with each attempt—a clinically relevant figure to convey to patients.

The single serious problem with the MFR lies in its inherent assumption: all menstrual cycles after surgery are of equal probability to result in a pregnancy. This may not be true under two circumstances. First, patients may have a variety of confounding factors that make lumping them together into a single cohort inappropriate. To remedy this, stratification of the patient population is required. Second and most important, only infrequently do subsequent attempts at conceiving in a woman carry the same rate of success as in the preceding cycle. For this to be the case, the assumption is that, given an infinite number of cycles, the pregnancy rate will approach 100%. Although this is true for parous women seeking therapeutic donor insemination (14), it is rarely true for other infertile women. Such a model initially underestimates the chance of conception but eventually overestimates the probability of occurrence (12,15).

Two-Parameter Exponential Models

Given the latter drawback of the MFR, a more precise means of describing a cumulative pregnancy curve numerically was needed. This has been achieved by mathematically deriving a two-parameter exponential model that fits well with the cumulative pregnancy curve (15). The underlying assumption of this model is that the observed cumulative pregnancy curve is really a weighted average of two curves: one for patients who will conceive (cured) and the other for those who will never conceive (not cured) (Fig. 4). In the latter instance, the curve is a horizontal line at 0%. As time advances and women from the cured group achieve pregnancy, the uncured group represents a larger and larger population of those remaining in the study; thus, the cumulative pregnancy curve appears to plateau well before 100% conception is achieved. Two clinically meaningful numbers describe this model: the "cure rate," which represents the percentage of women who conceive given an infinite length of follow-up, and the monthly probability of pregnancy (MPP) for those who do achieve conception. This model appears to correspond well with empirical data generated in fertility trials.

The greatest problem with this technique in the past has been its complexity. All too often the dataset is not large enough for an adequate calculation of the model parameters; this difficulty appears recently to have been solved by the development of a program for the microcomputer, which is adaptable to studies of varying sizes (Guzick DS, Bross DS, personal communication, 1990).

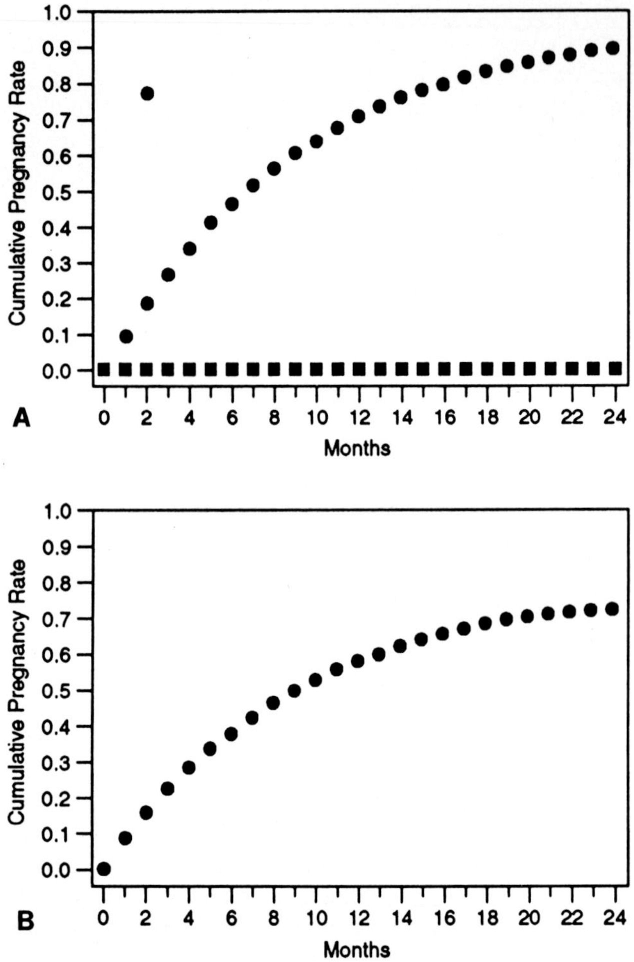

FIG. 4. Cumulative pregnancy graphic representation based on the two-parameter exponential model. **A:** *Solid circles* represent the cumulative pregnancy curve for the "cured" couples, who compose 80% of the total sample. *Solid squares* represent the cumulative pregnancy rate for the "uncured" couples, who compose 20% of the same. **B:** A weighted average, combining the two curves in panel A. Note the apparent plateau at a cumulative rate of 0.8. (From ref. 4.)

Regression Models

Many studies investigate the association of a number of different confounding variables on the outcome of surgical intervention. Regression models are used frequently in such situations. These models take a variety of forms, but their common aim is to study the individual and joint effect of a number of different factors on an outcome variable.

When the outcome is binary (pregnant vs. not pregnant) at a specifically defined time point without censoring of patients, multiple logistic regression modeling is the appropriate method (16). Details of the calculations involved are beyond the scope of this chapter. Suffice it to say that by performing logistic regression for a number of predictor variables, the effect of each on the chance of achieving pregnancy can be determined. Thus, this method is the desired approach when attempting to sort out the value of a treatment in the face of multiple confounding variables.

More often, however, the situation is such that the outcome is not a simple yes or no at a specified time point but rather a cumulative pregnancy curve across a wide span of time. In this situation, the Cox proportional hazards model (17) (an analog of multiple linear regression) corrects for confounding variables yet takes into account the overall structure of the pregnancy curve (18). The major advantages of this technique include the ability to correct for confounding influences and its independence from traditional exponential models of life tables. A major disadvantage of the technique is a greater sensitivity to rate of pregnancy than ultimate cure rate.

Dangers of Statistical Models

Although many well-known physical equations describe relationships exactly, statistical models use equations quite differently. The equation for a statistical model is not expected to be exactly true; instead, it represents a useful framework within which the statistician is able to study relationships that are of interest (19). There are often no biologically plausible reasons supporting statistical models: in general, they should be regarded simply as attempts to provide empirical summaries of observed data. Whenever such modeling is to be attempted, it is suggested that consultation with a statistician is appropriate to ensure proper handling and interpretation.

Comparing Data

Categorical Comparisons

With endpoints of pregnancy (yes/no), methodology used to compare treatment groups must deal with this categorical type of outcome. Categorical comparisons are appropriate for simple and corrected pregnancy rates and MFRs. In each case, the outcome may be expressed as falling into one of two categories. Two tests appropriate for comparing treatment with these endpoints include Fisher's test (20) and the χ^2 test (21).

Fisher's test is limited to data that can be summarized in a 2 × 2 table (22). Thus, no more than two groups can be compared and no more than two outcomes can be possible. Fisher's test is commonly referred to as Fisher's exact test, as it evaluates the exact significance level of the null hypothesis that the probability of success is the same in two distinct groups. In the past, studies with large numbers made calculations for the test quite formidable. Today, however, with the advent of the microcomputer for statistical analysis, it is clear than any 2 × 2 categorical comparison should be analyzed by Fisher's test rather than the χ^2 test with continuity correction. If, however, the comparison involves a grid larger than 2 × 2, χ^2 testing is indicated.

With either of the preceding tests, there are two important assumptions. First, the probability of success must be the same for each subject in a group. Second, the outcome of the experiment for any subject may not influence the outcome for any member of either group. When these requirements are overlooked or ignored, such analyses could mask important effects or generate spurious ones.

Comparing Cumulative Pregnancy Curves

When cumulative pregnancy curves are generated for two methods of surgical intervention, it is desirable to compare them to one another. One test, called the log rank of Mantel–Haenszel test (23,24), is frequently used to compare cumulative rates of two or more populations. The log-rank test is designed specifically to detect a difference between cumulative pregnancy curves that result when the pregnancy rate in one group is consistently higher than the corresponding rate in a second group, and the ratio of these two rates is constant over time, i.e., the pregnancy rate for treatment A may be 5%/month and that for treatment B may be 15%/month. In this case, the ratio is 1:3 for each month of observation, and the log-rank test would seem particularly appropriate.

Another method of comparing these curves is the Breslow formulation (25) of the Kruskal–Wallis test (26). This test is similar to the log-rank test, but its particular strength is in weighting points along a cumulative pregnancy curve. Thus, if a study contains large numbers of censored patients, the Breslow test may be optimal.

These tests are but two of those designed to compare cumulative curves. Under particular circumstances, more specialized testing may be required. All such calculations are carried out via computer.

Two-Parameter Exponential Model Comparisons

A likelihood ratio test has been devised to allow easy comparison of two populations modeled by the two-parameter exponential method described previously (27). In this test, the cure rate and MPP are estimated under varying assumptions about these parameters in the two curves, corresponding to four "models":

Model 1: Cure rate and MPP are both different
Model 2: Cure rates are the same but MPP are different
Model 3: Cure rates are different but MPP are the same
Model 4: Both cure rate and MPP are the same

For each model, the maximized value of the likelihood function is computed. The hypothesis that one or both of the parameters differ between groups is tested by comparing pairs of each of the models under consideration, with the comparison statistic providing a χ^2 distribution. The program for this testing is available on microcomputer.

Comparison by Regression

Logistic regression modeling can allow comparison of treatment modalities by making one of the predictor variables equal to treatment. If two treatments were attempted, the determinations can be made as to whether a change in treatment influences the outcome variable. If a significant relationship is determined, it can be concluded that one of the treatments is superior to the other in producing the desired outcome.

Sequential Changes of Treatment Status

The evaluation of comparative pregnancy data in surgical studies is subject to a variety of biases. One common bias is analysis of patients who transfer from one treatment group to another or even back and forth between two or more treatment groups.

The Mantel–Byar analysis method, an approach for constructing and comparing modified life tables that reflect sequential changes of treatment status, is applicable to these types of situations (28). The method can compensate for patient transfer from one comparison group to another (or even back and forth between groups). The analysis is nearly assumption-free, and stratification of patients to increase homogeneity is possible.

TREATMENT OF PELVIC PAIN

Trials investigating relief of pelvic pain warrant a different type of analytic consideration than do fertility trials. Whereas fertility trials have an objective outcome in pregnancy (either yes or no), pelvic pain can be highly variable, subjective, and subject to degrees of relief. Despite this, the variability in length of follow-up among study patients mandates techniques similar to those described above. However, two additional issues arise: how should pelvic pain be quantified, and how does a continuous outcome variable change an investigator's analytic approach?

Measurement of Pelvic Pain

Measuring the subjective effect of pain has been a research priority among investigators for over a decade. However, little work has been done specifically in the area of pelvic pain, and that which has been performed often is flawed and of little value. Comments such as "Well, of course, the subjective experience of pain cannot be measured" are used to justify nonvalidated and poorly reliable scales to demonstrate the degree of pelvic pain in study subjects. Such attitudes are unscientific. The physicist cannot measure tiny particles directly and must rely on instruments to attach numbers to indirect effects of the particles. The same approach to pain research can yield quantifiable results that are meaningful (29).

The minimum requirement for a pain scale is reliability and validity (29). A reliable measure has the property of yielding consistent results under varying circumstances. Test–retest reliability is particularly important if the measure is to be used repeatedly in a subject to assess response to therapy. Validity is a more difficult concept and is used to express the degree a measure approximates reality. In treatment trials of pelvic pain, reliability is much more important than validity.

A number of methods have been developed and found reliable for the measurement of pain. However, the worth of these scales may be highly variable when compared with one another, and it is incumbent on researchers and critics to evaluate the particular measurement scale in relation to the research being performed. Six pain intensity scales are shown in Fig. 5, and all have received extensive evaluation in the literature (30).

Generally, there are five criteria for judging pain intensity scales: ease of administration of scoring, relative rates of incorrect responding, sensitivity as defined by the number of available response categories, sensitivity of the scales in their ability to detect treatment effects, and magnitude of the relationship between each scale and a "best possible" measure of subjective pain intensity (30). In terms of correct response rate and predictive validity, all of the above scales perform similarly. However, in terms of sensitivity (especially to detect treatment differences), scales with greater response options, such as the 101-point Numerical Rating Scale (NRS-101) and the Visual Analog Scale (VAS), are optimal (28). An understanding of the strengths and limitations of scoring systems is essential to appropriate analysis of clinical pain trials.

Another issue that sets apart pain measurement from pregnancy outcome is the possibility of a placebo effect of surgery itself. The actual quantification of pain relief following sham surgery for pelvic pain has received little attention, although preliminary data would suggest that the effect is quite small (31). Consideration of this factor in uncontrolled trials is important to the overall conclusions to be drawn from the study.

Analysis of Pelvic Pain Treatment Trials

The use of continuous outcome variables for the measure of pelvic pain both simplifies and complicates the analysis. In an uncontrolled trial, there remains the paired preoperative to postoperative comparison; χ^2 analysis or a student's paired t test generally is used de-

The Visual Analogue Scale (VAS)

No pain ———————————— Pain as bad as it could be

The 101-point Numerical Rating Scale (NRS-101)

Please indicate on the line below the number between 0 and 100 that best describes your pain. A zero (0) would mean "no pain," and a one hundred would mean "pain as bad as it could be." Please only write one number.

____

The 11-point Box Scale (BS-11)

If a zero (0) means "no pain," and a ten (10) means "pain as bad as it could be," on this scale of 0 to 10, what is your level of pain? Put an "X" through that number.

0	1	2	3	4	5	6	7	8	9	10

The 6-point Behavioral Rating Scale (BRS-6)

- ☐ No pain.
- ☐ Pain present, but can easily be ignored.
- ☐ Pain present, cannot be ignored, but does not interfere with everyday activities.
- ☐ Pain present, cannot be ignored, interferes with concentration.
- ☐ Pain present, cannot be ignored, interferes with all tasks except taking care of basic needs such as toileting and eating.
- ☐ Pain present, cannot be ignored, rest or bedrest required.

The 4-point Verbal Rating Scale (VRS-4)

- ☐ No pain.
- ☐ Some pain.
- ☐ Considerable pain.
- ☐ Pain which could not be more severe.

The 5-point Verbal Rating Scale (VRS-5)

- ☐ Mild.
- ☐ Discomforting.
- ☐ Distressing.
- ☐ Horrible.
- ☐ Excruciating.

FIG. 5. Six pain intensity measures. (From ref. 30.)

pending on the number of response categories in the measurement scale. In situations with many response categories and oddly distributed data, nonparametric statistics may be required.

Two caveats to this type of analysis are the unknown placebo effect on pain relief and the timing of postoperative evaluation. The magnitude of placebo effect in an uncontrolled trial leaves considerable uncertainty as to the actual efficacy of the procedure—this point should always be made when discussing treatment results.

The timing of postoperative evaluation is also critical, as degree of pain relief may vary tremendously with length of follow-up. It is of foremost importance to ensure that all patients grouped for postoperative evaluation have been followed up for an identical amount of time after surgery. If there is considerable variability among subjects, construction of a time-related pain curve (analogous to the cumulative pregnancy curve) is appropriate; for example, see Fig. 6. One important distinction is worth noting, however: unlike cumulative pregnancy curves, which continually increase with time, time-related pain curves may increase or decrease as a function of time. This unique aspect has not been adequately dealt with for analytic purposes.

In controlled trials with multiple distinct time points for comparison, analysis of variance is appropriate, although it fails to utilize the full value of the data by not considering the paired nature of the information. A multiple range test can be applied to adequately determine which follow-up intervals differ from preoperative pain levels. Finally, to understand the pattern of pain relief as a function of time, various types of complex survival analysis procedures and trend analyses may be applied (32). A full discussion of these methods is beyond the scope of this chapter, and consultation with a statistician is recommended.

Comparing two or more groups in a treatment trial for pain relief can be similarly complex. Here, samples are no longer paired at each specific time point of comparison, yet they still are paired within a given treatment type for different time points, such as preoperative and 3 months postoperative. In this situation, the data may be compared in several ways. The simplest method is merely to compare all combinations of data groups: this would mean comparing the two groups preoperatively, comparing the two groups postoperatively, and comparing each of the groups preoperatively to postoperatively. The first two comparisons could be by Student's t test (33) or the Mann–Whitney U test; the third requires a paired t test or the Wilcoxon sign rank test (34). Although such multiple testing will give an idea of what the data is implying, it is not making complete use of the available data in a single test, and thus each result must be considered conceptually in relation to the others. Thus, there is no definitive analysis, only a set of impressions.

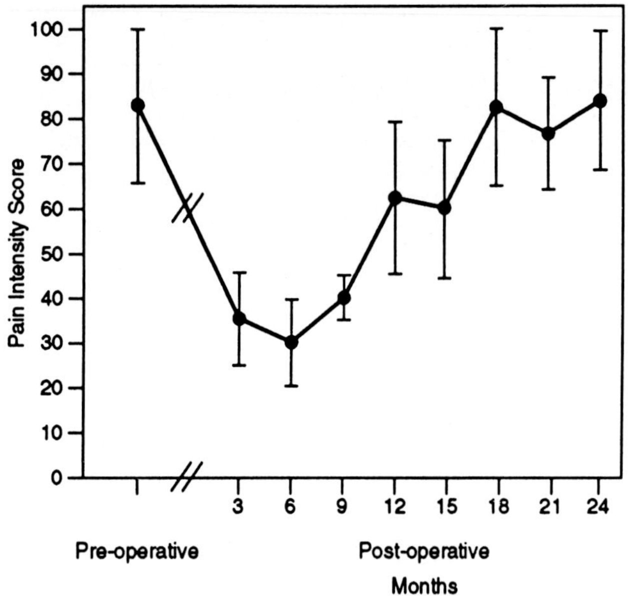

FIG. 6. Graphic representation of a time-related pain curve. Assessment is preoperative and at three-month intervals for 2 years. Error bars indicate the standard error of the mean.

Two more complete analytic techniques are available. A difference in pain level can be calculated for each patient, i.e., the preoperative level minus postoperative level, and this value can be compared for the two treatment groups by the methods listed above. More precise analysis can occur by use of regression models. Multiple linear regression can be performed with the outcome variable being the postoperative pain level and the predictor variables being preoperative pain level and treatment group. This type of analysis will provide the relative effect of treatment type and is amenable to input of additional confounding variables if they are identified.

When the outcome is not accrued at a specific time but across a wide time span, the comparison of time-related pain curves can be quite complex. Sophisticated survival analysis procedures are often required and statistical consultation necessary.

SIGNIFICANCE AND POWER

In the comparison of the results of two treatments (or one treatment vs. no therapy), absolutely conclusive results are not attainable. Instead, one must play the odds when trying to decide if success rates differ. The key to determining this is *statistical significance,* a concept which states that, given the available data, the odds overwhelmingly favor there being a real difference between two groups. Generally, statistical significance requires that, given an observed difference between two treatments, it will in fact be a *real* difference (rather than just a statistical fluke) at least 95% of the time.

Occasionally a study suggests a difference in success between treatments, yet in reality there is not one. This is called a type I statistical error. The rate for a type I error in a given experiment is termed the alpha value and is generally set at no more than 5%.

Some studies suggest no difference in pregnancy rates between treatments. However, occasionally a real difference will exist despite a failure to demonstrate this in a treatment trial. The chances of this occurring is called a type II statistical error. The rate for a type II error in a given experiment is termed the β value and a maximum chance is generally set at no more than 20%. In such a situation, the statistical *power* to avoid a type II error is $1-\beta$ (at least 80% in most settings) (35).

Significance and power are two critical concepts, which must be clearly delineated in a treatment trial. If a study presumes to show a difference between treatments, it is imperative to know whether statistical significance was achieved and, if so, what was the preset α value. If the authors claim no difference, one must ask if the study achieved reasonable power in avoiding a type II error given the sample size and significance threshold. It is all too often the case that a poorly conceived study fails to demonstrate a significant difference between treatments, yet is not of sufficient power to exclude with reasonable certainty that such a difference exists. These investigations are of little value to anyone and generally serve only to muddle the literature. This highlights the importance of thoroughly planning an investigation prior to its initiation, emphasizing the inherent value of the prospective approach.

HIGHLIGHTS

The need for continued research in the field of endoscopic surgery is apparent; we are constantly faced with unproven opinion in every facet of the field. Yet if endoscopic surgery is to become scientifically sound, the procedures utilized must be based on information obtained in well-designed, adequately analyzed studies. The poorly constructed research trial or the inappropriately analyzed study tends to mislead and confuse.

As endoscopic surgeons, we should insist on honest appraisal of developing techniques. This requires investigation into developing endosurgical techniques prior to their being heralded as the standard of care. It requires studies performed with foresight and full utilization of the available tools to answer the research questions posed. Finally, it requires honest and forthright reporting of findings, without deletion of patients or manipulation of data to present the best apparent picture. Only then can we apply these procedures in an intelligent manner that results in quality patient care.

REFERENCES

1. Feinstein AR. Clinical biostatistics. 44. A survey of the research architecture used for publications in general medical journals. *Clin Pharmacol Ther* 1978;24:117.

2. Feinstein AR. Clinical biostatistics. 48. Efficacy of different research structures in preventing bias in the analysis of causation. *Clin Pharmacol Ther* 1979;26:129.
3. Feinstein AR. Clinical biostatistics. 42. A glossary of neologisms in quantitative clinical science. *Clin Pharmacol Ther* 1981;30:564.
4. Olive DL: Analysis of clinical fertility trials: a methodologic review. *Fertil Steril* 1986;45:157.
5. Feinstein AR. Clinical biostatistics. 24. The role of randomization in sampling, testing, allocation, and credulous idolatry (conclusion). *Clin Pharmacol Ther* 1973;14:1035.
6. Student. The Lenarkshire milk experiment. *Biometrika* 1931;23:398.
7. Smithells RW, Sheppard S, Schorah CJ, et al. Possible prevention of neural-tube defects by peri-conceptional vitamin supplementation. *Lancet* 1980;1:339.
8. Berkson J, Gage RP: Calculation of survival rates for cancer. *Mayo Clin Proc* 1950;25:270.
9. Cutler SJ, Ederer F. Maximum utilization of the life-table method of analyzing survival. *J Chronic Dis* 1958;8:699.
10. Katayama KP. A method of analyzing data with incomplete follow-up. *Am J Obstet Gynecol* 1975;123:214.
11. Lamb EJ, Cruz AL. Data collection and analysis in an infertility practice. *Obstet Gynecol* 1972;23:310.
12. Olive DL. Analyzing results of the ovulation induction trial. *Inf Reprod Med Clin North Am* 1990;1:187.
13. Cramer DW, Walker AM, Schiff I. Statistical methods in evaluating the outcome of infertility therapy. *Fertil Steril* 1979;32:80.
14. Peek JC, Godfrey B, Matthews CD. Estimation of fertility and fecundity in women receiving artificial insemination by donor semen and in normal fertile women. *Br J Obstet Gynaecol* 1984;91:1019.
15. Guzick DS, Rock JA. Estimation of a model of cumulative pregnancy following infertility therapy. *Am J Obstet Gynecol* 1981;140:573.
16. Matthews DE, Farewell VT. Binary logistic regression. In: *Using and understanding medical statistics.* New York: S Karger; 1955:139.
17. Cox DR. Regression models and life tables. *J R Stat Soc* 1972;34(8):187.
18. Lee KL, McNeer JF, Starmer CF, et al. Clinical judgment and statistics. Lessons from a stimulated randomized trial in coronary artery disease. *Circulation* 1980;61:508.
19. Matthews DE, Farewell VT. Linear regression models for medical data. In: *Using and understanding medical statistics.* New York: S Karger; 1985:123.
20. Fisher RA. *Statistical methods for research workers.* 5th ed. Edinburgh: Oliver and Boyd; 1934.
21. Yates F. Contingency tables involving small numbers and the χ^2 test. Supplement, *J R Stat Soc* 1934;1:217–235.
22. Brown GW. 2 × 2 tables. *Am J Dis Child* 1985;139:410.
23. Mantel N. Evaluation of survival data and two new rank order statistics arising in its consideration. *Cancer Chemother Rep* 1966;50:163.
24. Peto R, Pike MC, Armitage P, et al. Design and analysis of randomized clinical trials requiring prolonged observation of each patient. II. Analysis and examples. *Br J Cancer* 1977;35:1.
25. Breslow N. A generalized Kruskal–Wallis test for comparing K samples subject to unequal patterns of censorship. *Biometrika* 1970;57:579.
26. Kruskal WH, Wallis WA. Use of ranks in one-criterion variance analysis. *Am J Stat Assoc* 1952;47:583.
27. Guzick DS, Bross DS, Rock JA. A parametric method for comparing cumulative pregnancy curves following infertility therapy. *Fertil Steril* 1982;37:503.
28. Mantel N, Byar DP. Evaluation of response-time data involving transient states: an illustration using heart-transplant data. *J Am Stat Assoc* 1974;69:81.
29. Williams RC. Toward a set of reliable and valid measures for chronic pain assessment and outcome research. *Pain* 1988;35:239.
30. Jensen MP, Karoly P, Braver S. The measurement of clinical pain intensity: a comparison of six methods. *Pain* 1986;27:117.
31. Tjaden B, Schlaff WD, Kimball A, Rock JA. The efficacy of presacral neurectomy for the relief of midline dysmenorrhea. *Obstet Gynecol* 1990;76:89.
32. Cox DR, Oakes D. *Analysis of survival data.* London: Chapman and Hall; 1984.
33. Student. The probable error of a mean. *Biometrika* 1908;6:1–25.
34. Wilcoxon F, Wilcox RA. *Some rapid approximate statistical procedures.* Pearl River: Lederle; 1964.
35. Cohen J. *Statistical power analysis for the behavioral sciences.* Hillsdale, NJ: Lawrence Erlbaum Associates; 1988.

Endoscopic Management of Gynecologic Disease,
edited by G.D. Adamson and D.C. Martin.
Lippincott-Raven Publishers, Philadelphia © 1996.

CHAPTER 38

Cost Effectiveness and Laparoscopic Surgery

D. Alan Johns

Until recently, the first and most important concern of the gynecologic surgeon was securing the optimum outcome for the patient. New technology was eagerly evaluated by the outcome it could produce. Cost was rarely a significant consideration as long as the surgical outcome was reasonable.

In the new medical world that has developed around physicians and hospitals over the past few years, cost and outcome are both considered important. It will be mandatory for gynecologic surgeons in this new world to evaluate the cost effectiveness of each endoscopic procedure. Those procedures producing the optimal outcome at minimal cost will be preferred, whether performed at laparoscopy or laparotomy.

The components of medical cost include frequency (number of procedures performed per capita) and the cost per procedure (including costs related to complications and postoperative disability). Cost effectiveness can be defined as producing optimum outcome for an expenditure. With the advent of managed care, numerous attempts have been made to measure outcome. These attempts have been variously labeled: medical technologies assessment, outcome studies, and quality indicators. Other buzz words will surely follow.

Unfortunately, as of 1995, the study of surgical outcome and quality indicators is in its infancy. This is primarily due to a very deficient database on which to base conclusions. The study of surgical outcomes in gynecology is extremely subjective and difficult. Unlike other surgical specialties, surgical outcome in gynecology often relates more to quality-of-life issues. These variables are extremely difficult to measure and quantify.

In addition, those qualities generally associated with laparoscopic surgery (shorter recovery time) are often difficult to measure due to their extremely subjective nature. Despite these limitations, it is generally accepted that laparoscopic surgery is associated with shorter recovery times than those associated with laparotomy. These databases and assessments will surely become more accurately defined in the near future.

The physician has been faced with an ever-increasing number of reimbursement systems. The traditional fee for service composes a decreasing proportion of insurance reimbursal systems. Taking its place has been an infinite variety of alphabet systems including discounted fee for service, health maintenance organization (HMO), preferred provider organization (PPO), allowable maximum, and relative base value unit (RBVU), to name only a few. Although extremely complex, these systems have had a significant impact on the private practice of medicine. Many physicians have seen the percentage of patients covered by "managed care" organizations rise from a small percentage of their practice to 80–90% of their patient base over the past 2–3 years. Simultaneously, hospital reimbursement has undergone an equally dramatic change. Currently, many large hospital systems are reimbursed according to a discounted formula by the majority of payors.

The end result of these massive changes has been tremendous pressure on hospitals and physicians to develop indicators for cost effectiveness in all specialties. As medical reimbursement moves increasingly toward capitation (the end game) in medical cost containment, cost effectiveness and quality containers will become the most important aspects of any reimbursal system. Since a capitated system of reimbursement produces the greatest physician incentive to maintain a quality and cost-effective surgical practice, it is likely that all gynecologic surgeons will carefully evaluate every new surgical advance from the standpoint of cost effectiveness as well as quality. New surgical gadgetry will no longer be tolerable in this system.

The health care financing administration defines *cost effective* in three ways: (a) "less costly and at least as

D. A. Johns: Richland Medical Center, Fort Worth, Texas 76180.

effective as an alternative covered technology"; (b) "more effective and more costly than a covered alternative, but improved health outcome justify additional expenditures"; and (c) "less effective and less costly than existing alternatives, but a viable alternative for some patients" (1).

The cost effectiveness of a surgical procedure can be evaluated by examination of four components of that procedure: applicability (the number of patients potentially benefiting from the surgical procedure), outcome of the surgical procedure (including complications), expenditures (including those related to complications and disability), and availability (is the procedure restricted to only a few large centers or is it widely available). These criteria will be examined with respect to six endoscopic procedures. Hopefully, this analysis will help in understanding the complex nature of evaluating cost effectiveness.

LAPAROSCOPIC TREATMENT OF ECTOPIC PREGNANCY

Several articles published in peer-reviewed journals have suggested that at least 80% of all patients with ectopic pregnancies are candidates for a laparoscopic approach (2–6). Reich and Johns reported successful laparoscopic treatment of 109 consecutive ectopic pregnancies, including 16 patients with ruptured tubal gestations. Every surgical procedure normally performed for treatment of ectopic pregnancy was accomplished laparoscopically in this group of 109 patients. This included salpingostomy (65), salpingectomy (21), partial salpingectomy (12), cornual resection (3), ovarian pregnancy (1), and salpingo-oophorectomy (1). Therefore, the applicability of a laparoscopic approach to ectopic pregnancy is extremely high.

It has been conclusively shown that persistent ectopic rates, subsequent pregnancy rates, tubal patency rates, and subsequent ectopic rates in patients treated with an endoscopic approach are identical to those attained when the ectopic pregnancy is treated at laparotomy (3,7,8). In addition, complications of the endoscopic approach are at least equal to if not less than those encountered at laparotomy (3,7,8). Reich reported no intraoperative or postoperative complications in his study and no patient required laparotomy.

With these studies in mind, the outcome of the laparoscopic approach to the treatment of ectopic pregnancy is at the very least equal to that attained at laparotomy.

Three studies have shown laparoscopic treatment of ectopic pregnancy to be associated with a decrease in hospitalization and recovery time (7,9,10). Furthermore, Mauri found that $105 million in savings would have been generated, had 80% of the ectopics diagnosed in 1987 been treated endoscopically rather than by laparotomy (11). Therefore, the expenditure associated with laparoscopic treatment of ectopic pregnancy is significantly less than that associated with treatment at laparotomy. When the shorter recovery time of the laparoscopic approach is considered, this savings is even greater.

It is assumed that every gynecologist is capable of performing a laparotomy for treatment of an ectopic pregnancy. At this time, however, an unknown number of gynecologic surgeons are capable of treating an ectopic pregnancy with an endoscopic approach. Since the majority of ectopic pregnancies in the United States are still treated by laparotomy, it would seem that the availability of laparoscopic treatment of ectopic pregnancy is not widespread. There is little doubt, however, that laparoscopic treatment of an ectopic pregnancy is more cost-effective than similar surgery performed at laparotomy.

LAPAROSCOPIC TREATMENT OF ENDOMETRIOSIS

Although an extremely large number of patients undergo surgical treatment of endometriosis each year, the surgical treatment varies tremendously from one surgeon to the next and one hospital to the next. Relatively few studies have evaluated the applicability of laparoscopic treatment of endometriosis in patients other than those suffering from infertility. Several authors, however, have indicated that laparoscopic treatment of the majority of patients with AFS stages III and IV endometriosis is possible (12–16). This assessment will therefore be limited to treatment of those infertility patients with stages III and IV endometriosis.

As previously stated, the majority of infertile patients with AFS stages III and IV endometriosis can be treated endoscopically by the surgeon skilled in these techniques (12–16). The applicability of this mode of therapy is therefore great. Adamson has shown that patients in these categories have experienced higher pregnancy rates than similar patients treated at laparotomy (15,16). Luciano et al. reported their experience in the laparoscopic treatment of endometriosis in infertile patients. He reported a 3-day reduction in hospital stay associated with operative laparoscopy vs. laparotomy. His patients experienced a 19-day shorter recovery time and decreased hospital costs ($1821 for laparoscopy as compared to $4068 for laparotomy) (13). Therefore, when outcomes (pregnancy) are considered, the laparoscopic treatment of endometriosis is preferable to that at laparotomy.

Although the laparoscopic treatment of endometriosis is associated with a shorter hospital stay than treatment at laparotomy, several authors have advocated the use of the laparoscopic CO_2 laser in the treatment of these patients (12–14). At a cost of approximately $50,000–

$100,000 per laser, approximately 300–600 patients with AFS stages III and IV endometriosis would have to be treated endoscopically to offset this cost. The expenditures for the endoscopic treatment of endometriosis therefore are questionable. Fewer than 40% of practicing gynecologists have access to a laser of any wavelength. Far fewer than this have the expertise and experience in the endoscopic techniques necessary to treat advanced endometriosis. Therefore, the availability of the laparoscopic treatment of advanced endometriosis is extremely limited. With the above in mind, laparoscopic treatment of advanced endometriosis in infertile patients produces pregnancy rates superior to those attained by laparotomy when adequate training and equipment are available. Unfortunately, the expenditure and availability considerations make the cost effectiveness of the endoscopic approach questionable except in high-volume centers with skilled surgeons.

LAPAROSCOPIC ADNEXECTOMY

Johns, Reich, Daniell, Mage, and Pittaway found that laparoscopic techniques are applicable in most patients undergoing adnexectomy for benign disease (17–20). Reich et al. reported 312 patients undergoing laparoscopic adnexectomy. The only patients excluded from a laparoscopic approach were those felt to have a significant risk of malignant ovarian disease. None of these patients required laparotomy for completion of their adnexectomy (17). The total number of patients undergoing adnexectomy for benign disease in any given year is unknown. Based on these authors' experiences, it would appear that laparoscopic techniques are applicable in most patients undergoing adnexectomy.

These same authors have shown complication rates for laparoscopic adnexectomy to be comparable with or less than those associated with the same procedure performed at laparotomy using laparoscopic techniques. These authors were able to successfully remove the adnexa in the overwhelming majority of their patients without resorting to laparotomy and without increasing complication rates.

Outcome studies evaluating adnexectomy by either laparoscopy or laparotomy do not exist. However, since complication rates for the two methodologies are comparable, it is unlikely that outcomes will be any different between the two methods of access. Based on data by Levine and Luciano, each patient undergoing laparoscopic adnexectomy as an outpatient will save the health care reimbursement system approximately $1500 (18). In addition, there is a decrease in recovery time of approximately 21 days when the endoscopic approach is used. With these factors in mind, the expenditures for laparoscopic adnexectomy are significantly less than those associated with the same procedure performed at laparotomy.

Every gynecologic surgeon is assumed to be capable of performing adnexectomy at laparotomy. However, the percentage of practicing gynecologists capable of performing laparoscopic adnexectomy is unknown. The availability of laparoscopic adnexectomy in the United States is therefore unknown.

The only conclusion that can be reached is that laparoscopic adnexectomy is cost effective in the hands of surgeons trained in the techniques of operative laparoscopy when electrosurgery and nondisposable laparoscopic technology are utilized. Widespread availability of this expertise and technology is questionable.

LAPAROSCOPIC TUBAL REANASTOMOSIS

The total number of patients undergoing tubal reanastomosis in a given year in the United States is unknown. It is assumed, however, that laparoscopic techniques could be employed in most of these patients undergoing microtubal reanastomosis. The applicability of the techniques is therefore extremely high.

Very few authors have reported on pregnancy rates following laparoscopic tubal reanastomosis. These authors have shown outcomes (pregnancy rates) to be between 35% and 50% (21,22). Microtubal reanastomosis done at laparotomy and minilaparotomy, however, are associated with pregnancy rates between 50% and 70% (23,24).

Complication rates associated with microtubal reanastomosis at laparotomy and minilaparotomy are well established. However, those complication rates associated with the endoscopic approach are unknown.

With these factors in mind, the outcome (pregnancy) associated with laparoscopic tubal reanastomosis falls well below that that can be attained by the same procedure performed at laparotomy or outpatient minilaparotomy.

Although laparoscopic tubal reanastomosis can be performed with a 4- to 6-hr hospital stay, surgeons have reported operating times to vary between 3 and 6 hr (22). The same procedure performed at laparotomy is associated with operating times between 1.5 and 2.5 hr (24).

With the advent of laparoscopic tubal reanastomosis at minilaparotomy a 24-hr hospital stay can be easily achieved (24). The recovery from tubal reanastomosis by minilaparotomy varies from 7 to 14 days. Laparoscopic tubal reanastomosis is associated with a 1- to 3-day recovery period.

In summary, the decreased expenditure associated with laparoscopic tubal reanastomosis is more than offset by a doubling of operating time. Therefore, published data do not support laparoscopic tubal reanastomosis over the same procedure performed by outpatient minilaparotomy.

LAPAROSCOPIC-ASSISTED VAGINAL HYSTERECTOMY

Although 75% of all hysterectomies (approximately 600,000 per year) in the United States are currently performed abdominally (25), it is felt that a minimum of 70% of these hysterectomies for benign disease can be completed vaginally or with laparoscopic assistance (26–28). With the majority of hysterectomies performed abdominally, the applicability of laparoscopic techniques to convert these to vaginal procedures is very high.

Numerous authors have reported complication rates associated with laparoscopic-assisted vaginal hysterectomy (LAVH) and vaginal hysterectomy to be lower than those complication rates associated with abdominal hysterectomy (28–31). Although the purpose of the operation (removal of the uterus) is accomplished in all cases, outcome studies of these patients will require further study. It is unlikely, however, that there will be any difference in the long-term outcome of the patient undergoing LAVH, vaginal hysterectomy, or total abdominal hysterectomy (TAH).

Each patient undergoing vaginal hysterectomy or LAVH instead of abdominal hysterectomy has a decrease in hospital stay of approximately 1.5 days and a decrease in recovery time of approximately 21 days.

In his report "Retrospective Analysis of 2,563 Hysterectomies," Johns reported an operating time for LAVH (102 min) to be only slightly longer than that for TAH (82 min). Hospital stay associated with LAVH (43 hr) was significantly less than that associated with TAH (68 hr). The average hospital charge for LAVH ($6431) was comparable to that for TAH ($6552). Using these data, it was concluded that when reusable equipment and electrosurgery are utilized, the cost associated with LAVH are equal to or less than those associated with abdominal hysterectomy (28). However, when disposable laparoscopic equipment and stapling devices are employed, LAVH is significantly more expensive than its abdominal counterpart (29,30).

If one-half of the 450,000 hysterectomies performed abdominally each year in the United States could be converted to vaginal hysterectomy or LAVH, an annual savings of $450,000,000 would be generated. The costs related to LAVH are equal to or less than those with abdominal hysterectomy. When complications or recovery are considered, expenditures are significantly less than for the abdominal approach.

Although one major retrospective study has shown a decrease in the abdominal hysterectomy rate over 2 years from 65% to 36% (28), the number of gynecologists nationally skilled in the techniques of LAVH is unknown. Since the percentage of hysterectomies performed abdominally has remained unchanged, it would be logical to assume that the availability of LAVH is rather limited. LAVH is therefore cost-effective in the appropriately selected patient (a patient who is not a candidate for vaginal hysterectomy) when reusable equipment and electrosurgery are utilized. The availability of LAVH is unknown.

HIGHLIGHTS

As demonstrated in this brief synopsis of a few endoscopic procedures, evaluation of the cost effectiveness of any surgical procedure is at best difficult and inexact. The availability of physicians skilled in cost-effective endoscopic techniques appears to be a key factor in recognizing the cost effectiveness of any laparoscopic procedure. This training must begin in residency and extend throughout the physician's surgical experience.

Numerous factors have contributed to the cost ineffectiveness often associated with laparoscopic surgical procedures. LAVH is a good example of a procedure that was promoted by industry supported programs. This resulted in widespread use of expensive disposable laparoscopic devices before their cost effectiveness had been properly and independently evaluated. Once the surgeon's skills and experiences have taken him or her beyond reliance on disposable equipment, many gynecologic procedures become cost-effective.

Additionally, hospitals and physicians must develop a team concept in the endoscopic suite. Physicians, surgeons, and hospitals must recognize that any surgical procedure (particularly laparoscopic procedures) is more efficiently and safely performed when everyone works in concert. This team concept of endoscopic surgery has been shown to be effective in minimizing the cost associated with major laparoscopic procedures.

In summary, the future of laparoscopic surgery lies in the hands of gynecologic surgeons who now realize the potential of this relatively new field. If those physicians are able to demonstrate the cost effectiveness of these new endoscopic procedures, these procedures will become the standard of care in gynecologic surgery during the next decade. This scenario was predicted by DeCherney (32) in 1985 when he wrote "the obituary of laparotomy for reconstructive pelvic surgery has been written, only its publication remains." However, should gynecologic surgeons show these endoscopic techniques to be less than cost-effective, they will be relegated to the status of an interesting footnote in future medical texts.

REFERENCES

1. Healthcare Financing Administration, Medicare Program, *Fed Reg* 1989;54:4302–4316.

2. Silva PD. A laparoscopic approach can be applied to most cases of ectopic pregnancy. *Obstet Gynecol* 1980;72:944–947.
3. Vermesh M, Silva PD, Rosen GF, Stein AL, Fossum GT, Sauer MV. Management of unruptured ectopic gestation by linear salpingostomy: a prospective, randomized clinical trial of laparoscopy versus laparotomy. *Obstet Gynecol* 1989;73–101.
4. Henderson SR. Ectopic tubal pregnancy treated by operative laparoscopy. *Am J Obstet Gynecol* 1989;160:1482–1489.
5. Dubuisson JB, Bruel D, Aubriot FX, de Joliniere JB, Foulot H, Mandellnot L. Reproductive outcome after laparoscopic salpingectomy for tubal pregnancy. *Fertil Steril* 1990;53:1004–1007.
6. Reich J, Johns DA, et al. Laparoscopic treatment of 109 consecutive ectopic pregnancies. *J Reprod Med* 1988;33:885–890.
7. Brumsted J, Kessler C, Gibson C, Nakajima S, Riccick DH, Gibson M. A comparison of laparoscopy and laparotomy for treatment of ectopic pregnancy. *Obstet Gynecol* 1988;71:889–892.
8. Zouves C, Urman H, Gomel V. Laparoscopic surgical treatment of tubal pregnancy. A safe, effective alternative to laparotomy. *J Reprod Med* 1992;37:205–209.
9. Levine RL. Economic impact of pelviscopic surgery. *J Reprod Med* 1985;30:653.
10. Azziz R, Steinkampf MP, Murphy A. Postoperative recuperation: relation to the extent of endoscopic surgery. *Fertil Steril* 1989;51:1061–1064.
11. Mauri F, Azziz R. Laparoscopic surgery for ectopic pregnancies; technology, assessment, and public health implications. *Fertil Steril* 1993;59:487–498.
12. Martin DC, et al. Excisional techniques of endometriosis with the CO_2 laser laparoscope. *J Reprod Med* 1987;32:753.
13. Luciano AA, Lowrey J, Jacobs SL. Endoscopic treatment of endometriosis-associated infertility. Therapeutic, economic, and social benefits. *J Reprod Med* 1992;32:573.
14. Adamson GD, Lu J, Subak LL. Laparoscopic CO_2 Laser vaporization of endometriosis compared with traditional treatments. *Fertil Steril* 1988;50:704–710.
15. Adamson GD, Hurd J, et al. Laparoscopic endometriosis treatment: is it better? *Fertil Steril* 1993;59:35–44.
16. Adamson GD, Pasta DJ. Surgical treatment of endometriosis-associated infertility: meta-analysis compared with survival analysis. *Am J Obstet Gynecol* 1994;171:1488–1505.
17. Reich H, Johns DA, Daves G, Diamond MP. Laparoscopic oophorectomy. *J Reprod Med* 1993;38:499–501.
18. Pittaway DE, Takacs P, et al. Laparoscopic adnexectomy: a comparison with laparotomy. *Am J Obstet Gynecol* 1995;171:385–392.
19. Daniell JF, Kurtz BR, Lee JY. Laparoscopic oophorectomy: comparative study of ligatures, bipolar coagulation, and autonomic stapling devices. *Obstet Gynecol* 1992;80:325–328.
20. Mage G, Canis M, et al. Laparoscopic management of adnexal cystic masses. *J Gynecol Surg* 1990;6:71.
21. Reich H, McGlynn F, Parente C, Sekel L, Levie M. Laparoscopic tubal anastomosis, *J Am Assoc Gynecol Laparoscopists,* 1993; vol 1, no 1.
22. Koh CH. Laparoscopic tubal reanastomosis. *MVP Video J Ob/Gyn,* 1993;6(6).
23. Gomel V. Microsurgical reversal of female sterilization: a reappraisal. *Fertil Steril* 1980;88, 6(1).
24. Silva PD, Schaper AM, Meisch JK, Schauberger CW. Outpatient microsurgical reversal of tubal sterilization by a combined approach of laparoscopy and minilaparotomy. *Fertil Steril* 1991;55(4):34–36.
25. Wilcox LS, Koonin LM, Pokras R, Strauss LT, Xia Z, Peterson HB. Hysterectomy in the United States, 1988–1990. *Obstet Gynecol* 1994;83(4):549–555.
26. Kovac SR, Cruikshank SH, Retto HF. Laparoscopy-assisted vaginal hysterectomy. *J Gynecol Surg* 1990;6(3):185–193.
27. Kovac SR. Guidelines to determine the route of hysterectomy. *Obstet Gynecol* 1995;85:18–23.
28. Johns DA. The medical and economic impact of laparoscopically-assisted vaginal hysterectomy (LAVH) in a large metropolitan not-for-profit hospital. Presented at the Central Association of Obstetricians and Gynecologists, 62nd Annual Meeting, October 13, 14, 15, 1994, Peabody Hotel, Memphis, Tennessee.
29. Nezhat F, Nezhat C, Gordon S, Wilkins E. Laparoscopic versus abdominal hysterectomy. *J Reprod Med* 1992;37(3):247–250.
30. Boike GM, Elfstrand EP, DelPriore G, Schumock D, Holley HS, Lurain JR. Laparoscopically assisted vaginal hysterectomy in a University Hospital: report of 82 cases and comparison with abdominal and vaginal hysterectomy. *Am J Obstet Gynecol* 168(6 Pt 1):1690–1701.
31. Querleu D, Cosson M, Parmentier D, Debodinance P. The impact of laparoscopic surgery on vaginal hysterectomy. *Gyn Endosc* 1993;2:89–91.
32. DeCherney AH. The leader of the band is tired. . . . *Fertil Steril* 1985·44:299–302.

Endoscopic Management of Gynecologic Disease,
edited by G.D. Adamson and D.C. Martin.
Lippincott-Raven Publishers, Philadelphia © 1996.

CHAPTER 39

Future Developments

William R. Keye, Jr.

The modern era of reconstructive pelvic surgery began in the 1960s with the introduction of the laparoscope for the evaluation of the pelvis in infertile women (1–3). With the information gained from laparoscopy, the reproductive surgeon was able to plan a rational and systematic approach to the management of the infertile couple.

However, the results of pelvic reconstructive surgery in the 1960s were poor. Authors described using 4-0 and 5-0 chromic gut suture, peritonealization of all denuded surfaces, dabbing of tissues with moist sponges, and the use of devices such as the silastic hood and Holter hood retractor (4). Given the poor results of reconstructive surgery, innovative and desperate approaches to treat tubal factor infertility, such as the use of artificial oviducts or the appendix as an oviductal substitute, were reported (5,6).

However, a big breakthrough came with the introduction of microsurgery to gynecology (7–11). The success of pelvic surgery to treat infertility improved dramatically with the use of microsurgery. For the past two decades, microsurgical pelvic surgery has been the gold standard against which all other surgical techniques should be measured.

As gynecologists were embracing microsurgery in the early 1980s, the next major addition to their surgical armamentarium—the laser—was being evaluated in small clinical trials (12–15). Soon thereafter the endoscopic delivery of laser energy was explored in the hope that it would provide the benefits of microsurgery without the morbidity of laparotomy (16). It was not long thereafter that operative laparoscopy in conjunction with the laser became a popular technique for the surgical treatment of infertility and endometriosis. By 1990, prominent gynecologic surgeons had predicted the demise of the laparotomy to treat pelvic diseases associated with infertility (17).

Encouraged by the popularity of lasers, manufacturers of electrosurgery devices and mechanical instruments that could be passed easily through the laparoscope and hysteroscope were turning out safer and more effective instrumentation at a fast pace. Gynecologists found that they could perform endoscopic pelvic surgery effectively using electrosurgery and mechanical instruments as well as lasers. The pace at which new techniques for reconstructive pelvic procedures are being developed has quickened greatly in the past couple of years.

As a result, it appears that the 1990s will see several new and exciting developments in the field of endoscopic surgery.

1. The first will be the miniaturization and increasing sophistication of endoscopes as well as of electrosurgery and mechanical instruments for endoscopic surgery.
2. New generation laser systems will be developed that will lead to a renewed interest in lasers for therapy.
3. New diagnostic endoscopes will become available that will use the principles of holography or fluorescence to detect subtle pelvic diseases, such as endometriosis or infections, which are not detectable by the unaided human eye.

However exciting these developments appear, there is a concern among some pelvic surgeons and endoscopists that, in our enthusiasm to perform complicated operations through the laparoscope, we may expose the patient to increased risk and poorer clinical results. There has also been concern as to whether we are training operative endoscopists in the most effective fashion. Finally, there has been little research to (a) determine the appropriate indications for pelvic endoscopy, (b) match the patient and the technique, and (c) determine which

W. R. Keye, Jr: Division of Reproductive Endocrinology, William Beaumont Hospital, Royal Oak, Michigan 48073.

endoscopic techniques yield the best clinical results with the least risk and cost. Thus the future of gynecologic endoscopy will include a concerted effort to develop better teaching techniques and develop and use objective methods of technology assessment and controlled clinical trials.

MINIATURIZATION OF ENDOSCOPES

For more than 20 years, standard endoscopes and hysteroscopes have been relatively large instruments because of the need for a large light bundle and an optical system capable of providing a panoramic view and a large image. However, the development of more efficient light sources and fiberoptic delivery systems have made it possible to create smaller and smaller endoscopes without sacrificing the view nor the brilliance of the image. In addition, the ability to couple very sensitive cameras with high-resolution capabilities to high-resolution monitors has made it possible to miniaturize endoscopes without sacrificing the quality of the image.

For example, a 3-mm minilaparoscope, also known as an optical fiber or minilaparoscope, is available for diagnostic laparoscopy (Fig. 1). These minilaparoscopes may make it possible to perform diagnostic office laparoscopy just as we now commonly perform diagnostic office hysteroscopy. Using these minilaparoscopes, the gynecologist may soon be able to evaluate the cul-de-sac, ovaries, and distal fallopian tubes in the office using a local anesthetic and a small volume of gas. Translaparoscopic gamete intrafallopian transfer (GIFT) may also become an office procedure.

For the past several years Grochmal and Lomano, as well as Dorsey, have been performing feasibility trials using these small minilaparoscopes or optical catheters for office laparoscopy under local anesthesia and intravenous sedation (18,19). These minilaparoscopes are made up of many 6-μm microfibers, which are capable of transmitting a video image as well as acting as a light bundle for illumination. After the local infiltration of the umbilicus with a local anesthetic and the administration of a sedative, a modified Veress cannula is introduced through a small subumbilical incision into the peritoneal cavity. The surgeon insufflates the abdominal cavity with 1–2 L of carbon dioxide or nitrous oxide and introduces a probe through a 3-mm suprapubic port. The gynecologist then performs an organ-by-organ examination of the pelvis maintaining a short distance between the end of the scope and each organ. Despite the limited field of vision, adhesions, endometriosis, myomata, and polycystic ovaries can be clearly visualized. In addition, the gynecologist can lyse adhesions, coagulate and vaporize endometriosis, and excise myomata using a neodymium:yttrium-aluminum-garnet (Nd:YAG) laser and contact fiber. GIFT also has been carried out in several patients.

The potential advantages of this technique are obvious. First, it can be performed with minimal anesthesia in an office setting. Second, surgeons who find it difficult to obtain operating time in a hospital or surgicenter would find an in-office procedure very appealing. Procedures such as laparoscopies to evaluate acute pain or GIFT could be scheduled on short notice and for the convenience of the surgeon and patient. Third, minilaparoscopy would probably require shorter convalescence than a standard laparoscopy. Finally it would encourage preinterventional screening and postsurgical second-look laparoscopy which could lead to more informed decision making.

Small endoscopes may also be of value in the future practice of obstetrics. A report by DeLia using a Nd:YAG laser fiber through a fetoscope to treat twin–twin transfusion syndrome illustrates the exciting possibilities for fetal surgery (20). After studying the ability of the fetoscopically delivered Nd:YAG laser energy to

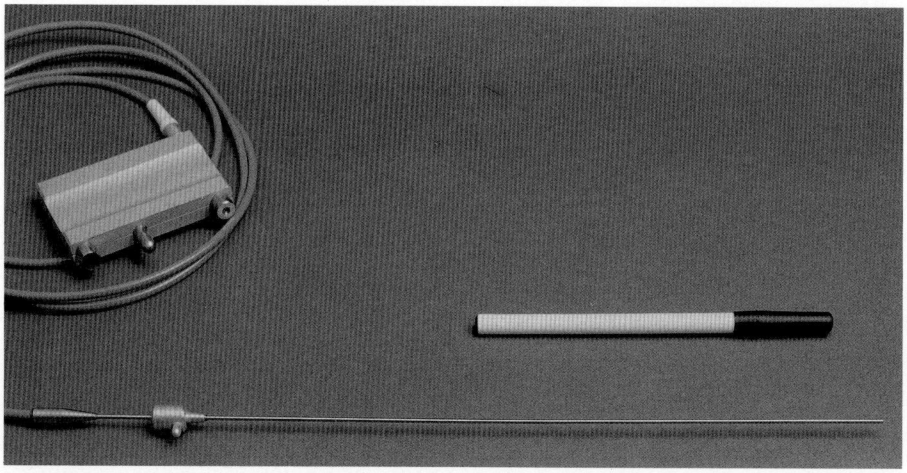

FIG. 1. A minilaparoscope (optical fiber) (Medical Dynamics, Englewood, CO).

occlude the placental vasculature in sheep and rhesus monkeys, he and his colleagues at the University of Utah performed fetoscopy on several patients with evidence of severe midtrimester twin–twin transfusion syndrome (acute onset of polyhydramnios with evidence of fetal compromise). The fetoscopy was performed at laparotomy through a hysterotomy incision under general anesthesia (Fig. 2). A fetoscope, modified to a length of 25 cm with a channel for the laser fiber, was used. After identification of the insertion of the umbilical cord of the polyhydramniotic twin, the vessels were followed toward the vascular equator. The vessels that were thought to communicate between the two twins were coagulated for 2–3 sec over a length of 1 cm with 60 W of energy at a distance of 0.5–1.0 cm through a 400-μm fiber. After coagulation of all apparent communicating vessels, the surgery was terminated and the patients were followed without additional therapy of the polyhydramnios.

Over the next several days serial ultrasounds demonstrated a decrease in fundal height, an increase in fluid around the smaller fetus, improved umbilical artery flow in the smaller twin, and appropriate internal growth. By 1993 DeLia had performed fetoscopy on 19 patients with a salvage rate of 56% (20 of 38) of all fetuses (21). Seventy-eight percent of the women delivered at least one live fetus. The future of this procedure looks promising.

The development of microendoscopes will also extend the surgeon's ability to evaluate the pelvis at endoscopy. For example, John Kerin and his colleagues described their experience with transcervical falloposcopy using such a microendoscope (22). Falloposcopy is a modification of a technique known as tuboscopy described by Henry-Suchet (23) and Brosens (24). In an attempt to detect intrauterine pathology, Henry-Suchet and Brosens performed translaparoscopic endoscopy of the ampullary portion of the fallopian tube with a rigid tuboscope with an outside diameter of 3 mm. They used this technique to diagnose tubal lesions not seen at hysterosalpingography or laparoscopy and to aid in the selection of patients for tubal microsurgery or assisted reproduction. Unfortunately, this procedure was limited to evaluation of the ampulla and required laparoscopy.

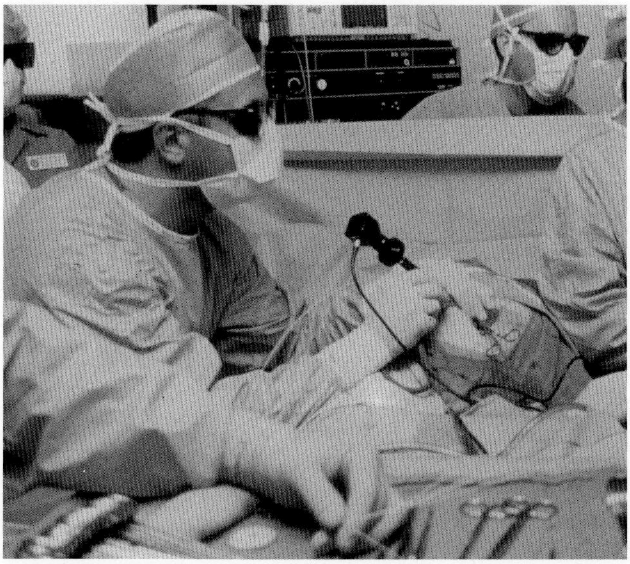

FIG. 2. The first Nd:YAG laser ablation of placental vessels at fetoscopy performed by Julian DeLia, University of Utah.

Falloposcopy, on the other hand, is a double-endoscopy technique in which a small flexible falloposcope is directed through the operating channel of a flexible hysteroscope into the proximal fallopian tube. The prototype falloposcope has an outside diameter of 0.5 mm. It has an atraumatic end and is flexible enough to minimize the chance of damage to the endosalpinx. The images are relayed to a microchip video camera and displayed on a high-resolution color monitor or stored on videotape or still photographs.

The technique of falloposcopy involves introducing a flexible hysteroscope into the uterine cavity and to a point within 1–2 mm of a tubia ostium. A small, steerable, platinum-tip, tapered guidewire is then directed into the proximal fallopian tube. These guidewires, which are 0.3–0.8 mm OD are designed to traverse the proximal tube without damaging the endosalpinx. Once the guidewire is passed 15 cm beyond the uterotubal junction, flexible Teflon cannulas, 1.2–1.3 mm OD, are introduced over the guidewires and into the proximal tube. The guidewire is then withdrawn and the falloposcope is passed into the fallopian tube and through the inside of the cannula. Hydrotubation is performed and the various segments of the fallopian tube are inspected. The visualization of the fallopian tube is best achieved by viewing the endosalpinx as the falloposcope is withdrawn back toward the uterus. Kerin and his colleagues were able to evaluate the entire length of the fallopian tube and, as a result, discovered that proximal occlusion may often be the result of mucous plugs and intraluminal debris. They also were able to dislodge the debris and establish patency through the falloposcope thus avoiding unnecessary segmental resection and end-to-end anastomosis of the tube. In the future, microendoscopy may become a standard part of the diagnostic evaluation of the infertile woman even prior to or in conjunction with laparoscopy. Microendoscopy may also be utilized for the transvaginal evaluation of ovarian cysts.

The next generation beyond these microendoscopes may involve ultrathin silica fibers, which have made it possible to squeeze 2000–6000 pixels into fibers with diameters of 0.2–0.5 mm. These ultrathin fibers may offer improved contrast, higher pixel density, and easier handling. In addition, they exhibit an interesting property known as "strong coloring," in which a particular wavelength or "color" is propagated more efficiently or strongly than another color. This property may be useful for fluorescent sensing in the detection of abnormal tissue within the reproductive tract. In fluorescent sensing, these ultrathin fibers would be used to transmit blue light, which in turn would excite fluorescent dyes within cancerous tumors, endometriosis, or infections. The fibers would then transmit this fluorescence back to a camera or other recording device for diagnosis and localization.

NEW GENERATION LASER SYSTEMS

The development of new laser systems may lead to a resurgence in the use of lasers for endoscopic surgery. For example, the carbon dioxide laser of the future may be no larger than an average household flashlight and much less expensive than the lasers currently available. The trend toward miniaturization of CO_2 lasers has already begun in the industrial arena. Currently, the smallest industrial CO_2 lasers that can deliver 750–1000 W have a laser head that weighs 300–400 kg and occupies a volume of more than 600 L. A prototype CO_2 laser that incorporates conduction cooling, radiofrequency excitation and a resonator has permitted the construction of a compact and portable high-powered laser that is one sixth the volume and weighs one quarter of the weight of currently available industrial CO_2 lasers. Thus, the prototype of a CO_2 laser capable of delivering 750 W is similar to the size of surgical CO_2 lasers that can deliver 60–80 W. The advances that have allowed the miniaturization of industrial lasers will certainly be applied to the medical laser field, thus making it possible to deliver significant laser energy from very small laser devices.

It is even possible that future laser devices, based on tiny diode lasers, may be small enough to incorporate within the endoscope itself. These high-powered microprocessor-controlled diode lasers are inexpensive ($50–$60 each), very small (approximately 1 cm in diameter), and capable of generating ultraviolet as well as visible light in the blue and green portion of the spectrum. Although these visible diode lasers are not commercially available, they may in the future be available and be powerful enough to activate solid state lasers that may be built into the endoscopes. Thus, a laser endoscope in the future may consist of a series of diode lasers built into the viewing end of the endoscope. The energy from these diode lasers would be transmitted through a fiber, which would activate a small Nd:YAG or other solid state laser, which would be built into the operating end of the endoscope. Alternatively, the laser of the future may consist of a small diode laser that "pumps" or powers a special optical fiber which is doped with holmium, erbium, thalium, or neodymium. The fiber thus acts as a laser capable of emitting infrared energy of a desired wavelength. A high-powered, continuous wave Nd:YAG laser pumped by four, 15-W continuous wave diode bars and capable of emitting 92 W was described at an optics meeting in April of 1993. These laser endoscopes would be simpler, smaller, and much less expensive than currently available laser systems.

The development of new lasers would also enhance endoscopy. At present, only the argon, Nd:YAG, frequency-doubled Nd:YAG, and CO_2 lasers are commonly used in gynecology. However, the next generation of lasers will provide new wavelengths and new lasers. For example, the titanium:sapphire laser is a solid-state laser that is tunable from approximately 690 to 1100 nm. This laser is capable of delivering both continuous wave and ultrashort pulses. An example of a nontunable solid-state laser that has recently been introduced is the holmium:yttrium-aluminum-garnet (Ho:YAG) laser with a wavelength of 2100 nm. This laser can be transmitted through silica fibers and creates very little thermal damage to tissue. It can cut through tissue very efficiently with little lateral thermal damage. Combining diode and solid-state lasers may be another means for greatly enhancing and miniaturizing endoscopes in the future.

Other new lasers may be developed through the use of the free electron laser (FEL) developed by Dr. John Madey (25). The FEL has made it possible to explore the biological impact of new wavelengths. It consists of a linear accelerator that generates a beam of free electrons that pass between two rows of powerful magnets referred to as wigglers. By modifying the polarity and strength of the magnetic field, one can create a tunable and very powerful laser. With the free electron laser it will be possible to evaluate many wavelengths as well as to evaluate the biological effect of very short (nanosecond) pulses and high energies on the order of giggiwatts. The information gained with the free electron laser may ultimately lead to the development of new lasers for clinical use.

These developments in the miniaturization of lasers and the development of new lasers may revive the somewhat stagnant laser market, for it will be the laser that will make microendoscopy a therapeutic as well as a diagnostic tool.

NEW DIAGNOSTIC ENDOSCOPES AND ENDOSCOPIC TECHNIQUES

The development of new fluorescent dyes that preferentially bind to specific tissues may make it possible for the early diagnosis of benign diseases such as endometriosis. At present, the diagnosis of endometriosis depends on the ability of the surgeon to detect gross abnormalities of the peritoneum. However, in the future, the diagnosis of endometriosis in its microscopic and more subtle forms may be made easier by the ability to deliver fluorescent dyes to the endometriosis and to visualize the fluorescence with special endoscopes and cameras.

It has long been known that certain dyes are capable

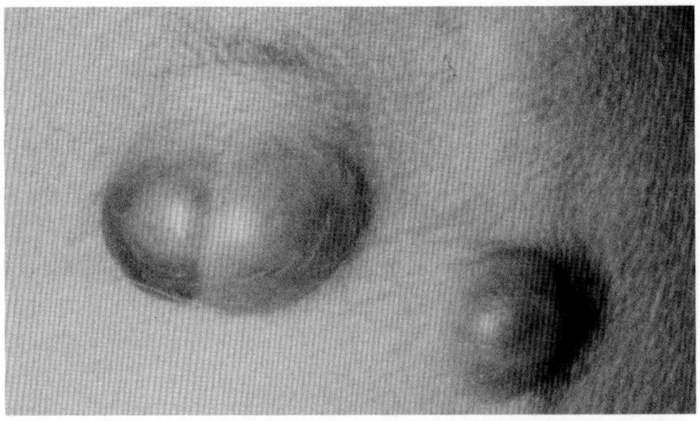

FIG. 3. Subcutaneous abdominal wall nodule of endometriosis in the rhesus monkey produced by William Brenner, Oregon Regional Primate Center.

of concentrating in abnormal tissues. A classic application of this principle has been in the photodynamic therapy of malignancies. In this technique, dyes that are administered to individuals with malignancies are selectively retained by the malignant tissue. When the dye is exposed to specific wavelengths of light, a biochemical reaction involving the dye takes place within the malignant tissue. As a result of this biochemical reaction, the formation of singlet oxygen destroys the malignant cells without damage to surrounding normal tissue. This technique is in wide use in the treatment of malignancies. However, photodynamic therapy has recently been explored for the treatment of endometriosis. At the University of Adelaide, Dr. Ozzie Petrucco has created an animal model of endometriosis in the rabbit (26). Following the intravenous administration of hematoporphyrin derivatives, the lesions were exposed to the gold vapor laser. Destruction of the lesions took place without damage to surrounding normal tissues.

Similarly the studies of experimental endometriosis in the monkey by Keye and his colleagues at the University of Utah have also demonstrated the specific and selective destruction of experimental endometriosis (unpublished observations). Working with scientists at the Regional Primate Center in Beaverton, Oregon, they used an experimental endometriosis created by Dr. William Brenner. In this model, endometrium was obtained from the

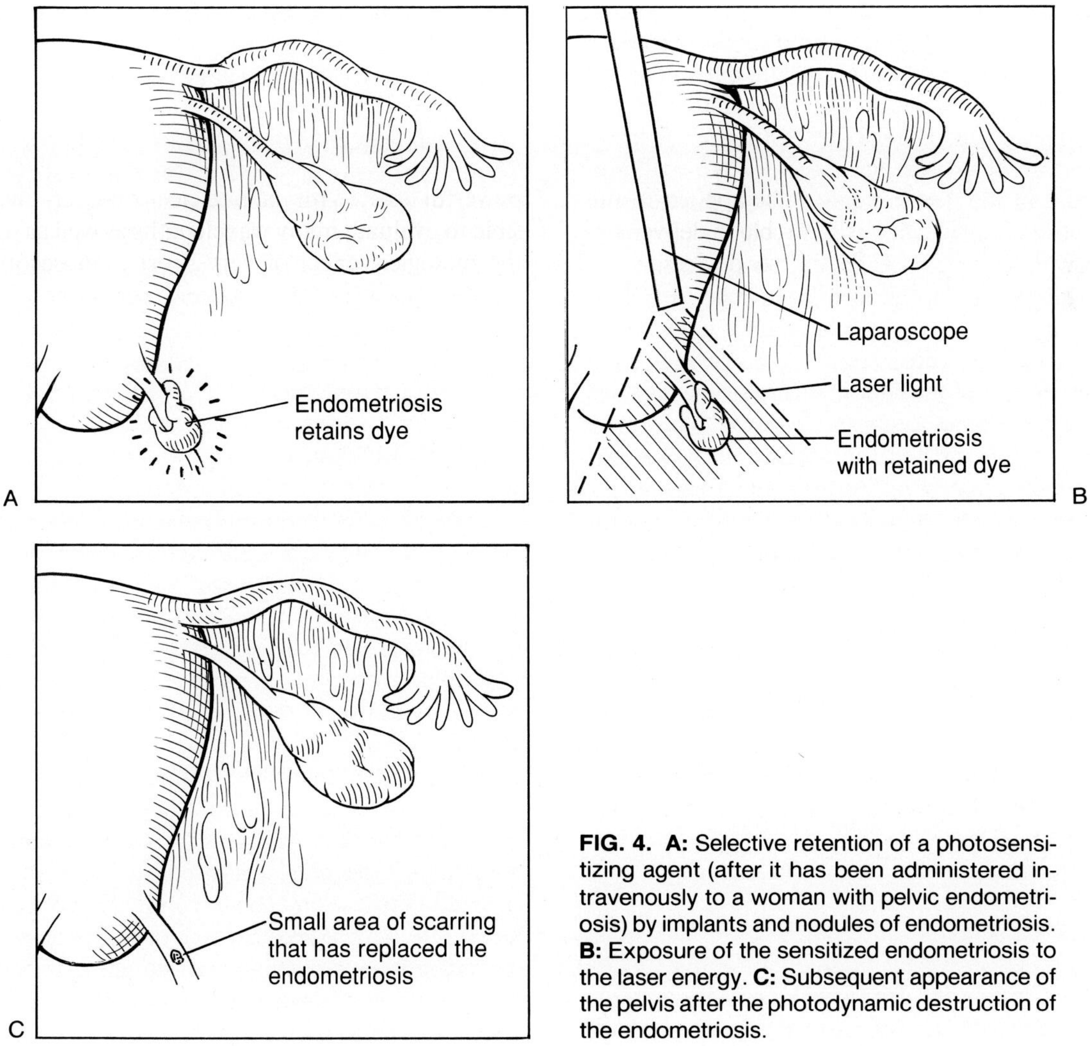

FIG. 4. A: Selective retention of a photosensitizing agent (after it has been administered intravenously to a woman with pelvic endometriosis) by implants and nodules of endometriosis. **B:** Exposure of the sensitized endometriosis to the laser energy. **C:** Subsequent appearance of the pelvis after the photodynamic destruction of the endometriosis.

uterus and was removed at laparotomy and injected subcutaneously under the abdominal skin of rhesus monkeys (Fig. 3). Following the administration of estrogen and progesterone to mature these experimental lesions, the animals each received an intravenous injection of hematoporphyrin derivative. Twenty-four hours later there was a fourfold increase in the concentration of the hematoporphyrin derivative within the lesions as compared to normal surrounding tissues. The presence of the dye within the implants rendered them sensitive to the effect of the energy of an argon-pumped dye laser. An illustration of how pelvic endometriosis could be treated by photodynamic therapy is seen in Fig. 4.

As the result of these studies, one can envision that future diagnosis and treatment of endometriosis will consist of administering a dye intravenously to a patient about to undergo laparoscopy. After several hours, laparoscopy would be performed and the pelvic cavity filled with a light-diffusing liquid medium consisting of a dilute lipid solution and the pelvic cavity would be illuminated with a cylindrical dispersion "light stick" attached to the end of an optical fiber. This optical fiber would deliver light of a specific wavelength, 630–800 nm, which would cause the dye that would be concentrated in the endometriotic lesions to fluoresce and to photoactivate, thereby destroying the lesions. This technique may allow for a more complete diagnosis and thus more effective therapy with a reduced chance for recurrence. With the development of new dyes that are activated at longer wavelengths and the development of new diode lasers, these techniques may become clinically practical.

Using new diagnostic endoscopes, the gynecologist of the future will be able to perform nondestructive diagnostic imaging. For example, holographic endoscopes will make it possible to project three-dimensional, near-microscopic images of the endometrium or the endosalpinx without removing tissue. As a result, the patient who undergoes in vitro fertilization in the future may have the transfer of embryos during a short and precise window of time as determined by the appearance of the endometrium by endoscopic holography. Similarly, surgeons will be able to determine in advance the functional status of the fallopian tube using a transcervically directed microsalpingoscope that can provide holographic images of the endosalpinx. As a result, the tubal surgeon will know in advance whether or not tubal surgery offers any hope of pregnancy to the patient. In a patient with an abnormal endosalpinx, the surgeon may recommend in vitro fertilization with embryo transfer instead of tubal surgery.

BETTER EDUCATION

Most of the recent developments of new endoscopic procedures and the training of endoscopic surgeons have taken place in community-based hospitals rather than in academic research centers. As a result, many recent residents have graduated from their training programs poorly equipped to utilize endoscopes fully in their gynecologic practices. Thus only a limited number of clinicians have been trained to perform advanced endoscopic surgery. In addition, the quality of training and research has been extremely variable and uncontrolled. Finally, many manufacturers of endoscopic equipment have played, what is in the opinion of some, too great a role in determining the content of the educational programs provided for the clinician. As a result, most training programs have emphasized how to use the equipment and have neglected the indications for and complications of endoscopic surgery.

Gynecologic residents of the future must be trained in these futuristic endoscopic procedures during their training. They must be trained in the preoperative evaluation of the patient, the selection of the appropriate procedure and instrumentation, and the postoperative management of complications. Although many endoscopic procedures are now experimental, they will eventually become a standard part of a specialist's practice and must become a standard part of gynecologic training programs.

Finally, the continuing education of the generalist who uses gynecologic endoscopy within a broader practice may be enhanced in the future by the use of telemedicine or remote endoscopy, in which the endoscopic image is transmitted via satellite or fiberoptics from the operating suite in the hospital of the operating surgeon to the office of the endoscopic specialist who may be located in a tertiary setting miles away. The endoscopic specialist would view the images, assist in making diagnostic decisions, and talk to the surgeon and perhaps to the patient.

CONCLUSIONS

The successful integration of endoscopes into gynecology will depend on several factors. First, the key to the effective and innovative use of endoscopes for the monitoring, diagnosis, and treatment of gynecologic diseases will be the interfacing of optics, laser technology, and computer software. Second, we must standardize the training of future endoscopists and encourage endoscopic research and education within our universities and tertiary health centers. Finally, we must narrow the gap between the innovators, educators, and experts and the generalist who uses but does not restrict his or her practice to gynecologic endoscopy.

Endoscopes will make a revolutionary change in medicine. Using these less invasive procedures, patients will not require hospitalization as often, medical costs may be lower, and medical space and personnel can be utilized for purposes other than acute postoperative care.

The earlier detection of disease by the use of the endoscope will hopefully simplify and shorten the course of treatment, thus conserving money, space, and personnel. As a result, endoscopic surgery will undoubtedly play an increasingly significant role in providing medical care in the face of limited medical resources.

REFERENCES

1. Semm K. Technique of gynecological pelviscopy. *Med Gynecol Social* 1962;4:62.
2. Behrman SJ, Kistner RW. A rational approach to the evaluation of infertility. In: *Progress in infertility.* Boston: Little, Brown; 1968:17.
3. Roland M. Culdoscopy and laparoscopy: competitive and complimentary techniques. *Fertil Steril* 1970;21:361.
4. Gracia C-R. Surgical reconstruction of the oviduct in the infertile patient. In: *Progress in infertility.* Boston: Little, Brown; 1968:255–272.
5. Charles AG, Labes JE, Cohen M, Fetch LB, Schoemaker WB. Techniques for substitution of the uterine tube. *Obstet Gynecol* 1962;20:174.
6. O'Neill JJ. The use of the vermiform appendix as a fallopian tube. *Am J Obstet Gynecol* 1966;95:218.
7. Garcia CR, Allen J. Surgical approach to tubal disease. *Clin Obstet Gynecol* 1974;17:102.
8. McCormick WG, Torres J. A method of Pomeroy tubal ligation anastomosis. *Obstet Gynecol* 1976;47:623.
9. Gomel V. Tubal reanastomosis by microsurgery. *Fertil Steril* 1977;28:59.
10. Winston RML. Microsurgical tubocornual anastomosis for reversal of sterilization. *Lancet* 1977;1:284.
11. Diamond E. Microsurgical reconstruction of the uterine tube in sterilized patients. *Fertil Steril* 1977;28:1203.
12. Baggish MS, Chong AP. Carbon dioxide laser microsurgery of the uterine tube. *Obstet Gynecol* 1981;58:111.
13. Bruhat MA, Mage G. Use of CO_2 laser in salpingoneostomy. In: Kaplan I, ed. *Laser surgery.* Vol 3. part 1. Jerusalem: Academic Press; 1979:271.
14. Bellina JH. Microsurgery of the fallopian tube with CO_2 laser: 82 cases with follow-up. *Laser Surg Med* 1982;36:129.
15. Kelly RW, Roberts DK. Experience with the CO_2 laser in gynecologic microsurgery. *Am J Obstet Gynecol* 1983;146:285.
16. Tadir Y, Ovadia J, Zuckerman Z. Laparoscopic applications of the CO_2 laser. In: Atsumi, Nimsakol J, eds. *Proceedings of the Fourth Congress of the International Society for Laser Surgery,* September 1981:25.
17. DeCherney AH. The leader of the band is tired. . . . *Fertil Steril* 1985;44:299–302.
18. Lomano JM, Grochmal S. Personal communication.
19. Dorsey JH, Tabb CR. Mini-laparoscopy and fiber optic lasers. *Obstet Gynecol Clin North Am* 1991;18:99–103.
20. DeLia JE, Cruikshank DP, Keye WR. Fetoscopic neodymium: YAG laser occlusion of placental vessels in severe twin–twin transfusion syndrome. *Obstet Gynecol* 1990;75:1046.
21. DeLia J, Kuhlmann R, Harstad T, Cruikshand D. Twin–twin transfusion syndrome treated by fetoscope neodymium: YAG laser occlusion of chorioangiopagus. *Am J Obstet Gynecol* 1993;168: Abstract 50.
22. Kerin JF, Surrey ES. Clinical applications of the falloposcope. Seminars in Reproductive Endocrinology, Vol. 10, No. 1, February, 1992. p 51.
23. Henry-Suchet J, Lofredo V, Tesquier I, Pez J. Endoscopy of the tube: its prognostic value for tuboplasties. *Acta Eur Fertil* 1985;16:139.
24. Brosens I, Boeckx W, Delattin PH, Puttemans P, Vasquez G. Salpingoscopy: a new preoperative diagnostic tool in tubal infertility. *Brit J Obstet Gynecol* 1987;94:768.
25. Christensen CP. New laser technology. *Science* 1984;224:117–123.
26. Petrucco OM, Sathananden M, Knowles S, McKenzie L, Forbes IJ, Cowles PM, Keye WR, Jr. Ablation of endometriotic implants in rabbits by haematoporphyrin derivative (HPD) photoradiation therapy using gold vapour laser. *Lasers in Med and Surgery,* 1990;10:344–348.

Endoscopic Management of Gynecologic Disease,
edited by G.D. Adamson and D.C. Martin.
Lippincott-Raven Publishers, Philadelphia © 1996.

Appendix: Suppliers of Endoscopic Equipment

Aesculap, Inc., 1000 Gateway Boulevard, South San Francisco, California 94080-7030

Allen Medical Systems, 5198 Richmond Road, Bedford Heights, Ohio 44146

American Hydro-Surgical Instruments, 430 Commerce Drive, Delray Beach, Florida 33065

American Medical Source/L.A.S.E.R., Inc., 14227 Sandy Lane, Tomball, Texas 77375

American Surgical Technologies Corporation, 300 Billerica Road, Chelmsford, Massachusetts 01824

Apple Medical Corporation, 580 Main Street, Bolton, Massachusetts 01740

Bard Gynecology, 13183 Harland Drive NE, Covington, Georgia 30209

BEI Medical Systems/Zinnanti Surgical, 83 Hobart Street, Hackensack, New Jersey 07601

Bioenterics Corporation, 1035 Cindy Lane, Carpinteria, California 93013

Cabot Medical Corporation, 2021 Cabot Boulevard West, Langhorne, Pennsylvania 19047

Circon Acmi, 300 Stillwater Avenue, Stamford, Connecticut 06902

Coherent, Inc., 3270 West Bayshore Road, Palo Alto, California 94303

Conceptus, Inc., 1021 Howard Avenue, San Carlos, California 94070

Cook OB/GYN, 1100 West Morgan Street, P.O. Box 271, Spencer, Indiana 47402

Cooper Surgical, 15 Forest Parkway, Shelton, Connecticut 06484

Electroscope, Inc., 4890 Sterling Drive, Boulder, Colorado 80301

Ellman International, Inc., 1135 Railroad Avenue, Hewlett, New York 11557

Elmed, Inc., 60 West Avenue, Addison, Illinois 60101

Ethicon Endo-Surgery, 4545 Creek Road, Cincinnati, Ohio 45242

Everest Medical Corporation, 13755 1st Avenue North, Minneapolis, Minnesota 55441

W. L. Gore & Associates, Inc., 3750 West Kiltie Lane, Flagstaff, Arizona 86001

Imagyn Medical, Inc., 27651 La Paz Road, Laguna Niguel, California 92656

Innerdyne Medical, Inc., 1244 Reamwood Avenue, Sunnyvale, California 94089

Johnson & Johnson Medical, Inc., 2500 Arbrook Boulevard, Arlington, Texas 76014

Lasersonics (A Division of Heraeus Surgical), 575 Cottonwood Drive, Milpitas, California 95030

Marlow Surgical Technologies, Inc., 1810 Joseph Lloyd Parkway, Willoughby, Ohio 44094

Microsurge, Inc., 150 A Street, Needham, Massachusetts 02194

Olympus America, Inc., 4 Nevada Drive, Lake Success, New York 11042

Origin Medsystems, 135 Constitution Drive, Menlo Park, California 94062

Reznik Instrument, Inc., 7337 N. Lawndale Avenue, Skokie, Illinois 60076

Sharplan Lasers, Inc., 1 Pearl Court, Allendale, New Jersey 07401

Siemens Medical Systems, Inc., Ultrasound Group, 22010 SE 51st Street, Issaquah, Washington 98027

Karl Storz Endoscopy-America, Inc., 600 Corporate Point, Culver City, California 90230

Stryker Endoscopy, 210 Baypointe Parkway, San Jose, California 95134

Sun Medical, Inc., 1179 Corporate Drive West, Suite 100, Arlington, Texas 76006

Surgical Laser Technologies, 200 Cresson Boulevard, Oaks, Pennsylvania 19456

Syntex Laboratories, Inc., 3401 Hillview Avenue, Palo Alto, California 94303

Tap Pharmaceuticals, Inc., 2355 Waukegan Road, Deerfield, Illinois 60015

Tetrad Corporation, 357 Inverness Drive South, Suite A, Englewood, Colorado 80112

Ultracision, 25 Thurber Boulevard, Smithfield, Rhode Island 02917

United Medical Network, 708 S. Third Street, Suite 400, Minneapolis, Minnesota 55415

United States Surgical Corporation, 150 Glover Avenue, Norwalk, Connecticut 06856

Valleylab, Inc., 5920 Longbow Drive, Boulder, Colorado 80301

Wisap/Market-Tiers, Inc., 8305 Melrose Drive, Lenexa, Kansas 66214

Richard Wolf Medical Instruments Corporation, 353 Corporate Woods Parkway, Vernon Hills, Illinois 60061

Carl Zeiss, Inc., One Zeiss Drive, Thornwood, New York 10594

Zimmer, 2801 Fortune Circle E, Suite F, Indianapolis, Indiana 46241

Subject Index

Subject Index

Page numbers followed by *f* indicate figures; page numbers followed by *t* indicate tables.